CLINICAL MANUAL OF

CHINESE HERBAL PREPARED MEDICINES

A guide to ethical and pure prepared medicines

Third Edition

Eastland Press
Seattle

Clinical Manual of Chinese Herbal Prepared Medicines
A Guide to Ethical and Pure Chinese Herbal Prepared Medicines

Eastland Press
P.O. Box 99749
Seattle, WA 98139
USA
www.eastlandpress.com

First published 2000
2nd Edition 2003
3rd Edition 2016; revised 2019

National Library of Australia Cataloguing-in-Publication data:
Maclean, William
Clinical Manual of Chinese Herbal Prepared Medicines

Bibliography
Includes Index
ISBN: 978-0-939616-90-9
1. Herbs – Therapeutic use
2. Medicine, Chinese – Handbooks, manuals.
3. Prepared medicines – Handbooks, manuals.
I. Title II. Title: Chinese Herbal Prepared Medicines

Illustrations: Karen Vance

Disclaimer

The recommendations and information in this book are intended for use by professionals and in no way substitute for professional advice. Any plant or animal substance intended for medicinal use has the potential to cause allergic reaction in sensitive individuals and unwanted effects may accrue from inaccurate prescription. Neither the author nor the publisher can be held responsible for claims arising from the inappropriate use of any remedy in this book. Do not attempt self diagnosis or self treatment for any chronic or serious illness without consulting a qualified professional.

Every effort has been made to ensure that the information contained in this volume is accurate and as up to date as possible. However, due to the rapidly changing nature of the industry, formulations, packaging and availability vary from time to time.

Acknowledgements

Thanks to all those who contributed in some way to this work, and to those who helped with the seemingly endless revisions, checking, double checking and proofing that are the lot of the author and publisher. My special appreciation to Bill Maclean for support above and beyond the call of duty. Thanks also to those friends and colleagues whose dedication and integrity remain an inspiration – David Legge, Greg Doyle, Dr Dai Wei Min, Dr Li Dong Sen, Christine Flynn, Jane Lyttleton, Clarence Tsang, Danny Wu, and most of all Kathryn. Dedicated to the memory of two gentlemen practitioners, mentors and good friends, Peter Townsend and Chris Madden.

Contents

Liver & Gallbladder

Tonics

Shén

Ear, Nose, Throat, Eyes

Introduction

Prepared medicines are medicines manufactured from raw or processed herbal materials into pills, powders or liquid extracts for ingestion, and plasters and liniments for external application. Most are available as 'over the counter' products in herb shops and supermarkets in the Chinatown's of the world. The Chinese have been manufacturing prepared medicines for centuries, indeed some of the most well known and best loved medicines, such as **7.9 Jin Gui Shen Qi Wan**, **7.1.1 Liu Wei Di Huang Wan** and **1.17 Gui Zhi Fu Ling Wan**, were originally produced in prepared medicine form. Prepared medicines have been a popular and convenient form of health care for centuries, and recent changes to the industry in terms of regulation and quality control, both in and out of China, have led to a resurgence in interest in this ancient system.

Large numbers of prepared medicines are produced in China and the range is continually growing. Many are developed from famous proven prescriptions, and are produced (with minor variations) by many different factories. Others may be unique to a single producer, perhaps a secret family recipe handed down through generations.

Dried herb prescriptions versus prepared medicines

The practitioner of Chinese herbal medicine has two methods of delivering herbal material to a patient, each with strengths and weaknesses. The first, and still most popular method in China, is the dispensing of dried herbs that are boiled and decocted into a tea. Dried herb prescriptions usually require a consultation and prescription from a qualified physician. The advantage of dried herb prescriptions is flexibility and strength, both of which are advantageous in acute or serious illnesses. The disadvantages of dried herb prescriptions are the inconvenience of daily decoction, poor compliance in prolonged illnesses, difficulties involved in maintenance of a dried herb pharmacy, the degree of expertise required to utilize dried herbs effectively, dubious quality control and the cost to the patient. Many practitioners in China and the Western world make use of both systems, starting patients on boiled decoction until a certain result is attained, then switching to prepared medicines to continue the treatment.

Advantages of prepared medicines

Prepared medicines offer some specific advantages to the modern practitioner. They are relatively cheap and easy to take, thereby encouraging patient compliance, and are easy to store with a long shelf life. Maintaining a comprehensive pharmacy is affordable and space efficient. Because prepared medicines are mostly mild in action, they are less likely to cause problems if incorrectly prescribed. Many of the classic prepared medicines have been used for centuries on countless patients and have proved themselves time and again to be effective and safe. New medicines are being produced on the basis of modern research findings, leading to an amalgamation of the best of science and tradition. Technology is being harnessed to improve extraction ratios and stability of some modern formulas.

In general, prepared medicines are not as strong or effective as dried herb decoction for acute and serious illnesses, although some prepared medicines are quite good at clearing toxic and damp heat or purging fire, etc., when taken correctly at the right dose. The main advantages of prepared medicines from a clinical point of view, are in treatment of chronic problems that make up the bulk of the modern Chinese medicine practice. In my opinion, prepared medicines are superior to dried herb prescriptions in several areas. The first is when prolonged and gentle rebuilding of yin or blood is desired. Similarly, dispersal of constrained qi and blood stasis is best achieved by persistently chipping away at the stagnation over a prolonged period, for which prepared medicines are ideal. These patterns require a gradual, persistent and prolonged treatment course. Rebuilding yin and blood, dispersing stagnant blood and harmonizing qi are processes that cannot be forced by using large and powerful dried herb prescriptions. They are better dealt with by slow and persistent encouragement of constitutional change, change that for the most part is better carried out by the gentle action of prepared medicines.

The other main advantage of prepared medicines is in the area of quality control. Dried herbs are not subject to the stringent quality control checks applied to medicines manufactured according to the principles of Good Manufacturing Practice (GMP, see p.xii), and may be contaminated with various residues. Occasional batches of dried herbs in the Australian market have been found to be contaminated by industrial pollutants, pesticide residues, heavy metals, molds and insects. There is no way of being completely sure of the origin, history or quality of any dried herb offered for sale in herb shops. Prepared medicines produced in GMP factories however, are guaranteed to be what they claim to be, and to contain only the ingredients listed on the label.

Prepared medicine formats

Pills and tablets

Pills and tablets (*wán* 丸, *piàn* 片) come in a number of different sizes and forms. They are made of finely ground up herbs or concentrated extracts that are bound by pressure, or by the addition of honey, water or some other sticky medium. When ingested the ingredients are released in the intestine and absorbed slowly at a constant rate. Depending on the binding medium and the size of the pill, absorption and metabolism rates can vary. For example, pills bound with a starch paste (usually rice or wheat flour) are absorbed more slowly than those bound with honey, and thus are used when a prolonged action is required. Pills are convenient for fast administration in acute disorders, but are best for chronic problems that require lengthy therapy. They are particularly suited for the long term tonification required to build yin and blood. They are also the preferred method when a formula requires herbs that are unsuitable for decoction.

Two common pill types appear in this book, the large traditional honey pill (also known as a bolus), usually sealed in a wax coated plastic ball, and smaller pills coated in licorice powder.

Tablets are produced by squeezing herb powder under pressure to form a uniform disc that can be coated with sugar or an enteric coating. This is an advantage if the herbal ingredients are bitter or distasteful, or if the acid environment of the stomach degrades some essential component of the medicine.

Powders

Powders (*sàn* 散) are finely ground herbs sifted through a uniform mesh. They can be taken directly, chased down with a liquid, or boiled and the resulting liquid taken as a draft. Powders are useful for long term administration in the treatment of chronic disorders, can be applied externally for skin diseases, blown into the nose or throat for local disorders or to resuscitate patients from unconsciousness. Powdered herbs are good for local application and are the format of choice for children.

Dissolvable granules

Dissolvable granules (*chōng jì* 冲剂) are made by decocting herbal ingredients until a thick concentrate is produced. A stabilizing excipient is then added, usually a starch of some type (commonly corn starch), in sufficient quantity to form a thick paste. The ground dregs of the decoction, powdered *Dioscorea opposita* root (shan yao) or *Poria cocos* (fu ling) are also used. The resulting paste is fed through a heated drum sieve that instantly dries it to uniform granules that can be reconstituted to decoction with hot water. The technology required to produced dissolvable granules has recently improved and current products are of excellent quality. Volatile elements are captured and reintroduced to the final product. Recent developments in low temperature processing (never more than 100°C) ensure that even highly sensitive components are not degraded.

A number of companies are producing individual herbs as dissolvable granules. The big advantage is that individual formulas can be constructed from the components. This format is gradually replacing traditional decoction in hospitals across China, and more formulas and individual herbs in dissolvable granules appear in the over the counter market each year.

Liquid extracts

Liquid extracts (*kǒu fú yè* 口服液) are a modern format that involves extraction and suspension of herbs in a liquid medium, usually sugar based. Packaged in sterilized single dose vials, they are good for children as the dose is usually small and the taste of the herbs disguised. Liquid extracts are absorbed and utilized quickly.

Plasters, syrups, ointments

Plasters (*gāo* 膏) are sheets of adhesive material with herbal extracts bound to the sticky surface. Applied locally for bruising and sprain, pain and arthritic conditions. In general, they warm the local area, invigorate local circulation and promote healing. Syrups are liquid extracts thickened with honey or sugar. Ointments are finely ground or decocted herbs suspended in a thick oil based medium. They are applied topically for skin conditions.

Liniments

Liniments are herbs or herbal oils extracted and suspended in an oil base for long action, or alcohol medium for fast absorption. They are used topically for pain, trauma or skin diseases. Liniments are similar to plasters in action.

QUALITY CONSIDERATIONS

Good Manufacturing Practice

The majority of the prepared medicines presented in this volume are produced by Good Manufacturing Practice compliant companies. Good Manufacturing Practice (GMP) is an internationally agreed upon set of principles and procedures which, when followed by manufacturers of medicines and medical devices, helps ensure that the products manufactured will have the required pharmaceutical grade quality. The basic concept of GMP is that quality must be built into each batch of product during all stages of the manufacturing process. It involves quality control and checking at all stages of production, including selection of the herbs and testing for active ingredients and contaminants, extraction and binding methods, and packaging and labeling. GMP has become the standard against which all pharmaceutical practices are judged.

The role of the Therapeutic Goods Administration (TGA)

The Australian Therapeutic Goods Administration (TGA) is responsible for administering the provisions of the Therapeutic Goods Act. The TGA carries out a range of assessment and monitoring activities to ensure therapeutic goods available in Australia conform to GMP standards. Quality control of herbal medicine products is determined in the following ways:

Premarket assessment

Products assessed as having a higher level of risk (prescription medicines and some nonprescription medicines) are evaluated for quality, safety and efficacy. Once approved for marketing in Australia these products are included in the Australian Register of Therapeutic Goods as 'registered' products and are identified by an AUST R number.

Products assessed as being lower risk (many nonprescription medicines and most prepared medicines) are assessed for quality and safety. Once approved for marketing in Australia, these products are included in the Australian Register of Therapeutic Goods as 'listed' products and are identified by an AUST L number.

In assessing the level of risk, factors such as the strength of a product, side effects, potential harm through prolonged use, toxicity and the seriousness of the medical condition for which the product is intended to be used, are all taken into account.

Licensing of manufacturers

Manufacturers of therapeutic goods must be licensed and their manufacturing practices must comply with principles of good manufacturing practice. The aim of licensing and standards is to protect public health by ensuring that medicines and medical devices meet definable standards of quality assurance and are manufactured in conditions that are clean and free of contaminants.

Overseas manufacturers of therapeutic goods supplied to Australia must provide evidence that the goods are manufactured to a standard of GMP equivalent to that expected of Australian manufacturers of similar goods. What this means in practice is that representatives of the TGA inspect and personally approve any factory that applies for GMP status. Inspection and audit of herbal manufacturing facilities can last up to seven days and involve thorough examination of all aspects of the manufacturing process. The rigor of the inspection process ensures that factories that attain Australian GMP status are among the best in the world

Monitoring compliance

Once all government requirements of GMP are met and a factory obtains GMP status, on site inspections are carried out every two years. Any factory that fails to maintain full compliance with GMP standards can lose its certification at any time. In addition, the TGA investigates reports of problems and performs random testing of products on the market to ensure ongoing compliance with the legislation.

Unregistered products

A number of products presented in this manual are not registered by the TGA, although they may be manufactured by a GMP compliant company. This is usually because they are not currently offered for sale in Australia, but are available in Asia, the

US or Europe. A relatively large selection of classical formulas, manufactured by the reputable Lanzhou Foci Pharmaceutical Factory, are currently available as practitioner only products in the US and UK. See Selection of Formulas, p.xiv.

A few formulas that are not manufactured by GMP companies are included. This is usually because they are classified as food products and therefore not subject to TGA registration.

The issue of contamination

It has long been suspected, and recently shown, that some Chinese prepared medicines not produced in GMP compliant factories are contaminated with heavy metals and/or unlisted pharmaceutical drugs. The problem is further complicated by differing definitions of what constitutes a contaminant.

Heavy metals have traditionally been used in prepared medicines, but almost all are now considered obsolete and are not included in products for sale outside China, and less and less often within China as regulations tighten. Heavy metal contamination not listed as an ingredient presumably results from industrial pollution on the herbs in the field or as an consequence of the manufacturing process.

Other substances considered contaminating in one country may not be thought so in another. For example, berberine and borneol are listed as contaminants in the US, whereas these substances are therapeutically acceptable to the TGA in Australia and appear in listed products.

When in doubt, only use products that are registered or listed with the TGA, or that are produced in a GMP compliant facility.

ETHICAL CONSIDERATIONS

Endangered species

A number of the medicines described in this volume contain substances derived from animals. In general, items such as the moulted shell of the summer cicada, earthworms, various beetles or other insects and shells are used. These products are abundant and therapeutically useful in the correct context.

Unfortunately however, Chinese medicine has a long history of using parts from now rare animals. There are, in the Chinatowns of the world, medicines claiming to contain tiger bone, rhino and saiga antelope horn, as well as seahorse and musk deer gland. In China, these substances have been prized for centuries for their strength (in many cases dubious) and their rarity (and thus high price and the implied status that goes along with being able to afford such items). The practice of listing endangered species on medicine labels continues even though tests have shown that the substance may not be present or that some other product has been substituted (for example cat or dog bone for tiger bone, water buffalo horn for rhino horn). An expensive animal product on the label implies a superior product.

Even though endangered species are probably not being used (both hard to get and wildly expensive), the labeling practice continues to generate an illegal market and encourages poaching of remaining populations. We feel very strongly that no medicine listing an endangered species as an ingredient should be used under any circumstance. None of the medicines in this volume contains parts of endangered species.

SELECTION OF FORMULAS

Medicines are selected primarily on the basis of their availability over the counter in the Australian market, listing with the TGA or because they are produced in factories that comply with the principles of GMP. In addition to the new medicines available in the Australian market, the text includes numerous medicines that are not currently available in Australia, but which can be obtained in North America and Europe. The reason for this is the desire to make this manual a more practical companion to the Clinical Handbook of Internal Medicine series (University of Western Sydney) for those readers outside Australia.

The author of this book practices in Australia and so has an Australian slant, and relies upon the Australian regulatory authority of the TGA. However, the formulas described are essentially the traditional, sometimes ancient, Chinese formulas and are of universal application. Accordingly, the author considers that the information contained in this volume applicable to countries such as the USA and European Union which have a similar approach to Chinese medicine as that practiced in Australia.

THE FACTORIES

There are literally hundreds of factories producing prepared medicines in China. Of these hundreds of factories, only a relatively small proportion are deemed to be of sufficient quality to qualify for certification by the Australian TGA.

The majority of prepared medicines in this book are produced in just five factories. Of these factories, three are famous throughout China and the orient and between them produce hundreds of products for domestic and export consumption. These are the Lanzhou Foci Pharmaceutical Factory, Beijing Tong Ren Tang Pharmaceutical Factory and Tianjin Drug Manufactory. The other two, Guangzhou Qixing Pharmaceutical Factory and the Jing Xian Pharmaceutical Co., also in Guangzhou, are examples of the new and substantial investments in standards of quality and technology that are occurring as China develops and modernizes.

Lanzhou Foci Pharmaceutical factory

Lanzhou Foci Pharmaceutical factory in Gansu Province, Western China was founded in 1929. The majority of pills described in the text are produced by this factory. Lanzhou Foci produces more than 100 kinds of products, including pills, tablets, ointments, granules, liquid extracts, syrups and capsules. Their products were exported to Southeastern Asian countries as early as 1930, and now are found in over forty countries including the United States, Japan, Singapore, Thailand, Malaysia, Indonesia, Canada, Australia, the United Kingdom, Hong Kong, Macao and Taiwan.

Lanzhou Foci manufactures a wide range of classical and unique formulas, the pill forms being most commonly available outside China. The trademark for concentrated pills sold outside China is the "Minshan" (Mountain Minshan) brand. The popularity of this factory's products has inspired numerous imitators and fakes.

Beijing Tong Ren Tang Pharmaceutical Factory

Situated in Beijing, this massive company with 11000 employees has been famous for over 300 years. It was established in 1669 by Yue Zunyu who worked in the imperial hospital. Because of its great reputation and effective prescriptions, Tong Ren Tang was able to gain the privilege of providing medicines for the imperial court pharmacy during the years of Emperor Yong Zheng (1723-1735). In 1861, Tong Ren Tang was ordered to prepare medicines for the imperial family directly. Tong Ren Tang specializes in the large honey pill format, although recently it has begun to manufacture increasing numbers of granulated products. Tong Ren Tang produces hundreds of different products in all formats which are revered throughout China for their high quality.

Tianjin Drug Manufactory

Tianjin Drug Manufactory in Shandong province is a large and well respected herb manufacturer specializing in the traditional format of honey pills, as well as tablets.

ARRANGEMENT OF CATEGORIES

I have grouped the medicines according to the most common conditions for which we use them. This arrangement is, however, arbitrary and dependent on clinical experience and personal bias. Many medicines could appear in several groups. For example, **1.9 Gui Pi Wan** is effective for qi and blood deficiency type gynecological and postpartum disorders, however it is also widely used for *shén* disturbances, fatigue patterns and bleeding syndromes. It is found in the gynecological section, but could just as easily fall into the *shén* calming or tonic section.

LAYOUT OF THE TEXT

All the information needed to quickly prescribe is described under the relevant headings. In the graphical representation of the pattern identifying features, the bold text indicates an important symptom of the relevant pattern, or the features which differentiate the formula from those with similar action.

Terminology

Terminology follows the Eastland Press term set used by Bensky et al. in the standard works, Chinese Herbal Medicine Materia Medica and Formulas and Strategies. Chinese medically defined organs systems are capitalized. Other technical terms defined in the glossary.

Icons

The icons at the edge of the page are a quick summary of certain key features that define a prepared medicine, such as whether or not the medicine is listed with the TGA or produced in a GMP compliant factory, available as a practitioner only product, the typical duration of use, pregnancy contraindication, inclusion of animal products and any potential for herb drug interactions. The icon key appears on the inside back cover.

Alternative names

Some prepared medicines have traditionally been known by certain common names or by alternative transliterations of Chinese (*pīn yīn* or Wade Giles), for example **1.1 Ba Zhen Wan** has long been known as Women's Precious Pills, **1.9 Gui Pi Wan** as Kwei Be Wan, and so on. These alternatives are noted at the top of each page. The main name given is the one common in the Australian market or the standard *pīn yīn* name, and may vary in other countries.

Factory

The specified factory is important to note as many factories produce medicines of the same name. We recommend only the products of the factories listed in the text.

Indications

The indications are the range of conditions and patterns for which a certain medicine can be used. I have included both Chinese and biomedically defined diseases and syndromes, where appropriate. I have tried to be as comprehensive and practical as possible, but be aware that making comparisons between Chinese medical patterns and biomedical diseases is fraught with danger and the potential for misunderstanding. As long as the underlying Chinese medical pattern is diagnosed correctly, the specific biomedical disease the patient has is irrelevant, except from a prognostic point of view. The logic of diagnosis must proceed from the Chinese medical pattern so as to avoid the trap of directly equating a disease with a particular pattern, so often a source of clinical failure. Thus hepatitis is not damp heat in the Liver but may in some circumstances appear as that pattern. Always check the pattern identifying features before prescribing.

Pattern identifying features

The pattern identifying features are the symptoms denoting the appropriate pattern for the use of a particular formula. Not all symptoms will, or need be, present to make the diagnosis. Bold text indicates the most important features.

Combinations

Many formulas can be combined to produce a stronger therapeutic effect or to treat a condition for which neither alone is indicated. Suggestions for combinations are drawn from clinical experience and are by no means exhaustive. When combining small pills (from Lanzhou Foci), it is usually convenient to mix them in a generic container, rather than give them separately to the patient. We use opaque plastic jars of various sizes, upon which we fix our clinic label and specific directions for use. This assists in keeping the dosage instructions as simple as possible and avoids any potential confusion. The random selection of pills from the combined jar will ensure the correct mix over the period of treatment.

The proportions in which formulas are mixed depends on the clinical assessment of the individual being treated, the symptom picture and the weighting the practitioner wants to give to the elements in the mix. In general, the higher weighting (and thus higher proportion in a mix) is given to the formula targeting the constitutional elements of a pattern, with formulas for symptomatic relief or secondary patterns in a lower proportion. For many applications, the standard ratio is 2:1, primary constitutional formula to symptomatic or secondary pattern formula. For example, when treating a patient with reflux esophagitis of a Liver qi invading the Stomach type, a good combination is **6.3 Chai Hu Shu Gan Wan** and **2.26 Xiang Lian Wan**. In this case the **6.3 Chai Hu Shu Gan Wan** is the constitutional formula, aimed at correcting the underlying pathology, the Liver qi constraint, while the **2.26 Xiang Lian Wan** is added to provide symptomatic relief of the reflux. Depending on the severity of the reflux, proportionately more **2.26 Xiang Lian Wan** can be added, and as the patient improves the proportion can be reduced. The typical mix of this combination is 2:1 (**6.3 Chai Hu Shu Gan Wan** to **2.26 Xiang Lian Wan**) but 1:1 or even 1:2 may be used in the early stages of treatment to bring quick symptomatic relief. The dose of combined formulas is usually the same as for either formula alone, not doubled.

Dosage

The dosages listed are guides for average sized individuals under common clinical conditions. Dosage must be flexibly applied, and tends to be weight dependent with larger individuals requiring larger doses in general than small individuals. Dose also depends on the severity of the condition being treated. With a few exceptions (noted in the text), the doses of most of the prepared medicines in this volume can be experimented with to find the optimum range for the individual being treated. Clinical experience is the ultimate guide.

Children present a special challenge to the delivery of prepared medicines. Doses that are too small will be ineffective, while those that are too large may damage the child's delicate qi. Often, simply getting the child to ingest the medicine is trouble enough. The following guidelines may be used to determine the correct dose and the frequency of administration. When using medicines not specifically designed for children, one third of the adult dose is given to children 3-7 years old; one half the adult dose for children 7-13 years old. These guidelines should be flexibly applied, and body weight may be a more useful indicator if the child is large or small for his or her age. For children younger than three, special pediatric medicines in powder and granule form are used.

Before attempting to administer any medicine, the importance of the medicine to the child's wellbeing should be clearly communicated to the child. Parents should be advised to remain calm and not force the child against his or her will. Pills should be crushed or cut into small pieces before ingestion. They can also be softened in hot water, and the resulting liquid taken. Medicines for children can be disguised in a palatable medium such as honey or apple sauce. For infants, medicine can be mixed with water or milk and delivered in an eye-dropper or on the nipple. If a child vomits after taking a medicine, reduce the amount given in each dose and give more frequently. Gentle pressure on PC–6 (*nèi guān*) or LI–4 (*hé gǔ*) may also assist.

Contraindications

There are certain important contraindications for some of the medicines; these are noted in the text. The main one is pregnancy. Medicines contraindicated during pregnancy are usually blood invigorating or purgative and can cause uterine contractions, threatening the developing fetus.

Certain herbs and formulas are known to interact with pharmaceutical drugs, either potentiating or negating their activity and thus creating side effects. In addition, new drugs are appearing all the time, so the potential for new interactions is ongoing. Ensure a complete history with all current medications is taken before prescribing. Always exercise appropriate caution when a patient is taking other medications. See possible herb drug interactions for more information.

USING A SPECIFIC MEDIUM TO TAKE THE MEDICINE

Although all medicines can be washed down with water, the therapeutic effect of some prepared medicines is enhanced when they are taken with a specific liquid.

Ginger

Ginger can be brewed as a tea and used to wash down prepared medicines. Ginger is useful if a medicine causes stomach upsets, nausea, bloating or flatulence. It can be used to protect the stomach when cooling medicines are used, and to enhance the mucolytic action of medicine for Phlegm damp patterns. To prepare, boil a knob of ginger (about 10-20 grams) for ten minutes in 1-2 cups of water.

In large doses (20-30 grams) ginger is diaphoretic and warming to the internal organs. It is useful to enhance the effects of any medicine used to dispel wind cold or treat cold type pain.

Wine, alcohol

Alcohol is used to enhance the ability of a medicine to promote the circulation of qi and blood, and alleviate pain. Medicines for painful obstruction syndrome and other chronic pain or stagnation patterns are often taken with wine or steeped and extracted in wine, which is then taken. Alcohol is also used with some tonic medicines, in particular those used to warm yang.

Usually either a neutral spirit such as vodka or a mild wine such as sherry or sake is suitable. The Chinese favor white or yellow wines made from sorghum or millet. The best come from Shaoxing in Jiangsu province. Shaoxing wines are widely available in the Chinatowns and oriental supermarkets found in most major cities. Shaoxing wines are very similar to sherry in alcohol content and flavor. The dose is 25-50 mls (1-2 ounces), at room temperature or slightly warmed.

Rice porridge

Rice porridge, a common Chinese breakfast food, is sometimes given with diaphoretic medicines to encourage sweating. Usually some shallots (scallions) or ginger will be added as well. Also good for convalescents recovering from a serious illness or surgery in combination with an appropriate tonifying medicine. When used for convalescents the rice porridge is usually prepared with chicken stock for extra nutrition.

Chicken soup

Chicken soup tonifies qi and blood and is an excellent nutritive liquid and immune stimulant. It can be used to enhance the effect of any qi and/or blood tonic medicine.

Honey

Honey is frequently employed as a binding agent in the large traditional pills (boluses). It is a mild Spleen tonic in its own right and is usually used with tonifying medicines. It can also moisten the lungs to alleviate dry cough, and lubricate the intestines to promote bowel movement. Honey is excellent for making sometimes unpleasant medicines palatable.

Brown sugar

Brown sugar dispels cold, moves and nourishes blood. It is especially useful combined with medicines for gynecological conditions associated with blood deficiency and cold accumulation.

Cinnamon sticks

Cinnamon sticks warm the channels and dispel cold. As a tea, they assist medicines aimed at expelling wind cold damp from the channels and joints for the treatment of *bi* syndrome, and can warm the uterus to alleviate dysmenorrhea.

Chrysanthemum flowers

Chrysanthemum flowers cool the Liver and disperse wind heat. Good for inflammatory eye conditions and Liver heat patterns. They can also be used as an eyewash for red sore eyes, in which case they must be boiled for ten minutes, then cooled before application.

Peppermint tea

Peppermint tea disperses wind heat and moves Liver qi. Used to enhance any medicine for clearing wind heat or alleviating qi stagnation.

GENERAL RULES FOR TAKING PREPARED MEDICINES

1. Prepared medicines are usually best taken on an empty stomach, thirty minutes before eating or one hour after eating, except when they cause gastric irritation or upset, in which case they can be taken on a full stomach,
2. Avoid taking prepared medicines with substances that may interact with and bind active ingredients, possibly taking them out of the body through the bowel. These include the tannins found in ordinary tea, bulking agents such as psyllium husks and other fibre containing materials.
3. Use qi and yang tonic medicines, those that strengthen the Spleen and Stomach, and those with stimulant herbs (like ginseng and deer velvet which can upset sleep) earlier in the day. Sedatives and *shén* calming medicines should be taken towards the end of the day.
4. It is better to ensure the daily dose is taken rather than be too concerned about timing. If taking prepared medicines three time daily proves inconvenient for your patients, it is better for them to take more medicine in fewer doses, rather than less overall.
5. For acute problems, take the appropriate dose of the medicine at frequent intervals (every 2-3 hours).
6. Persistence pays off. Prepared medicines are mostly mild and slow acting, so with the exception of acute disorders, it is usually unrealistic to expect quick results. Many chronic patterns, in particular chronic deficiencies like yin and blood deficiency, and blood stasis, may take some months or longer to correct. If diagnosis is reasonable, continue therapy for 6 weeks before making a judgment about whether the treatment is working or not. If a medicine does not seem to be working reassess the diagnosis and make sure the patient is taking the medicine, taking it correctly and in the right dose.

BUYING PREPARED MEDICINES

Make sure the prepared medicine you purchase is produced in the factory specified. Read the label and check the trademark if in doubt. Many factories manufacture formulas with the same name, especially the classic formulas and there is always the incentive in retail outlets to try to sell a substitute if the desired product is unavailable. We cannot attest to the quality or efficacy of prepared medicines produced by companies other than those we have specified in this book.

Beware of fakes

There is, unfortunately, a flourishing fake medicine industry with formulas made to look like their GMP produced counterparts, so buyer beware. The products of good quality factories are often copied. In particular, the popularity of the products manufactured by the Lanzhou Foci Pharmaceutical Factory has singled it out for mass imitation. The copies may look similar, but are clearly inferior in effect. Look for the Min Shan trademark.

Pill labeling

Many medicines list a narrow range of indications, or even misleading indications. This is due to the restricted nature of statements that the Therapeutic Goods Administration allows. The range of allowable statements are designed for over the counter pharmacy products, and are structured so that people with serious illnesses are not tempted to self prescribe. What suppliers are left with are bland and often incorrect statements such as 'Assists in blood circulation', 'For maintenance of peripheral circulation' and 'Helps provide stamina and endurance'.

Availability

Not all the medicines described in this volume are available at all times. Due to the current flux in the industry worldwide, new listed and registered medicines appear and some old favorites disappear. Products without TGA registration are not generally available in Australia, but are readily available in North America, the United Kingdom and Europe. We have made every effort to be as comprehensive and up to date as possible. Packaging changes from time to time, and standard formulations may be altered for no apparent reason.

Products available outside Australia

The original intent of this book was to record the commonly available and TGA listed over the counter medicines available in Australia. However, to expand the range of the text and to make it a more useful companion volume to the **Clinical Handbook of Internal Medicine** (2018 Maclean et al., Eastland Press), I have included a range of products not currently available in Australia. Many of these formulas are practitioner only products available from companies in America and the United Kingdom. These companies supply prepared medicines manufactured in GMP compliant facilities in China, and include Mayway Corporation (Plum Flower Brand), Bio Essence Corporation (Bio Essence Brand) and Nuherbs Co. (Herbal Times and Jade Dragon Brand). These formulas are manufactured under license by the same Chinese manufacturers represented extensively in this book. For example, the Plum Flower Brand is made by the Lanzhou Foci Pharmaceutical Factory in Gansu, maker of the famous Minshan Brand. Because their products are manufactured by Lanzhou Foci, I have chosen Plum Flower as representative of quality products available outside Australia and thus without official TGA listing.

A number of these formulas are available from several companies. Because of the variation in composition and proportions of herbs of some formulas with the same name supplied by different companies, the herbs listed are those of Plum Flower Brand. These formulas generally follow the classical prescription.

When a formula is available in the US or UK under different names, the suppliers are noted as follows: Plum Flower Brand – (PF), Bio Essence Brand – (BE), Herbal Times Brand – (HT), Jade Dragon Brand – (JD).

Given the fluidity and changes in regulation within the Chinese medicine market in the US, Europe and Australia (let alone China), products come and go, or are altered to meet legislative requirements with surprising rapidity. The products listed in this text are available at the time of printing, but may change formulation or be discontinued without notice.

妇科 1

Gynecological

1.1 BA ZHEN WAN

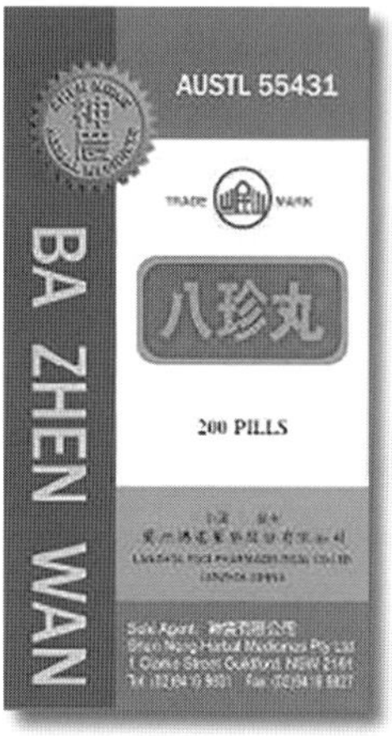

八珍丸

Lanzhou Foci Pharmaceutical Factory (Gansu)
'Eight Precious Pills'
Ba Zhen Wan is packaged in bottles of 200 pills
Also available as: Women's Precious Pills, Women's Precious Teapills (PF), Nu Ke Ba Zhen Wan, Tangkuei and Ginseng Eight Combination (conc. extract)

Chinese medical action

Tonifies qi and blood, regulates menstruation and the *chōng mài* and *rèn mài*

Biomedical action

Energy tonic and stimulant, promotes metabolism, hematinic, regulates menstruation, galactagogue

INDICATIONS

- Qi and blood deficiency. Widely used for menstrual disorders, and with the appropriate identifying features, **1.1 Ba Zhen Wan** can be used to treat a large variety of conditions associated with systemic qi and blood deficiency, including scanty menstrual periods or amenorrhea, infertility, habitual miscarriage, mild abnormal uterine bleeding, long menstrual cycle or irregular menstruation, postpartum weakness or insufficient lactation and weakness during pregnancy. Also useful for dull dysmenorrhea and lower abdominal pain that responds favorably to warmth and pressure.
- For non-gynecological conditions associated with qi and blood deficiency, including general fatigue and exhaustion, anemia, postural dizziness, visual weakness, floaters before the eyes, chronic hepatitis, debility, post surgical or post hemorrhage weakness, restless leg syndrome and malnutrition associated with deprivation or anorexia.
- Chronic muscle spasm, neck and shoulder pain aggravated by physical therapy like massage. There may be dull headaches that are worse when fatigued. The muscles feel firm or tense upon initial palpation but lack tone when palpated deeply.
- Chronic yin sores or ulcers that are slow to heal, such as bedsores, tropical ulcers, diabetic ulcers and chronic abscesses.

Composition (each pill contains powdered)

Angelica sinensis (dang gui, chinese angelica) 22mg, *Rehmannia glutinosa* (shu di, processed rehmannia) 22mg, *Paeonia alba* (bai shao, white peony) 15mg, *Atractylodes macrocephala* (bai zhu, atractylodes) 15mg, *Codonopsis pilosula* (dang shen, codonopsis) 15mg, *Poria cocos* (fu ling, hoelen) 15mg, *Ligusticum wallichi* (chuan xiong, ligusticum) 11mg, *Glycyrrhiza uralensis* (gan cao, licorice) 7mg

Pattern identifying features

- **qi and blood deficiency**
- **fatigue**
- anemia
- poor appetite

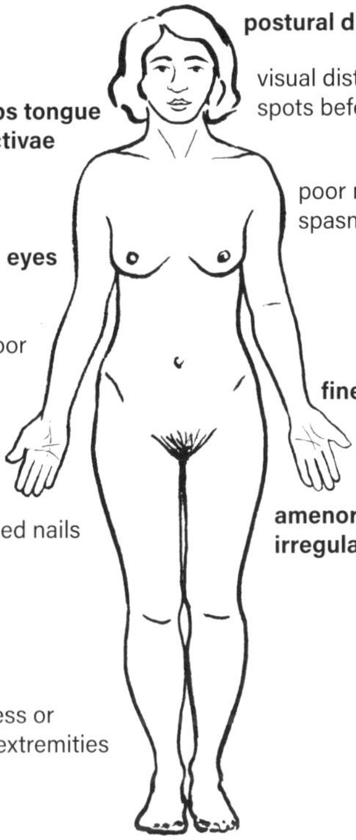

Combine with

- **7.12 Lu Rong Jiao** for yang deficient infertility, characterized by weak progesterone (yang) phase of the menstrual cycle (*see* pp.605, 606)
- **13.14 Ching Wan Hung** topically for chronic bedsores or tropical ulcers

Dosage and method of administration

8-12 pills three times daily on an empty stomach. The dose can be spread out, or taken in two lots of 12-18 pills, morning and evening. In severe cases or during the early stages of treatment (the first few weeks), a 50% increase in dose can be used, then reduced as treatment takes effect.

Cautions and contraindications

Contraindicated during the early phase of acute illness such as colds and flu. Care should be taken in patients with a tendency to abdominal bloating, loose stools or general digestive weakness. Some patients may find **1.1 Ba Zhen Wan** aggravates these symptoms. This can usually be alleviated by taking the pills with a small dose (3-6 pills at the same time) of **2.18 Bao He Wan** or **2.9 Xiang Sha Liu Jun Wan**.

1.2 SI WU WAN

四物丸

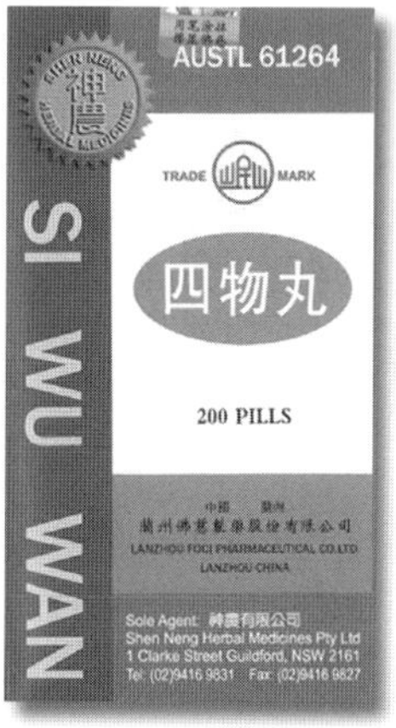

Lanzhou Foci Pharmaceutical Factory (Gansu)
'Four Ingredient Pills'
Si Wu Wan is packaged in bottles of 200 pills.
Also available as: Four Substances for Women Teapills (PF), Tangkuei Four Combination (conc. extract)

Chinese medical action

Tonifies blood, regulates menstruation and the *chōng mài* and *rèn mài*

Biomedical action

Hematinic, tones the uterus and muscles, galactagogue

INDICATIONS

- Blood deficiency. The base formula for tonifying blood and regulating menstruation, and the fundamental unit from which all blood tonic formulas are built. Especially good for menstrual disorders and Heart and Liver blood deficiency patterns. Used to augment other formulas where increased blood tonification is desired.
- Widely used for conditions associated with blood deficiency, such as anemia, visual weakness, dryness of the skin and eyes, chronic itchy dry skin diseases (such as eczema, dermatitis and psoriasis), and chronic sores or ulcers that are slow to heal, including diabetic ulcers, bedsores and tropical ulcers.
- With the appropriate identifying features, this formula can be used to treat conditions such as irregular menstruation, scanty periods, amenorrhea, insufficient corpus luteum function, postpartum convalescence, weakness during pregnancy, postpartum weakness and dizziness, postural dizziness, mild dysmenorrhea, infertility and insufficient lactation.

Composition (each pill contains powdered)

Rehmannia glutinosa (shu di, processed rehmannia) 60mg, *Angelica sinensis* (dang gui, chinese angelica) 60mg, *Paeonia alba* (bai shao, white peony) 60mg, *Ligusticum wallichi* (chuan xiong, ligusticum) 20mg

Combine with

- **14.1 Huang Lian Jie Du Wan** for stubborn skin diseases with inflammation, redness and thickening of the dermis (such as psoriasis)
- **13.14 Ching Wan Hung** topically for chronic bedsores or tropical ulcers
- **6.1 Xiao Chai Hu Wan** for acute or lingering colds and flu in run down women, or the same associated with the menstrual period
- **13.2 Xiao Feng Wan** for skin diseases with itching and dryness
- **7.22 Shen Qi Da Bu Wan** with a degree of qi deficiency

Pattern identifying features

- **blood deficiency**
- palpitations
- forgetfulness
- abdominal masses
- dysmenorrhea

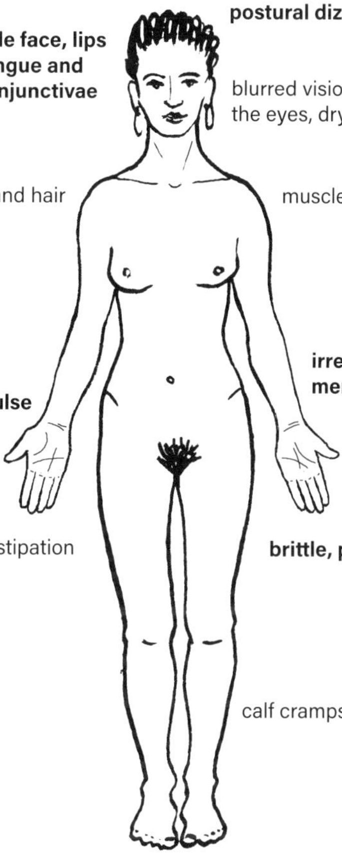

Dosage and method of administration

8-12 pills three times daily on an empty stomach. The dose can be spread out, or taken in two lots of 12-18 pills, morning and evening. In severe cases or during the early stages of treatment (the first few weeks), a 50% increase in dose can be used, then reduced as treatment takes effect.

Cautions and contraindications

Contraindicated during the early phase of acute illness such as colds and flu. Care should be taken in patients with a tendency to abdominal bloating, loose stools or general digestive weakness. Some patients may find **1.2 Si Wu Wan** aggravates these symptoms. This can usually be alleviated by taking the pills with a small dose (3-6 pills at the same time) of **2.18 Bao He Wan** or **2.9 Xiang Sha Liu Jun Wan**.

1.3 BA ZHEN YI MU WAN

八珍益母丸

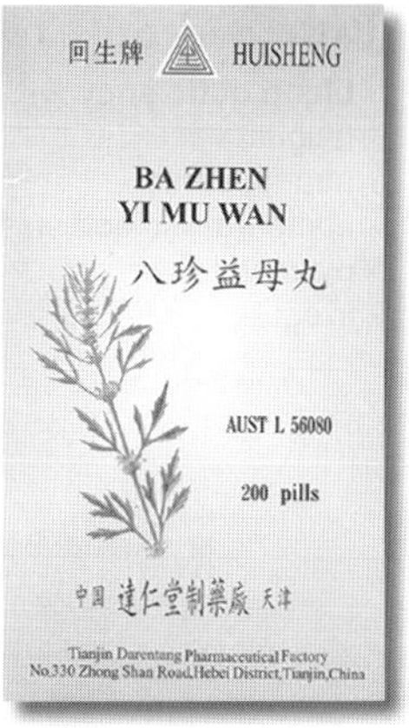

Tianjin Darentang Pharmaceutical Factory (Shandong)
'Eight Precious Pills with Motherwort'
Ba Zhen Yi Mu Wan is packaged in bottles of 200 pills

Chinese medical action

Tonifies qi and blood, regulates blood, menstruation and the *chōng mài* and *rèn mài*

Biomedical action

Energy tonic and stimulant, promotes metabolism, hematinic, stimulates blood circulation, regulates menstruation, emmenagogue

INDICATIONS

- Qi and blood deficiency with mild blood stasis. As a variation of **1.1 Ba Zhen Wan**, this formula has similar action and indications. The difference is the addition of *Leonurus sibirica* (yi mu cao, motherwort) which gently invigorates static blood and promote urination. **1.3 Ba Zhen Yi Mu Wan** is better when there is a mild degree of blood stasis in addition to qi and blood deficiency. Motherwort also assists in regulating menstruation, and is especially good for postpartum recovery, encouraging complete expulsion of birth products and quick contraction of the uterus back to normal.
- With the appropriate identifying features, this formula can be used to treat conditions such as postpartum blood stagnation, placental retention, scanty menstrual periods or amenorrhea, mild dysmenorrhea, infertility, habitual miscarriage, premenstrual fluid retention, mild abnormal uterine bleeding with clotting, long menstrual cycle, irregular menstruation, bedsores, tropical ulcers, diabetic ulcers and chronic abscesses.

Composition (each pill contains powdered)

Leonurus sibirica (yi mu cao, motherwort) 46mg, *Angelica sinensis* (dang gui, chinese angelica) 24mg, *Rehmannia glutinosa* (shu di, processed rehmannia) 24mg, *Paeonia alba* (bai shao, white peony) 11mg, *Atractylodes macrocephala* (bai zhu, atractylodes) 11mg, *Poria cocos* (fu ling, hoelen) 11mg, *Ligusticum wallichi* (chuan xiong, ligusticum) 11mg, *Glycyrrhiza uralensis* (gan cao, licorice 6mg), *Codonopsis pilosula* (dang shen, codonopsis) 11mg

Dosage and method of administration

8-12 pills three times daily on an empty stomach. The dose can be spread out, or taken in two lots of 12-18 pills, morning and evening. In severe cases, for placental retention, or in the early stages of treatment (the first few weeks), a 50% increase in dose can be used, then reduced as treatment takes effect.

Pattern identifying features

- **blood deficiency with mild blood stasis**
- fatigue
- poor appetite
- postpartum blood stasis
- placental retention
- irregular menstruation

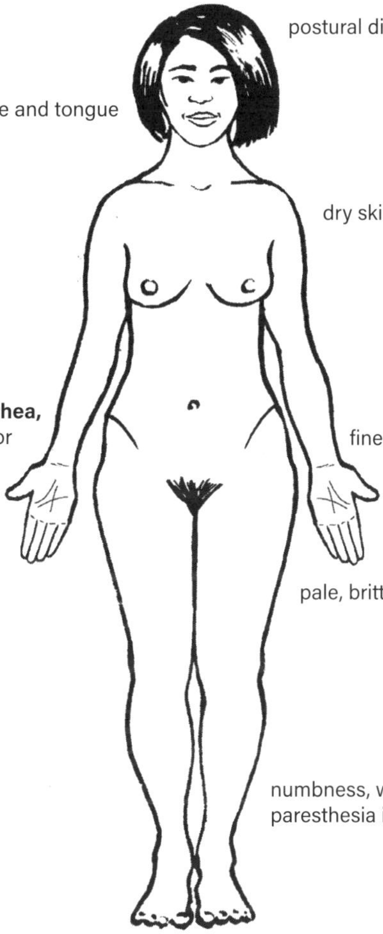

Cautions and contraindications

Contraindicated during the early phase of acute illness such as colds and flu. Care should be taken in patients with a tendency to abdominal bloating, loose stools or general digestive weakness. Some patients may find **1.3 Ba Zhen Yi Mu Wan** aggravates these symptoms. This can usually be alleviated by taking the pills with a small dose (3-6 pills at the same time) of **2.18 Bao He Wan** or **2.9 Xiang Sha Liu Jun Wan**.

1.4 YI MU TIAO JING TABLET

益母调经片

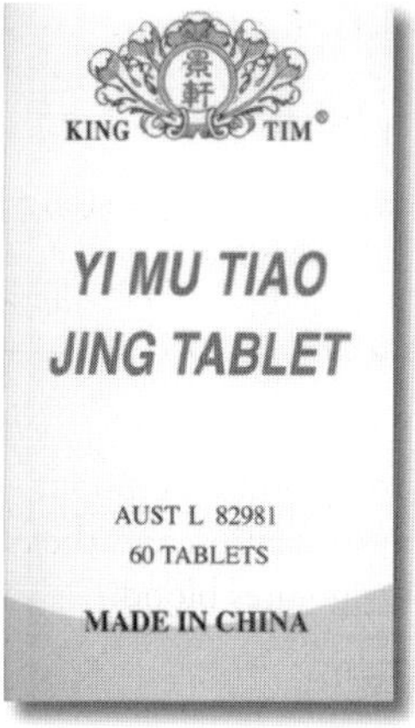

(*Yi Mu Tiao Jing Pian*)
Jing Xian Pharmaceutical Co. (Guangzhou)
'Motherwort Pills to Regulate Menstruation'
Yi Mu Tiao Jing Tablets are packaged in bottles of 60 tablets

Chinese medical action

Tonifies qi and blood, regulates qi and invigorates blood, regulates menstruation and the *chōng mài* and *rèn mài*

Biomedical action

Energy tonic and stimulant, promotes metabolism, hematinic, stimulates blood circulation, regulates menstruation, emmenagogue

INDICATIONS

- Blood deficiency with mild blood stasis causing irregular menstruation, and dysmenorrhea.
- Incomplete expulsion of birth products following labor. Enhances contraction of the uterus back to normal following childbirth.

Composition (each tablet contains extracts equivalent to dry)

Leonurus sibirica (yi mu cao, motherwort) 325mg, *Salvia miltiorrhiza* (dan shen, salvia) 325mg, *Cyperus rotundus* (xiang fu, cyperus) 325mg, *Rehmannia glutinosa* (shu di, processed rehmannia) 225mg, *Atractylodes macrocephala* (bai zhu, atractylodes) 225mg, *Angelica polymorpha* (dang gui, chinese angelica) 175mg, *Ligusticum wallichi* (chuan xiong, ligusticum) 175mg, *Paeonia lactiflora* (bai shao, white peony) 200mg

Dosage and method of administration

3-5 tablets, three times daily on an empty stomach.

Cautions and contraindications

Contraindicated during pregnancy and during the early phase of acute illness such as colds and flu. Care should be taken in patients with a tendency to abdominal bloating, loose stools or general digestive weakness. Any discomfort can usually be alleviated by taking the pills with a small dose (3-6 pills at the same time) of **2.18 Bao He Wan** or **2.9 Xiang Sha Liu Jun Wan**.

1.5 BU XUE TIAO JING TABLET

补血调经片

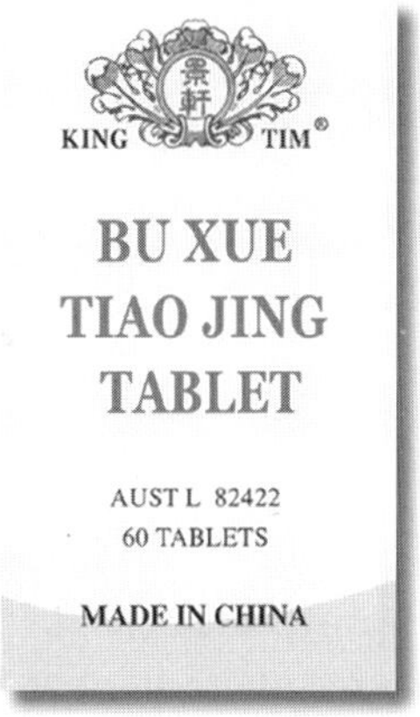

(*Bu Xue Tiao Jing Pian*)
Jing Xian Pharmaceutical Co. (Guangzhou)
'Tonify Blood and Regulate Menstruation Pills'
Bu Xue Tiao Jing Tablets are packaged in bottles of 60 tablets

Chinese medical action

Tonifies qi and blood, warms Kidney yang, regulates menstruation and the *chōng mài* and *rèn mài*, regulates qi and invigorates blood.

Biomedical action

Energy tonic and stimulant, promotes metabolism, hematinic, stimulates blood circulation, regulates menstruation, emmenagogue.

INDICATIONS

- Blood deficiency with mild blood stasis. Similar to **1.4 Yi Mu Tiao Jing Tablet**, with more emphasis on blood tonification. Useful for patterns with a greater component of blood deficiency, for example for women following a relatively severe hemorrhage during labor.

Composition (each tablet contains extracts equivalent to dry)

Rehmannia glutinosa (shu di, processed rehmannia) 450mg, *Angelica polymorpha* (dang gui, chinese angelica) 325mg, *Cyperus rotundus* (xiang fu, cyperus) 325mg, *Spatholobus suberectus* (ji xue teng, spatholobus) 325mg, *Leonurus sibirica* (yi mu cao, motherwort) 125mg, *Salvia miltiorrhiza* (dan shen, salvia) 125mg, *Atractylodes macrocephala* (bai zhu, atractylodes) 125mg, *Ligusticum wallichi* (chuan xiong, ligusticum) 125mg, *Dipsacus asper* (xu duan, dipsacus) 125mg, *Zizyphus jujuba* (da zao, chinese dates) 100mg

Dosage and method of administration

3-5 tablets, three times daily on an empty stomach.

Cautions and contraindications

Contraindicated during pregnancy and during the early phase of acute illness such as colds and flu. Care should be taken in patients with a tendency to abdominal bloating, loose stools or general digestive weakness. Any discomfort can usually be alleviated by taking the pills with a small dose (3-6 pills at the same time) of **2.18 Bao He Wan** or **2.9 Xiang Sha Liu Jun Wan**.

1.6 BAI FENG WAN

白凤丸

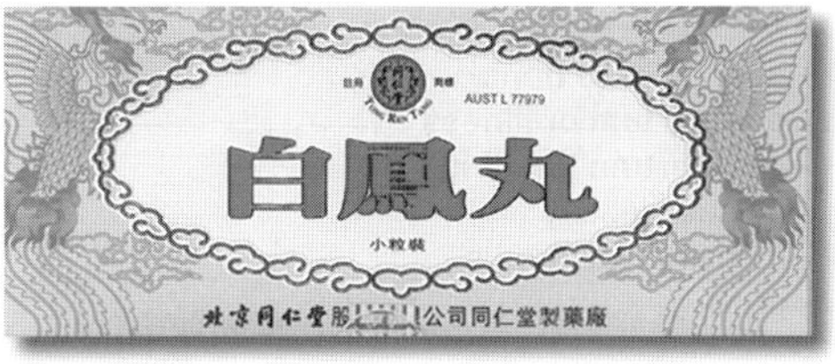

Tong Ren Tang (Beijing)
'White Phoenix Pills'

Bai Feng Wan is packaged either as small peppercorn sized honey pills or as a single large honey pill sealed inside a wax ball, ten balls per box

Chinese medical action

Tonifies qi and blood, nourishes Kidney yin, clears heat from deficiency, regulates menstruation and the *chōng mài* and *rèn mài*, stops leukorrhea

Biomedical action

Hematinic, tones the uterus and muscles, galactagogue

INDICATIONS

- Qi and blood deficiency patterns with mild Liver qi constraint. This version of **Bai Feng Wan** is very similar to **1.1 Ba Zhen Wan**, with the addition of ginseng and astragalus to tonify qi and strengthen the Spleen, and cyperus and salvia to regulate Liver qi and blood. The black boned chicken makes this a richer tonic, excellent for relatively severe blood deficiency. However, its gentle qi and blood moving qualities allow it to tonify without cloying and potentially aggravating stagnation.
- Traditionally used in China following menstruation to rebuild blood and qi, and to nourish blood to keep the skin healthy, soft and elastic.
- With the appropriate identifying features, this formula can be used to treat conditions such as profuse leukorrhea, irregular menstruation, premenstrual backache, scanty periods, amenorrhea, postpartum convalescence, weakness during pregnancy, postpartum weakness and dizziness, postural dizziness, infertility and insufficient lactation. Good for convalescence following major illness, chemotherapy or surgery.

Composition (each dose [50 small pills] contains)

Black boned chicken 550mg, *Rehmannia glutinosa* (sheng di, rehmannia) 570mg, *Angelica polymorpha* (dang gui, chinese angelica) 210mg, *Panax ginseng* (ren shen, ginseng) 190mg, *Paeonia lactiflora* (bai shao, white peony) 190mg, *Dioscorea opposita* (shan yao, dioscorea) 190mg, *Cyperus rotundus* (xiang fu, cyperus) 190mg, *Salvia miltiorrhiza* (dan shen, salvia) 190mg, *Ostrea gigas* (mu li, oyster shell) 140mg, *Ligusticum wallichi* (chuan xiong, ligusticum) 70mg, *Glycyrrhiza uralensis* (gan cao, licorice) 70mg, *Asparagus lucidius* (tian dong, asparagus) 70mg, *Astragalus membranaceous* (huang qi, astragalus) 70mg, *Stellaria dichotoma* (yin chai hu, stellaria root) 55mg, honey 1.9g

Dosage and method of administration

One pill (or a plastic ball of small pills) twice daily on an empty stomach.

Pattern identifying features

- **qi and blood deficiency with heat from deficiency**
- **postpartum or illness convalescence**
- **postpartum flushing or heat**
- fatigue, debility
- menstrual disorders
- poor memory, vision

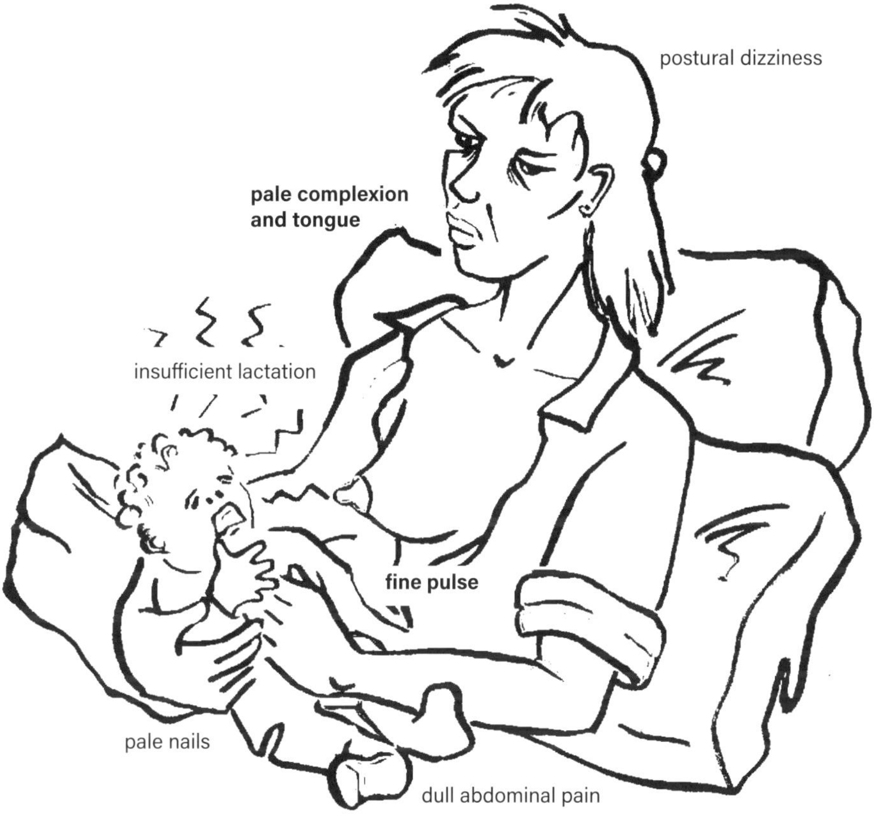

Cautions and contraindications

Contraindicated during the early phase of acute illness such as colds and flu. Care should be taken in patients with a tendency to abdominal bloating, loose stools or general digestive weakness. Some patients may find **1.6 Bai Feng Wan** aggravates these symptoms. This can usually be alleviated by taking the appropriate dose with a small quantity (3-6 pills at the same time) of **2.18 Bao He Wan** or **2.9 Xiang Sha Liu Jun Wan**.

1.7 WU JI BAI FENG WAN

乌鸡白凤丸

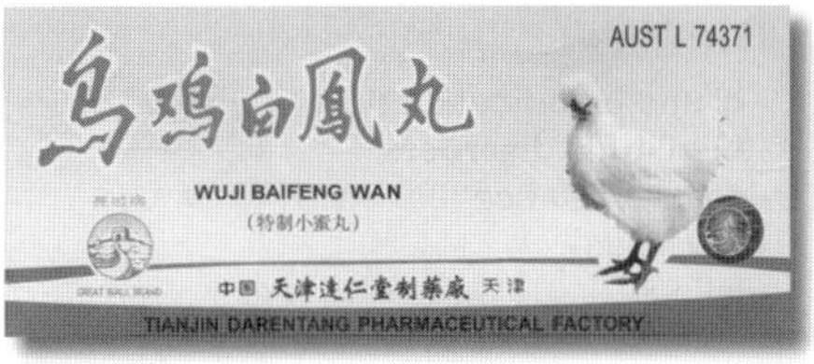

1-3/12

Tianjin Darentang Pharmaceutical Factory (Shandong)
'Black Chicken White Phoenix Pills'
Wu Ji Bai Feng Wan is packaged as small peppercorn sized honey pills inside a wax ball, ten balls per box

Chinese medical action

Tonifies qi, blood and Kidney yin and yang, regulates menstruation and the *chōng mài* and *rèn mài*, invigorates blood

Biomedical action

Energy tonic and stimulant, promotes metabolism, hematinic, regulates menstruation, galactagogue, emmenagogue

INDICATIONS

- Blood deficiency with Liver and Kidney deficiency. The black boned chicken is a special and nourishing tonic for the Liver and Kidneys, especially indicated for postpartum and severe blood deficiency. Similar to **1.6 Bai Feng Wan**, this version incorporates deer horn resin to enhance warming of Kidney yang and aid the transformation of food qi into blood. Well balanced and widely popular, **1.7 Wu Ji Bai Feng Wan** is able to strongly tonify without causing stagnation. Traditionally used in China following menstruation to rebuild blood and qi, and to nourish blood to keep the skin healthy, soft and elastic.
- With the appropriate identifying features, this formula can be used to treat conditions such as infertility, anovulation, scanty periods, amenorrhea, postpartum weakness and postural dizziness, mild dysmenorrhea and insufficient lactation. In addition, it is useful for severe or refractory anemia, to protect bone marrow during chemotherapy or radiotherapy and for chronic sores and ulcers that are slow to heal, such as bedsores, diabetic ulcers and tropical ulcers.

Composition (each dose [50 small pills] contains)

Black boned chicken 1.5g, *Rehmannia glutinosa* (shu di, processed rehmannia) 600mg, *Cervus japonicus* (lu jiao jiao, deer horn resin) 450mg, *Angelica polymorpha* (dang gui, chinese angelica) 335mg, *Paeonia lactiflora* (bai shao, white peony) 300mg, *Panax ginseng* (ren shen, ginseng) 300mg, *Dioscorea opposita* (shan yao, dioscorea) 300mg, *Cyperus rotundus* (xiang fu, cyperus) 300mg, *Salvia miltiorrhiza* (dan shen, salvia) 300mg, *Asparagus lucidius* (tian dong, asparagus) 150mg, *Ligusticum wallichi* (chuan xiong, ligusticum) 150mg, *Euryale ferox* (qian shi, euryale seed) 150mg, *Ostrea gigas* (mu li, oyster shell) 110mg, *Scutellaria baicalensis* (huang qin, scute) 85mg, *Glycyrrhiza uralensis* (gan cao, licorice) 75mg, *Stellaria dichotoma* (yin chai hu, stellaria root) 60mg, honey 2.3g

Pattern identifying features

- **qi and blood deficiency, Liver and Kidney deficiency**
- **menstrual disorders**
- cold intolerance
- low libido
- fatigue

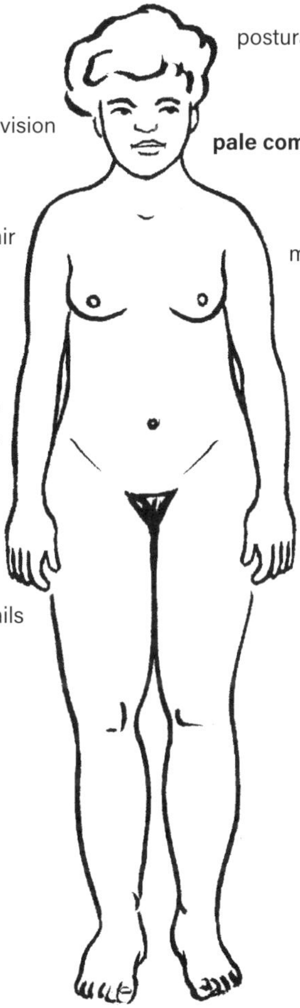

Combine with

– With **13.14 Ching Wan Hung** topically for bedsores or tropical ulcers

Dosage and method of administration

50 small pills (the contents of one wax ball) twice daily, on an empty stomach.

Cautions and contraindications

Contraindicated during the early phase of acute illness such as colds and flu. Generally well tolerated, however some sensitive patients may find **1.7 Wu Ji Bai Feng Wan** causes abdominal bloating, loose stools or general digestive upset. This can usually be alleviated by taking the dose with a small quantity (3 6 pills at the same time) of **2.18 Bao He Wan** or **2.9 Xiang Sha Liu Jun Wan**.

1.8 TONG REN WU JI BAI FENG WAN

同仁乌鸡白凤丸

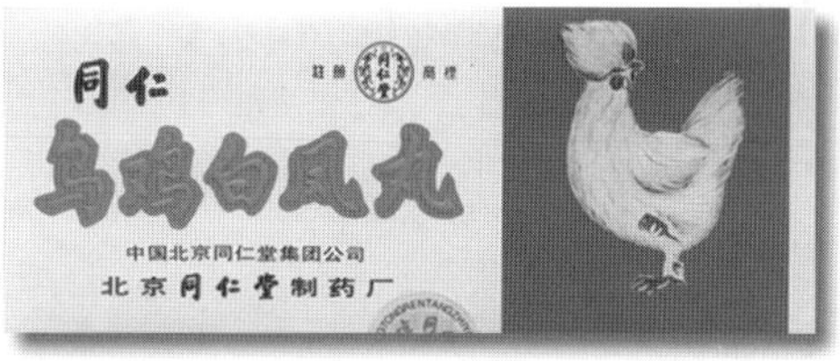

Tong Ren Tang (Beijing)
'Black Chicken White Phoenix Pills from Tong Ren Tang'

Tong Ren Wu Ji Bai Feng Wan is packaged as large 9 gram honey pills sealed inside a wax ball, ten balls per box

Chinese medical action

Tonifies qi, blood and Kidney yin, regulates qi and menstruation, clears heat from deficiency

Biomedical action

Energy tonic and stimulant, hematinic, regulates menstruation

INDICATIONS

- Qi and blood deficiency, with mild depletion of yin resulting in heat from deficiency and sweating. Similar to **1.6 Bai Feng Wan**, with an emphasis on clearing heat.
- Postpartum problems such as blood deficiency, anemia, low grade afternoon or bone steaming fever and night sweats.
- Irregular menstruation, mild abnormal uterine bleeding, leukorrhea and mild dysmenorrhea associated with deficiency.

Composition

Black bone chicken, *Panax ginseng* (ren shen, ginseng), *Angelica sinensis* (dang gui, chinese angelica) *Rehmannia glutinosa* (shu di, processed rehmannia), *Cyperus rotundus* (xiang fu, cyperus), *Ostrea gigas* (mu li, oyster shell), *Stellaria dichotoma* (yin chai hu, stellaria root)

Dosage and method of administration

One pill chewed twice daily on an empty stomach.

Cautions and contraindications

Contraindicated during the early phase of acute illness such as colds and flu. Generally well tolerated, however some sensitive patients may find **1.8 Tong Ren Wu Ji Bai Feng Wan** causes abdominal bloating, loose stools or general digestive upset. This can usually be alleviated by taking the dose with a small quantity (3-6 pills at the same time) of **2.18 Bao He Wan** or **2.9 Xiang Sha Liu Jun Wan**.

Pattern identifying features

- **qi and blood deficiency with heat from deficiency**
- low grade fever, bone steaming fever
- facial flushing, malar flush
- night sweats, easy sweating
- exhaustion, fatigue
- insomnia
- insufficient lactation

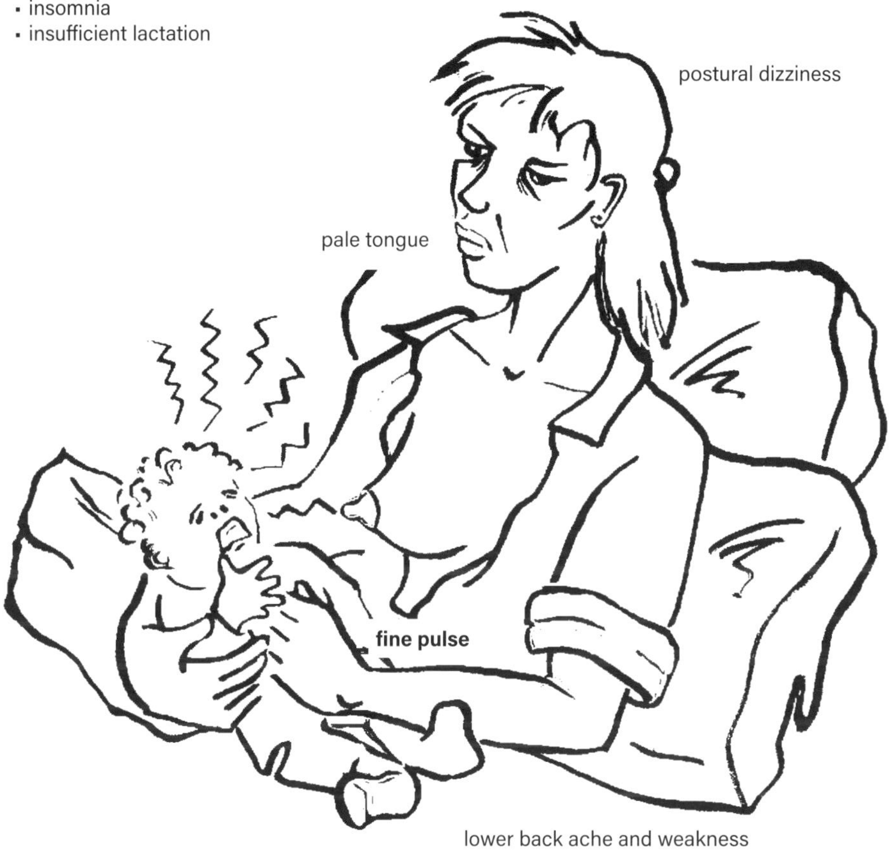

1.9 GUI PI WAN

归脾丸

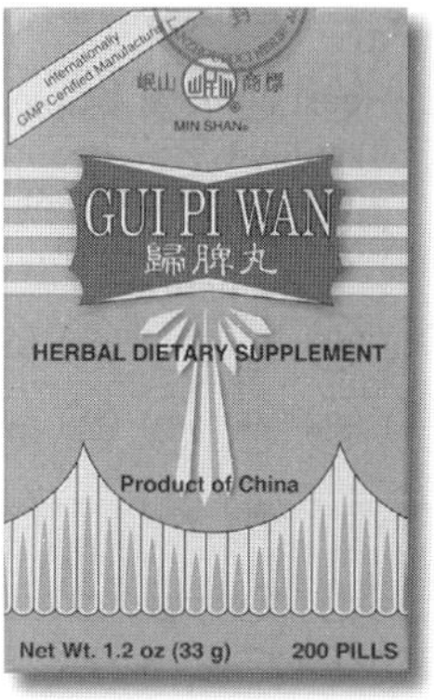

Lanzhou Foci Pharmaceutical Factory (Gansu)
'Return the [Health of] Spleen Pills'
Gui Pi Wan is packaged in bottles of 200 pills.
Also available as: Kuei Be Wan, Gui Pi Teapills (PF), Ginseng and Longan Combination (conc. extract)

Chinese medical action

Tonifies qi and blood, strengthens the Spleen and Heart, calms the *shén*, strengthens the Spleen's function of keeping blood in the vessels

Biomedical action

Enhances digestive functions, hematinic, hemostatic, sedative for anxiety and mild neurosis, nervine

INDICATIONS

- Spleen qi and Heart blood deficiency. The focus of this important formula is to nourish qi and blood, strengthen the Spleen's blood holding capacity, and calm the *shén*.
- Menstrual disorders associated with qi and blood deficiency, such as scanty periods or amenorrhea, irregular menstruation, infertility and premenstrual syndrome with insomnia and anxiety.
- For a wide variety of bleeding disorders resulting from the Spleen qi failing to hold blood in the vessels, including uterine bleeding, intermenstrual bleeding, menorrhagia, continuous spotting, easy bruising, rectal bleeding, bleeding hemorrhoids, purpura and clotting disorders.
- Heart and *shén* disorders associated with qi and blood deficiency, and blood failing to anchor the *shén*, including insomnia, palpitations, poor concentration and memory, anxiety, panic attacks, phobias, mental obsession and obsessive compulsive disorder.
- Postpartum disorders from qi and blood deficiency with weakness, fatigue, anxiety, depression, breathlessness, postural dizziness and anemia.
- With the appropriate identifying features, this formula can be used to treat conditions such as thrombocytopenic or allergic purpura, Henoch Schönlein purpura, supraventricular tachycardia, cardiac arrhythmia, anemia, neurosis, hypoproteinemia, chronic gastroenteritis, chronic fatigue syndrome and some mild psychiatric disorders.

Composition

Angelica sinensis (dang gui, chinese angelica), *Poria cocos* (fu ling, hoelen), *Polygala tenuifolia* (yuan zhi, polygala), *Atractylodes macrocephala* (bai zhu, atractylodes), *Euphoriae longana* (long yan rou, longan), *Zizyphus spinoza* (suan zao ren, zizyphus), *Saussurea lappa* (mu xiang, saussurea), *Astragalus membranaceous* (huang qi, astragalus), *Glycyrrhiza uralensis* (gan cao, licorice)

Pattern identifying features

- **Heart blood and Spleen qi deficiency**
- **insomnia**
- **anxiety**, panic attacks
- **bleeding disorders**
- poor memory, forgetfulness
- poor appetite
- fatigue, weakness
- visual disturbances

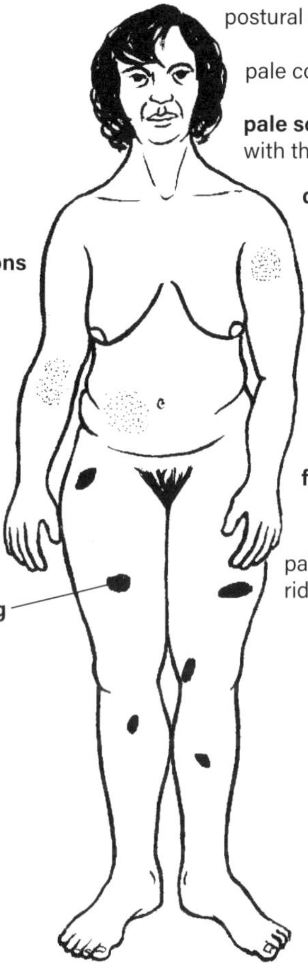

Combine with

– **6.4 Xiao Yao Wan** (taken day 15-28 to regulate qi and the yang phase), and **1.9 Gui Pi Wan** taken following menstruation until mid-cycle (day 4-14, to nourish blood and yin) for irregular menstruation, infertility and other menstrual disorders

Dosage and method of administration

8-12 pills three times daily on an empty stomach. The dose can be spread out, or taken in two lots of 12-18 pills, morning and evening. In severe cases or during the early stages of treatment (the first few weeks), a 50% increase in dose can be used, then reduced as treatment takes effect.

Cautions and contraindications

Contraindicated during the early phase of acute illness such as colds and flu. Care in patients with a tendency to damp or phlegm, abdominal bloating or loose stools. This can usually be alleviated by combining with a small dose (3-6 pills at the same time) of **2.18 Bao He Wan** or **2.9 Xiang Sha Liu Jun Wan**.

GMP

1.10 DANG GUI JING

1-3/12

当归精

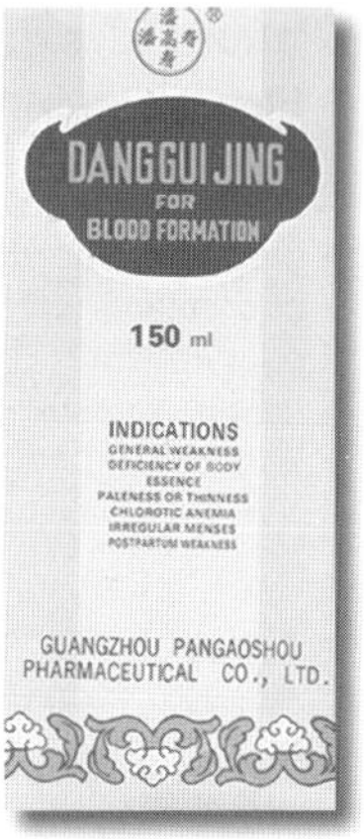

(*Dang Gui Jing*)
Guangzhou Pangaoshou Pharmaceutical Company (Guangzhou)
'Essence of *Angelica sinensis*'
Dang Gui Jing is packaged as liquid in bottles of 150ml

Chinese medical action

Tonifies qi and blood, regulates menstruation and the *chōng mài* and *rèn mài*

Biomedical action

Energy tonic and stimulant, promotes metabolism, hematinic, regulates menstruation, galactagogue

INDICATIONS

- Qi and blood deficiency. Used to treat a wide variety of conditions associated with qi and blood deficiency, including gynecological conditions such as scanty menstrual periods, amenorrhea, infertility, habitual miscarriage, long menstrual cycle or irregular menstruation, postpartum weakness or insufficient lactation and weakness during pregnancy.
- Also used for non-gynecological conditions associated with qi and blood deficiency, including general fatigue and exhaustion, anemia, postural dizziness, visual weakness, floaters before the eyes, generalized weakness, post surgical or post hemorrhage weakness, restless leg syndrome and malnutrition associated with deprivation or anorexia.

Composition

Angelica sinensis (dang gui, chinese angelica), *Codonopsis pilosula* (dang shen, codonopsis), *Rehmannia glutinosa* (shu di, processed rehmannia), *Paeonia alba* (bai shao, white peony), *Poria cocos* (fu ling, hoelen), *Ligusticum wallichi* (chuan xiong, ligusticum), *Astragalus membranaceous* (huang qi, astragalus), *Glycyrrhiza uralensis* (zhi gan cao, honey fried licorice root)

Dosage and method of administration

10mls, three times daily on an empty stomach.

Pattern identifying features

- **blood deficiency**
- anemia
- postpartum or post hemorrhage weakness
- fatigue

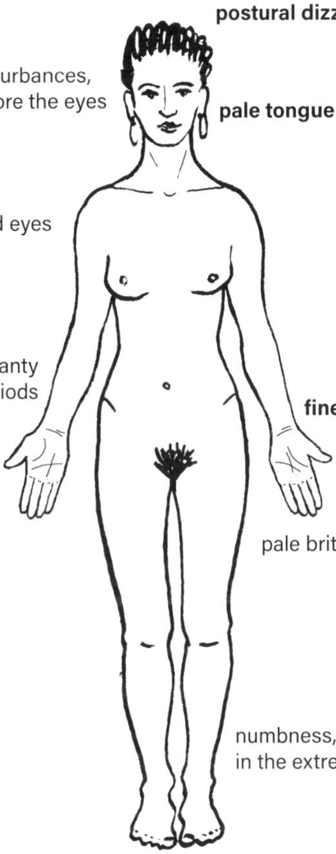

Cautions and contraindications

Contraindicated during the early phase of acute illness such as colds and flu. Care in patients with a tendency to dampness or phlegm, abdominal bloating or loose stools. This can usually be alleviated by taking the formula with a small dose (3-6 pills at the same time) of **2.18 Bao He Wan** or **2.9 Xiang Sha Liu Jun Wan**.

1.11 DANG GUI WAN

当归丸

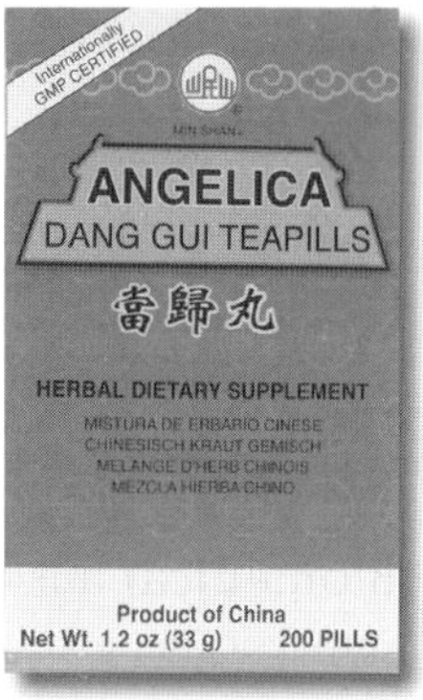

Lanzhou Foci Pharmaceutical Factory (Gansu)
'Dang Gui Pills'
Dang Gui Wan is packaged in bottles of 200 pills
Also available as: Angelica Dang Gui Teapills (PF)

Chinese medical action

Tonifies qi and blood, regulates menstruation

Biomedical action

Hematinic

INDICATIONS

- Blood and qi deficiency. Especially good for menstrual disorders, such as mild dysmenorrhea, amenorrhea, scanty menstruation, fatigue following menstruation, infertility, postpartum abdominal pain and dizziness, anemia and insufficient lactation.
- Dizziness, insomnia, poor memory, anxiety, tics and tremors from Heart and Liver blood deficiency.
- Traumatic injury, superficial suppurative sores, wind damp painful obstruction, and postpartum abdominal pain from sluggish blood circulation or stasis.
- Chronic constipation in the elderly and postpartum women.
- Can be added to other constitutional formulas when enhanced qi and blood tonification is desired.

Composition

Angelica sinensis (dang gui, chinese angelica), *Ligusticum wallichi* (chuan xiong, ligusticum), *Atractylodes macrocephala* (bai zhu, atractylodes), *Zizyphus jujuba* (da zao, chinese date)

Dosage and method of administration

4-6 pills three times daily on an empty stomach. The dose can be spread out, or two lots of 6-9 pills taken morning and evening.

Cautions and contraindications

Contraindicated during the early phase of acute illness such as colds and flu, and during pregnancy. Very occasionally a sensitive patient may experience mild nausea, diarrhea or loose stools in the early days of treatment. This can be alleviated by reducing the dose or by adding a few pills of **2.18 Bao He Wan** or **2.9 Xiang Sha Liu Jun Wan**.

1.12 SHI XIAO WAN

失效丸

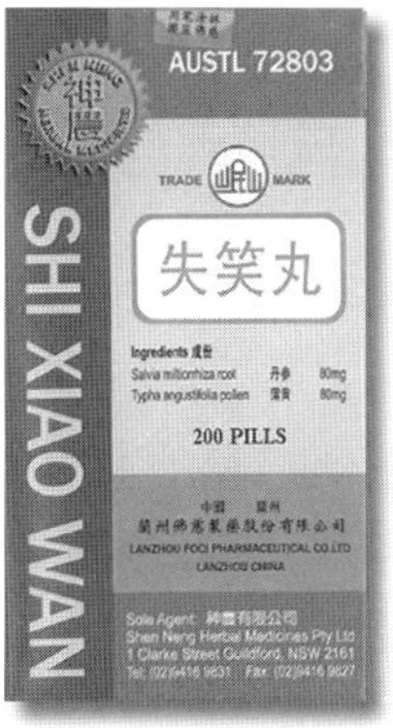

Lanzhou Foci Pharmaceutical Factory (Gansu)
'Break Into a Smile Pills'
Shi Xiao Wan is packaged in bottles of 200 pills

Chinese medical action

Invigorates blood, disperses stagnant blood, stops pain

Biomedical action

Analgesic, improves circulation

INDICATIONS

- Blood stasis pain. Mostly used for gynecological pain, but can be used for pain originating from other sites such as the stomach, hypochondrium and head. Usually added to a constitutional formula where a degree of blood invigorating action is desired.
- May be used prior to and during menstruation when pain is anticipated, to enhance the analgesic affect of any other treatments.

Composition (each pill contains powdered)

Salvia miltiorrhiza (dan shen, salvia) 80mg, *Typhae angustifolia* (pu huang, bulrush pollen) 80mg

Combine with

– **6.4 Xiao Yao Wan** for dysmenorrhea from qi and blood stasis
– **6.3 Chai Hu Shu Gan Wan** for focal epigastric pain from Liver qi invading the Stomach

Dosage and method of administration

The recommended dose if used alone is 8-12 pills three times daily before meals. However, this formula is usually combined with a constitutional formula, in which case the dose can be reduced by 50-75%.

Cautions and contraindications

Contraindicated during pregnancy. Caution in patients taking warfarin or other blood thinning agents as clotting time may be reduced.

GMP

1.13 WOO GARM YUEN MEDICAL PILLS

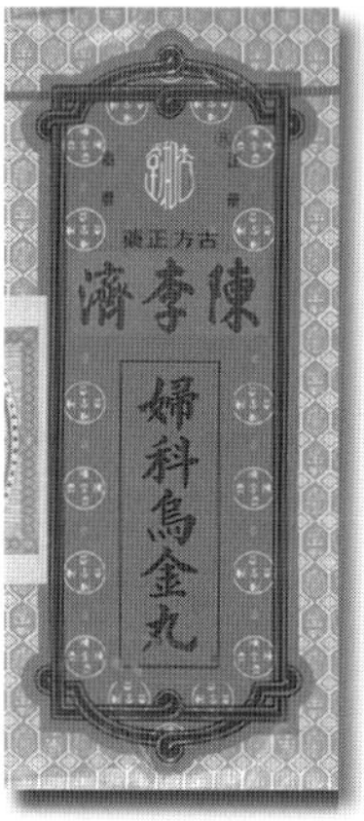

妇科乌金丸

(*Fu Ke Wu Jin Wan*)
Chan Li Chai Medical Factory (Hong Kong)
'Black and Gold Pills for Gynecological Disorders'
Woo Garm Yuen Medical Pills are packaged as large honey pills in a yellow wax ball, ten pills per box

Chinese medical action

Invigorates qi and blood, disperses stagnant blood, dispels cold, warms the uterus, nourishes blood

Biomedical action

Emmenagogue, regulates menstruation, improves circulation, stops pain, relieves stagnation in the uterus

INDICATIONS

- Dysmenorrhea, fibroids, endometriosis or cysts from blood and qi stagnation with cold accumulation in the uterus or other structures of the lower burner. Also for uterine bleeding and bleeding fibroids from blood stasis. The primary mechanism is cold accumulation causing poor movement and subsequent pooling of blood in the pelvic basin. A well balanced formula that equally addresses the blood stasis and the cold; best for excess patterns with little deficiency.
- With the appropriate identifying features, this formula can be used to treat primary dysmenorrhea, mittlesmertz, gynecological masses, chronic pelvic inflammatory disease, polycystic ovaries, amenorrhea, intermenstrual bleeding, infertility, irregular menstrual cycle (especially long cycle) and postpartum placental retention. It can also be used for prostatic masses and prostatic hypertrophy in men from blood stasis, cold and qi deficiency.

Composition

Artemesia vulgaris (ai ye, mugwort) 13.6%, *Cyperus rotundus* (xiang fu, cyperus) 13.6%, *Atractylodes macrocephala* (bai zhu, atractylodes) 12.5%, *Angelica sinensis* (dang gui, chinese angelica) 8.2%, *Cinnamomum cassia* (rou gui, cinnamon bark) 8.2%, *Curcuma ezhu* (e zhu, curcuma) 7%, *Typhae angustifolia* (pu huang, bulrush pollen) 6.8%, *Solidago virdaurea* (liu ji nu, solidago) 6.8%, *Scutellaria baicalensis* (huang qin, scute) 6.8%, *Citrus reticulata* (qing pi, immature citrus) 5.5%, *Citrus aurantium* (zhi ke, aurantium) 5.5%, *Zingiber officinalis* (gan jiang, dry ginger) 5.5%

Combine with

- **1.1 Ba Zhen Wan** or **1.16 Tao Hong Si Wu Wan** during the first half of the menstrual cycle for women with heavy periods with lots of pain and clotting; start **1.13 Woo Garm Yuen Medical Pills** after mid-cycle, or just before if there is ovulation pain

Pattern identifying features

- **blood stasis and cold in the Uterus and lower burner**
- **dark menstrual blood with significant clotting**
- **lower abdominal masses**
- spider veins around the medial ankle and knee
- cold intolerance, cold extremities
- low abdomen feels cool to the touch

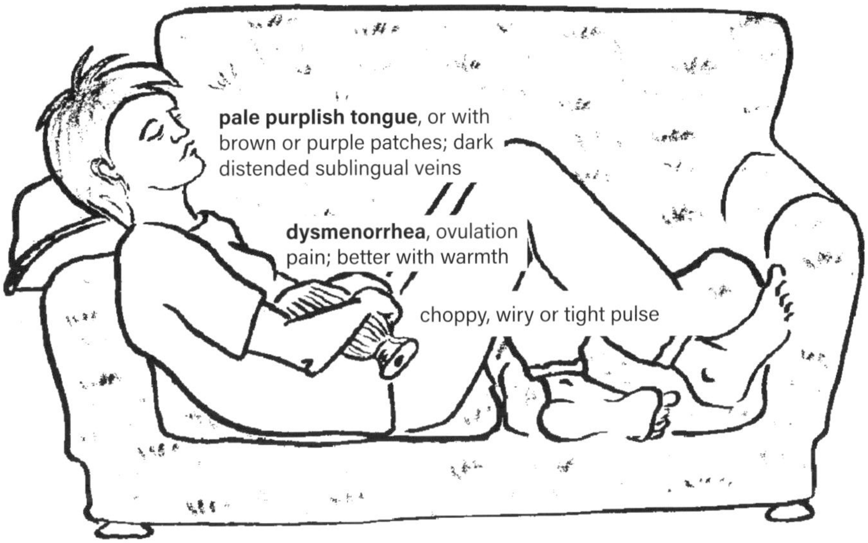

- **1.34 Hai Zao Jing Wan** or **1.35 Nei Xiao Luo Li Wan** for phlegm type gynecological cysts and masses
- **7.9 Jin Gui Shen Qi Wan** or **7.10 You Gui Wan** for patients with significant yang deficiency
- **11.1 Qian Lie Xian Capsule** or **11.2 Prostate Gland Pills** for male urinary disturbances from prostate swelling

Dosage and method of administration

One or two pills per day with warm water, yellow wine (*shào xīng jiǔ* 绍兴酒) or ginger tea, on an empty stomach. Can be taken through a menstrual period to take advantage of the extra movement of blood during that time. The pills are quite hard and need to be softened in boiling water for 10 minutes before ingestion.

Cautions and contraindications

Contraindicated during pregnancy and in women with menorrhagia without dark blood or clotting. Some women will experience heavier (and possibly more painful) periods once or twice as the stagnation is moved. Caution in patients on anticoagulant therapy. Watch for bruising or increased tendency to bleeding.

GMP

1.14 WEN JING WAN

温经丸

1-3/12

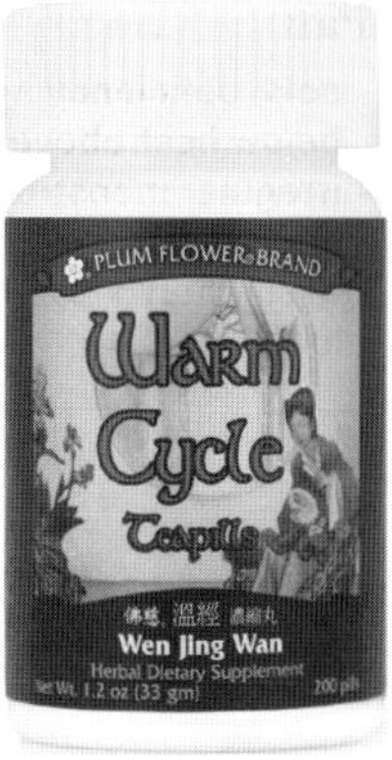

Lanzhou Foci Pharmaceutical Factory (Gansu)
'Pills to Warm Menses'
Wen Jing Wan is packaged in bottles of 200 pills
Also available as: Tangkuei and Evodia Combination (conc. extract)

Chinese medical action

Tonifies qi and blood, warms the Uterus, regulates *chōng mài* and *rèn mài* invigorates blood and dispels static blood

Biomedical action

Regulates menstruation, stops pain

INDICATIONS

- Deficiency and cold patterns of the Uterus, *chōng mài* and *rèn mài*, with cold congealing blood and blood stasis. The main focus is to strengthen qi and blood while warming and dispelling cold from the Uterus, and gently dispersing static blood. Cold displaces the natural warmth of the lower burner; the heat is forced to the periphery as fever, dry mouth and warm palms. The key features are the unpredictably of length and volume of the menstrual period, the coldness of the lower abdomen which is significantly relieved by warmth, and pain which is somewhat alleviated by pressure, or at least not made significantly worse. Compared to **1.18 Shao Fu Zhu Yu Wan** and **1.13 Woo Garm Yuen Medical Pills**, used when the pattern is primarily excess, this formula is best for patterns of mixed excess and deficiency. A common pattern of older women experiencing menopausal symptoms and infertility.
- Impotence, erectile dysfunction, sperm disorders (motility problems, low count), testicular pain, prostate pain and swelling and urinary disorders from yang deficiency with mild blood stasis in the lower burner.
- With the appropriate identifying features, this formula may assist in the treatment of conditions such as irregular menstruation, uterine bleeding, persistent bleeding following termination or miscarriage, infertility, chronic pelvic inflammatory disease, primary dysmenorrhea and amenorrhea.

Composition

Evodia rutacarpae (wu zhu yu, evodia), *Angelica sinensis* (dang gui, chinese angelica), *Paeonia lactiflora* (chao bai shao, dry fried white peony), *Equus asinus* (e jiao, donkey skin gelatin), *Codonopsis pilosula* (dang shen, codonopsis), *Pinellia ternata* (zhi ban xia, processed pinellia), *Ophiopogon japonicus* (mai dong, ophiopogon), *Cinnamomum cassia* (gui zhi, cinnamon twigs), *Paeonia suffruticosa* (mu dan pi, moutan), *Glycyrrhiza uralensis* (gan cao, licorice), *Ligusticum wallichi* (chuan xiong, ligusticum), *Zingiber officinale* (sheng jiang, ginger)

Pattern identifying features

- **cold, deficiency and blood stasis affecting the Uterus and *chōng mài* and *rèn mài*; cold below heat above**
- **irregular menstruation**
- **infertility**
- **dysmenorrhea**
- low grade fever at dusk

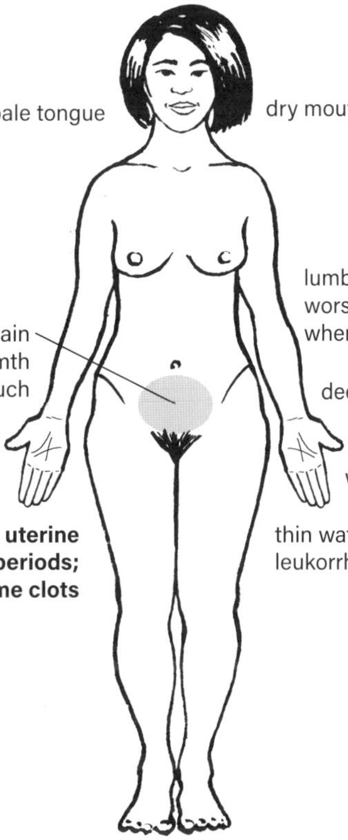

Combine with

- **2.13 Li Zhong Wan** for more severe cold
- **10.2 Raw Tienchi Tablets** for persistent bleeding
- **11.4 Tian Tai Wu Yao Wan** with qi constraint

Dosage and method of administration

8-12 pills three times daily on an empty stomach. The dose can be spread out, or taken in two lots of 12-18 pills, morning and evening. Can be taken through the entire period, including during the bleed, to gently encourage the expulsion of static blood.

Cautions and contraindications

Contraindicated during pregnancy, in women with menorrhagia without dark blood or clotting, and in cases where the excess, i.e. blood stasis and cold is the primary pathogen (*see* **1.18 Shao Fu Zhu Yu Wan** or **1.13 Woo Garm Yuen Medical Pills** for that problem).

1.15 TONG JING WAN

痛经丸

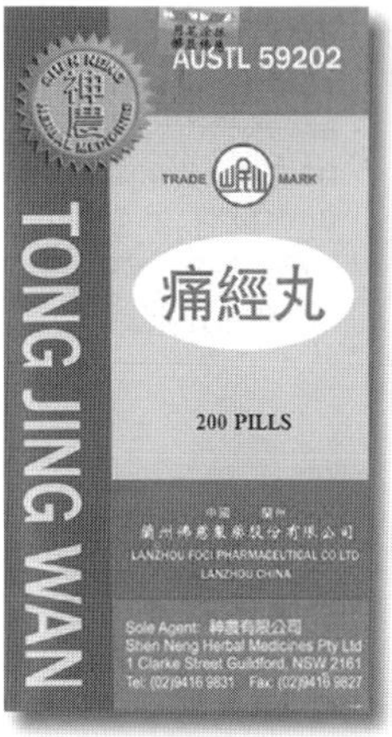

Lanzhou Foci Pharmaceutical Factory (Gansu)
'Dysmenorrhea Pills'
Tong Jing Wan is packaged in bottles of 200 pills
Also available as: Calm in the Sea of Life Teapills (PF), Period Ease Pills (BE)

Chinese medical action

Invigorates qi and blood in the lower burner, disperses stagnant blood, stops pain

Biomedical action

Regulates menstruation, improves circulation, stops pain, relieves stagnation in the uterus

INDICATIONS

- Relatively severe blood stasis causing dysmenorrhea or amenorrhea. This is a strong blood moving and analgesic formula, suitable for robust patients with little or no deficiency. Can be used during and prior to menstruation for pain associated with gynecological masses and endometriosis.
- Used for blood stasis patterns and masses in other structures of the lower burner in women and men, such as in the prostate, testicles, or urinary bladder causing dysuria or hematuria.
- Post surgical blood stasis and pain.

Composition (each pill contains powdered)

Paeonia lactiflora (bai shao, white peony) 24.5mg, *Prunus persica* (tao ren, peach seed) 24.1mg, *Salvia miltiorrhiza* (dan shen, salvia) 20.4mg, *Lindera strychnifolia* (wu yao, lindera) 20.4mg, *Corydalis turtschaninovii* (yan hu suo, corydalis) 20.4mg, *Cyperus rotundus* (xiang fu, cyperus) 16.4mg, *Angelica polymorpha* (dang gui, chinese angelica) 16.4mg, *Ligusticum wallichi* (chuan xiong, ligusticum) 14.4mg, *Carthamus tinctorius* (hong hua, carthamus) 12.4mg, *Panax pseudoginseng* (tian qi, pseudoginseng) 10.2mg

Combine with

- **1.12 Shi Xiao Wan** or **10.21 Yan Hu Suo Zhi Tong Wan** to enhance the analgesic action during episodes of pain
- **1.2 Si Wu Wan** for patients with blood deficiency
- **1.13 Woo Garm Yuen Medical Pills** for relatively dysmenorrhea associated with fibroids or endometriosis
- **11.1 Qian Lie Xian Capsules** or **11.2 Prostate Gland Pills** for prostate swelling and perineal pain from blood stasis

Pattern identifying features

- **blood stasis pain**
- lower abdominal pain and distension, worse with pressure
- palpable masses
- dark or clotted menstrual blood
- usually younger women < 35

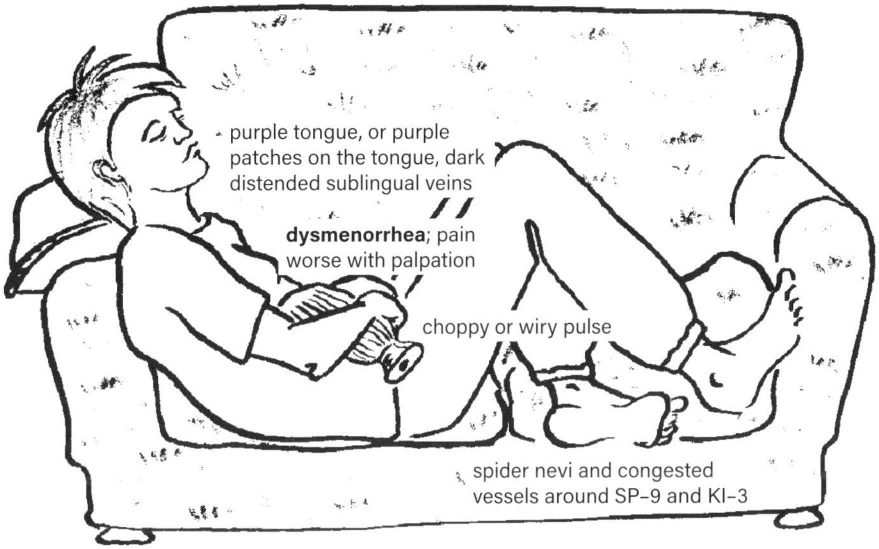

Dosage and method of administration

8-12 pills three times daily, on an empty stomach. The dose can be spread out, or taken in two lots of 12-18 pills, morning and evening. An increased dose can be used in the week prior to an expected painful period. Can be taken through a period to promote movement of blood.

Cautions and contraindications

Contraindicated during pregnancy and in women with menorrhagia without dark blood or clotting. Caution in patients who are very run down or fatigued. Some women will experience heavier, and possibly more painful periods once or twice as the stagnation is moved. Caution in patients taking warfarin or other blood thinning agents as clotting time may be reduced.

1.16 TAO HONG SI WU WAN

桃红四物丸

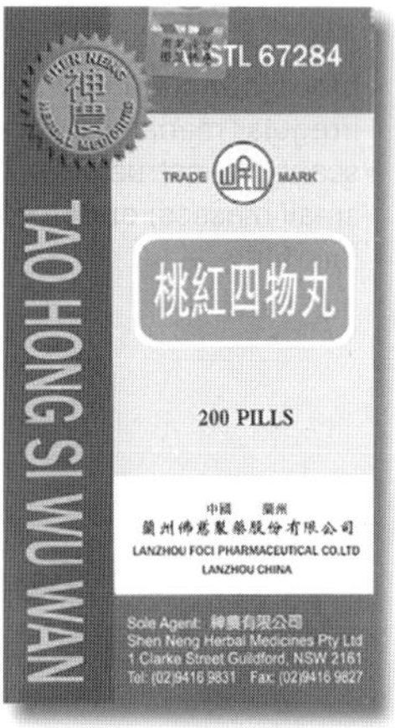

Lanzhou Foci Pharmaceutical Factory (Gansu)
'Four Ingredient Pills with Safflower and Peach Seed'
Tao Hong Si Wu Wan is packaged in bottles of 200 pills
Also available as: Tao Hong Si Wu Tang Teapills (PF), Tangkuei Four, Persica and Carthamus Combination (conc. extract)

Chinese medical action

Tonifies and invigorates blood, gently disperses static blood

Biomedical action

Emmenagogue, regulates menstruation, improves circulation, stops pain, relieves mild stasis in the uterus

INDICATIONS

- Menstrual disorders from mild blood stasis and blood deficiency affecting the Uterus or other structures of the lower burner. Widely used to treat dysmenorrhea, amenorrhea, irregular menstruation, shortened periods with heavy or clotted bleeding, menorrhagia, infertility, chronic pelvic inflammatory disease and masses such as fibroids, endometriosis, fallopian tube blockage or cysts.
- To encourage expulsion of retained birth products and lochia following birth.
- To assist recovery of bruising and contusions following traumatic injury, especially when there has been significant hemorrhage associated with the trauma. Helpful for preventing adhesions and alleviating constipation after abdominal surgery.
- Post traumatic stress disorder, chronic depression. These conditions frequently have a component of blood stasis, and a gentle blood invigorating approach can help initiate movement without forcing it, and assist in recovery.
- This formula has broad application, and although mostly used for gynecological problems, any condition characterized by blood deficiency with mild blood stasis can be treated. With the appropriate identifying features, these include circulatory, cardiovascular, cerebrovascular, dermatological and hepatic disorders such as varicose and spider veins, chronic phlebitis, peripheral neuropathy, post stroke hemiplegia, tics and tremors, chronic eczema, psoriasis and dermatitis, purplish discoloration of the limbs, mild angina, hepatosplenomegaly and anemia.

Composition (each pill contains powdered)

Rehmannia glutinosa (shu di, processed rehmannia) 36mg, *Angelica sinensis* (dang gui, chinese angelica) 36mg, *Paeonia lactiflora* (bai shao, white peony) 36mg, *Prunus persica* (tao ren, peach seed) 36mg, *Carthamus tinctorius* (hong hua, carthamus) 18mg, *Ligusticum wallichi* (chuan xiong, ligusticum) 18mg

Combine with

- **6.4 Xiao Yao Wan** for depression or post traumatic stress with Liver qi constraint
- **13.2 Xiao Feng Wan** for chronic itchy skin diseases with purplish or painful lesions

Pattern identifying features

- **blood deficiency with mild blood stasis**
- irregular menstrual cycle (short or long)
- scanty menstrual flow, amenorrhea
- small masses; endometriosis, fibroids
- infertility

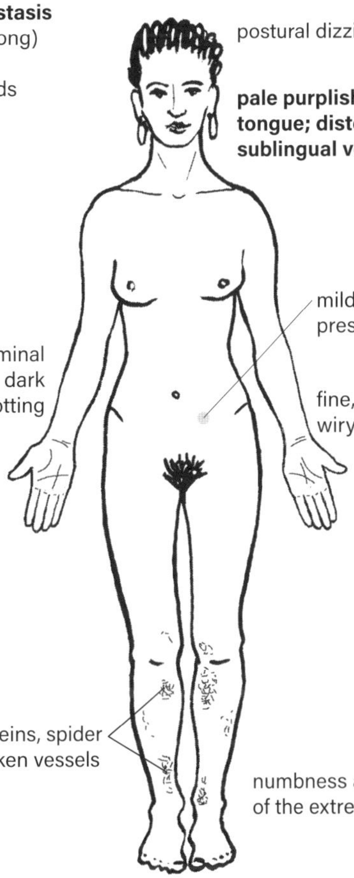

- **5.7 Sunho Multi Ginseng Tablets** for small gynecological masses and circulatory and peripheral vascular disorders
- **1.12 Shi Xiao Wan** for severe dysmenorrhea
- **2.22 Er Chen Wan** for numbness in the extremities from blood and phlegm stagnation following wind-stroke

Dosage and method of administration

8-12 pills three times daily on an empty stomach. The dose can be spread out, or taken in two lots of 12-18 pills, morning and evening. In severe cases or during the early stages of treatment (the first few weeks), a 50% increase in dose can be used, then reduced as treatment takes effect. Can be taken through a menstrual period to promote movement of blood.

Cautions and contraindications

Contraindicated during pregnancy and in women with menorrhagia without dark blood or clotting. Some women will experience heavier (and possibly more painful) periods once or twice as stagnation is moved.

1.17 GUI ZHI FU LING WAN

桂枝茯苓丸

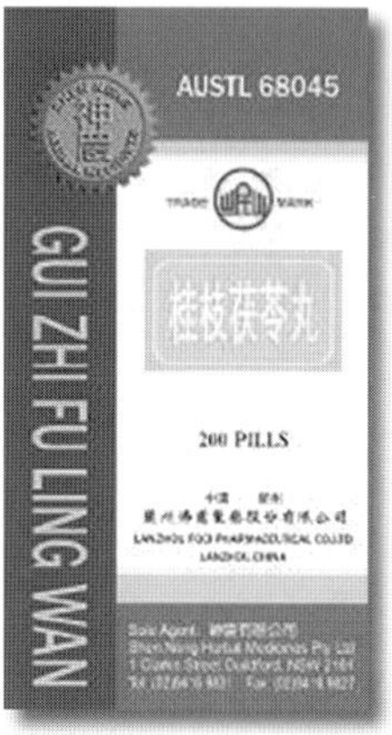

Lanzhou Foci Pharmaceutical Factory (Gansu)
'Cinnamon Twig and Hoelen Pills'
Gui Zhi Fu Ling Wan is packaged in bottles of 200 pills
Also available as: Cinnamon and Poria Teapills (PF), Cinnamon and Poria Formula (conc. extract)

Chinese medical action

Invigorates blood and gradually disperses static blood, warms the uterus, and dissipates abdominal masses

Biomedical action

Emmenagogue, regulates menstruation, improves circulation, stops pain, relieves stagnation in the uterus

INDICATIONS

- Blood stasis masses affecting the reproductive system and lower burner. Used for small benign gynecological masses such as fibroids, cysts, endometriosis and chronic inflammatory masses.
- Blood stasis in the prostate or testicles, with pain that may radiate to the groin or lower abdomen, masses and lumps, or blood stagnation affecting sperm quality. Useful following vasectomy reversal.
- With the appropriate identifying features, this formula can be used to treat disorders such as mild primary dysmenorrhea, fibroids, ovarian cysts, chronic pelvic inflammatory disease, cervical erosion, chronic salpingitis, endometriosis and postpartum placental retention, testicular varicosities or varicocele, hemospermia, non-liquefaction of sperm, antisperm antibodies (immunological infertility, especially following vasectomy reversal), aspermia, post traumatic, surgical or idiopathic testicular pain and mild uncomfortable prostatic swelling.

Composition (each pill contains powdered)

Poria cocos (fu ling, hoelen) 36mg, *Cinnamomum cassia* (gui zhi, cinnamon twigs) 36mg, *Prunus persica* (tao ren, peach seed) 36mg, *Paeonia suffruticosa* (mu dan pi, peony root bark) 36mg, *Paeonia veitchii* (chi shao, red peony) 36mg

Combine with

- **1.2 Si Wu Wan** to nourish blood and regulate menstruation. If a stronger blood moving action is desired, combine with **1.16 Tao Hong Si Wu Wan**
- Other formulas to encourage the movement of qi and blood in the lower burner, such as **7.9 Jin Gui Shen Qi Wan** or **7.16 Shi Quan Da Bu Wan** if blood stasis is due to weak circulation of yang and pooling of blood; with **7.1 Liu Wei Di Huang Wan** or **1.23 Zhi Bai Di Huang Wan** if due to congealing of blood from increased viscosity associated with yin deficiency

Pattern identifying features

- **small blood stasis type masses**
- amenorrhea
- infertility

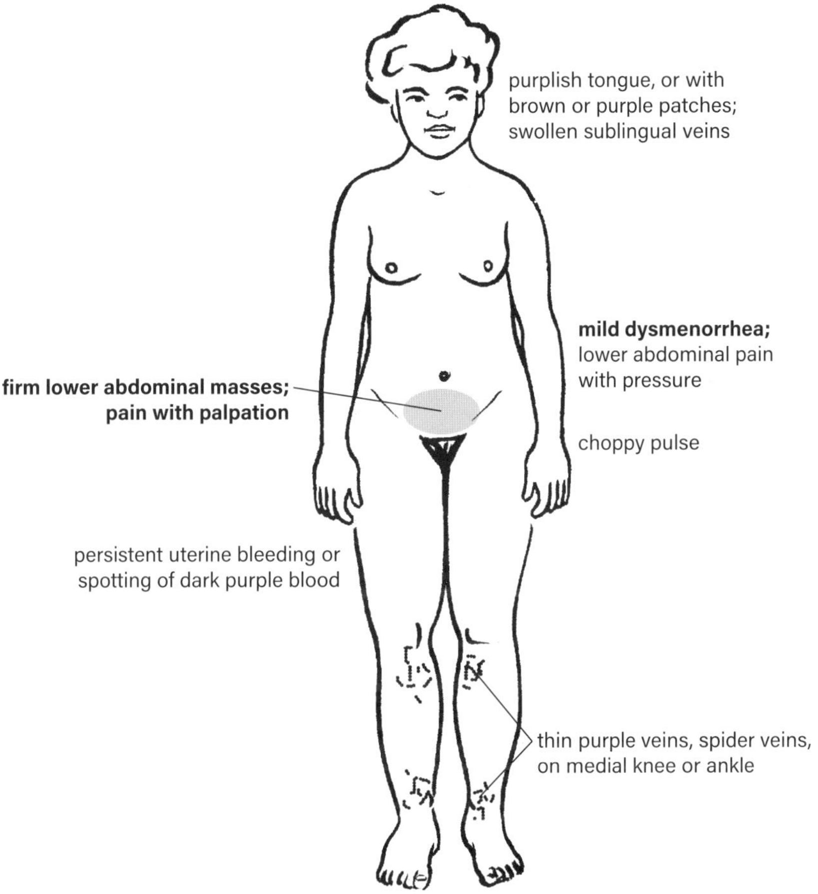

Dosage and method of administration

8-12 pills three times daily on an empty stomach. The dose can be spread out, or taken in two lots of 12-18 pills, morning and evening. Can be taken through the entire menstrual cycle, including the period to encourage the expulsion of static blood.

Cautions and contraindications

Extreme caution during pregnancy. **1.17 Gui Zhi Fu Ling Wan** was originally designed for bleeding during pregnancy accompanied by abdominal pain, and thus is quite a gentle formula. It is rarely used during pregnancy today, and only by very experienced practitioners.

GMP

1.18 SHAO FU ZHU YU WAN

少腹逐瘀丸

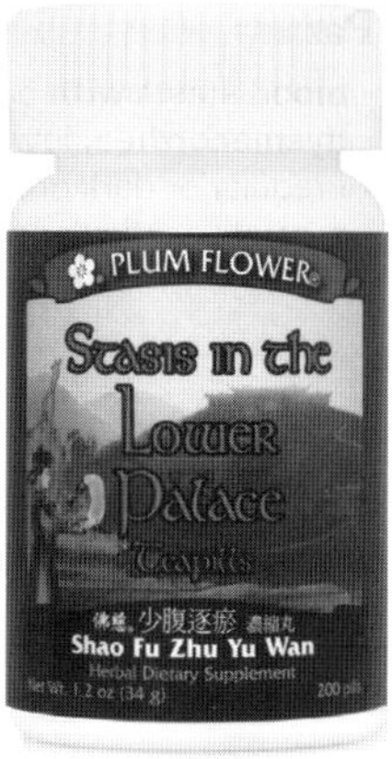

3+/12

Lanzhou Foci Pharmaceutical Factory (Gansu)
'Remove Stagnant Blood from the Lower Abdomen Pills'
Shao Fu Zhu Yu Wan is packaged in bottles of 200 pills
Also available as: Fennel Seed and Corydalis Combination (conc. extract)

Chinese medical action

Invigorates blood, breaks up stagnant blood, warms the Uterus and lower burner, dispels cold, stops pain

Biomedical action

Vasodilator, analgesic, anti-platelet action, softens and resolves masses

INDICATIONS

- Blood stasis with cold in the lower burner. The main features are lower abdominal pain alleviated by heat, and/or palpable masses which may or may not be painful. A variation of **5.1 Xue Fu Zhu Yu Wan**, specifically targeted at dispelling cold and dispersing stagnant blood from the lower burner.
- Gynecological disorders with dark clotted bleeding and pain, or palpable masses. The main feature is the nature of the pain – fixed, sharp, focal, worse with palpation, but alleviated somewhat by heat.
- Cold and blood stasis patterns of the lower burner in men, including disorders such as chronic prostatic and testicular swelling and discomfort, and pelvic pain syndrome.
- With the appropriate identifying features, this formula may assist in the treatment of conditions such as endometriosis, fibroids, ovarian cysts, dysmenorrhea, premenstrual backache, mittlesmertz, amenorrhea, menorrhagia, uterine bleeding, irregular menstruation, infertility, prostatic hypertrophy or early dysplasia, bladder pain, varicocele or painful testicular masses.

Composition

Angelica sinensis (dang gui, chinese angelica), *Typhae angustifolia* (pu huang, bulrush pollen), *Paeonia veitchii* (chi shao, red peony), *Corydalis turtschaninovii* (yan hu suo, corydalis), *Ligusticum wallici* (chuan xiong, ligusticum), *Commiphora myrrha* (mo yao, myrrh), *Cinnamomum cassia* (rou gui, cinnamon bark), *Foeniculum vulgarae* (chao xiao hui xiang, dry fried fennel seed), *Zingiber officinale* (gan jiang, dry ginger), *Boswellia carterii* (ru xiang*, frankincense) [*substituted for the restricted* Trogopterus xanthipes *(wu ling zhi, flying squirrel feces) of the original formula*]

Combine with

– **1.16 Tao Hong Si Wu Wan** for patients with a greater degree of blood deficiency

Pattern identifying features

- **blood stasis with cold in the lower burner**
- **dysmenorrhea, lower abdominal pain**
- irregular or dark or purple and clotted menses, abnormal uterine bleeding
- prostate, testicular and bladder pathology

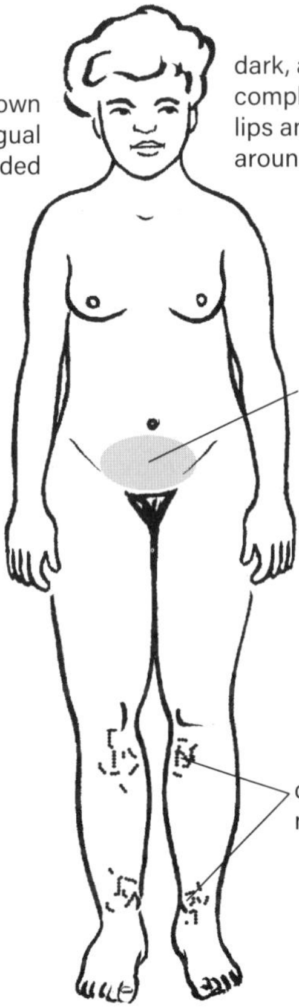

Dosage and method of administration

8-12 pills three times daily on an empty stomach. The dose can be spread out, or taken in two lots of 12-18 pills, morning and evening. In severe cases or during the early stages, a 50% increase in dose can be used, then reduced as treatment takes effect. Can be taken through a menstrual period to promote movement of blood.

Cautions and contraindications

Contraindicated during pregnancy, in women with menorrhagia (other than that associated with blood stasis), and with bleeding disorders. Caution in patients on anticoagulant therapy. Watch for bruising or increased tendency to bleeding. Prolonged use can deplete qi and blood, so a break every 2-3 months, with a change to a simple qi and blood tonic for a few weeks, is recommended.

GMP

1.19 YANG RONG WAN

养荣丸

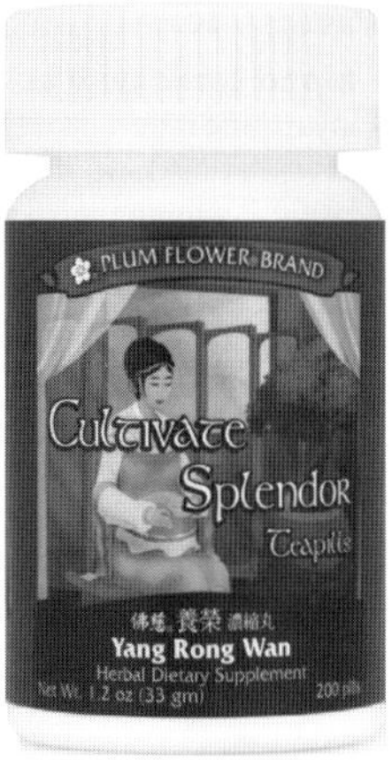

3+/12

Lanzhou Foci Pharmaceutical Factory (Gansu)
'Luxuriantly Nourishing Pills'
Yang Rong Wan is packaged in bottles of 200 pills

Chinese medical action

Warms and tonifies qi and blood, warms the Uterus and Kidney yang, regulates menstruation and the *chōng mài* and *rèn mài*

Biomedical action

Energy tonic and stimulant, promotes metabolism, hematinic, regulates menstruation, emmenagogue

INDICATIONS

- Menstrual disorders and infertility from qi and blood deficiency, cold accumulation in the Uterus, and Spleen and Kidney yang deficiency. Used to regulate and strengthen *chōng mài* and *rèn mài*, thus promoting healthy menses and fertility. Typical features include irregular periods (usually long cycles), scanty periods, dull dysmenorrhea improved with warmth, watery leukorrhea, premenstrual backache and infertility.
- Persistent uterine bleeding, menorrhagia or spotting from cold in the Uterus with underlying Spleen and Kidney deficiency.
- For the post ovulation (progesterone) phase of a cyclical treatment (days 15-28, *see* glossary) to warm and maintain Kidney yang.

Composition

Angelica sinensis (dang gui, chinese angelica), *Rehmannia glutinosa* (shu di, processed rehmannia), *Atractylodes macrocephala* (bai zhu, atractylodes), *Paeonia lactiflora* (bai shao, white peony), *Ligusticum wallichi* (chuan xiong, ligusticum), *Cyperus rotundus* (xiang fu, cyperus), *Leonurus heterophylla* (yi mu cao, motherwort), *Eucommia ulmoides* (du zhong, eucommia), *Astragalus membranaceous* (huang qi, astragalus), *Artemesia argyi* (ai ye, mugwort), *Poria cocos* (fu ling, hoelen), *Equus asinus* (e jiao, donkey skin gelatin), *Ophiopogon japonicus* (mai dong, ophiopogon), *Citrus reticulata* (chen pi, citrus), *Glycyrrhiza uralensis* (gan cao, licorice), *Amomum villosum* (sha ren, cardamom)

Combine with

- A Liver and Kidney and blood tonic, such as a mixture of **7.1 Liu Wei Di Huang Wan** and **1.2 Si Wu Wan**, or qi and blood tonic such as **1.9 Gui Pi Wan** or **7.16 Shi Quan Da Bu Wan**) during the first half of a menstrual cycle to strengthen the Kidneys and tonify qi and blood, with **1.19 Yang Rong Wan** given in the second half to support yang and the progesterone phase

Pattern identifying features

- **qi and blood deficiency, cold in the Uterus, Spleen and Kidney yang deficiency**
- **infertility**
- irregular menstruation
- fatigue, weakness, exhaustion
- cold intolerance

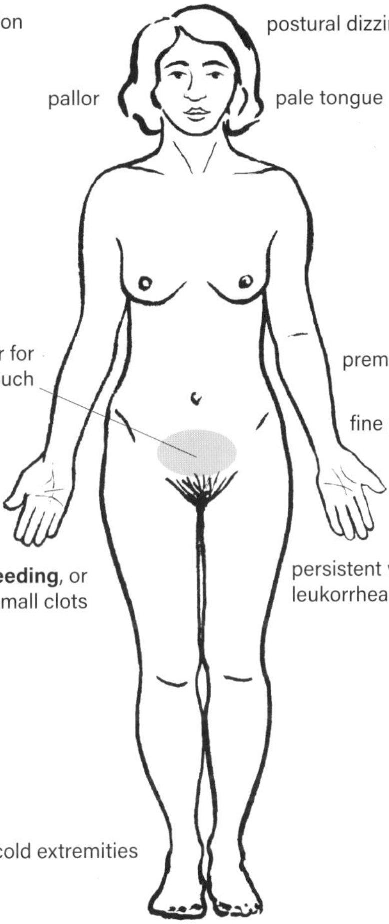

Dosage and method of administration

8-12 pills three times daily on an empty stomach. The dose can be spread out, or taken in two lots of 12-18 pills, morning and evening. In severe cases or during the early stages of treatment (the first few weeks), a 50% increase in dose can be used, then reduced as treatment takes effect.

Cautions and contraindications

Contraindicated during the early phase of acute illness such as colds and flu. Care in patients with a tendency to dampness or phlegm, abdominal bloating or loose stools, although the cardamom and citrus in this formula generally mean it is well tolerated.

1.20 CU YUN YU TAI CAPSULE

促孕育胎丸 [妇女宝]

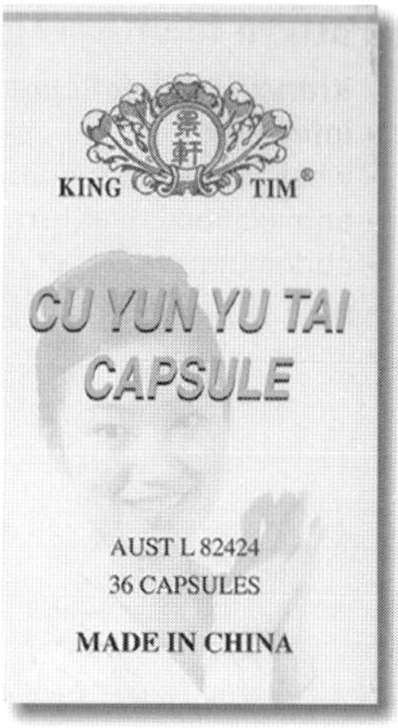

(*Cu Yun Yu Tai Wan*, also listed in Chinese as *Fu Nu Bao*)
'Promote Pregnancy Pills'
Cu Yun Yu Tai Capsules are packaged in bottles of 36 capsules

Chinese medical action

Tonifies the Liver and Kidneys, warms the Uterus and Kidney yang, regulates the *chōng mài* and *rèn mài*, strengthens the Spleen, regulates qi and invigorates blood, promotes transformation of yin into yang

Biomedical action

Strengthens the progesterone phase of the menstrual cycle, thermogenic, stimulant, promotes ovulation

INDICATIONS

- Infertility associated with Kidney yang qi deficiency, *chōng mài* and *rèn mài* dysfunction, and cold accumulation in the Uterus. This is usually reflected in the basal body temperature chart – the post ovulation progesterone (yang) phase fails to rise sufficiently or to maintain an adequate rise long enough. Supports the yang phase of the menstrual cycle and promotes transformation of yin into yang at mid-cycle to encourage ovulation.
- Used to strengthen yang in those women prone to recurrent miscarriage due to yang deficiency. Also for low libido and impotence from weak Kidney yang.
- With the appropriate identifying features, this formula may be used for primary and secondary infertility, irregular menstruation, long menstrual cycle, low or short progesterone phase of the menstrual cycle, copious thin watery leukorrhea, weakness in the lower back, knees and legs, loss of libido, dizziness and general debility.

Composition (each capsule contains extract equivalent to dry)

Astragalus membranaceous (huang qi, astragalus) 248mg, *Paeonia lactiflora* (bai shao, white peony) 248mg, *Cuscuta hygrophila* (tu su zi, cuscuta) 248mg, *Lycium barbarum* (gou qi zi, lycium fruit) 223mg, *Salvia miltiorrhiza* (dan shen, salvia) 223mg, *Rehmannia glutinosa* (shu di, processed rehmannia) 173mg, *Dioscorea opposita* (shan yao, dioscorea) 173mg, *Epimedium brevicornu* (xian ling pi, epimedium) 124mg, *Curculigo orchioides* (xian mao, curculigo) 124mg, *Dipsacus asper* (xu duan, dipsacus) 124mg, *Panax ginseng* (ren shen, ginseng) 22.5mg

Combine with

- A blood tonic such as **1.2 Si Wu Wan**, **1.9 Gui Pi Wan** or **7.16 Shi Quan Da Bu Wan** during the first half of the menstrual cycle to replenish qi and blood, followed by **1.20 Cu Yun Yu Tai Capsule** after ovulation to regulate qi and blood, support Kidney yang and the progesterone phase
- **1.2 Si Wu Wan** for a greater degree of blood deficiency

Pattern identifying features

- **Kidney yang deficiency, *chōng mài* and *rèn mài* deficiency; cold in the Uterus**
- **infertility**
- weak yang (progesterone) phase of menstrual cycle
- anovulation
- abdominal pain, better for warmth
- poor appetite
- loss of libido

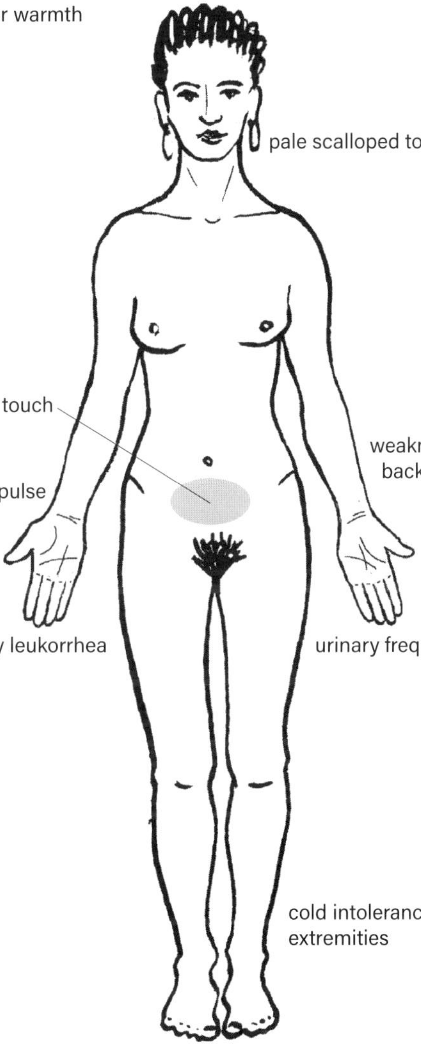

Dosage and method of administration

3-4 capsules, three times daily on an empty stomach.

Cautions and contraindications

Contraindicated during the early phase of acute illness such as colds and flu, and infertility associated with yin deficiency or heat patterns. Caution during pregnancy. Caution for patients on anticoagulant therapy; watch for bruising or increased tendency to bleeding.

1.21 TIAO JING CU YUN WAN

调经促孕丸

Tong Ren Tang (Beijing)
'Regulate Menses, Promote Pregnancy Pills'
Tiao Jing Cu Yun Wan Pills are packaged in vials of 50 pills, ten vials per box

Chinese medical action

Warms and tonifies Kidney and Spleen yang, invigorates blood, warms the Uterus, promotes transformation of yin into yang

Biomedical action

Regulates the hypothalamic-ovarian axis, regulates menstruation, strengthens the progesterone phase of the menstrual cycle, promotes ovulation

INDICATIONS

- Infertility, long menstrual cycles, scanty periods or amenorrhea associated with Kidney and Spleen yang deficiency. Quite a warm formula, specifically designed to promote ovulation and to maintain the yang phase of the menstrual cycle once ovulation has occurred. Astragalus and salvia are used to assist ovulation by mobilizing and elevating yang qi and moving blood.
- With the appropriate identifying features, this formula can be used to treat conditions such as primary or secondary infertility, amenorrhea, irregular menstruation, anovulation and corpus luteum failure.

Composition

Cervus japonicus (lu rong, deer velvet), *Epimedium brevicornu* (xian ling pi, epimedium), *Cuscuta hygrophila* (tu su zi, cuscuta), *Lycium barbarum* (gou qi zi, lycium fruit), *Dioscorea opposita* (shan yao, dioscorea), *Poria cocos* (fu ling, hoelen), *Salvia miltiorrhiza* (dan shen, salvia), *Astragalus membranaceous* (huang qi, astragalus)

Combine with

– A blood tonic such as **1.2 Si Wu Wan**, **1.9 Gui Pi Wan** or **7.16 Shi Quan Da Bu Wan** during the first half of the menstrual cycle to replenish qi and blood, followed by **1.21 Tiao Jing Cu Yun Wan** after ovulation to regulate qi and blood, support Kidney yang and the progesterone phase

Dosage and method of administration

Fifty pills (one vial) twice daily, on an empty stomach. The dose can be spread out, taking a few pills at frequent intervals throughout the day. When used as part of a cyclical treatment, the appropriate dose is taken from mid-cycle onwards until menstruation occurs. In the case of amenorrhea, the pills can be taken continually for three months before review.

Pattern identifying features

- **Spleen and Kidney yang deficiency**
- **infertility**
- weak yang phase of menstrual cycle
- anovulation
- long menstrual cycle, amenorrhea
- cold intolerance
- fatigue, weakness, lassitude
- poor appetite
- loss of libido

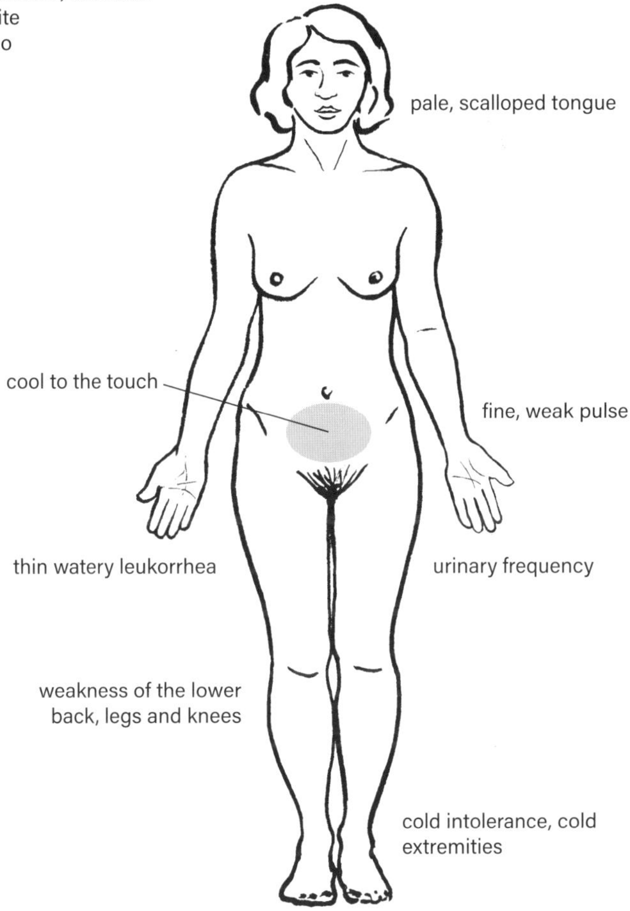

Cautions and contraindications

Contraindicated during the early phase of acute illness such as colds and flu, and in patients with yin deficiency patterns with heat. Caution during pregnancy. Caution for patients on anticoagulant therapy. Watch for bruising or increased tendency to bleeding. This formula is quite warming and may cause some patients to overheat, especially if they are using other warming medications or substances (such as B vitamins).

1.22 REHMANNIA GLUTINOSA COMPOUND PILLS

妇科种子丸

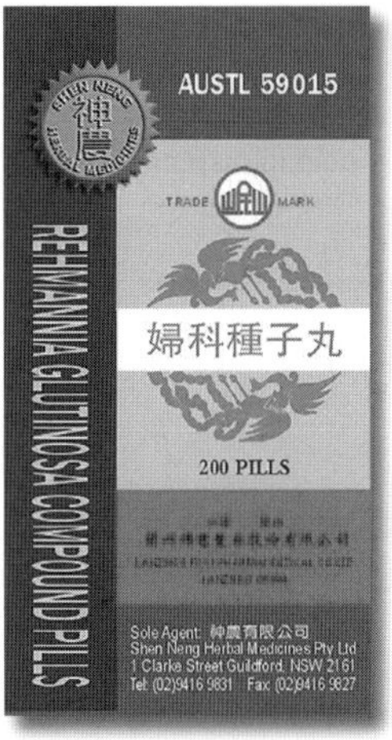

(*Fu Ke Zhong Zi Wan*)
Lanzhou Foci Pharmaceutical Factory (Gansu)
'Women's Cultivation (of Fertility) Pills'
Rehmannia Glutinosa Compound Pills are packaged in bottles of 200 pills
Also available as: Fertile Field Teapills (PF)

Chinese medical action

Nourishes and invigorates blood, tonifies and warms Kidney yang, warms the Uterus, strengthens the *chōng mài* and *rèn mài*.

Biomedical action

Energy tonic and stimulant, promotes metabolism, hematinic, regulates menstruation.

INDICATIONS

- Infertility, dysmenorrhea, amenorrhea, premenstrual backache and other menstrual disorders from Kidney yang qi deficiency, blood deficiency and cold accumulation in the Uterus. Similar in scope and action to **1.19 Yang Rong Wan**.
- Chronic uterine bleeding, spotting or menorrhagia from cold and yang deficiency.
- Promotes transformation of yin into yang at mid-cycle to encourage ovulation. Warms yang and supports the yang phase of the menstrual cycle (as measured by the basal body temperature [BBT] chart, *see* glossary).
- Recurrent miscarriage from Kidney yang and blood deficiency (used in between pregnancies).

Composition

Rehmannia glutinosa (shu di, processed rehmannia), *Eucommia ulmoides* (du zhong, eucommia), *Cyperus rotundus* (xiang fu, cyperus), *Angelica sinensis* (dang gui, chinese angelica), *Ligusticum wallichi* (chuan xiong, ligusticum), *Dipsacus asper* (xu duan, dipsacus), *Artemesia argyi* (ai ye, mugwort), *Scutellaria baicalensis* (huang qin, scute), *Equus asinus* (e jiao, donkey skin gelatin), *Paeonia lactiflora* (bai shao, white peony)

Combine with

- **7.12 Lu Rong Jiao** or **7.11 Deer Velvet** prior to ovulation to increase yang transformation

Dosage and method of administration

8-12 pills three times daily on an empty stomach. The dose can be spread out, or taken in two lots of 12-18 pills, morning and evening. In severe cases a 50% increase in dose can be used. Usually used in the two weeks prior to menstruation.

Pattern identifying features

- **Kidney yang deficiency, blood deficiency, cold in the Uterus**
- **infertility**
- cold intolerance

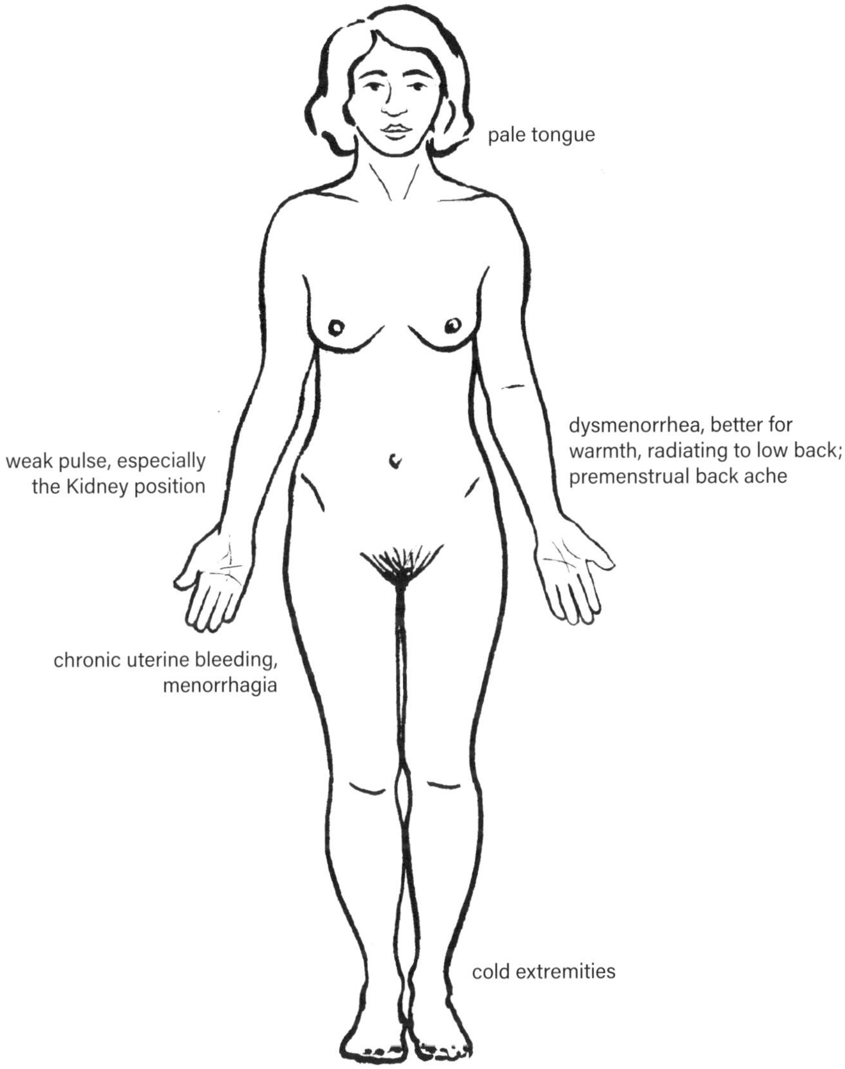

Cautions and contraindications

Contraindicated during the early phase of acute illness such as colds and flu. Caution during pregnancy. Care in patients with a tendency to abdominal bloating, loose stools or general digestive weakness. Some patients may find **1.22 Rehmannia Glutinosa Compound Pills** aggravates these symptoms. This can be alleviated by reducing the dose or by adding a few pills of **2.9 Xiang Sha Liu Jun Wan** or **2.18 Bao He Wan**.

1.23 ZHI BAI DI HUANG WAN

知柏地黄丸

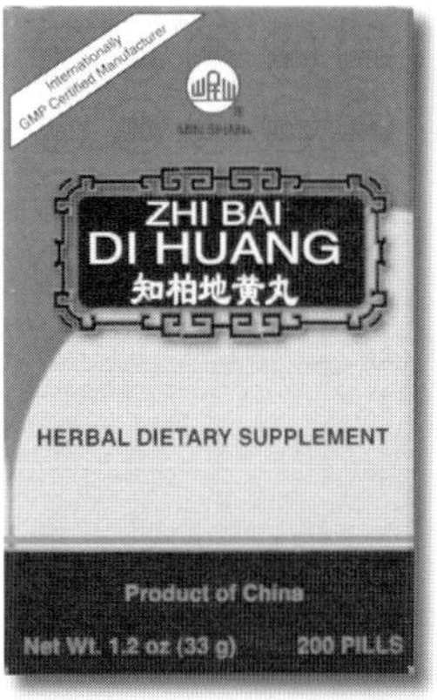

Lanzhou Foci Pharmaceutical Factory (Gansu)
'Anemarrhena, Phellodendron and Rehmannia Pills'
Zhi Bai Di Huang Wan is packaged in bottles of 200 pills
Also available as: Eight Flavor Rehmannia Teapills (PF), Chih Pai Pa Wei Wan, Anemarrhena, Phellodendron and Rehmannia Formula (conc. extract)

Chinese medical action

Tonifies Kidney yin, moistens dryness, clears heat and fire from deficiency

Biomedical action

Demulcent febrifuge, hematinic, hypoglycemic, improves kidney function, soothes the urinary tract, reduces excessive perspiration

INDICATIONS

- Kidney yin deficiency with heat or fire. Widely used for gynecological conditions such as menopausal syndrome with heat and/or dryness, chronic or recurrent cystitis, interstitial cystitis, vaginal dryness or irritation, chronic vaginitis and chronic pelvic inflammatory disease.
- Chronic consumptive disorders with low grade fevers and emaciation.
- To alleviate the side effects of long term corticosteroid use (which damages yin).
- Chronic sore throat that is worse in the afternoon and evening, and when fatigued (in a patient with heat signs).
- Kidney yin deficiency with damp heat in the lower burner, Bladder, prostate or Uterus. The combination of yin deficiency and damp heat is quite common, with the Kidney deficiency making the pelvic basin vulnerable to a lingering pathogen, or the initial damp heat pathogen damaging yin by its presence.
- With the appropriate identifying features, this formula can be used to treat disorders such as those noted above, also chronic tonsillitis, post streptococcal glomerulonephritis, chronic nephritis, fever of unknown origin, sperm viscosity disorders, diabetes, hyperthyroidism and sore dry or irritated eyes.

Composition

Rehmannia glutinosa (shu di, processed rehmannia), *Cornus officinalis* (shan zhu yu, cornus), *Dioscorea opposita* (shan yao, dioscorea), *Poria cocos* (fu ling, hoelen), *Alisma orientalis* (ze xie, alisma), *Paeonia suffruticosa* (mu dan pi, moutan), *Anemarrhena aspheloides* (zhi mu, anemarrhena), *Phellodendron amurense* (huang bai, phellodendron)

Combine with

- **1.35 Nei Xiao Luo Li Wan** or **11.2 Prostate Gland Pills** for men with a yin deficient constitution, prostate swelling and/or elevated prostate specific antigen
- **7.4 Da Bu Yin Wan** or **3.41 Xu Han Ting** for severe sweating

Pattern identifying features

- **Kidney deficiency with heat or fire from deficiency**
- **heat intolerance, low grade fevers, afternoon and tidal fever**
- **facial or malar flushing**
- **night sweats**
- **hot hands and feet**
- **dryness of skin, hair and eyes**
- tiredness and exhaustion

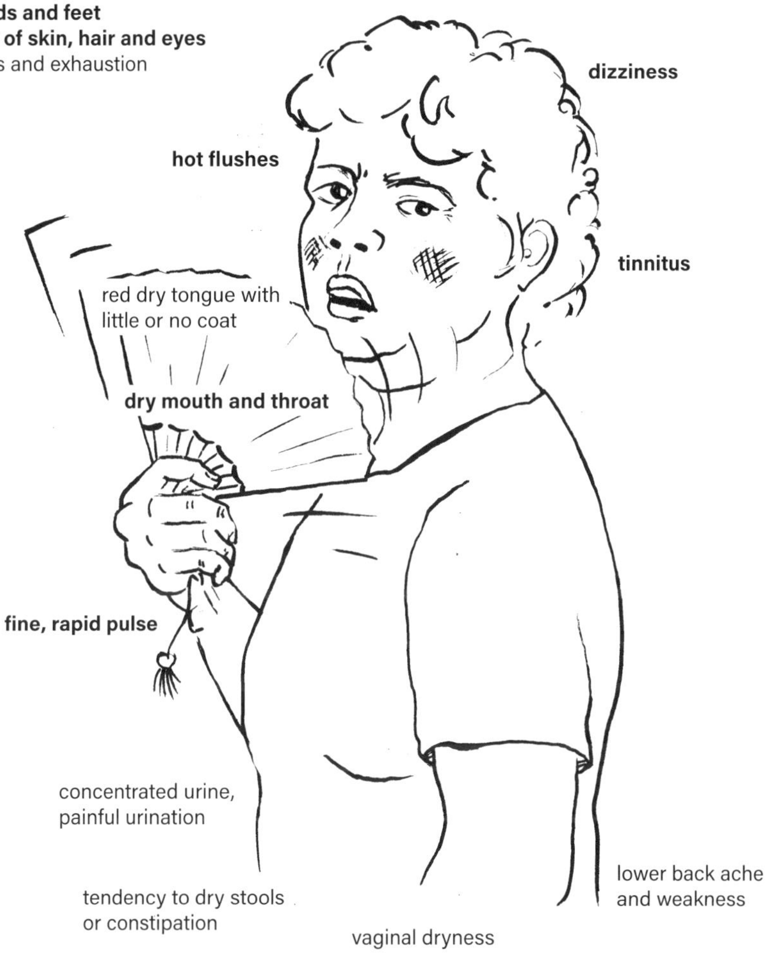

Dosage and method of administration

8-12 pills three times daily, on an empty stomach. The dose can be spread out, or taken in two lots of 12-18 pills, morning and evening. In severe cases or during the early stages of treatment (the first few weeks), a 50% increase in dose can be used, then reduced as treatment takes effect.

Cautions and contraindications

Contraindicated during the early phase of acute illness such as colds and flu. Care should be taken in patients with a tendency to abdominal distension, loose stools or mucus accumulation. This is a cooling formula and overuse can weaken the Spleen.

1.24 SHENG HUA WAN

生化丸

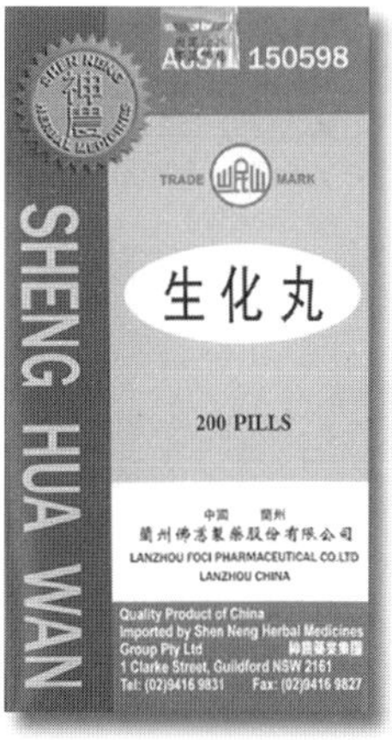

Lanzhou Foci Pharmaceutical Factory (Gansu)
'Generation and Transformation Pill'
Sheng Hua Wan is packaged in bottles of 200 pills
Also available as: Tangkuei and Ginger Combination (conc. extract)

Chinese medical action

Regulates blood and gently disperses blood stasis, warms the uterus, stops pain

Biomedical action

Regulates menstruation, stimulates uterine contraction and tones the uterus

INDICATIONS

- Postpartum uterine blood stasis with blood deficiency and cold. This is the blood stasis in the days following childbirth, especially when birth was long or traumatic. Any stasis present is always accompanied by blood deficiency, both from the birth process and from the blood invested in making the baby. In addition, the uterus is usually in a relative state of cold and deficiency following the warmth and fullness of gestation. The aim of the formula is to gently move any residual stasis, encourage blood circulation and promote uterine tone and return to normal size. Can also assist in preventing complications following termination of pregnancy or miscarriage.
- With the appropriate identifying features, this formula can be used to treat postpartum disorders such as abdominal pain, retained placenta, persistent lochia or bleeding, constipation and urinary retention.

Composition

Angelica sinensis (dang gui, chinese angelica), *Ligusticum wallichi* (chuan xiong, ligusticum), *Prunus persica* (tao ren, peach seed), *Zingiber officinalis* (gan jiang, dry ginger), *Glycyrrhiza uralensis* (zhi gan cao, honey fried licorice root)

Dosage and method of administration

8-12 pills three times daily on an empty stomach. The dose can be spread out, or taken in two lots of 12-18 pills, morning and evening. In severe cases, a 50% increase in dose can be used, then reduced as treatment takes effect. Traditionally taken with 15-30ml of rice or sorghum wine (*shào xīng jiù* 绍兴酒), but this is not essential. The patient should be advised to expect increased bleeding or discharge for a few days. Once pain is relieved and stasis cleared, usually in the form or clots or fleshy material, the formula is continued for a day or two to make sure all stasis is cleared, then stopped. Generally only used for a few days in the week following childbirth, and only if required. Routine use in all postpartum women, as occurs in some parts of China is not recommended.

Pattern identifying features

- **Postpartum blood stasis**

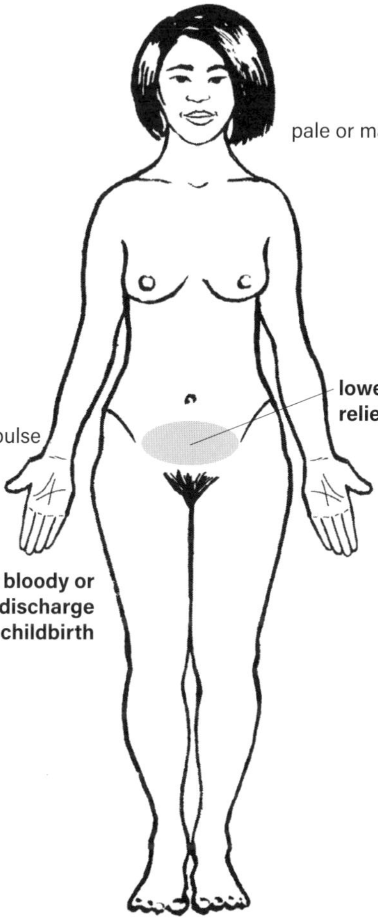

Cautions and contraindications

Contraindicated during pregnancy. Not suitable for women with bleeding from pathology other than blood stasis. Dang gui can pass through breast milk and may upset babies stomach. Contraindicated when there is heat (toxic heat, damp heat, heat from constraint) causing postpartum fever, night sweats, malodorous discharge and restlessness. Postpartum abdominal pain from blood stasis should be differentiated from pain due to other causes such as qi, blood or yang deficiency with no stasis.

GMP

1.25 ER XIAN WAN

二仙丸

3+/12

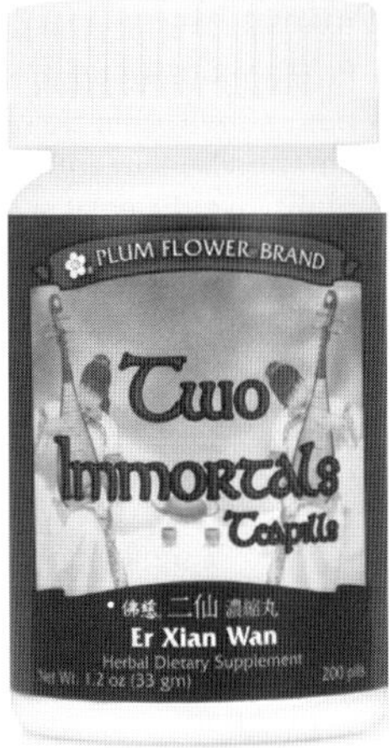

Lanzhou Foci Pharmaceutical Factory (Gansu)
'Two Immortals Pill'
Er Xian Wan is packaged in bottles of 200 pills
Also available as: Curculigo and Epimedium Combination (conc. extract)

Chinese medical action

Warms Kidney yang, benefits and tonifies yin and essence, nourishes blood, clears deficient heat, regulates the *chōng mài* and *rèn mài*

Biomedical action

Febrifuge, reduces excessive perspiration, regulates and balances the hormones associated with menopause, anti-hypertensive

INDICATIONS

- Kidney yin and yang deficiency with heat. The weakness of the Kidneys fails to support normal functioning of *chōng mài* and *rèn mài*, leading to reduction or cessation of menstruation. A modern formulation for the treatment of the symptoms of menopause, in particular when associated with heat and high blood pressure. Because yang is also deficient, many patients while feeling uncomfortably hot in the upper body, display symptoms of cold in the lower body. While primarily designed for women, this formula can also be used in men presenting with Kidney yin and yang deficiency patterns.
- With the appropriate identifying features, this formula can assist in the treatment of the symptoms of menopausal syndrome, hypertension associated with menopause, hyperthyroidism and chronic nephritis.

Composition

Curculigo orchioides (xian mao, curculigo), *Epimedium brevicornu* (xian ling pi, epimedium), *Morinda officinalis* (ba ji tian, morinda), *Anemarrhena aspheloides* (zhi mu, anemarrhena), *Phellodendron amurense* (huang bai, phellodendron), *Angelica sinensis* (dang gui, chinese angelica)

Combine with

- **7.1 Liu Wei Di Huang Wan** for relatively severe Kidney yin deficiency
- **6.5 Jia Wei Xiao Yao Wan** with elements of Liver qi constraint with heat
- **1.2 Si Wu Wan** for patients with a greater degree of blood deficiency

Pattern identifying features

- **Kidney yin and yang deficiency, deficient heat**
- **heat above, cold below**
- **amenorrhea, irregular menstrual period**
- **night sweats**, easy sweating
- **hypertension**
- insomnia, palpitations
- irritability, depression, anxiety
- poor thermo-regulation
- fatigue

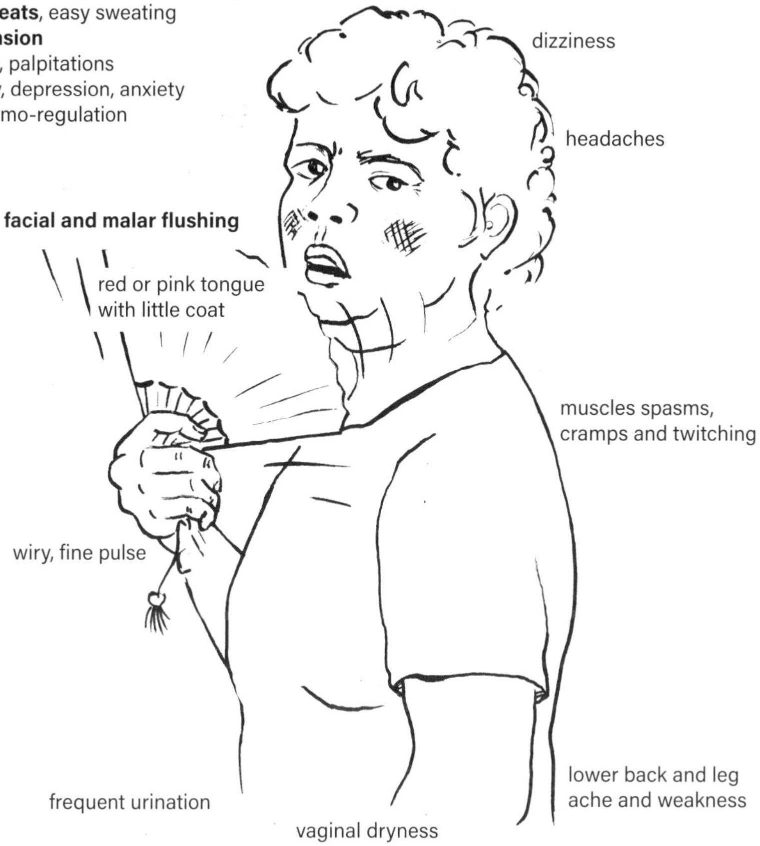

Dosage and method of administration

8-12 pills three times daily, on an empty stomach. The dose can be spread out, or taken in two lots of 12-18 pills, morning and evening. In severe cases or during the early stages of treatment (the first few weeks), a 50% increase in dose can be used, then reduced as treatment takes effect.

Cautions and contraindications

Contraindicated during the early phase of acute illness such as colds and flu. Care should be taken in patients with a tendency to abdominal distension, loose stools or mucus accumulation. This is a cooling formula and overuse can weaken the Spleen.

1.26 KUN BAO WAN

坤宝丸

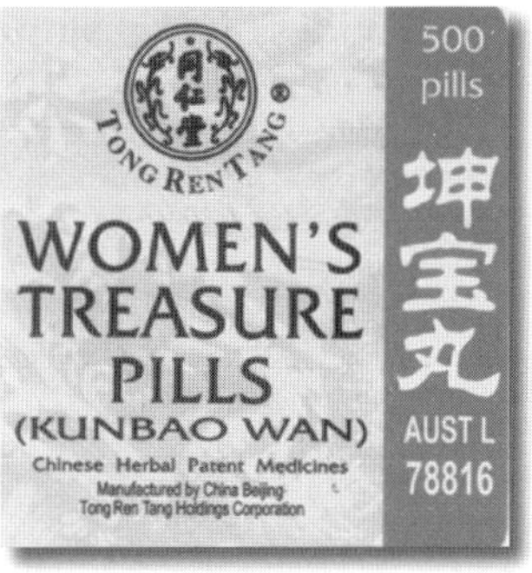

Tong Ren Tang (Beijing)
Kun Bao Wan are packaged in bottles of 500 tiny pills, or in vials of 50 tiny pills, ten vials per box

Chinese medical action

Tonifies Liver and Kidney yin, restrains yang, calms the *shén*, nourishes and cools the blood, clears heat from deficiency, opens the channels

Biomedical action

Regulates the hormones associated with the menstrual cycle, demulcent febrifuge, sedative

INDICATIONS

- Liver, Heart and/or Kidney yin deficiency with heat from deficiency and hyperactive yang type menopausal syndrome. Used for menopausal hypertension, dry scratchy eye disorders, vaginal dryness, headaches and dizziness associated with yin deficiency with ascendant yang.
- For the emotional aspects and for the generalized aches and pains that accompany menopause or yin deficiency patterns.

Composition (50 pills contains)

Spatholobus suberectus (ji xue teng, spatholobus) 315mg, *Paeonia veitchii* (chi shao, red peony) 315mg, *Paeonia lactiflora* (bai shao, white peony) 260mg, *Angelica acutiloba* (dang gui, chinese angelica) 250mg, *Eclipta prostrata* (han lian cao, eclipta) 210mg, *Dendrobium nobile* (shi hu, dendrobium) 160mg, *Ligustrum lucidum* (nu zhen zi, privet fruit) 160mg, *Lycium chinense* (di gu pi, lycium root bark) 160mg, *Rehmannia glutinosa* (sheng di, rehmannia) 160mg, *Chrysanthemum indicum* (ye ju hua, wild chrysanthemum) 160mg, *Scutellaria baicalensis* (huang qin, scute) 160mg, *Cynanchum atratum* (bai wei, swallowwort root) 160mg, *Adenophora tetraphylla* (sha shen, adenophora) 160mg, *Anemarrhena aspheloides* (zhi mu, anemarrhena) 160mg, *Cuscuta europea* (tu su zi, cuscuta) 105mg, *Rubus chingii* (fu pen zi, rubus) 105mg, *Polygonum multiflorum* (he shou wu, polygonum) 105mg, *Lycium barbarum* (gou qi zi, lycium fruit) 105mg, *Ophiopogon japonicus* (mai dong, ophiopogon) 105mg, *Morus alba* (sang ye, mulberry leaf) 105mg, *Zizyphus jujuba* (da zao, chinese date) 50mg

Combine with

- **8.3 An Shen Ding Zhi Wan** or **8.5 Shuian Capsule** for emotional turmoil and mood swings
- **7.1 Liu Wei Di Huang Wan** to enhance the Kidney yin enriching quality of the treatment
- **15.4 Tian Ma Gou Teng Wan** for severe headaches and dizziness associated with menopause

Pattern identifying features

- **Liver and Kidney yin deficiency with ascendant yang and heat**
- **mood swings, forgetfulness, irrational tears**
- **night sweats, heat at night**
- dry skin, mouth, throat
- insomnia

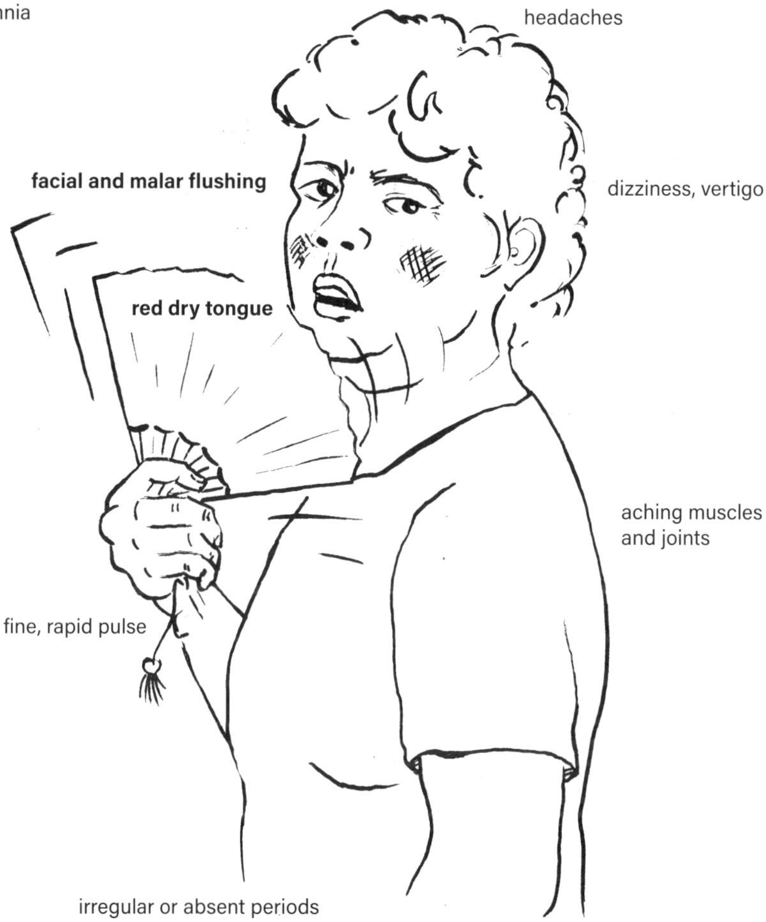

Dosage and method of administration

25-50 pills twice daily, on an empty stomach. The dose can also be spread out, taking a few pills at frequent intervals throughout the day.

Cautions and contraindications

Contraindicated during the early phase of acute illness such as colds and flu.

1.27 JING AN ORAL LIQUID

静安口服液

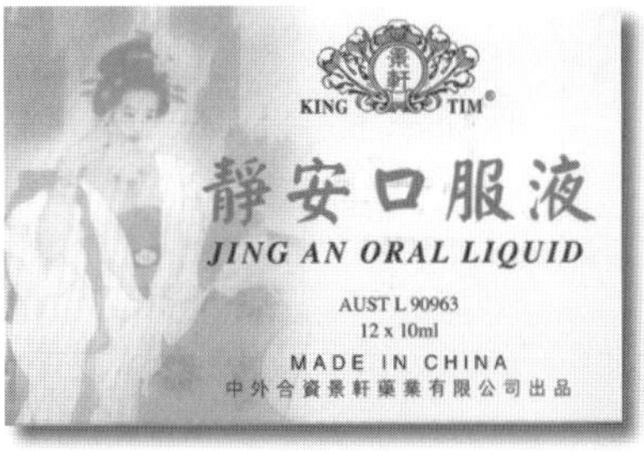

(*Jing An Kou Fu Ye*)
'Peace and Quiet Drink'
Jing Xian Pharmaceutical Co. (Guangzhou)
Jing An Oral Liquid is packaged in vials of 10ml liquid, 12 vials per box

Chinese medical action

Tonifies the Liver and Kidney, nourishes and invigorates blood

Biomedical action

Nutritive, tonic

INDICATIONS

- Menstrual disorders from Liver and Kidney yin and blood deficiency, including menopausal syndrome, amenorrhea, irregular menstruation, leukorrhea, uterine bleeding and menorrhagia. This formula is mild and gentle, suitable for all yin and blood deficiency patterns. Also suitable for patients with a mild degree of deficient heat, with symptoms such as flushing, low grade fever, sweating, anxiety, palpitations, dizziness and insomnia or restless sleep with vivid dreams.
- Yin and blood deficiency type visual weakness, dry eyes, excessive lacrimation in wind or red, sore, irritated eyes.
- Dry, flaky or scaly skin; dry, lusterless hair.

Composition (each vial contains extracts equivalent to dry)

Lycium barbarum (gou qi zi, lycium fruit) 8.4g, *Sesamum indicum* (hei zhi ma, sesame seed) 5.6g, *Morus alba* (sang zi, mulberry fruit) 5.6g, *Carthamus tinctorius* (hong hua, carthamus) 5.6g, *Zizyphus jujuba* (da zao, chinese dates) 4.2g, *Chrysanthemun sinense* (ju hua, chrysanthemum flower) 4.2g, *Citrus reticulata* (chen pi, citrus) 1.4g

Dosage and method of administration

1 vial, two or three times daily.

Cautions and contraindications

Contraindicated during the early phase of acute illness such as colds and flu.

1.28 LADY ORAL LIQUID

女士口服液

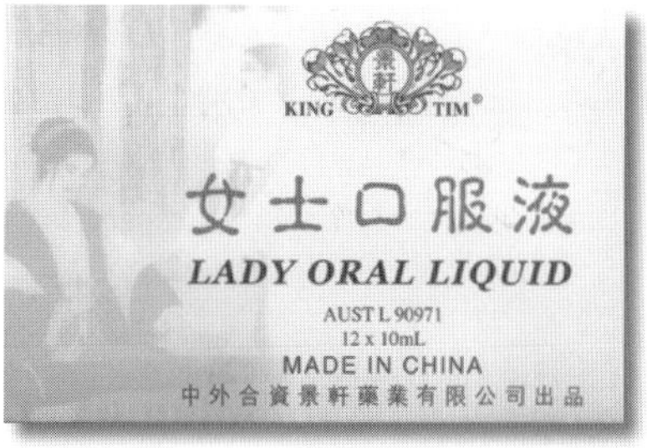

(*Nu Shi Kou Fu Ye*)
'Woman's Drink'
Jing Xian Pharmaceutical Co. (Guangzhou)
Lady Oral Liquid is packaged in vials of 10ml liquid, 12 vials per box

Chinese medical action

Tonifies qi and blood, nourishes yin and supports yang, regulates menstruation, settles the Heart and calms the *shén*

Biomedical action

Nutritive, tonic, regulates menstruation

INDICATIONS

- Qi and blood deficiency menstrual and *shén* disorders. Typical features include fatigue and tiredness, pallor, pale, ridged or brittle nails, insomnia and palpitations, vivid dreaming or dream disturbed sleep, irregular menses (especially long cycles, scanty periods or missed periods), mild dysmenorrhea, leukorrhea, lower back ache, premenstrual back ache and numbness in the extremities.
- Dry, flaky or scaly skin; dry, lusterless hair.

Composition (each vial contains extracts equivalent to dry)

Zizyphus jujuba (da zao, chinese dates) 4g, *Astragalus membranaceous* (huang qi, astragalus) 3.7g, *Lycium barbarum* (gou qi zi, lycium fruit) 3.7g, *Morus alba* (sang zi, mulberry fruit) 3g, *Juglans regia* (hu tao ren, walnut) 3g, *Zizyphus spinoza* (suan zao ren, zizyphus) 2.7g, *Polygonum multiflorum* (he shou wu, polygonum root) 2.7g, *Coix lachryma-jobi* (yi yi ren, coix) 2.7g, *Nelumbus speciosum* (lian zi, lotus seed) 2.2g, *Glycyrrhiza uralensis* (gan cao, licorice) 540mg, *Ostrea gigas* (mu li, oyster shell) 18mg

Dosage and method of administration

1 vial, two or three times daily.

Cautions and contraindications

Contraindicated during the early phase of acute illness such as colds and flu.

1.29 GENG NIAN LING

更年灵

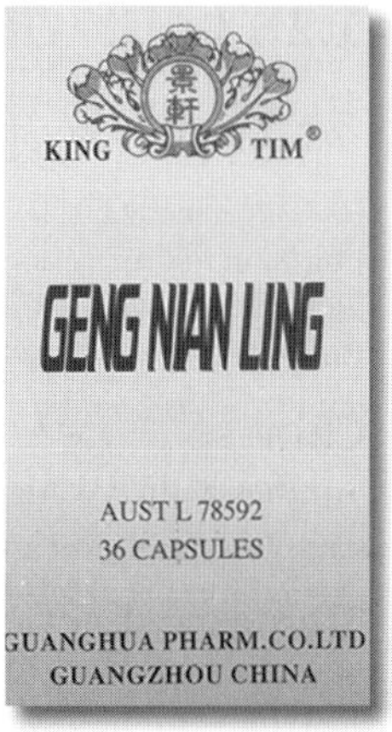

Guanghua Pharmaceutical Co. (Guangzhou)
'Miraculous [Pills for] Menopause'
Geng Nian Ling is packaged in bottles of 36 capsules

Chinese medical action

Warms Kidney yang, nourishes Kidney and Liver yin, clears heat from deficiency

Biomedical action

Regulates the hormones associated with the menstrual cycle, demulcent febrifuge, sedative, nervine

INDICATIONS

- Symptoms of menopause, in particular irregular and waning menstruation, intermenstrual spotting and uterine bleeding, facial flushing, sweats, vaginal dryness, palpitations, insomnia or frequent waking, forgetfulness and irritability. A modern formulation specifically tailored to be similar in action to **1.25 Er Xian Wan**, combining herbs of opposing natures to facilitate yin and yang tonification and clearance of deficiency heat symptoms.

Composition (each capsule contains)

Ligustrum lucidum (nu zhen zi, privet fruit) 800mg, *Epimedium brevicornu* (xian ling pi, epimedium) 550mg, Thiamine hydrochloride (Vitamin B1) 10mg, Pyridoxine hydrochloride (Vitamin B6) 10mg

Dosage and method of administration

1-2 capsules, two to three times daily on an empty stomach, to a maximum of 5 capsules daily

Cautions and contraindications

None noted.

1.30 BU GAI ZHUANG GU CAPSULE

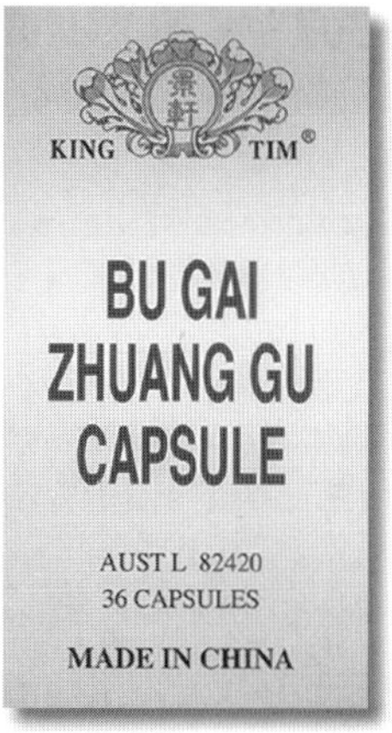

补钙壮骨丸

(*Bu Gai Zhuang Gu Wan*)
Jing Xian Pharmaceutical Co. (Guangzhou)
'Pills to Tonify Calcium and Strengthen Bones'
Bu Gai Zhuang Gu Capsule is packaged in bottles of 36 capsules

Chinese medical action

Tonifies Kidney yang, nourishes Kidney and Liver yin, strengthens sinews and bones, tonifies qi and blood

Biomedical action

Stimulant and tonic, supports thermogenesis and osteogenesis

INDICATIONS

- Osteoporosis associated with Kidney yang deficiency. Used to support and promote osteogenesis in those with, or at risk of, osteoporosis. In combination with weight bearing exercise, assists the Kidneys in maintenance of strong bones. Assists healing of bones following trauma or surgery. Used after blood moving herbs (such as **10.3 Die Da Zhi Tong Capsule**) have been applied for about two weeks to clear any blood stagnation.
- Also used for Kidney yang deficiency type infertility or impotence, urinary disorders, wind cold damp painful obstruction, chronic lower back ache and hypertension.

Composition (each capsule contains extracts equivalent to dry)

Epimedium brevicornu (xian ling pi, epimedium) 450mg, *Dioscorea opposita* (shan yao, dioscorea) 350mg, *Angelica polymorpha* (dang gui, chinese angelica) 320mg, *Rehmannia glutinosa* (shu di, processed rehmannia) 270mg, *Eucommia ulmoides* (du zhong, eucommia) 250mg, *Lycium barbarum* (gou qi zi, lycium fruit) 200mg, *Morinda officinalis* (ba ji tian, morinda) 180mg, *Curculigo orchioides* (xian mao, curculigo) 150mg, *Cornus officinalis* (shan zhu yu, cornus) 135mg, *Ostrea gigas* (mu li, oyster shell powder) 25mg

Dosage and method of administration

2 capsules, three times daily on an empty stomach.

Cautions and contraindications

This formula is quite warming and may overheat some patients. Contraindicated unmodified in patients with yin deficiency and internal heat patterns.

1.31 TANGKWEI ESSENCE OF CHICKEN

当归鸡精

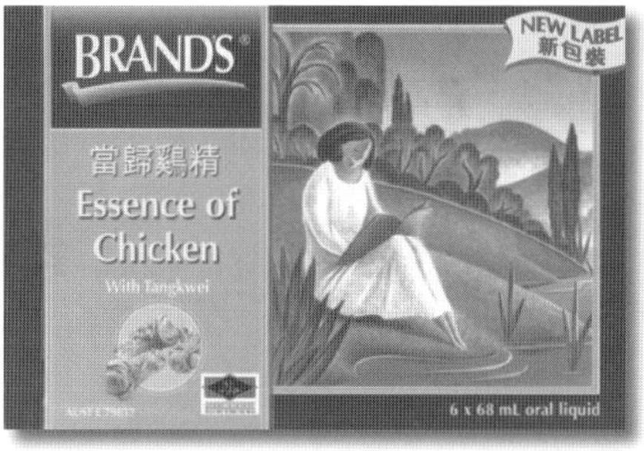

(*Dang Gui Ji Jing*)
Cerebos Thailand Ltd (Thailand)
Tangkwei Essence of Chicken is packaged in 68ml jars of liquid extract, six jars to a box

Chinese medical action

Tonifies qi and blood, promotes transformation of blood into mothers milk

Biomedical action

Powerfully nourishes qi blood, tones the uterus and muscles, galactagogue

INDICATIONS

- Postpartum weakness and insufficient lactation from blood and qi deficiency. Based on **1.1 Ba Zhen Wan**, the black boned chicken makes this formula a rich and fast acting tonic, ideal for all mothers. In addition to its main use to strengthen postpartum women, it can be used to treat a wide range of qi and blood deficiency problems such as fatigue and exhaustion, dizziness, anemia, weight loss and lusterless or falling hair.
- As support in patients with significant convalescent or nutritional needs, for example patients with cancer or other severe illness.

Composition (each jar contains extracts equivalent to dry)

Black bone chicken, *Angelica sinensis* (dang gui, chinese angelica) 13.3g, *Codonopsis pilosula* (dang shen, codonopsis) 2g, *Ligusticum wallichi* (chuan xiong, ligusticum) 1.1g, *Paeonia alba* (bai shao, white peony) 880mg, *Atractylodes macrocephala* (bai zhu, atractylodes) 880mg, *Poria cocos* (fu ling, hoelen) 880mg, *Rehmannia glutinosa* (shu di, processed rehmannia) 880mg, *Glycyrrhiza uralensis* (gan cao, licorice) 475mg

Dosage and method of administration

In the early days following childbirth, one jar can be taken daily, either neat or diluted with warm water. As energy or milk improves, one jar every second or third day is sufficient. For prolonged breast feeding, or in women with other extensive demands on their energy, one or two jars weekly are useful for maintenance. **1.31 Tangkwei Essence of Chicken** can also be used as a base for blood enriching soups and stews.

Pattern identifying features

- **qi and blood deficiency**
- **postpartum fatigue, exhaustion**
- weight loss
- poor appetite
- anemia

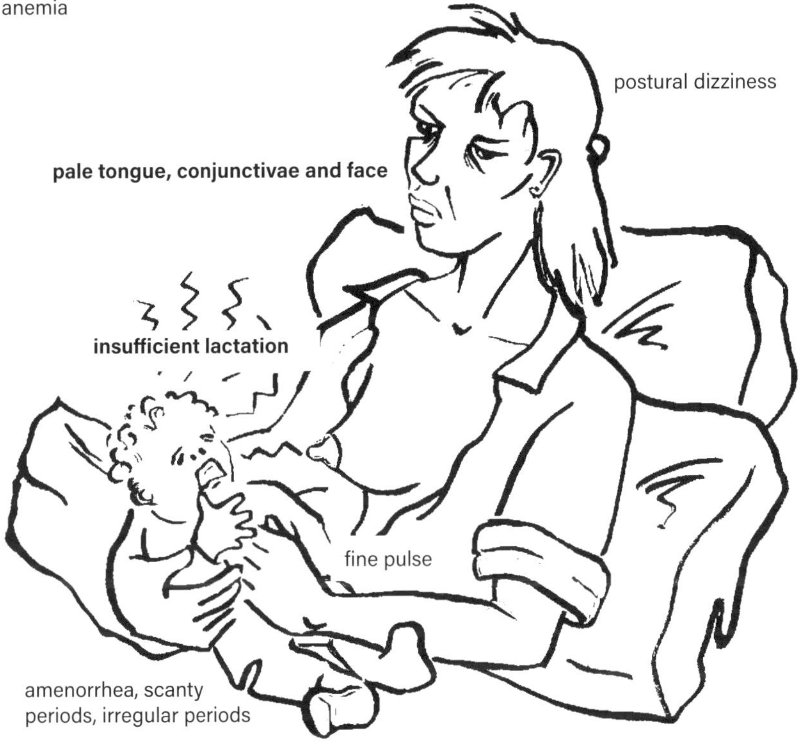

Cautions and contraindications

Contraindicated during the early phase of acute illness such as colds and flu. Caution in women with adequate milk production, as the extra milk stimulated can overwhelm the childs' feeding capacity and predispose to mastitis by congesting the milk ducts. Contraindicated during mastitis. Care should be taken in patients with a tendency to abdominal distension, loose stools or nausea. Some patients may find **1.31 Tangkwei Essence of Chicken** aggravates these symptoms. This can usually be alleviated by diluting it with a strong ginger root tea or taking it after food.

GMP

1.32 SHIH SAN TAI PAO WAN

1-3/52

十三太保丸

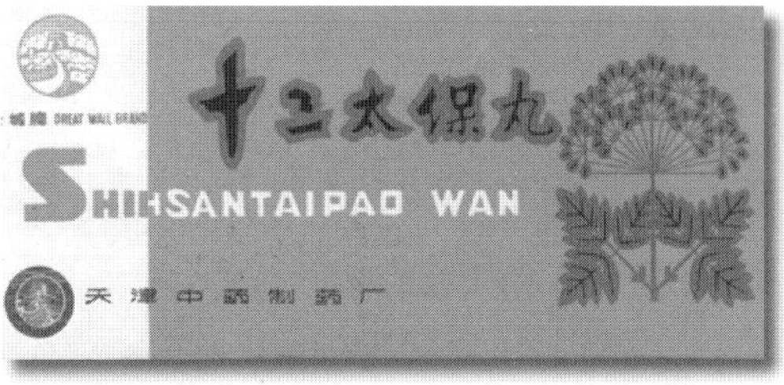

(*Shi San Tai Bao Wan*)
Tianjin Drug Manufactory (Shandong)
'Pills to Powerfully Protect [during the first] Thirteen [weeks of pregnancy]'
Shih San Tai Pao Wan is packaged as large honey pills sealed in wax balls

Chinese medical action

Tonifies qi and blood, alleviates food stagnation, dries damp, regulates qi and blood, strengthens the Kidneys and restores the qi dynamic

Biomedical action

Hematinic, energy stimulant

INDICATIONS

- Used to prepare for labor, especially in women having their first child, by relaxing the muscles of the uterus and pelvic basin. Fetal qi (and thus the structures enveloping the fetus) can be overly consolidated and tight in new or anxious mothers, so by relaxing the pelvic basin and thereby opening up the birth canal the process of giving birth is facilitated and eased. Used from the eighth month of pregnancy onwards for this purpose.
- Assists in turning breech or malpositioned fetus.
- Gastrointestinal problems during pregnancy associated with disruption to the qi dynamic (*see* glossary). Symptoms include nausea and vomiting, abdominal distension and discomfort, sluggish stools or constipation, belching and loss of appetite. The mode of action of this formula is aimed at re-establishing the correct flow of Spleen and Stomach qi, which is easily disrupted by physiological stagnation of the developing fetus and the obstruction to the normal descent of *chōng mài* qi. The descending action of the magnolia bark and immature citrus is balanced by the ascending nature of the astragalus and notopterygium, the four acting together to drive the dynamo of middle burner qi movement.
- Wind cold common cold during menstruation or pregnancy. Also for acute or recurrent headaches and lower back and leg pain during pregnancy and menstruation, or in a patient with blood deficiency.

Composition

Angelica sinensis (dang gui, chinese angelica) 18.18%, *Ligusticum wallichi* (chuan xiong, ligusticum) 18.18%, *Cuscuta chinensis* (tu su zi, cuscuta) 18.18%, *Paeonia lactiflora* (bai shao, white peony) 13.63%, *Fritillaria cirrhosa* (chuan bei mu, fritillaria) 12.10%, *Astragalus membranaceous* (huang qi, astragalus) 6.10%, *Magnolia officinalis* (hou po, magnolia bark) 5.30%, *Citrus aurantium* (zhi ke, immature citrus) 4.54%, *Notopterygium incisum* (qiang huo, notopterygium) 3.79%

Pattern identifying features

- **blood deficiency with disruption to the qi dynamic**
- to relax the uterus to facilitate labor
- turn breech presentation
- abdominal distension and discomfort
- nausea, morning sickness

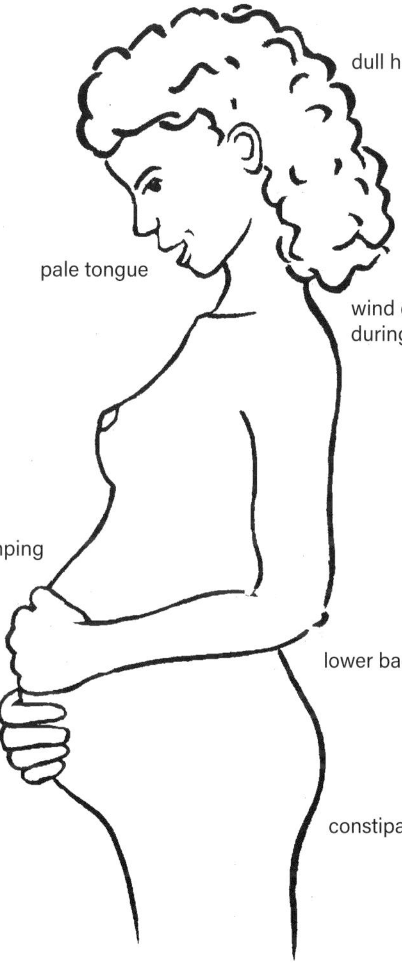

Dosage and method of administration

One pill twice daily on an empty stomach for a week or so in the eighth month, then again a week or two before the due date.

Cautions and contraindications

Any medicine used during pregnancy must be used with caution.

1.33 RU JIE XIAO TABLET

乳结消

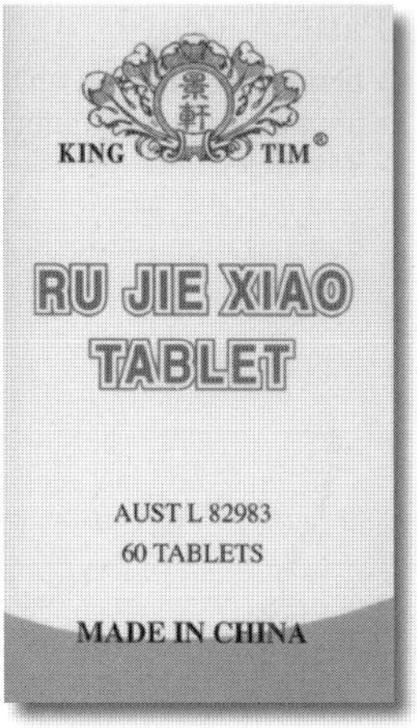

(Ru Jie Xiao)
Jing Xian Pharmaceutical Co. (Guangzhou)
'Reduce Accumulation in the Breast'
Ru Jie Xiao Tablets are packaged in bottles of 60 sugar coated tablets

Chinese medical action

Invigorates and regulates Liver qi, invigorates blood, disperses static blood, transforms phlegm, dissipates nodules and swellings

Biomedical action

Softens and reduces masses and lumps, benefits circulation, assists in regulating menstrual hormones

INDICATIONS

- Breast cysts, lumps and masses from Liver qi constraint, phlegm accumulation and/or blood stasis. The masses typically have a cyclical pattern, proliferating towards the end of the menstrual cycle. They are generally well defined and may or may not be tender. In addition, they are generally not inflammatory or suppurative, or associated with fever. This formula is also useful for other benign gynecological masses, such as ovarian cysts, fibroids and endometriosis of the same etiology.
- With the appropriate identifying features, this formula can be used to treat breast cysts, fibrocystic breast disease, hyperplasia of breast tissue, uterine fibroids and ovarian cysts.

Composition (each tablet contains extract equivalent to dry)

Bupleurum falcatum (chai hu, bupleurum) 377mg, *Salvia miltiorrhiza* (dan shen, salvia) 377mg, *Paeonia lactiflora* (bai shao, white peony) 293mg, *Citrus aurantium* (zhi ke, aurantium) 293mg, *Prunella vulgaris* (xia ku cao, prunella) 260mg, *Ranunculus ternatus* (mao zhua cao, ranunculus) 234mg, *Curcuma longa* (yu jin, curcuma) 202mg, *Angelica polymorpha* (dang gui, chinese angelica) 176mg, *Epimedium brevicornu* (xian ling pi, epimedium) 117mg, *Glycyrrhiza uralensis* (gan cao, licorice) 117mg

Combine with

– **6.4 Xiao Yao Wan** or **6.3 Chai Hu Shu Gan Wan** for fibrocystic breast disease from constrained Liver qi with phlegm accumulation
– **1.34 Hai Zao Jing Wan** to enhance the phlegm softening and transforming action of the formula
– **1.13 Woo Garm Yuen Medical Pills** or **1.14 Wen Jing Wan** for ovarian cysts from cold and yang deficiency

Pattern identifying features

- **Liver qi constraint, phlegm and blood stasis**
- premenstrual symptoms
- irritability

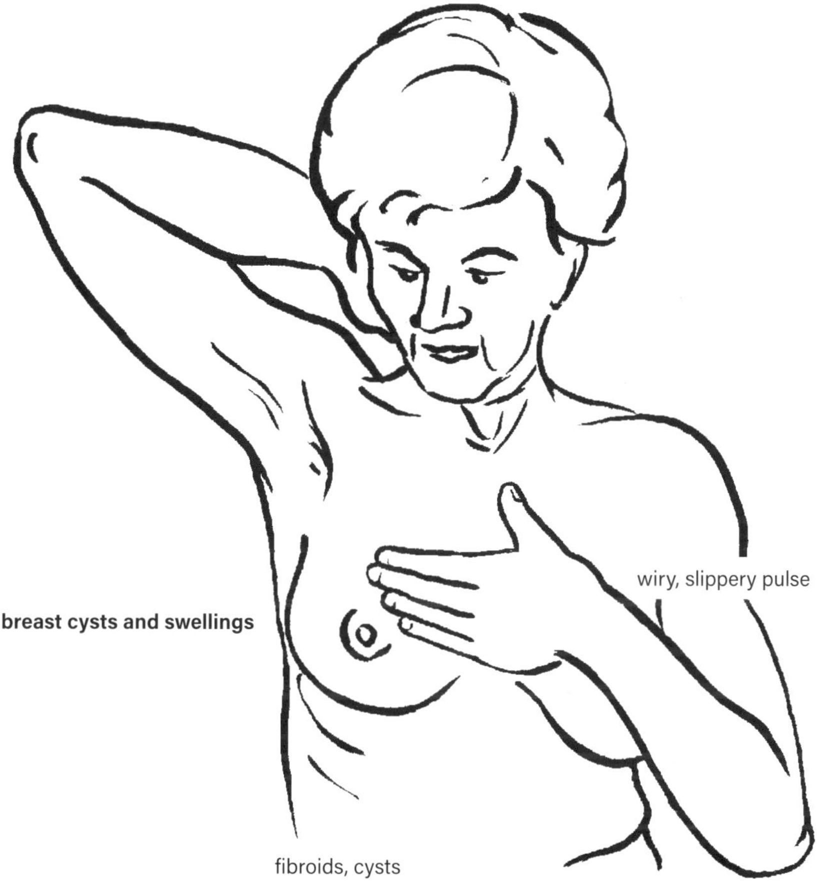

Dosage and method of administration

3-5 tablets, three times daily on an empty stomach. Patients should expect to see some reduction in the size of the lump within one or two months.

Cautions and contraindications

Caution during pregnancy, in women with menorrhagia, and in patients with bleeding disorders. Caution in patients on anticoagulant therapy (aspirin, warfarin, coumarin). Watch for bruising or increased tendency to bleeding.

1.34 HAI ZAO JING WAN

海藻晶丸

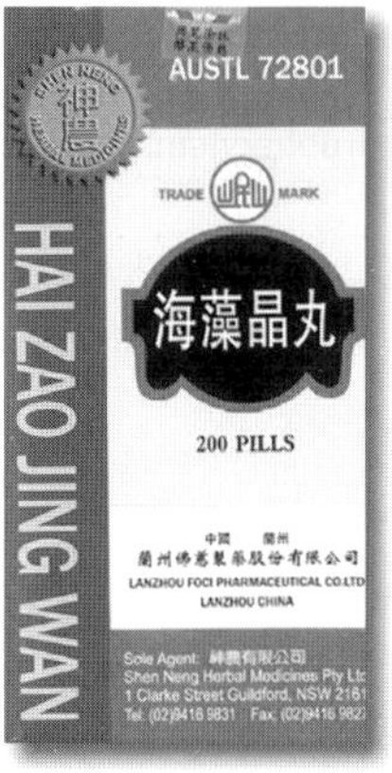

Lanzhou Foci Pharmaceutical Factory (Gansu)
'Crystalline Sargassum Pills'
Hai Zao Jing Wan is packaged in bottles of 200 pills

Chinese medical action

Disperses phlegm, softens hardness, reduces swelling

Biomedical action

Softens and reduces masses and lumps

INDICATIONS

- Phlegm type masses, nodules and lumps, that is, those that are soft or rubbery and well defined. Most commonly used for benign masses in the neck, such as thyroid nodules and goitre.
- Can assist in the treatment of breast cysts, parotid adenomas, lipomas, sebaceous cysts, ovarian cysts and fibroids, glandular and lymphatic congestion, lymphadenopathy, and testicular swellings such as varicocele and hydrocele.

Composition (each pill contains powdered)

Sargassum pallidum (hai zao, sargassum seaweed) 160mg

Combine with

- **1.33 Ru Jie Xiao Tablet**, **6.4 Xiao Yao Wan** or **6.3 Chai Hu Shu Gan Wan** for thyroid swelling or fibrocystic breast disease arising from constrained Liver qi with phlegm accumulation
- **8.1 Tian Wang Bu Xin Dan** for thyroid swelling or nodules, insomnia and palpitations associated with Heart and Kidney yin deficiency and phlegm accumulation
- **6.3 Chai Hu Shu Gan Wan** or **6.2 Si Ni Wan** for swelling in the neck associated with qi and phlegm stagnation
- **11.3 Ji Sheng Ju He Wan** or **11.4 Tian Tai Wu Yao Wan** for testicular swellings from phlegm accumulation
- **1.13 Woo Garm Yuen Medical Pills** for ovarian cysts
- **2.9 Xiang Sha Liu Jun Wan** or **2.23 Ping Wei San** for chronic lymphatic congestion from poor fluid metabolism
- **6.4 Xiao Yao Wan** for lymphatic congestion associated with Liver qi constraint
- **3.34 Bai He Gu Jin Wan** for chronic swollen lymph glands and other nodules that form in patients with Lung yin deficiency
- **8.8 Wen Dan Wan** or **14.1 Huang Lian Jie Du Wan** for nodules and masses associated with phlegm heat

Pattern identifying features

- **phlegm type nodules and swellings**
- rubbery, smooth well defined swellings

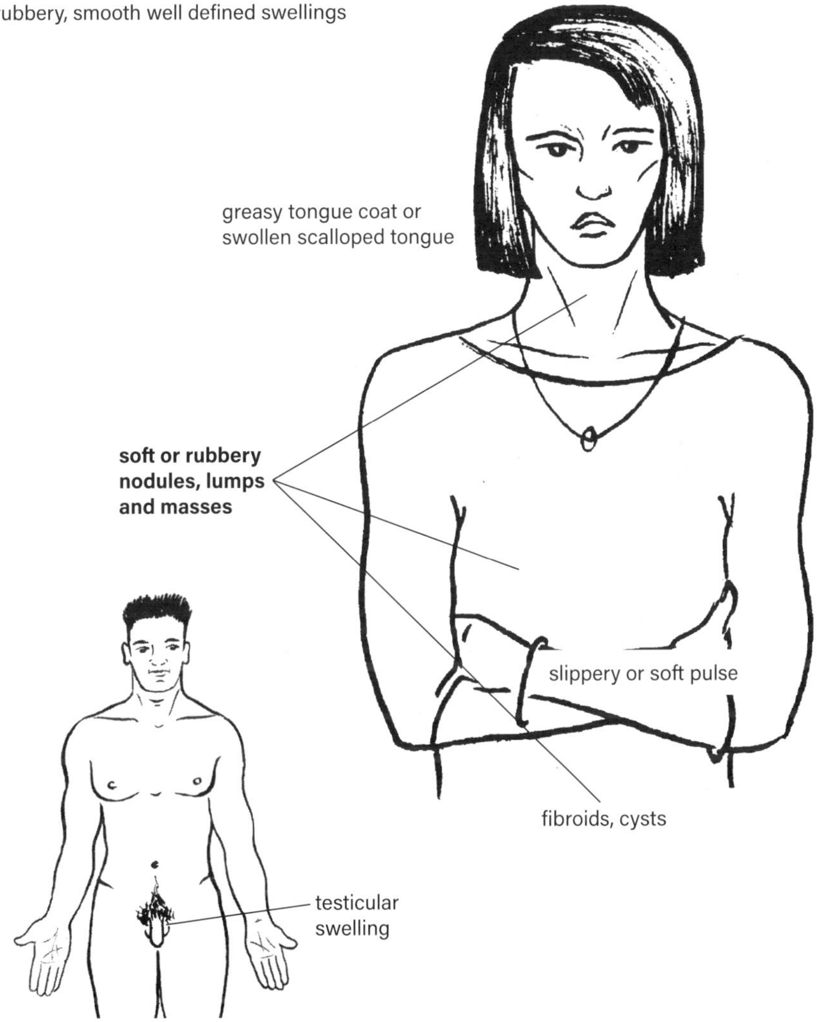

Dosage and method of administration

When used alone, the dose is 8-12 pills three times daily on an empty stomach. The dose can be spread out, or taken in two lots of 12-18 pills, morning and evening. This herb is usually combined with a constitutional formula so the dose can be reduced by 50-75% depending on the dose of the primary formula.

Cautions and contraindications

1.34 Hai Zao Jing Wan (and any preparation containing iodine) should be used cautiously in patients with a hyperthyroid condition as there is a possibility of aggravation.

1.35 NEI XIAO LUO LI WAN

内消瘰疬丸

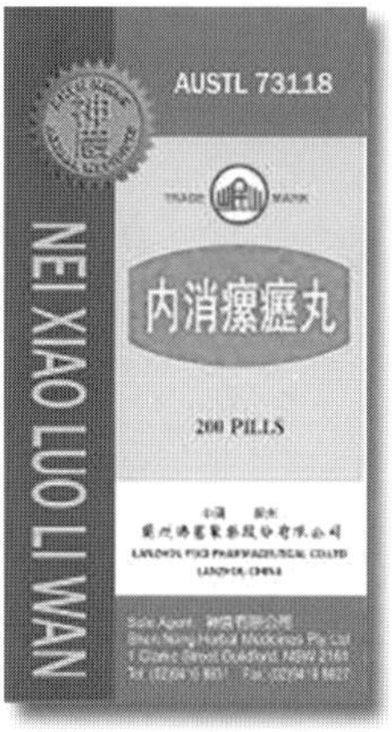

Lanzhou Foci Pharmaceutical Factory (Gansu)
'Internally Reducing Cervical Lymphadenitis Pills'
Nei Xiao Luo Li Wan is packaged in bottles of 200 pills
Also available as: Nei Xiao Luo Li Teapills (PF)

Chinese medical action

Softens and disperses phlegm, softens hardness, reduces masses, clears heat

Biomedical action

Softens and reduces masses and lumps, anti-inflammatory

INDICATIONS

- Benign masses, nodules and lumps associated with phlegm, hard phlegm and/or mild blood stasis. These masses are rubbery and well defined, or firm, tender and irregular. Most commonly used for swollen tender cervical lymph nodes, thyroid nodules, hyperthyroidism, thyroiditis and goitre. Even though this formula is focused on softening and dispersing phlegm and phlegm heat nodules, it can be used for blood masses as it can soften hardness and assist the breakdown of the mass.
- As an adjunct formula to assist in the softening and dispersal of masses such as endometriosis, ovarian cysts and fibroids, breast masses, inflammatory nodules, glandular and lymphatic congestion, hepatosplenomegaly, adenoma, testicular swellings (including post surgical) and chronic boils. Also used for internal inflammatory masses such as chronic diverticulitis and appendicitis.

Composition (each pill contains powdered)

Prunella vulgaris (xia ku cao, prunella) 40.2mg, *Scrophularia ningpoensis* (xuan shen, scrophularia) 25mg, *Fritillaria thunbergii* (zhe bei mu, fritillaria) 10mg, *Angelica sinensis* (dang gui, chinese angelica) 9.15mg, *Mentha haplocalycis* (bo he, mint) 9.15mg, *Citrus aurantium* (zhi ke, aurantium) 9.15mg, *Rheum palmatum* (da huang, rhubarb) 9.15mg, *Forsythia suspensa* (lian qiao, forsythia) 9.15mg, *Platycodon grandiflorum* (jie geng, platycodon) 9.15mg, *Ampelopsis japonica* (bai lian, ampelopsis) 5mg, *Trichosanthes kirilowii* (tian hua fen, trichosanthes root) 5mg, *Rehmannia glutinosa* (sheng di, raw rehmannia) 5mg, *Glycyrrhiza uralensis* (gan cao, licorice) 5mg

Combine with

- **6.3 Chai Hu Shu Gan Wan**, **6.1 Xiao Chai Hu Wan**, or **6.4 Xiao Yao Wan** for patients with qi and phlegm stagnation masses, such as hypochondriac pain from early liver cirrhosis, or fibrocystic breast disease
- **6.1 Xiao Chai Hu Wan** for chronic breast abscess

Pattern identifying features

- **phlegm, hard phlegm and/or mild blood stasis**
- rubbery, painless or tender masses, nodules and lumps; inflammatory masses

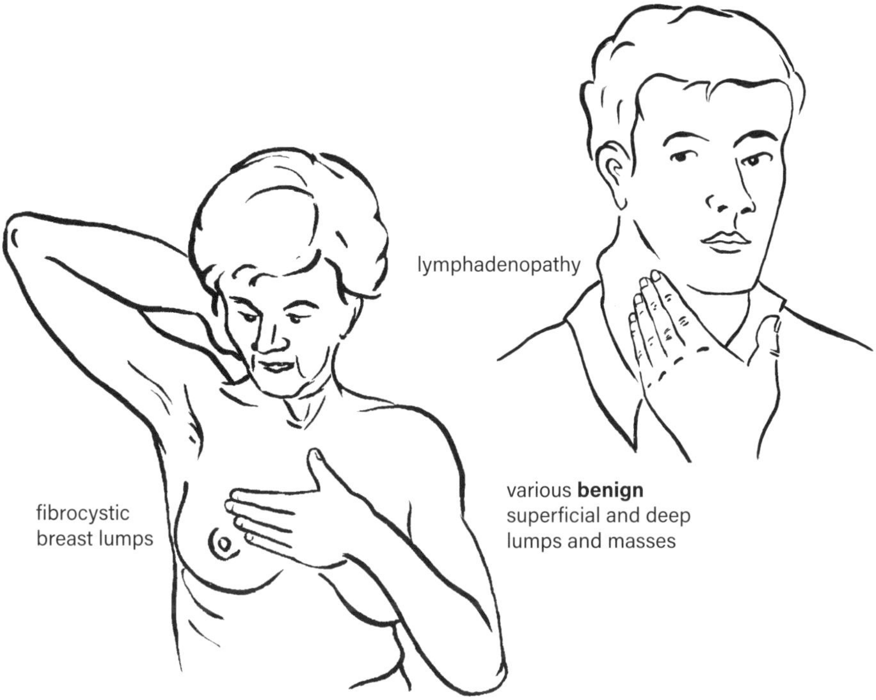

- **7.1 Liu Wei Di Huang Wan** or **1.23 Zhi Bai Di Huang Wan** for hard phlegm accumulations or nodules in patients with a yin deficient constitution
- **1.2 Si Wu Wan** for endometriosis and fibroids with blood deficiency
- **11.1 Qian Lie Xian Capsule** or **11.2 Prostate Gland Pills** for phlegm type prostate swelling from chronic prostatitis
- **6.6 Long Dan Xie Gan Wan** for inflamed and tender lymph nodes in the neck, or acute thyroid swelling

Dosage and method of administration

8-12 pills three times daily on an empty stomach. The dose can be spread out, or taken in two lots of 12-18 pills, morning and evening. In severe cases or during the early stages of treatment (the first few weeks), a 50% increase in dose can be used, then reduced as treatment takes effect.

Cautions and contraindications

Contraindicated during pregnancy.

1.36 FU YAN QING TABLET

妇炎清

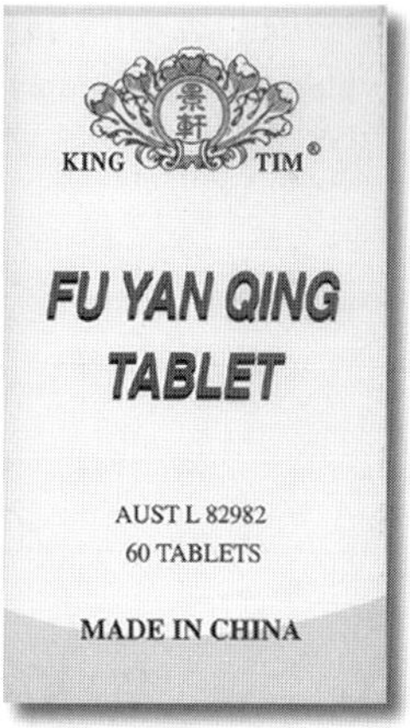

(*Fu Yan Qing*)
Jing Xian Pharmaceutical Co. (Guangzhou)
'Clear Female Inflammation'
Fu Yan Qing Tablets are packaged in bottles of 60 tablets

Chinese medical action

Clears damp heat and toxic heat, and drains damp from the lower burner, nourishes blood, stops pain

Biomedical action

Anti-inflammatory, diuretic, disinfectant

INDICATIONS

- Uterine and lower burner damp heat and/or toxic heat patterns presenting with colored malodorous leukorrhea, heat and pain.
- Infection and inflammation of the urinary tract, painful urination syndrome associated with heat, damp heat and toxic heat.
- With the appropriate identifying features, the formula can assist in the treatment of disorders such as endometritis, inflammation of the cervix, vulvitis, acute pelvic inflammatory disease, salpingitis, adnexitis, pruritus vulvae, genital herpes, *Trichomonas*, *Chlamydia*, thrush, anal fissure and fistula.

Composition (each tablet contains extracts equivalent to dry)

Lygodium japonicum (hai jin sha, lygodium spore) 325mg, *Plantago asiatica* (che qian zi, plantago) 325mg, *Poria cocos* (fu ling, hoelen) 225mg, *Polyporus umbellatus* (zhu ling, polyporus) 225mg, *Scutellaria baicalensis* (huang qin, scute) 225mg, *Angelica polymorpha* (dang gui, chinese angelica) 225mg, *Paeonia lactiflora* (bai shao, white peony) 225mg, *Phellodendron amurense* (huang bai, phellodendron) 175mg, *Polygonum aviculare* (bian xu, knotweed) 150mg, *Viola yedoensis* (zi hua di ding, viola) 100mg

Combine with

- **14.5 Chuan Xin Lian Antiphlogistic Tablets** for marked toxic heat and infection by *Trichomonas*
- **14.1 Huang Lian Jie Du Wan** for severe damp heat
- **13.13 Fu Yin Tai Liniment** for vulvitis and itch

Pattern identifying features

- **damp heat/toxic heat in the lower burner**
- infection of the genitourinary system
- urinary tract infection

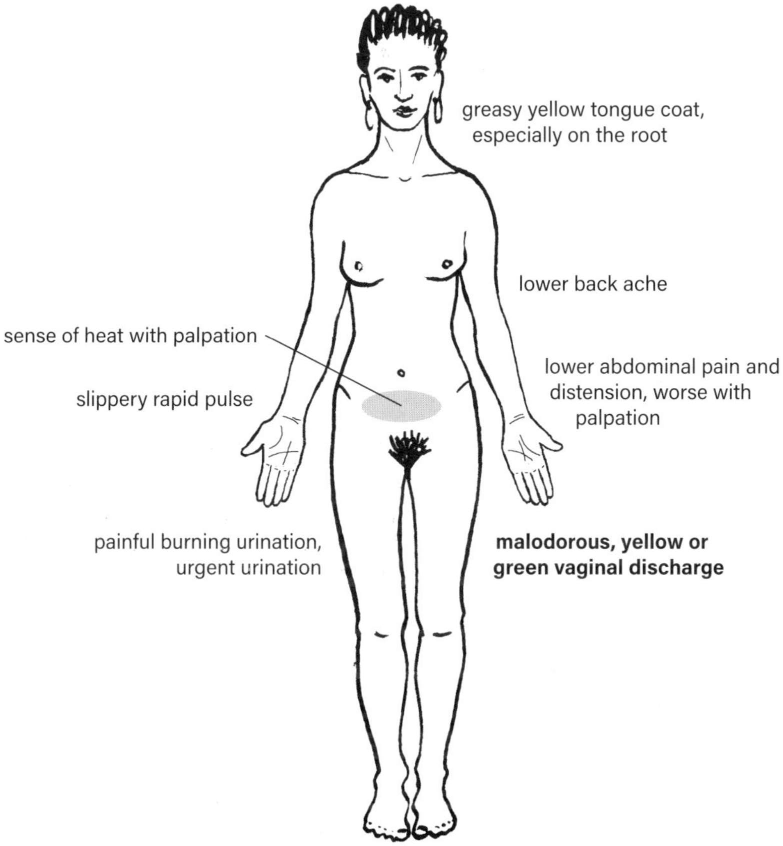

Dosage and method of administration

3-5 tablets, three times daily on an empty stomach. Double the dose in severe cases.

Cautions and contraindications

Contraindicated in patients with cold damp chronic vaginal discharge and with urinary pain and vaginal irritation from yin deficiency.

1.37 BI XIE SHENG SHI WAN

萆薢胜湿丸

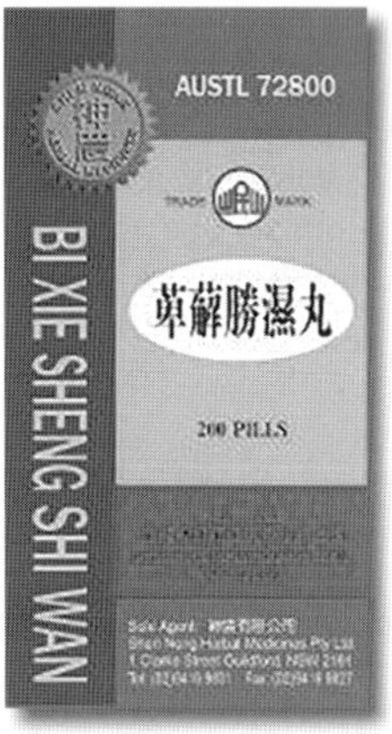

Lanzhou Foci Pharmaceutical Factory (Gansu)
'Fish Poison Yam Pills to Overcome Damp'
Bi Xie Sheng Shi Wan is packaged in bottles of 200 pills
Also available as: Subdue the Dampness Teapills (PF)

Chinese medical action

Clears damp heat from the lower burner (damp greater than heat), promotes urination, cools the blood

Biomedical action

Anti-inflammatory, diuretic, disinfectant

INDICATIONS

- Damp heat in the Uterus and lower burner. For persistent presentations of lower burner damp heat, with damp the dominant feature. A good alternative to **6.6 Long Dan Xie Gan Wan** for recurrent outbreaks of damp heat type genital sores and lower burner discharges in women and men, suitable for prolonged use.
- Damp heat type painful urination with cloudy or concentrated urine and dysuria. Good for chronic recurrent urinary tract infection.
- Damp heat in the skin with weeping, red, itchy lesions, mostly seen in the lower body, including eczema, dermatitis, chronic boils and vesicular skin diseases.
- With the appropriate identifying features, this formula can assist in the treatment of disorders such as pelvic inflammatory disease, pruritus vulvae, vulvitis, genital herpes, genital infection by organisms including *Trichomonas*, *Chlamydia*, and *Candida* (thrush), anal fissure and fistula and thick colored leukorrhea.

Composition (each pill contains powdered)

Coix lachryma-jobi (yi yi ren, coix), 24mg, *Poria cocos* (fu ling, hoelen) 19.2mg, *Dioscorea hypoglauca* (bei xie, fish poison yam) 16mg, *Phellodendron amurense* (huang bai, phellodendron) 16mg, *Dictamnus albus* (bai xian pi, dictamnus) 16mg, *Tetrapanax papyriferae* (tong cao, tetrapanax) 16mg, *Alisma orientale* (ze xie, alisma) 14mg, *Atractylodes lancea* (cang zhu, red atractylodes) 12.8mg, *Paeonia suffruticosa* (mu dan pi, moutan) 12.6mg, *Gardenia florida* (shan zhi zi, gardenia fruit) 12.8mg

Combine with

- **13.4 Ke Yin Wan** for severe damp heat in the skin
- **14.1 Huang Lian Jie Du Wan** for severe damp heat in the reproductive system
- **1.35 Nei Xiao Luo Li Wan** for painful palpable inflammatory masses in the lower abdomen (e.g. salpingitis) from damp heat
- **14.5 Chuan Xin Lian Antiphlogistic Tablets** for acute prostatitis

Pattern identifying features

- **damp heat in the lower burner and lower body**
- damp > heat
- pelvic infection
- urinary tract infections
- vesicular skin lesions

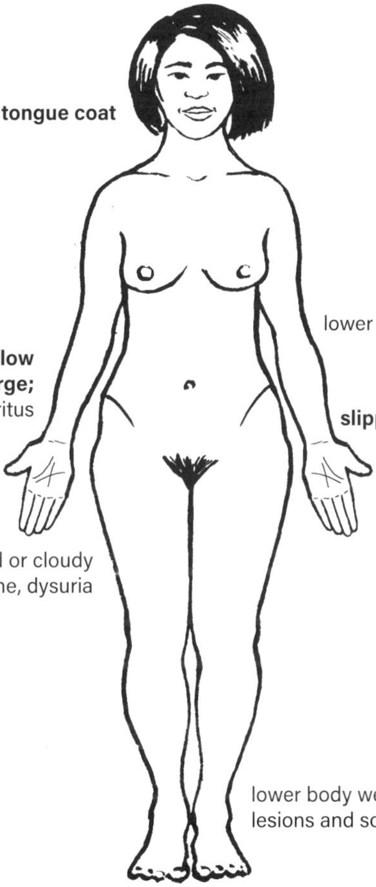

Dosage and method of administration

8-12 pills three or four times daily on an empty stomach, however in most acute cases this can be safely doubled. The dose should be spread out evenly, and in severe cases can be taken every two hours. When used to gradually leach out residual damp heat, a lower dose (~18-24 pills per day) is generally sufficient.

Cautions and contraindications

Generally well tolerated, but can weaken the Spleen and cause digestive upsets if overused.

1.38 YU DAI WAN

愈带丸

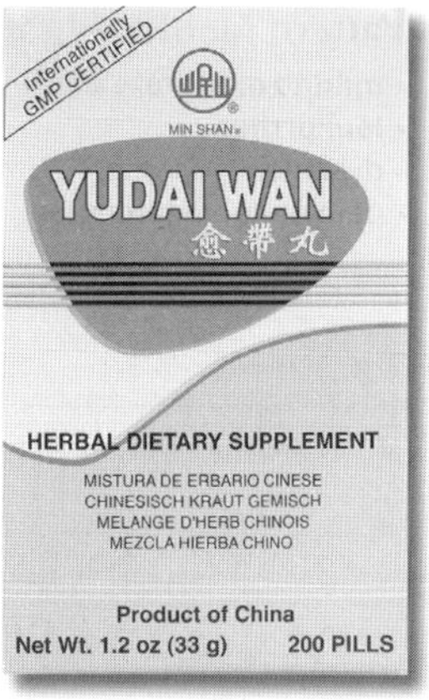

Lanzhou Foci Pharmaceutical Factory (Gansu)
'Pills to Resolve Vaginal Discharge'
Yu Dai Wan is packaged in bottles of 200 pills
Also available as: Yu Dai Teapills (PF)

Chinese medical action

Clears damp heat from the Uterus, stops leukorrhea, nourishes and tonifies blood

Biomedical action

Diuretic, disinfectant, hematinic

INDICATIONS

- Leukorrhea with thick, yellow or green, malodorous, vaginal itch and irritation from mild to moderate damp heat in the Uterus . There may be streaks of blood. The main ingredient, ailanthus, is especially effective in this condition because it not only clears damp heat but astringes discharge at the same time. Can be used for both mild acute and chronic cases. Being based on **1.2 Si Wu Wan** it is suitable for vaginal discharge from damp heat with underlying Liver blood deficiency that enables the damp heat to linger.
- Dysenteric disorder from damp heat.
- With the appropriate identifying features, this formula can assist in the treatment of conditions such as pelvic inflammatory disease, acute or chronic vaginitis, infection by pathogens such as *Trichomonas* and *Candida*, salpingitis, vaginitis, cervicitis and dysentery.

Composition (each pill contains powdered)

Ailanthus altissima (chun gen pi, ailanthus), *Paeonia lactiflora* (bai shao, white peony), *Rehmannia glutinosa* (shu di, processed rehmannia), *Angelica polymorpha* (dang gui, chinese angelica), *Ligusticum wallichi* (chuan xiong, ligusticum), *Phellodendron amurense* (huang bai, phellodendron), *Alpinia officinarum* (gao liang jiang, galangal)

Combine with

- **14.8 Wu Wei Xiao Du Wan**, **14.5 Chuan Xin Lian Antiphlogistic Tablets**, **14.2 Huang Lian Su Tablets** or **14.6 Fu Fang Nan Ban Lan Gen** for severe infection
- **6.6 Long Dan Xie Gan Wan** when accompanied by Liver fire

Dosage and method of administration

8-12 pills three times daily on an empty stomach. The dose can be spread out, or taken in two lots of 12-18 pills, morning and evening. In the early stages of treatment or in severe cases a 50% increase in dose can be used, then reduced as treatment takes effect.

Pattern identifying features

- **mild to moderate acute or chronic damp heat in the uterus**
- **leukorrhea**
- dysenteric disorder
- pain during intercourse

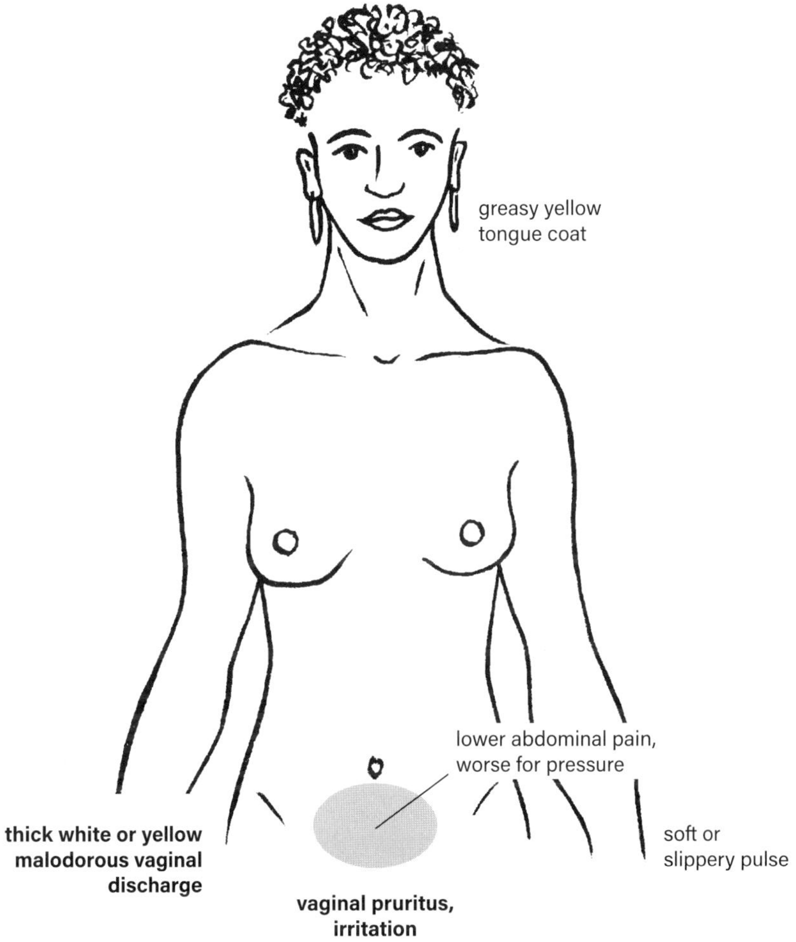

Cautions and contraindications

Not suitable for cold damp leukorrhea. Care should be taken in patients with a tendency to abdominal bloating, loose stools or general digestive weakness. Some patients may find the rehmannia and Chinese angelica in **1.38 Yu Dai Wan** aggravates these symptoms. This can usually be alleviated by taking the pills with a small dose (3-6 pills at the same time) of **2.22 Er Chen Wan** or **2.18 Bao He Wan**.

GMP

1.39 CHIEN CHIN CHIH TAI WAN

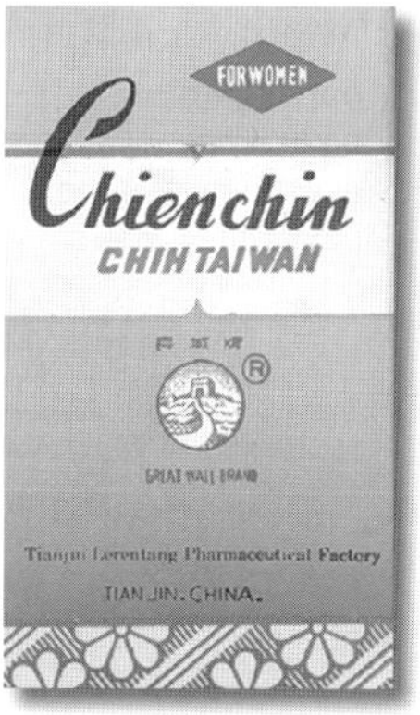

千金止带丸

1-3/12

(*Qian Jin Zhi Dai Wan*)
Tianjin Lerentang Pharmaceutical Factory (Shandong)
'Thousand Gold Pieces Pills to Stop Discharge'
Chien Chin Chih Tai Wan is packaged in bottles of 120 pills

Chinese medical action

Clears damp heat from the lower burner, stops leukorrhea and pain, strengthens the Spleen

Biomedical action

Anti-inflammatory, disinfectant

INDICATIONS

- Mild recurrent damp or damp heat in the Uterus and lower burner causing yellow or creamy leukorrhea. Suitable for deficiency, excess or mixed patterns. This formula is interesting in that it contains warming, tonifying, astringent and damp heat clearing herbs and is thus best for a variety of complex and chronic conditions, as well as recurrent or latent problems. The focus of the formula is the salty cold indigo, which has damp and toxic heat clearing ability (antibiotic and anti-inflammatory action). Therefore, even though the damp heat aspects are the primary focus, the formula recognizes the importance of deficiency (here Spleen qi, blood and Kidney yang) in enabling damp heat to linger and stagnate.
- With the appropriate identifying features, this formula can be used to treat conditions such as leukorrhea, *Candida* (thrush), chronic pelvic inflammatory disease, salpingitis, oophoritis, chronic prostatitis, chronic pyelonephritis, chronic or cloudy urinary problems (such as turbid or milky painful urination syndrome), albuminuria and chyluria.

Composition

Indigo Pulverata Levis (qing dai, indigo) 16%, *Angelica sinensis* (dang gui, chinese angelica) 10%, *Atractylodes macrocephala* (bai zhu, atractylodes) 5%, *Codonopsis pilosula* (dang shen, codonopsis) 12%, *Dipsacus asper* (xu duan, dipsacus) 10%, *Saussurea lappa* (mu xiang, saussurea) 10%, *Ostrea gigas* (mu li, oyster shell) 12%, *Foeniculum vulgarae* (xiao hui xiang, fennel seed) 5%

Combine with

- **7.1 Liu Wei Di Huang Wan** or **1.23 Zhi Bai Di Huang Wan** for chronic or recurrent urinary discomfort from damp heat and Kidney deficiency
- **11.1 Qian Lie Xian Capsules** or **11.2 Prostate Gland Pills** for chronic prostatitis from damp heat

Pattern identifying features

- **damp heat in the lower burner with Spleen and Kidney deficiency**
- pain during intercourse

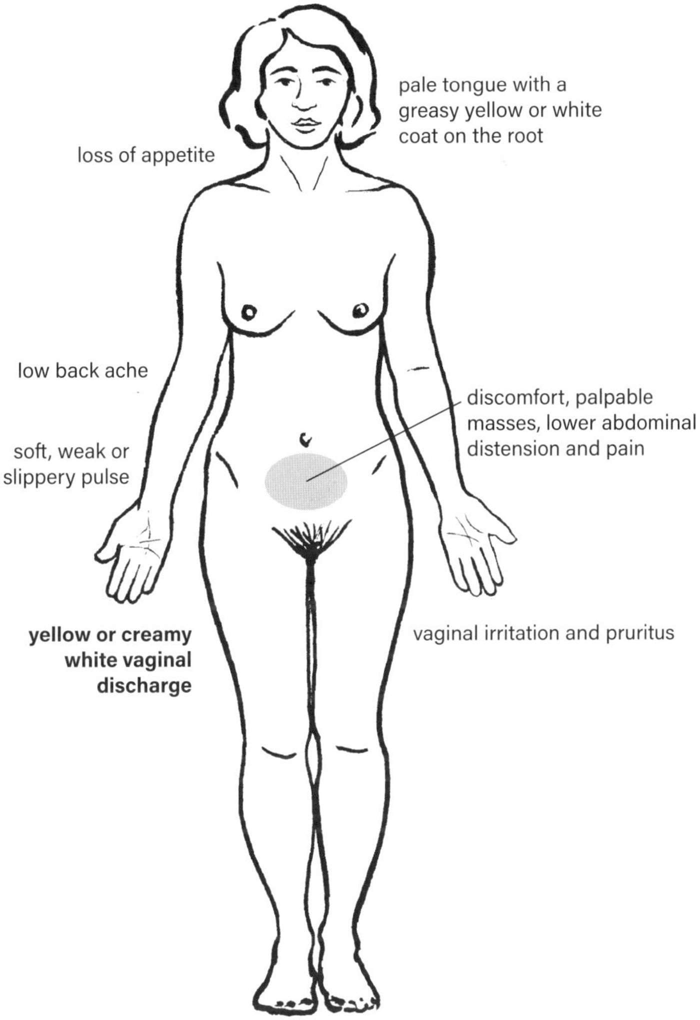

Dosage and method of administration

5 pills, three times daily on an empty stomach.

Cautions and contraindications

Not recommended for severe or acute damp heat or toxic heat discharges with no underlying deficiency (*see* **6.6 Long Dan Xie Gan Wan** or **1.36 Fu Yan Qing Tablet**).

1.40 YANG YAN QU BAN TABLET

养颜去斑片

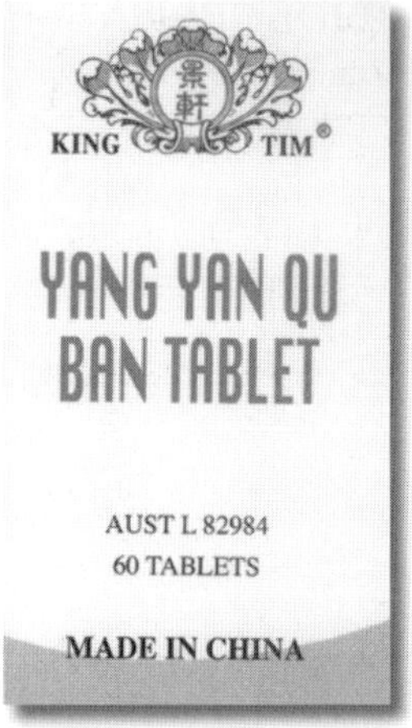

(*Yang Yan Qu Ban Pian*)
Jing Xian Pharmaceutical Co. (Guangzhou)
'Tablets to Nourish the Face and Eliminate Spots'
Yang Yan Qu Ban Tablets are packaged in bottles of 60 sugar coated tablets

Chinese medical action

Regulates qi and invigorates blood, tonifies blood, strengthens the Spleen

Biomedical action

Hematinic, regulates menstruation

INDICATIONS

- Hyperpigmentation of the skin (melasma, chloasma, melasma gravidarum), especially the face associated with Liver qi constraint, Liver and Spleen disharmony, blood deficiency and/or blood stasis. Features include coffee colored spots or patches on the face, trunk and abdomen, the hyper pigmentation of pregnancy (used postpartum) and pigmentation that complicates hormonal disorders and use of the oral contraceptive pill.

Composition (each tablet contains extracts equivalent to dry)

Codonopsis pilosula (dang shen, codonopsis) 325mg, *Vitex trifolia* (man jing zi, vitex fruit) 325mg, *Salvia miltiorrhiza* (dan shen, salvia) 250mg, *Curcuma longa* (yu jin, curcuma) 250mg, *Cyperus rotundus* (xiang fu, cyperus) 250mg, *Atractylodes macrocephala* (bai zhu, atractylodes) 250mg, *Paeonia lactiflora* (bai shao, white peony) 250mg, *Ligusticum wallichi* (chuan xiong, ligusticum) 225mg

Dosage and method of administration

3-5 tablets, three times daily on an empty stomach.

Cautions and contraindications

Contraindicated during pregnancy.

脾胃肠病 2

Gastrointestinal

External Invasion
2.1 Xing Jun San
2.2 Huo Hsiang Cheng Chi Pien
2.3 So Hup Yuen Medical Pills
2.4 Fu Ke An
2.5 Bao Ji Pills
2.6 Po Chai Pills

Spleen qi tonifying
2.7 Si Jun Zi Wan
2.8 Liu Jun Zi Wan
2.9 Xiang Sha Liu Jun Wan
2.10 Xiang Sha Yang Wei Wan
2.11 Bu Zhong Yi Qi Wan
2.12 Shen Ling Bai Zhu Wan

Spleen yang tonifying
2.13 Li Zhong Wan
2.14 Li Chung Yuen Medical Pills
2.15 Xiao Jian Zhong Wan

Food stagnation, Indigestion, weight loss
2.16 Zi Sheng Wan
2.17 Jian Pi Wan
2.18 Bao He Wan
2.19 Shen Chu Cha
2.20 Bojenmi Chinese Tea
2.21 Keep Fit Capsule

Phlegm damp
2.22 Er Chen Wan
2.23 Ping Wei San

Liver Spleen/Stomach disharmony
2.24 Shu Gan Wan
2.25 Tong Xie Yao Fang Wan
2.26 Xiang Lian Wan
2.27 Wei Te Ling
2.28 Wei Tong Ding

Large Intestine, constipation
2.29 Mu Xiang Shun Qi Wan
2.30 Chen Xiang Hua Qi Wan
2.31 Run Chang Wan
2.32 Wu Ren Wan
2.33 Da Huang Jiang Zhi Wan
2.34 Cong Rong Bu Shen Wan

Sugar and fat metabolism
2.35 Yu Quan Wan
2.36 Sugarid

Rectum, hemorrhoids
2.37 Huai Jiao Di Yu Wan
2.38 Hua Zhi Ling Tablet
2.39 Fargelin for Piles
2.40 Hemorrhoids Ointment

See also
6.2 Si Ni Wan
6.3 Chai Hu Shu Gan Wan
6.7 Da Chai Hu Wan
6.8 Yi Guan Jian Wan
6.9 Jigucao Wan
6.10 Qing Gan Li Dan Tablets
6.11 Li Dan Tablets
14.1 Huang Lian Jie Du Wan

2.1 XING JUN SAN

行军散

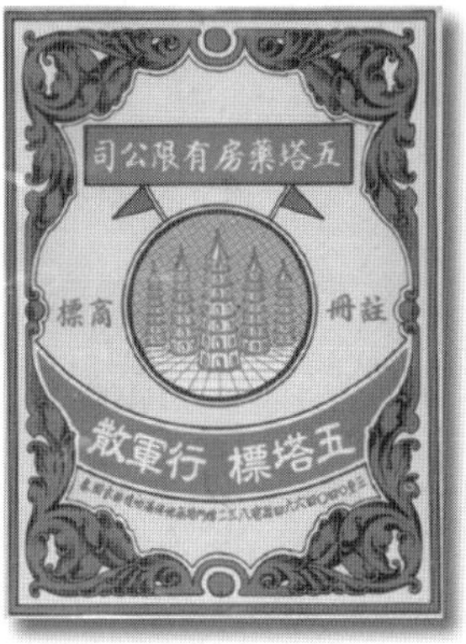

Five Pagodas Pharmacy Co. (Thailand)
'Marching Powder'
Xing Jun San is a highly aromatic green powder packaged in small 10 gram or large 25 gram jars

Chinese medical action

Fragrantly dispels and disperses summerdamp and deeply rooted damp, regulates the Stomach and Intestines, stops nausea and vomiting

Biomedical action

Eliminates pathogens from the digestive system, anti-emetic, anti-diarrheal

INDICATIONS

- Acute nausea and vomiting, abdominal cramps and diarrhea associated with summerdamp invasion, sudden turmoil disorder and gastrointestinal upsets. A powerful, fragrant and dispersing formula, when used correctly it generally works quickly. In acute situations, it should not be used for long, usually no longer than 3-5 days. If patients fail to improve in that time they should be reassessed.
- Given in small doses when patients with Spleen deficiency diarrhea fail to improve, or get worse with Spleen tonic formulas, an outcome suggesting hidden or deeply rooted damp.
- With the appropriate identifying features, this formula may be used to treat disorders such as acute viral or bacterial gastroenteritis, food poisoning, summer flu, stomach flu, acute colitis, travelers diarrhea, 'Bali belly' and motion sickness.

Composition (each 100 grams of powder contains)

Magnolia officinalis (hou po, magnolia bark) 11.8g, *Ligusticum wallichi* (chuan xiong, ligusticum) 9.3g, *Atractylodes lancea* (cang zhu, red atractylodes) 9.3g, *Agastache rugosa* (huo xiang, agastache) 7.1g, *Citrus reticulata* (chen pi, citrus) 7.1g, *Eugenia caryophyllata* (ding xiang, cloves) 7.1g, *Saussurea lappa* (mu xiang, saussurea) 7.1g, *Aquilaria agallocha* (chen xiang, aquilaria) 7.1g, *Cinnamomum cassia* (gui zhi, cinnamon) 7.1g, *Glycyrrhiza uralensis* (gan cao, licorice) 4.8g, Menthol 4.7g, *Acorus gramineus* (shi chang pu, acorus) 3.5g, *Angelica dahurica* (bai zhi, angelica) 3.5g, *Mentha haplocalycis* (bo he, mint) 3.5g, *Lysimachiae foeni-graeci* (ling ling xiang) 3.3g, *Asarum seiboldi* (xi xin*, asarum) 2.3g, *Dryobalanops camphora* (bing pian, borneol) 1.4g [**Restricted use in some jurisdictions; may be subject to substitution*]

Dosage and method of administration

- Summerdamp: Half to one teaspoon of powder in a little water every 2-3 hours in the acute phase. If the patient does not improve (especially nausea) within 30 minutes, the dose can be repeated. It is useful to continue treatment for 1-2 days following resolution of the symptoms (at a smaller dose) to ensure that all dampness has been cleared

Pattern identifying features

- **summerdamp invasion**
- acute gastric upset
- lethargy
- heaviness

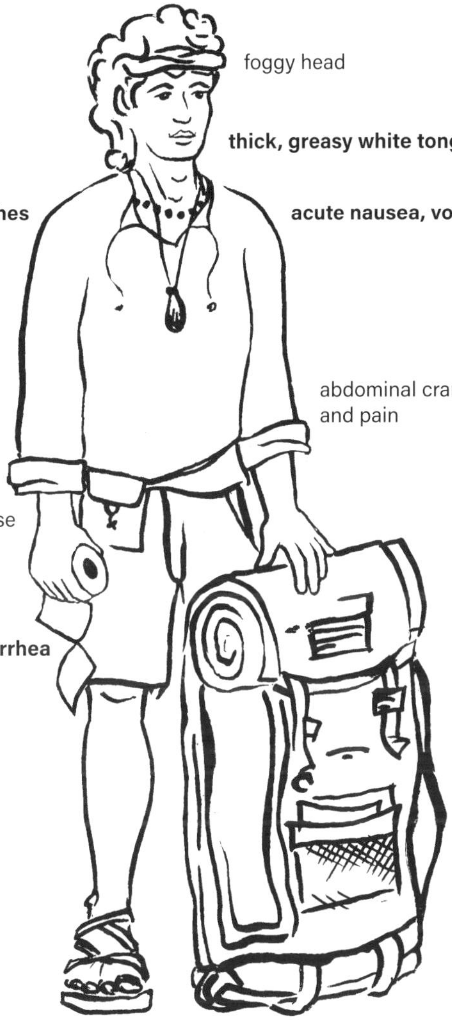

– For leaching hidden damp: ¼ teaspoon 2-3 times daily for two or so weeks
– For motion sickness: ⅛ teaspoon every hour or so as needed

Cautions and contraindications

Contraindicated during pregnancy. Not suitable for prolonged use. For acute conditions, satisfactory result should be observed within 24-72 hours If improvement is not apparent, review the patient and reconsider the prescription. Not suitable for patients with high fever and thirst.

2.2.1 HUO HSIANG CHENG CHI PIEN

TGA

1-3/52

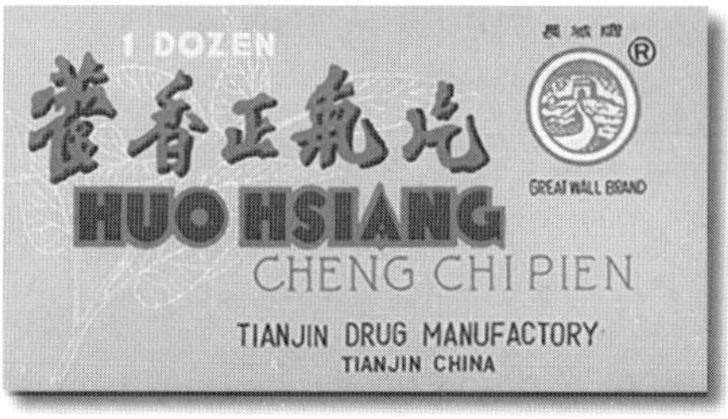

藿香正气片

(*Huo Xiang Zheng Qi Pian*)
Tianjin Drug Manufactory (Shandong)
'Agastache Qi Correcting Tablets'
Huo Hsiang Cheng Chi Pien is packaged in vials of 8 uncoated pills, 12 vials per box
Also available as: Agastache Formula (conc. extract)

Chinese medical action

Dispels dampness, regulates and harmonizes the Stomach and Intestines, stops vomiting and diarrhea

Biomedical action

Anti-emetic, anti-diarrheal, stomachic, alleviates acute gastric conditions

INDICATIONS

- Acute wind cold invasion with internal damp, with damp preexisting or carried in with wind. This pattern is commonly seen towards the end of summer and typically appears in clusters, sweeping through offices and schools.
- Summerdamp attack and sudden turmoil disorder (*see* glossary) without exterior symptoms.
- For patients with a tendency to internal damp manifested in digestive symptoms such as borborygmus, abdominal distension, nausea, loss of appetite and abdominal pain. Also prescribed for patients who get worse with Spleen qi tonic herbs. May also be useful, in short bursts, for children with acute exacerbation of an underlying damp condition, such as chronic sinus or ear congestion, or abdominal pain that is stirred up in windy weather.
- With the appropriate identifying features, this formula can be used to treat conditions such as acute viral or bacterial gastroenteritis, food poisoning, summer flu, stomach flu, travelers diarrhea, influenza, acute colitis and motion sickness.

Composition

Agastache rugosa (huo xiang, agastache) 13.32%, *Poria cocos* (fu ling, hoelen) 13.25%, *Areca catechu* (da fu pi, betel husk) 13.25%, *Angelica dahurica* (bai zhi, angelica) 13.25%, *Perilla frutescens* (zi su ye, perilla) 13.25%, *Magnolia officinalis* (hou po, magnolia bark) 9.4%, *Atractylodes lancea* (cang zhu, red atractylodes) 9.4%, *Citrus reticulata* (chen pi, citrus) 9.4%, *Glycyrrhiza uralensis* (gan cao, licorice) 5.5%

Pattern identifying features

- **summerdamp invasion; wind cold with internal damp**
- **acute gastric upsets**
- chills and fever (chills may be greater than fever)
- lethargy
- heaviness

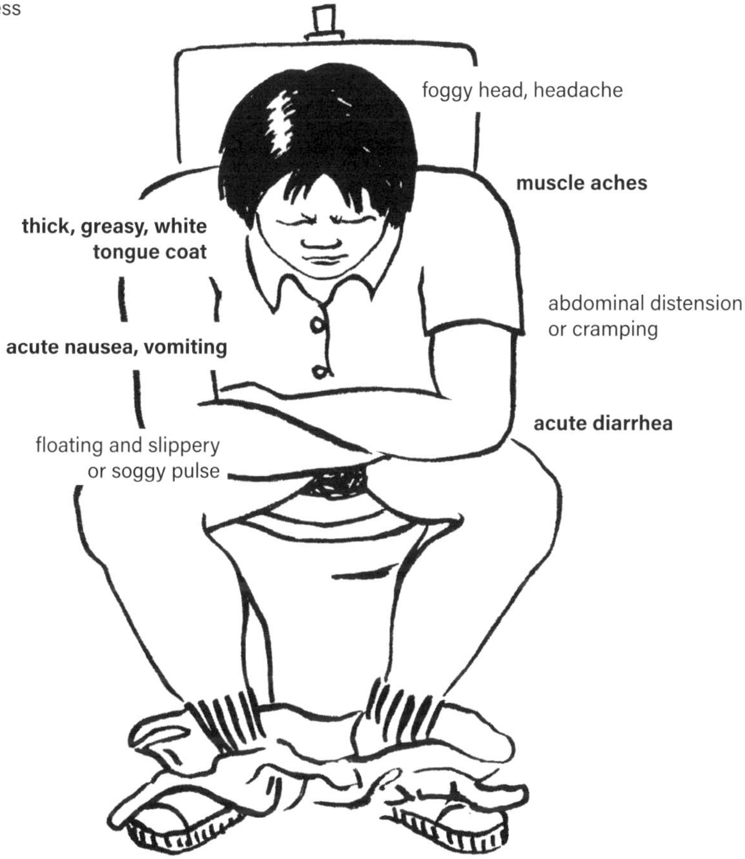

Dosage and method of administration

For acute cases, 4-8 tablets every 2 hours. For longer use (2-3 weeks maximum) in leaching deep lying damp, reduce the dose by 50-75%. Not suitable for small children due to the dimensions of the tablet.

Cautions and contraindications

Not suitable for digestive upsets due to heat or damp heat, (those with thirst, constipation, yellow tongue coat, fever with no chills, etc.).

2.2.2 HUO XIANG ZHENG QI WAN

藿香正气丸

Lanzhou Foci Pharmaceutical Factory (Gansu)
'Agastache Qi Correcting Pills'
Huo Xiang Zheng Qi Wan is packaged in bottles of 200 pills

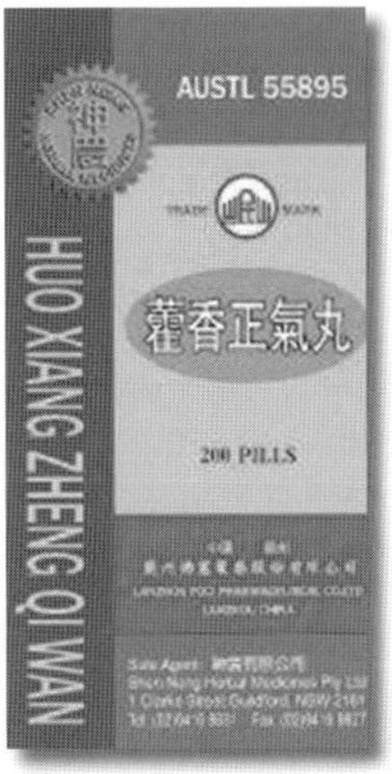

Chinese medical action

Dispels dampness, regulates and harmonizes the Stomach and Intestines, stops vomiting and diarrhea

Biomedical action

Anti-emetic, anti-diarrheal, stomachic, alleviates acute gastric conditions

INDICATIONS

- As for **2.2.1 Huo Hsiang Cheng Chi Pien**

Composition (each pill contains powdered)

Agastache rugosa (huo xiang, agastache) 23mg, *Magnolia officinalis* (hou po, magnolia bark) 15mg, *Platycodon grandiflorum* (jie geng, platycodon) 15mg, *Citrus reticulata* (chen pi, citrus) 15mg, *Glycyrrhiza uralensis* (gan cao, licorice) 15mg, *Pinellia ternata* (zhi ban xia, processed pinellia) 15mg, *Atractylodes macrocephala* (bai zhu, atractylodes) 15mg, *Angelica dahurica* (bai zhi, angelica) 8mg, *Perilla frutescens* (zi su ye, perilla) 8mg, *Poria cocos* (fu ling, hoelen) 8mg, *Zingiber officinale* (sheng jiang, ginger) 29mg, *Zizyphus jujuba* (da zao, chinese dates) 47mg

Dosage and method of administration

12-15 pills three times daily on an empty stomach. The dose may be spread out, or two lots of 18-22 pills taken morning and evening. In severe cases, take a dose every two hours or so.

Cautions and contraindications

As for **2.2.1 Huo Hsiang Cheng Chi Pien**.

2.2.3 COLD AND ABDOMINAL DISCOMFORT RELIEVER

藿香正气片

(*Huo Xiang Zheng Qi Pian*)
Tong Ren Tang (Beijing)
'Agastache Qi Correcting Tablets'
Cold and Abdominal Discomfort Reliever is packaged in bottles of 60 sugar coated tablets

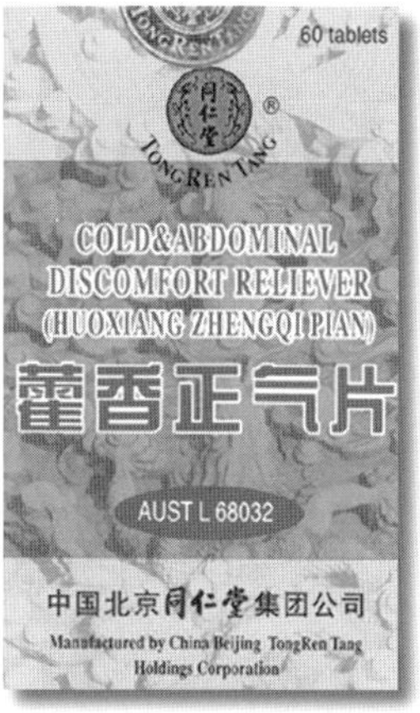

Chinese medical action

Dispels dampness, regulates and harmonizes the Stomach and Intestines, stops vomiting and diarrhea

Biomedical action

Anti-emetic, anti-diarrheal, stomachic, alleviates acute gastric conditions

INDICATIONS

- As for **2.2.1 Huo Hsiang Cheng Chi Pien**

Composition (each tablet contains)

Pinellia ternata (zhi ban xia, processed pinellia) 186mg, *Platycodon grandiflorum* (jie geng, platycodon) 160mg, *Areca catechu* (da fu pi, betel husk) 97mg, *Glycyrrhiza uralensis* (gan cao, licorice) 97mg, *Perilla frutescens* (zi su ye, perilla) 97mg, *Poria cocos* (fu ling, hoelen) 94mg, *Angelica dahurica* (bai zhi, angelica) 94mg, *Agastache rugosa* (huo xiang, agastache essential oil) 2.8mg, *Citrus reticulata* (chen pi, citrus essential oil) 1.9mg

Dosage and method of administration

4 tablets three times daily. In severe cases a dose can be taken every 2 hours or so.

Cautions and contraindications

As for **2.2.1 Huo Hsiang Cheng Chi Pien**.

GMP

2.3 SO HUP YUEN MEDICAL PILLS

追风苏合丸

1-3 / 12

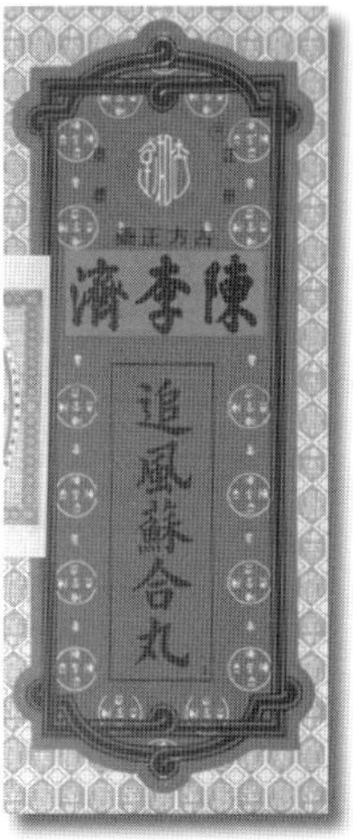

(*Zhui Feng Su He Wan*)
Chan Li Chai Medical Factory (Hong Kong)
'Chase Away Wind and Make Complete Pills'
So Hup Yuen Medical Pills are packaged as large honey pills in a yellow wax ball, ten pills per box

Chinese medical action

Fragrantly dispels and dries deeply rooted damp, warms and regulates the Stomach and Intestines, stops nausea and vomiting

Biomedical action

Eliminates pathogens from the digestive system, anti-emetic, anti-diarrheal

INDICATIONS

- Cold damp in the gastrointestinal system. Similar in action to **2.1 Xing Jun San**, this formula is fragrant, warming and dispersing, and used for locating and dispelling deep lying and hidden damp. Useful for unusual or resistant gastrointestinal complaints such as abdominal distension and chronic diarrhea that fail to respond to standard approaches. Can assist in the treatment of *gu* syndrome (*see* glossary).
- For acute wind cold invasion with gastrointestinal upset.
- With the appropriate identifying features, the formula can be used for conditions such as chronic infections of the gastrointestinal tract, chronic candidiasis, leaky gut syndrome, acute gastroenteritis (either viral or bacterial), summer flu, travelers diarrhea, influenza and acute colitis.

Composition

Agastache rugosa (huo xiang, agastache) 6.72%, *Eugenia caryophyllata* (ding xiang, cloves) 6.72%, *Piper longum* (bi ba, long pepper) 6.72%, *Santalum album* (tan xiang, sandalwood) 6.72%, *Myristica fragrans* (rou dou kou, nutmeg) 6.72%, *Notopterygium incisum* (qiang huo, notopterygium) 6.72%, *Ledebouriella divaricata* (fang feng, siler) 6.72%, *Mentha haplocalycis* (bo he, mint) 6.72%, *Glycyrrhiza uralensis* (gan cao, licorice) 6.72%, *Cyperus rotundus* (xiang fu, cyperus) 6.72%, *Terminalia chebula* (he zi, terminalia) 6.72%, *Atractylodes macrocephala* (bai zhu, atractylodes) 6.72%, *Aquilaria agallocha* (chen xiang, aquilaria) 6.72%, *Saussurea lappa* (mu xiang, saussurea) 6.72%, *Asarum seiboldi* (xi xin*, asarum) 4.52%, *Dryobalanops camphora* (bing pian, borneol) 1.4% [**Restricted use in some jurisdictions; may be subject to substitution*]

Pattern identifying features

- **cold damp in the gastrointestinal system**
- physical and mental exhaustion
- gastrointestinal symptoms worse with tonifying formulas
- loss of appetite, ravenous hunger or odd food cravings

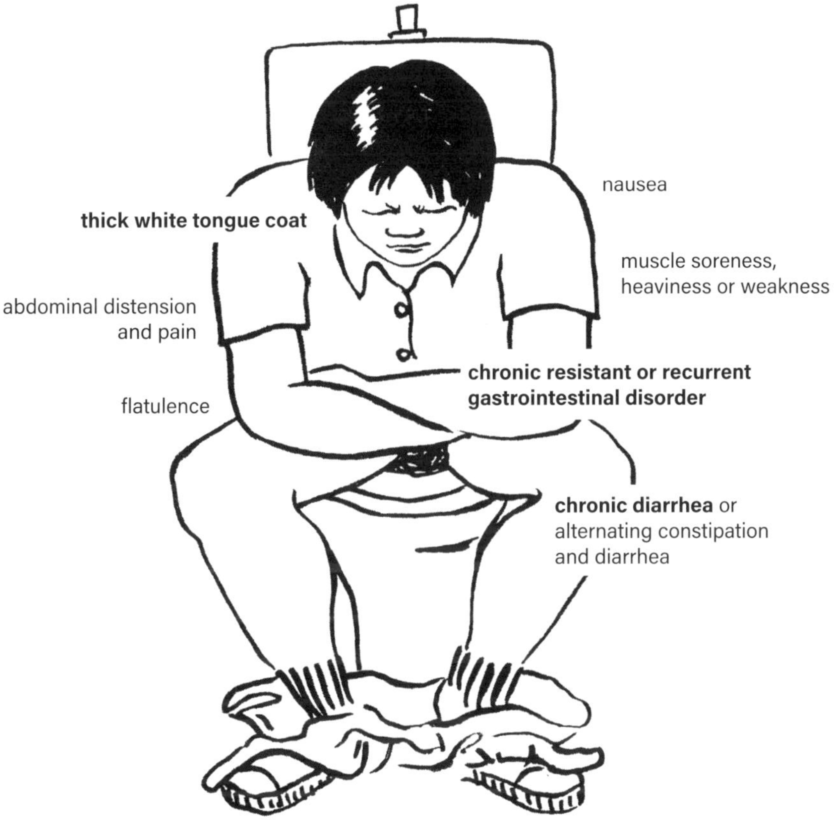

Combine with

– A small dose of **14.2 Huang Lian Su Tablets** for *gu* syndrome

Dosage and method of administration

One pill twice daily, on an empty stomach. These pills are often very hard and need to be softened in boiling water for 10 minutes before ingestion.

Cautions and contraindications

Not suitable for digestive upsets due to heat or damp heat, with thirst, constipation, yellow tongue coat and fever without chills.

2.4 FU KE AN

腹可安

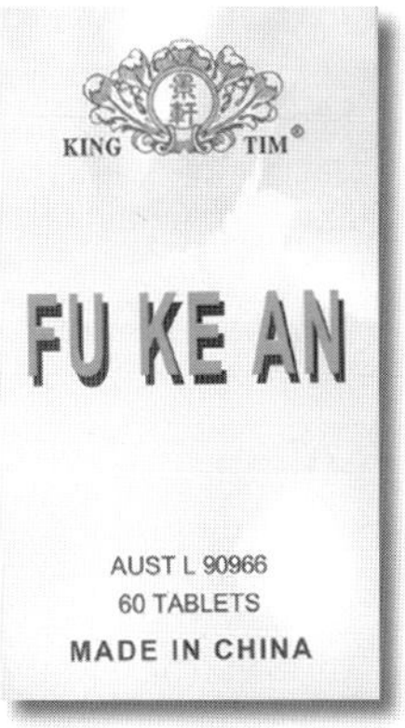

Jing Xian Pharmaceutical Co. (Guangzhou)
'Calm the Abdomen'
Fu Ke An is packaged in bottles of 60 sugar coated tablets

Chinese medical action

Clears damp heat, astringes the Intestines and stops diarrhea, stops pain

Biomedical action

Anti-diarrheal, alleviates acute gastric conditions

INDICATIONS

- Acute and chronic diarrhea associated with damp heat invasion of the Large Intestine. The first two herbs in this formula, chinese polygonum and iron holly bark, have specific activity against the common organisms that cause acute diarrhea. The main features are indigestion with spasmodic cramping abdominal or epigastric pain, acid reflux, nausea and vomiting, diarrhea, rectal and anal pain, fever and malaise. This medicine can be used to treat gastroenteritis, dysentery and colitis.

Composition (each tablet contains extracts equivalent to dry)

Polygonum chinense (huo tan mu, chinese polygonum) 872mg, *Ilex rotunda* (jiu bi ying, iron holly bark) 722mg, *Plantago asiatica* (che qian zi, plantago) 448mg, *Punica granatum* (shi liu pi, pomegranate skin) 448mg

Combine with

- **14.1 Huang Lian Jie Du Wan** for severe damp heat
- **14.5 Chuan Xin Lian Antiphlogistic Tablets** for dysentery from *Shigella* sp.

Dosage and method of administration

3-4 tablets, three times daily. In severe cases the dose can be increased to 3-4 tablets every 2 hours.

Cautions and Contraindications

Not suitable for acute diarrhea from summerdamp or cold damp invasion (*see* **2.1 Xing Jun San**, **2.2.1 Huo Hsiang Cheng Chi Pien**, or **2.23 Ping Wei San**).

2.5 BAO JI PILLS

保济丸

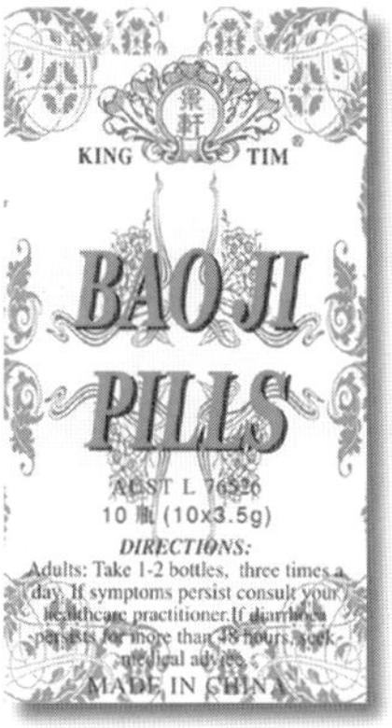

(*Bao Ji Wan*)
Jing Xian Pharmaceutical Co. (Guangzhou)
'Protect and Relieve Pills'
Bao Ji Pills are packaged in vials of tiny pills, 3.5 grams per vial

Chinese medical action

Clears damp heat from the Intestines, stops diarrhea

Biomedical action

Anti-diarrheal, anti-emetic, stomachic, alleviates acute gastric conditions

INDICATIONS

- Acute diarrhea and/or nausea and vomiting from damp heat invading the Large Intestine. Usually occurs during hot and humid weather, especially late summer when heat and humidity are the prevailing climatic features. Similar in action and indication to **2.6 Po Chai Pills**, this version has fewer astringent and anti-diarrheal herbs.
- With the appropriate identifying features (*see* illustration, p.85), this medicine may be used to treat acute gastroenteritis (either viral or bacterial), summer flu, travelers diarrhea, hangover, overindulgence in rich food and food poisoning.

Composition (each bottle [3.5g] contains extracts equivalent to dry)

Uncaria rhyncophylla (gou teng, gambir) 2.9g, *Magnolia officinalis* (hou po, magnolia bark) 2.9g, *Trichosanthes kirilowi* (tian hua fen, trichosanthes root) 2.9g, *Angelica dahurica* (bai zhi, angelica) 2.9g, *Agastache rugosa* (huo xiang, agastache) 2.9g, *Atractylodes lancea* (cang zhu, red atractylodes) 2.9g, *Saussurea lappa* (mu xiang, saussurea) 2.4g, *Citrus reticulata* (chen pi, citrus) 2.4g, *Setaria italica* (gu ya, sprouted rice) 2.4g, *Mentha haplocalycis* (bo he, mint) 1.4g

Dosage and method of administration

1-2 bottles, three times daily. In severe cases a dose can be taken every 2 hours.

Cautions and contraindications

None noted.

2.6 PO CHAI PILLS

TGA

保济丸

1/52

(*Bao Ji Wan*)
Li Chung Shing Tong Ltd (Hong Kong)
'Protect and Relieve Pills'
Po Chai Pills are packaged in vials of 100 tiny pills, eight vials to a box

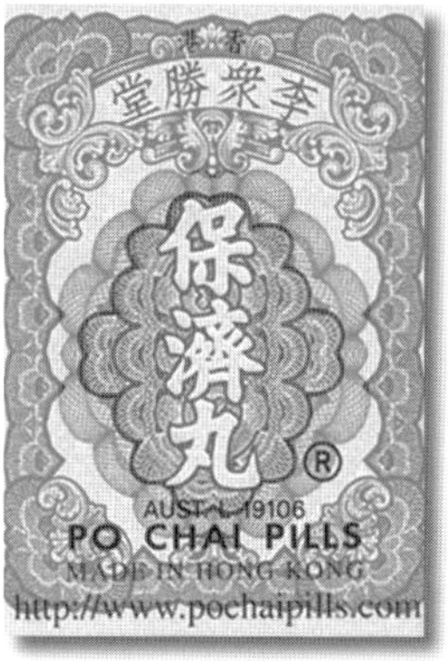

Chinese medical action

Clears damp heat from the Intestines, stops diarrhea

Biomedical action

Anti-diarrheal, anti-emetic, stomachic, alleviates acute gastric conditions

INDICATIONS

- Acute diarrhea and/or nausea and vomiting from damp heat invasion of the Large Intestine. Usually occurs during hot and humid weather, especially late Summer when heat and humidity are the prevailing climatic features. The difference between this formula and **2.1 Xing Jun San** and **2.2.1 Huo Hsiang Cheng Chi Pien**, is that this formula is best for the lower intestinal manifestations and diarrhea. Also used for digestive upsets (diarrhea, abdominal distension and pain) resulting from overindulgence in rich food and alcohol.
- With the appropriate identifying features, this formula may be used to treat acute gastroenteritis (either viral or bacterial), summer flu, travelers diarrhea, hangover, overindulgence and food poisoning.

Composition (w/v)

Poria cocos (fu ling, hoelen) 14%, *Saussurea lappa* (mu xiang, saussurea) 8%, *Atractylodes lancea* (cang zhu, red atractylodes) 8%, *Agastache rugosa* (huo xiang, agastache) 8%, *Angelica dahurica* (bai zhi, angelica) 8%, *Pueraria lobata* (ge gen, kudzu) 7%, *Magnolia officinalis* (hou po, magnolia bark) 7%, *Coicis lachryma-jobi* (yi yi ren, coix) 7%, Sun Kook Tea 7%, *Trichosanthes kirilowi* (gua lou, trichosanthes) 5.5%, *Hordeum vulgare* (mai ya, sprouted barley) 5.5%, *Mentha haplocalycis* (bo he, mint) 4.5%, *Halloysitum rubrum* (chi shi zhi, kaolin) 3.5%, *Chrysanthemum morifolium* (ju hua, chrysanthemum) 3.5%, *Citrus reticulata* (chen pi, citrus) 3.5%

Combine with

– **14.5 Chuan Xin Lian Antiphlogistic Tablets** or **14.1 Huang Lian Jie Du Wan** for damp heat with pus or blood in the stool

Pattern identifying features

- **acute damp heat invasion of the Large Intestine**
- **travellers diarrhea**
- headache, hangover
- fever

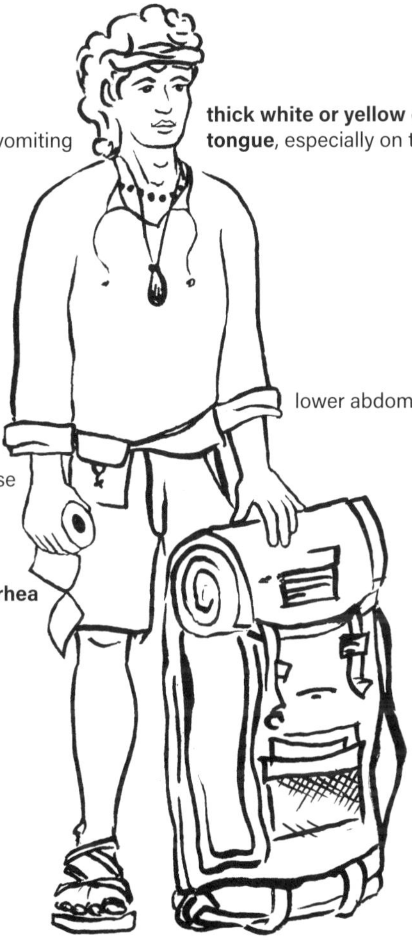

Dosage and method of administration

1-2 vials every two hours. Half dose for children. Continue the formula for a couple of days following the resolution of symptoms to ensure all damp heat is leached from the system.

Cautions and contraindications

None noted.

GMP

2.7 SI JUN ZI WAN

四君子丸

3+/12

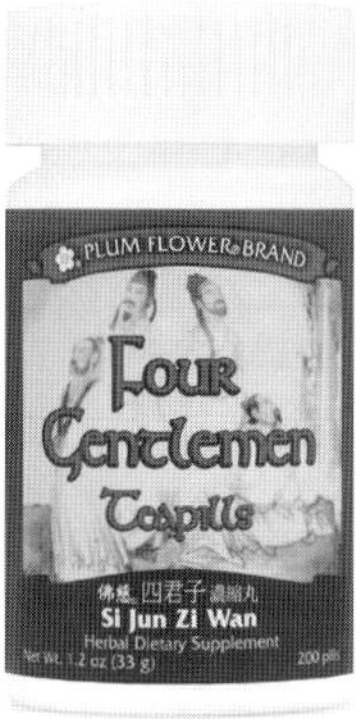

Lanzhou Foci Pharmaceutical Factory (Gansu)
'Four Gentlemen Pills'
Also available as: Four Major Herb Combination (conc. extract)

Chinese medical action

Strengthens the Spleen and tonifies qi

Biomedical action

Enhances and regulates digestive functions, strengthens immunity and resistance

INDICATIONS

- Digestive weakness, loss of appetite, abdominal distension and loose stools from Spleen qi deficiency. The base formula from which all qi tonic and Spleen strengthening formulas are built. For all Spleen and Lung qi deficiency patterns, with fatigue, weakness, pallor, a pale scalloped tongue and a weak pulse.
- Can be used alone or combined with another formula when a greater qi tonifying effect is desired.

Composition

Codonopsis pilosula (dang shen, codonopsis), *Poria cocos* (fu ling, hoelen), *Atractylodes macrocephala* (bai zhu, atractylodes), *Glycyrrhiza uralensis* (gan cao, licorice)

Combine with

- **6.4 Xiao Yao Wan** for Liver qi constraint with pronounced qi deficiency
- **4.3 Wu Pi Yin Wan** for mild edema during pregnancy
- **7.23 Yu Ping Feng Wan** for Spleen and Lung qi deficiency

Dosage and method of administration

8-12 pills three times daily on an empty stomach. The dose can be spread out, or taken in two lots of 12-18 pills, morning and evening. In severe cases or the early stages of treatment (the first few weeks), a 50% increase in dose can be used, then reduced as treatment takes effect. For the same problem in children *see* **12.6 Healthy Child Tea**.

Cautions and contraindications

Contraindicated during the early phase of acute illness such as colds and flu.

2.8 LIU JUN ZI WAN

GMP

3+/12

六君子丸

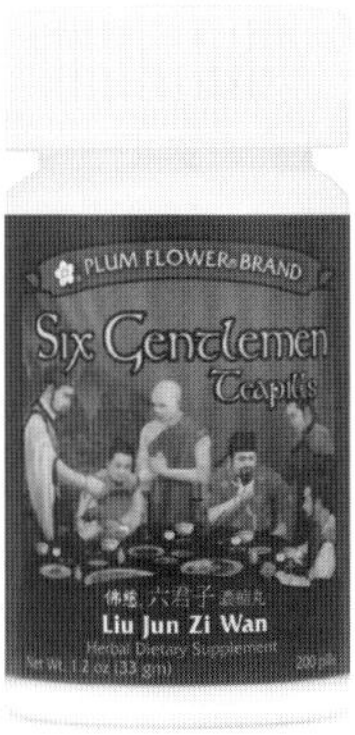

Lanzhou Foci Pharmaceutical Factory (Gansu)
'Six Gentlemen Pills'
Also available as: Major Six Herb Combination (conc. extract)

Chinese medical action

Strengthens the Spleen and tonifies qi, transforms phlegm damp, stops vomiting

Biomedical action

Enhances and regulates digestive functions, strengthens immunity and resistance, mucolytic, anti-emetic

INDICATIONS

- Spleen qi deficiency with phlegm damp. A variation of **2.7 Si Jun Zi Wan**, with the addition of processed pinellia and citrus to transform the phlegm damp that commonly complicates Spleen qi deficiency. In addition to the basic Spleen qi deficient symptom picture, there are signs of phlegm damp, such as pronounced abdominal distension, nausea or vomiting, diarrhea, mucus congestion and a pale scalloped tongue with a thick greasy tongue coat.
- For morning sickness from deficiency, chronic gastrointestinal weakness and chronic cough from Spleen qi deficiency with phlegm damp.

Composition

Codonopsis pilosula (dang shen, codonopsis), *Atractylodes macrocephala* (bai zhu, atractylodes), *Poria cocos* (fu ling, hoelen), *Pinellia ternata* (zhi ban xia, processed pinellia), *Citrus reticulata* (chen pi, citrus), *Glycyrrhiza uralensis* (gan cao, licorice), *Zingiber officinalis* (sheng jiang, ginger), *Zizyphus jujuba* (da zao, chinese dates)

Dosage and method of administration

8-12 pills three times daily on an empty stomach. The dose can be spread out, or taken in two lots of 12-18 pills, morning and evening. In severe cases or the early stages of treatment (the first few weeks), a 50% increase in dose can be used, then reduced as treatment takes effect. For the same problem in children *see* **12.6 Healthy Child Tea**.

Cautions and contraindications

Contraindicated during the early phase of acute illness such as colds and flu.

2.9 XIANG SHA LIU JUN WAN

香砂六君丸

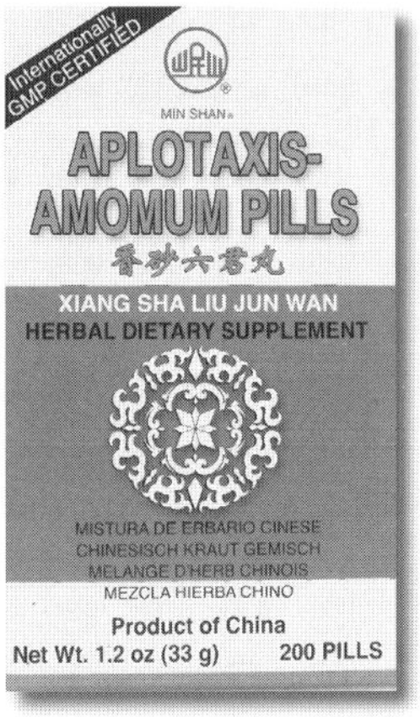

Lanzhou Foci Pharmaceutical Factory (Gansu)
'Six Gentlemen Pills with Cardamom and Saussurea'
Xiang Sha Liu Jun Wan is packaged in bottles of 200 pills
Also available as: Six Gentlemen Plus Teapills (PF), Aplotaxis Amomum Pills, Vladmiria and Amomum Combination (conc. extract)

Chinese medical action

Strengthens the Spleen, tonifies and regulates qi, transforms phlegm damp

Biomedical action

Enhances and regulates digestive functions, strengthens immunity and resistance, mucolytic, stomachic, anti-emetic

INDICATIONS

- Spleen qi deficiency with phlegm damp and qi stagnation. A variation of **2.8 Liu Jun Zi Wan**, this formula adds saussurea and cardamom to regulate middle burner qi. Its action is focused in the upper digestive tract – the Stomach and epigastrium. As the complications of Spleen qi deficiency addressed by this formula are so common, it is generally preferred over **2.7 Si Jun Zi Wan** or **2.8 Liu Jun Zi Wan.**
- Patients prone to mucus congestion, and those who suffer from recurrent sinus congestion, allergies, sore throats, ear infections or, in children, glue ear. Can be used for both adults and children.
- Chronic respiratory weakness and congestion with cough or wheezing and copious white sputum that collects in the lungs or sinuses.
- With the appropriate identifying features, this formula may be used to treat conditions such as peptic ulcer disease, chronic gastritis, dyspepsia, chronic colitis, chronic diarrhea, irritable bowel syndrome, morning sickness, hypoglycemia, general debility, narcolepsy, chronic bronchitis, chronic sinus congestion and poor concentration.

Composition (each pill contains powdered)

Atractylodes macrocephala (bai zhu, atractylodes), *Poria cocos* (fu ling, hoelen), *Zizyphus jujuba* (da zao, chinese dates), *Codonopsis pilosula* (dang shen, codonopsis), *Pinellia ternata* (zhi ban xia, processed pinellia), *Citrus reticulata* (chen pi, citrus), *Amomum villosum* (sha ren, cardamom), *Saussurea lappa* (mu xiang, saussurea), *Glycyrrhiza uralensis* (gan cao, licorice), *Zingiber officinalis* (sheng jiang, ginger)

Combine with

- A small dose of **2.18 Bao He Wan** for severe indigestion, bad breath, foul belching or undigested food in the stools from food stagnation
- **2.22 Er Chen Wan** for persistent nausea or vomiting

Pattern identifying features

- **Spleen qi deficiency with phlegm damp, qi and food stagnation**
- **loss of appetite**
- nausea, vomiting
- sleepiness after eating
- flatulence, belching, borborygmus
- loose stools, chronic diarrhea
- fatigue, heaviness in head and body
- indigestion
- early satiety

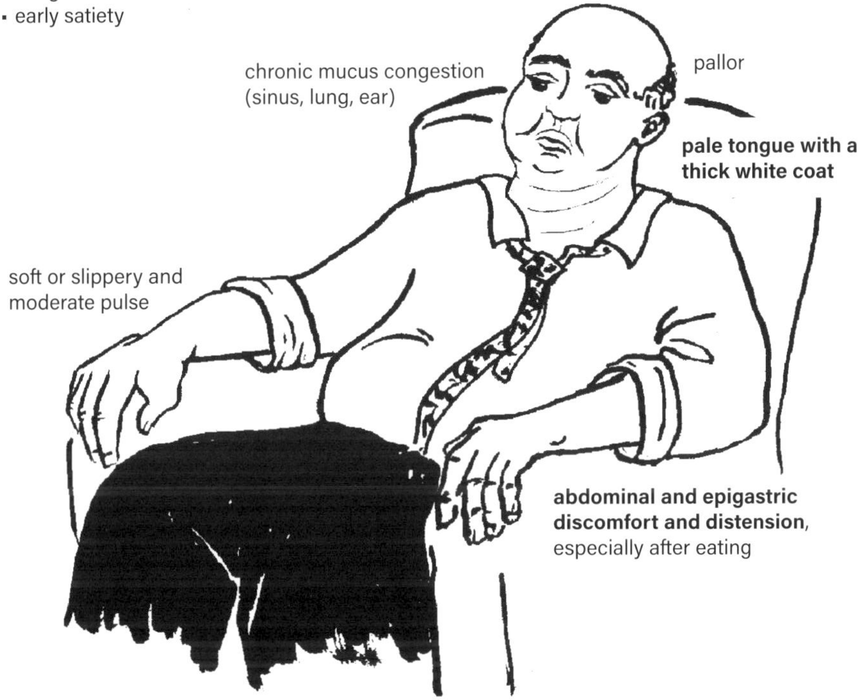

- **2.26 Xiang Lian Wan** for reflux and heartburn
- **2.23 Ping Wei San** for severe damp
- **7.23 Yu Ping Feng Wan** for allergies and frequent colds
- **9.18 Xin Yi San** for chronic sinus congestion from phlegm damp

Dosage and method of administration

8-12 pills three times daily on an empty stomach. The dose can be spread out, or two lots of 12-18 pills may be taken morning and evening. In severe cases or during the first few weeks of treatment, a 50% increase in dose may be used, then reduced as the treatment takes effect. For the same problem in children *see* **12.6 Healthy Child Tea**.

Cautions and contraindications

Contraindicated during the early phase of acute illness such as colds and flu.

2.10 XIANG SHA YANG WEI WAN

香砂养胃丸

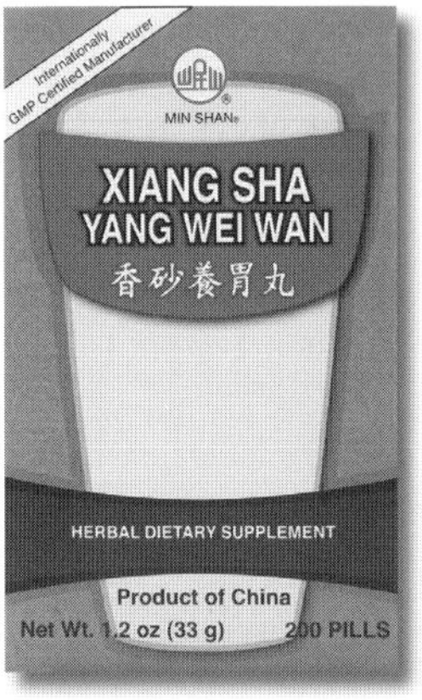

Lanzhou Foci Pharmaceutical Factory (Gansu)
'Cardamom and Saussurea Pills to Nourish the Stomach'
Xiang Sha Yang Wei Wan is packaged in bottles of 200 pills
Also available as: Appetite and Digestion Pill, Hsiang Sha Yang Wei Pien, Cyperus and Cardamom Combination (conc. extract)

Chinese medical action

Regulates qi in the middle burner, alleviates food stagnation, disperses damp, warms and strengthens the Spleen, harmonizes the Stomach and directs Stomach qi downward

Biomedical action

Enhances and regulates digestive functions, eases spasms in the gastrointestinal system, alleviates indigestion

INDICATIONS

- Acid reflux, heartburn, abdominal bloating, nausea or vomiting (including morning sickness) and variable bowel habits from stagnation of qi and damp in the Spleen and Stomach with a mild degree of Spleen deficiency. The main focus of this formula is on moving qi, drying the damp and redirecting qi downwards. Particularly good when Stomach qi fails to descend causing. Good for chronic indigestion and dyspepsia in an otherwise apparently robust individual.
- For mental cloudiness, poor concentration, forgetfulness, foggy head, depression and heaviness of spirit from a 'mist' of phlegm damp enveloping and obscuring the Heart and mind.

Composition (each pill contains powdered)

Atractylodes macrocephala (bai zhu, atractylodes), *Poria cocos* (fu ling, hoelen), *Citrus reticulata* (chen pi, citrus), *Pinellia ternata* (zhi ban xia, processed pinellia), *Saussurea lappa* (mu xiang, saussurea), *Agastache rugosa* (huo xiang, agastache), *Cyperus rotundus* (xiang fu, cyperus), *Alpinia katsumadai* (cao dou kou, katsumadai cardamom), *Magnolia officinalis* (hou po, magnolia bark), *Amomum villosum* (sha ren, cardamom), *Citrus aurantium* (zhi shi, aurantium), *Glycyrrhiza uralensis* (gan cao, licorice), *Zizyphus jujuba* (da zao, chinese dates), *Zingiber officinalis* (sheng jiang, ginger)

Combine with

- **2.26 Xiang Lian Wan** for acid reflux from Liver and Stomach qi stagnation with Spleen deficiency
- **2.27 Wei Te Ling** for marked hyper acidity
- **6.3 Chai Hu Shu Gan Wan** when there is a significant emotional component and obvious Liver qi constraint
- **2.23 Ping Wei San** for patients with severe damp
- **8.11 Jian Nao Yi Zhi Capsule** for mental cloudiness

Pattern identifying features

- **Spleen damp and qi stagnation; Spleen deficiency**
- poor appetite
- reduced sense of taste
- early satiety

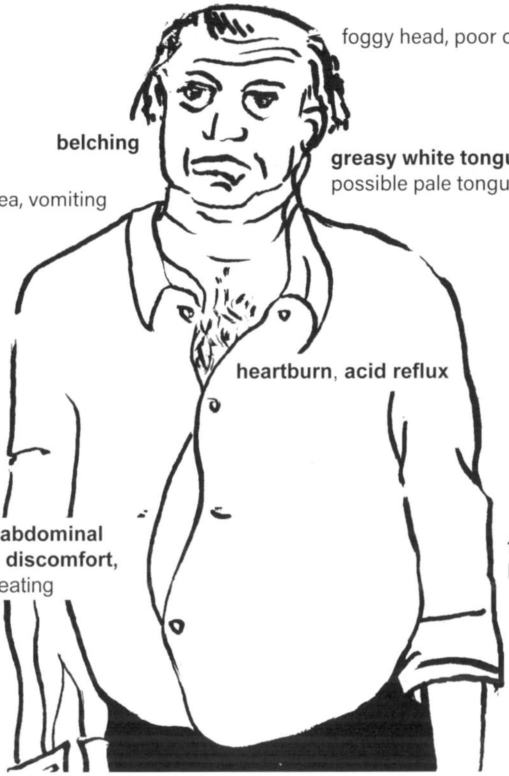

Dosage and method of administration

8-12 pills three times daily, on an empty stomach. The dose may be spread out, or two lots of 12-18 pills may be taken morning and evening. In severe cases or during the early stages of treatment (the first few weeks), a 50% increase in dose may be used, then reduced as the treatment takes effect.

Cautions and contraindications

Not suitable for indigestion from heat or phlegm heat in the Stomach.

2.11 BU ZHONG YI QI WAN
补中益气丸

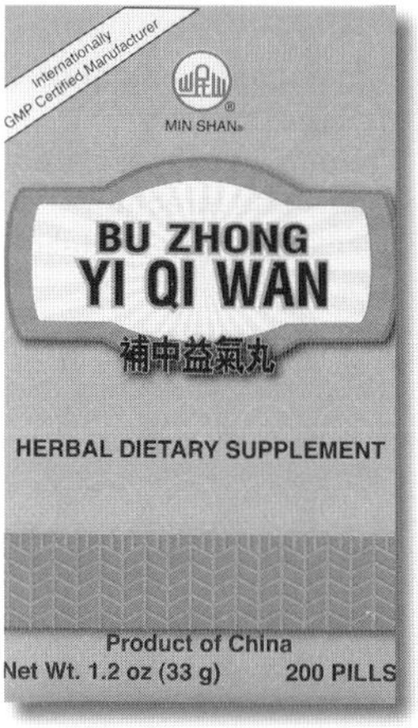

Lanzhou Foci Pharmaceutical Factory (Gansu)
'Tonify the Middle and Augment Qi Pills'
Bu Zhong Yi Qi Wan is packaged in bottles of 200 pills
Also available as: Central Chi Teapills (PF), Tonify the Middle Formula (JD), Tonify the Middle and Qi Pill (BE), Ginseng and Astragalus Combination (conc. extract)

Chinese medical action

Tonifies qi and strengthens the Spleen, Lung and defensive qi, elevates the yang energy of the body

Biomedical action

Tonic, digestive stimulant, elevates and tones weakened or prolapsed structures, stimulates and protects the immune system

INDICATIONS

- Spleen and Lung qi deficiency patterns with sinking qi. Improves muscle tone, elevates yang qi and lifts prolapsed organs; used for conditions where poor muscle tone and weak qi that is unable to resist the pull of gravity leads to various types of prolapse and lax tissue, including the eyelid (ptosis), hemorrhoids, rectum, uterus, bladder and soft palate (sleep apnoea). Used for poor tone and weakness of smooth and skeletal muscles. Strengthens the Spleen and elevates qi to alleviate chronic diarrhea, recurrent miscarriage and bleeding disorders.
- To strengthen defensive qi and boosting the immune system in those prone to frequent colds or infection, chronic fatigue syndrome and post-viral syndrome (of a pure deficiency type; for mixed patterns *see* **6.1 Xiao Chai Hu Wan**).
- Protects and stimulates the immune system and bone marrow in patients undergoing chemotherapy or radiotherapy.
- Recurrent low grade fever that rises in the morning, following exertion and when fatigued.
- With the appropriate identifying features, this formula may assist in the treatment of conditions such as first or second degree prolapse of the uterus, bladder or rectum, incompetent cervix, immune weakness, recurrent miscarriage, functional uterine bleeding, postpartum urinary incontinence, hypotension, hypoglycemia, post viral syndrome, chronic hepatitis, corneal ulcers, pernicious anemia, leukopenia, fever of unknown origin, myasthenia gravis and multiple sclerosis.

Composition (each pill contains powdered)

Astragalus membranaceous (huang qi, astragalus), *Glycyrrhiza uralensis* (gan cao, licorice), *Codonopsis pilosula* (dang shen, codonopsis), *Angelica sinensis* (dang gui), *Atractylodes macrocephala* (bai zhu, atractylodes), *Bupleurum falcatum* (chai hu, bupleurum), *Cimicifuga foetida* (sheng ma, cimicifuga), *Citrus reticulata* (chen pi, citrus), *Zizyphus jujuba* (da zao, chinese dates), *Zingiber officinalis* (sheng jiang, ginger)

Pattern identifying features

- **Spleen and Lung qi deficiency with sinking qi**
- **fatigue, debility**
- **immune weakness, frequent colds and infection**
- weakness, lack of vitality
- low grade fever
- symptoms initiated or aggravated when fatigued or with exertion

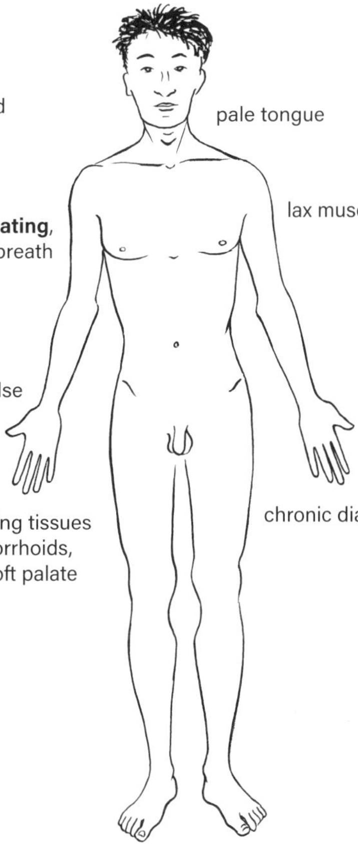

Combine with

– **7.26 Reishi Mushroom** as an adjunct to chemotherapy or radiotherapy
– **7.9 Jin Gui Shen Qi Wan** for prolapses with a degree of Kidney deficiency

Dosage and method of administration

8-12 pills three times daily on an empty stomach. The dose can be taken in two lots of 12-18 pills, morning and evening. In severe cases or during the early stages of treatment (the first few weeks), a 50% increase in dose can be used, then reduced as treatment takes effect. A double or treble dose is recommended for patients having chemotherapy or radiotherapy.

Cautions and contraindications

Contraindicated during the early phase of acute illness such as colds and flu or any other acute infection. This formula has an elevating tendency and in some patients can cause headaches and nausea. Some patients with Spleen deficiency (and hidden damp) patterns may find symptoms initially aggravate while taking **2.11 Bu Zhong Yi Qi Wan**. A few weeks of **2.1 Xing Jun San** or **2.2 Huo Hsiang Cheng Chi Pien** may be used first to clear the damp.

2.12 SHEN LING BAI ZHU WAN

参苓白术丸

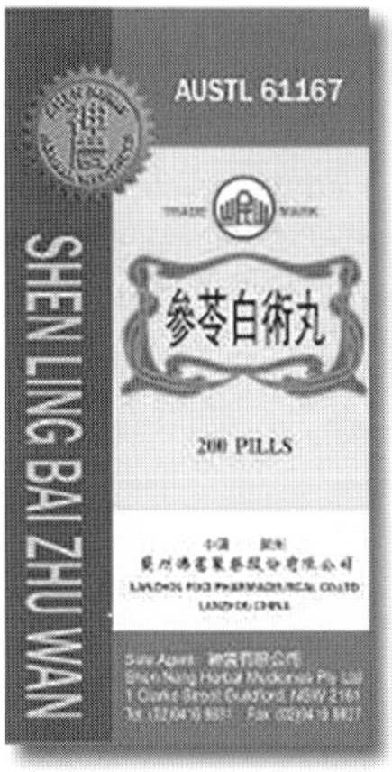

Lanzhou Foci Pharmaceutical Factory (Gansu)
'Ginseng, Poria and Atractylodes Pills'
Shen Ling Bai Zhu Wan is packaged in bottles of 200 pills
Also available as: Absorption and Digestion Pill (BE), Shen Ling Bai Zhu Pian (PF), Ginseng and Atractylodes Formula (conc. extract)

Chinese medical action

Tonifies qi, strengthens the Spleen, leaches damp, stops diarrhea

Biomedical action

Tonic, stimulant, strengthens digestive function and absorption of fluids and nutrients

INDICATIONS

- Spleen and Stomach qi deficiency with damp. For digestive weakness with various types of damp discharge, such as chronic loose stools, diarrhea and excessive vaginal discharge. Also used for diarrhea associated with consumption of uncooked or otherwise hard to digest food, diarrhea during pregnancy and preceding or accompanying menstruation. Used to alleviate diarrhea that can result from Spleen depleting medicines such as antibiotics and bitter cold herbs.
- Edema from Lung and Spleen qi deficiency; chronic and predominantly affecting the fingers, eyes and abdomen.
- Copious, persistent, watery or mucoid leukorrhea.
- Good to strengthen pale children over 5 years old (*see* **12.1 Bo Ying Compound** or **12.6 Healthy Child Tea** for children under 5), who are picky eaters, prone to loose stools, chronic diarrhea, are underweight and lacking vitality.
- Can improve regulation of blood glucose, and assist in prediabetic states. Can be used for both high and low blood glucose problems.
- Indefinable epigastric discomfort from Spleen and Stomach qi and yin deficiency. A well balanced formula which gently strengthens Spleen qi and leaches damp without drying and damaging yin.
- With the appropriate identifying features, this formula can assist in the treatment of disorders such as chronic gastroenteritis, chronic colitis, gastritis, peptic ulcer disease, malabsorption syndrome, leaky gut syndrome, malnutrition, hypoglycemia, diabetes mellitus, chronic nephritis, coeliac disease and anemia.

Composition (each pill contains powdered)

Codonopsis pilosula (dang shen, codonopsis) 24mg, *Poria cocos* (fu ling, hoelen) 24mg, *Atractylodes macrocephala* (bai zhu, atractylodes) 24mg, *Dioscorea officinalis* (shan yao, dioscorea) 24mg, *Nelumbus speciosum* (lian zi, lotus seed) 16mg, *Coicis lachryma-jobi* (yi yi ren, coix) 14.4mg, *Dolichos lablab* (bian dou, hyacinth bean) 14.4mg, *Platycodon grandiflorum* (jie geng, platycodon) 9.6mg, *Glycyrrhiza uralensis* (gan cao, licorice) 4.8mg, *Amomum villosum* (sha ren, cardamom) 4.8mg

Pattern identifying features

- **Spleen qi deficiency with damp, diarrhea and leukorrhea**
- nausea, vomiting
- edema, puffiness of the eyes and fingers
- weight loss, emaciation
- fatigue, weakness

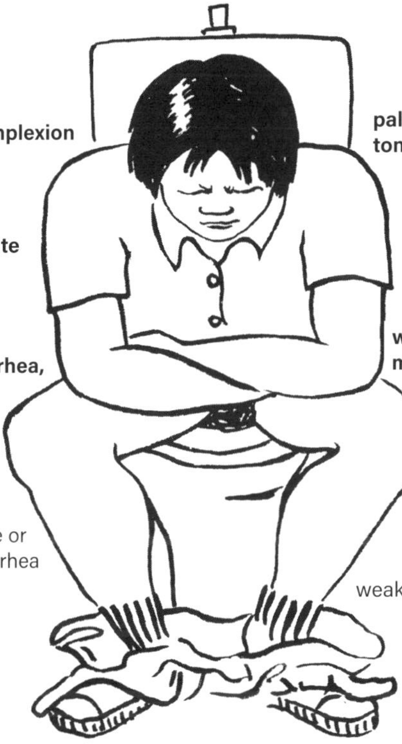

Combine with

– **4.14 Chin So Ku Ching Wan** or **4.2 Wu Ling Wan** for incessant diarrhea
– **2.23 Ping Wei San** or **4.5 Bi Xie Fen Qing Wan** for copious cold damp leukorrhea
– **4.2 Wu Ling Wan** for pathological fluid accumulation and edema

Dosage and method of administration

8-12 pills three times daily on an empty stomach. The dose can be spread out, or taken in two lots of 12-18 pills, morning and evening. In severe cases or during the early stages of treatment (the first few weeks), a 50% increase in dose can be used, then reduced as treatment takes effect.

Cautions and contraindications

Contraindicated during the early phase of acute illness such as colds and flu. Avoid cold raw foods and dairy products while using this formula.

2.13 LI ZHONG WAN

理中丸

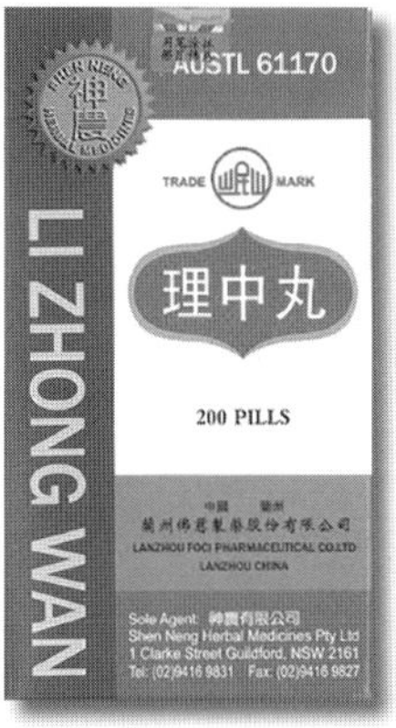

Lanzhou Foci Pharmaceutical Factory (Gansu)
'Regulate the Middle [Burner] Pills'
Li Zhong Wan is packaged in bottles of 200 pills
Also available as: Ginseng and Ginger Combination (conc. extract)

Chinese medical action

Tonifies and warms Spleen and Stomach yang, dispels cold, relieves *tài yīn* syndrome, dries damp and transforms phlegm

Biomedical action

Tonic, digestive stimulant, strengthens digestive function

INDICATIONS

- Spleen yang deficiency. For chronic digestive weakness and hypofunction with cold. Used for marked abdominal distension, loss of appetite and persistent, frequent diarrhea. Diarrhea is watery, with undigested food, and may wake the patient from sleep in the early hours of the morning (also known as cockcrow or fifth watch diarrhea). Symptoms are aggravated by ingestion of cold or raw foods and iced fluids.
- Productive cough and chronic respiratory weakness with copious thin watery sputum. Also used for chronic drooling or hypersalivation.
- Chronic bleeding from Spleen yang deficiency, typically low grade and persistent – uterine, menorrhagia and rectal.
- Chronic or recurrent mouth ulcers of a cold or yang deficient type.
- Chronic childhood convulsions in a cold emaciated child.
- Can also be used for acute vomiting and diarrhea (a type of sudden turmoil disorder), that causes rapid deterioration and damage to yang qi.
- With the appropriate identifying features, this formula may be used to treat disorders such as chronic gastroenteritis, chronic colitis, chronic dysentery, gastritis, peptic ulcer disease, malabsorption syndromes, leaky gut syndrome, cholera, chronic bleeding disorders, apthous ulcer, oral herpes, irritable bowel syndrome and chronic bronchitis.

Composition

Codonopsis pilosula (dang shen, codonopsis), *Zingiber officinale* (gan jiang, dry ginger), *Atractylodes macrocephala* (bai zhu, atractylodes), *Glycyrrhiza uralensis* (gan cao, licorice)

Combine with

- **7.9 Jin Gui Shen Qi Wan** for Spleen and Kidney yang deficiency
- **2.33 Cong Rong Bu Shen Wan** for chronic atonic constipation from failure of yang movement through the Intestines.
- **2.26 Xiang Lian Wan** for chronic dysenteric disorder

Pattern identifying features

- **Spleen yang deficiency**
- fatigue, exhaustion
- chronic digestive weakness
- loss of appetite

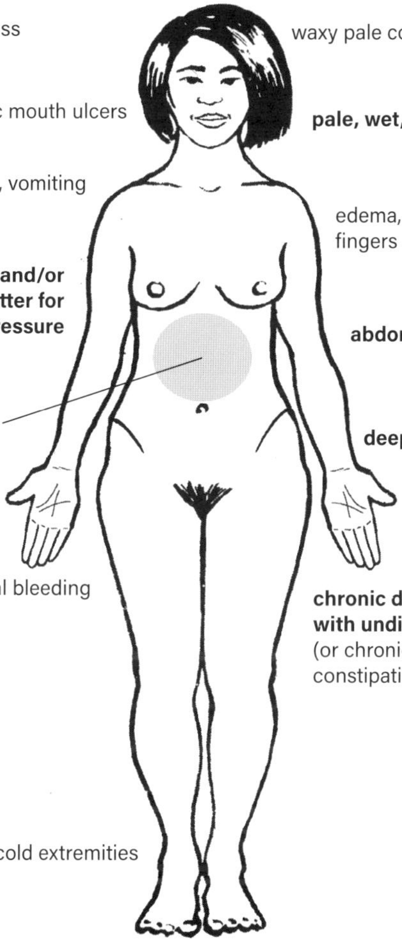

Dosage and method of administration

8-12 pills three times daily on an empty stomach. The dose can be spread out, or taken in two lots of 12-18 pills, morning and evening. In severe cases or during the early stages of treatment (the first few weeks), a 50% increase in dose can be used, then reduced as it takes effect. When used for sudden turmoil disorder, a dose may be taken every 2 hours until the symptoms subside.

Cautions and contraindications

Contraindicated during the early phase of acute illness such as colds and flu. It is essential that patients with Spleen yang deficiency minimize or omit raw and cold foods from their diet.

GMP

2.14 LI CHUNG YUEN MEDICAL PILLS

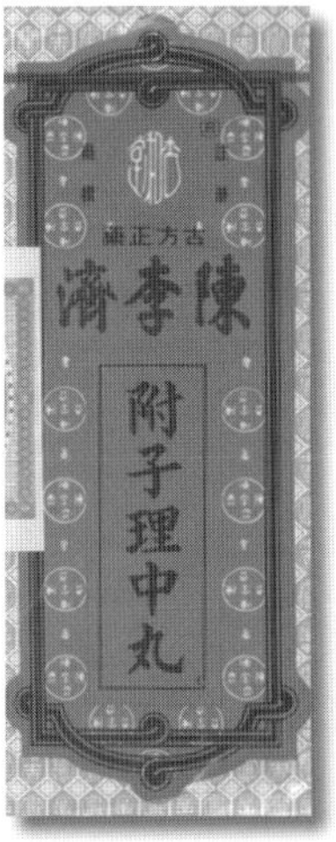

附子理中丸

(*Fu Zi Li Zhong Wan*)
Chan Li Chai Medical Factory (Hong Kong)
'Aconite Pills to Regulate the Middle [Burner]'
Li Chung Yuen Medical Pills are packaged as large honey pills sealed in wax balls, 10 pills per box
Also available as: Fu Zi Li Zhong Teapills (PF), Fu Tzu Li Chung Wan, Aconite, Ginseng and Ginger Combination (conc. extract)

Chinese medical action

Tonifies, and warms Spleen and Stomach yang, dispels cold, relieves *tài yīn* syndrome

Biomedical action

Tonic, digestive stimulant, strengthens digestive function

INDICATIONS

- Spleen yang deficiency. A variation of **2.13 Li Zhong Wan**, with the addition of aconite to increase its yang warming and mobilizing power. Similar in overall action and indications, but considerably warmer. Good for a range of chronic digestive problems associated with relatively severe weakness, cold and hypofunction of the Spleen and Stomach. Especially good for chronic diarrhea, loss of appetite or anorexia, relentless abdominal distension, indigestion, severe cold intolerance, cramping abdominal pain that feels better for warmth and pressure, nausea and severe vomiting.
- Chronic respiratory problems with copious thin watery sputum.
- Chronic or recurrent mouth ulcers of a cold deficient type.
- Chronic childhood convulsions resulting from deficient yang.
- Acute vomiting and diarrhea (a type of sudden turmoil disorder, *see* glossary), that causes rapid deterioration and damage to yang qi.
- With the appropriate identifying features, this formula may assist in the treatment of disorders such as chronic gastroenteritis, chronic colitis, chronic dysentery, gastritis, peptic ulcer disease, malabsorption syndromes, leaky gut syndrome, cholera, ascites, apthous ulcer, oral herpes, irritable bowel syndrome and chronic bronchitis.

Composition

Atractylodes macrocephala (bai zhu, atractylodes), *Codonopsis pilosula* (dang shen, codonopsis), *Zingiber officinale* (gan jiang, dry ginger), *Glycyrrhiza uralensis* (gan cao, licorice), *Aconite carmichaeli* (zhi fu zi, processed aconite)

Combine with

– **4.2 Wu Ling Wan** with significant edema
– **3.41 Xu Han Ting** for continuous sweating

Pattern identifying features

- **Spleen yang deficiency with marked cold**
- **cold intolerance**
- nausea, vomiting of watery, inoffensive material
- anorexia

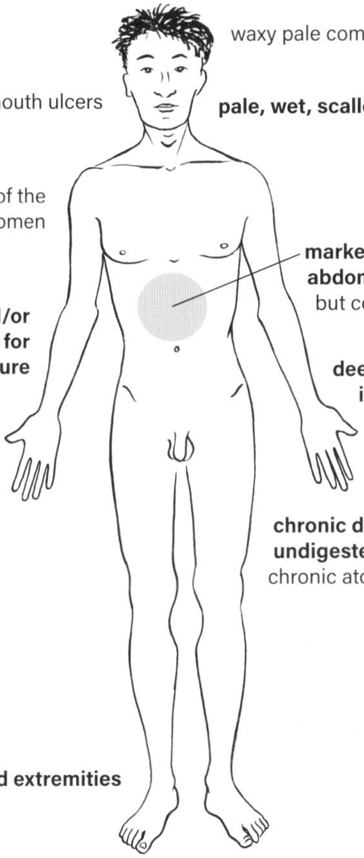

Dosage and method of administration

One or two pills per day, with warm water or ginger tea on an empty stomach. These pills can be quite hard and may need to be softened in hot water before ingestion. If one pill is prescribed, take half morning and evening.

Once the patient begins to warm up the dose can be reduced. Be careful not to overheat the patient.

Cautions and contraindications

Contraindicated during pregnancy and during the early phase of acute illness such as colds and flu. This formula is hot and drying, and not suitable for any heat pattern, or false cold, true heat pattern.

GMP

2.15 XIAO JIAN ZHONG WAN

小建中丸

1-3/12

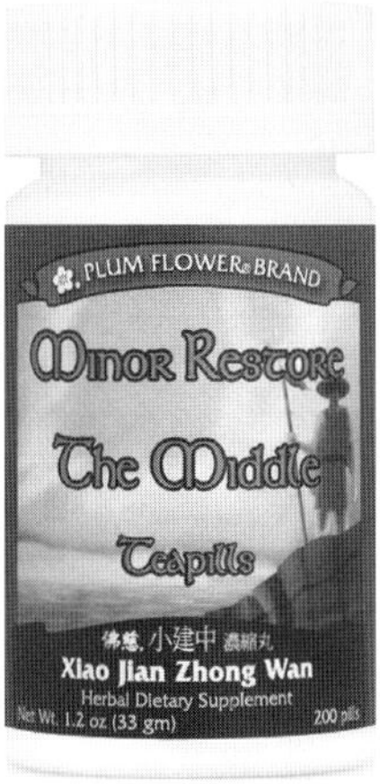

Lanzhou Foci Pharmaceutical Factory (Gansu)
'Minor Strengthen the Middle [Burner] Pills'
Xiao Jian Zhong Wan is packaged in bottles of 200 pills
Also available as: Minor Cinnamon and Peony Combination (conc. extract)

Chinese medical action

Warms the Spleen and Stomach, tonifies qi, alleviates abdominal spasm and pain

Biomedical action

Antispasmodic, digestive and energy stimulant

INDICATIONS

- Colicky epigastric and abdominal pain from Spleen and Stomach qi and/or yang deficiency with cold accumulation. As a variation of **3.6 Gui Zhi Wan**, with the simple addition of malt sugar and increased proportion of white peony, the focus of this formula is shifted to warming and strengthening the digestive system and alleviating spasmodic pain. The pain tends to be dull and persistent, or colicky, initiated or aggravated by cold raw or hard to digest foods.
- Pale, weak, thin children with little appetite and listlessness.
- Low grade fever from yang deficiency. This type of fever is more apparent early in the day (soon after waking) as the patient starts to move around, and is also aggravated when overtired or fatigued.
- Assist convalescence in patients with Spleen qi deficiency, those recovering from a major illness or abdominal surgery.
- With the appropriate identifying features, this formula may be used to treat disorders such as gastric and duodenal ulcers, chronic atrophic gastritis, chronic hepatitis, chronic peritonitis, anemia, and fever of unknown origin.

Composition

Saccharum Granorum (yi tang, malt sugar), *Paeonia lactiflora* (bai shao, white peony), *Zizyphus jujuba* (da zao, chinese dates), *Cinnamomum cassia* (gui zhi, cinnamon twigs), *Zingiber officinale* (sheng jiang, ginger), *Glycyrrhiza uralensis* (zhi gan cao, honey fried licorice)

Combine with

– **10.22 Shao Yao Gan Cao Wan** for intense colicky pain
– **7.22 Shen Qi Da Bu Wan** for more severe qi deficiency

Pattern identifying features

- **Spleen and Stomach qi and/or yang deficiency**
- possible low grade morning fevers
- drooling, hypersalivation
- picky eater

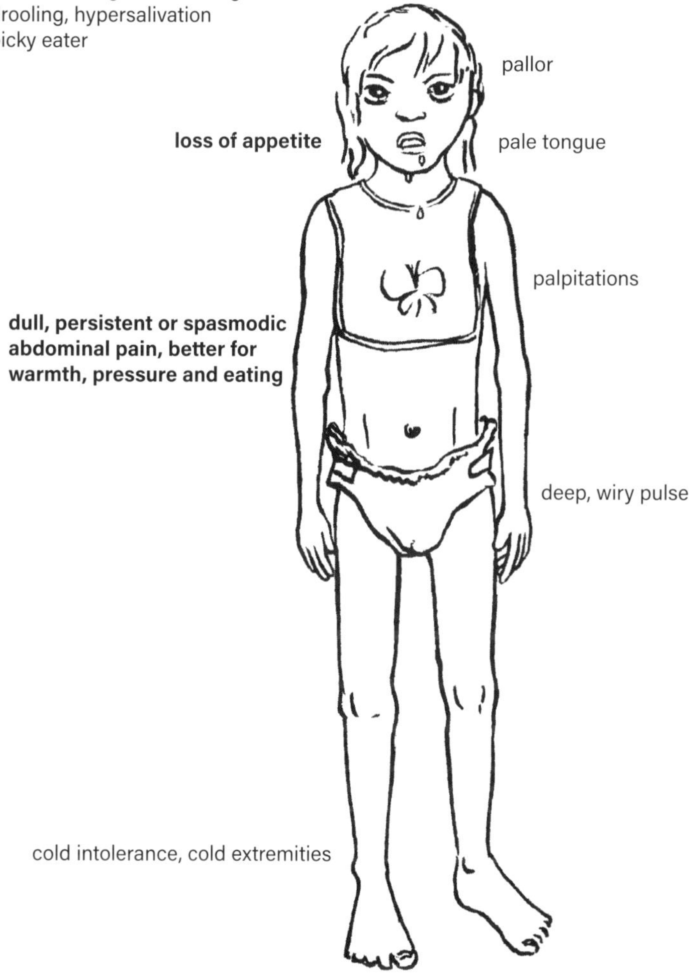

Dosage and method of administration

8-12 pills, three times daily on an empty stomach. For children, reduce the dose by half to one third. The pills can also be crushed up, decocted and delivered as a slurry in an eye-dropper for children.

Cautions and contraindications

Contraindicated in yin deficiency patterns, yin deficient fevers and internal heat patterns.

2.16 ZI SHENG WAN

资生丸

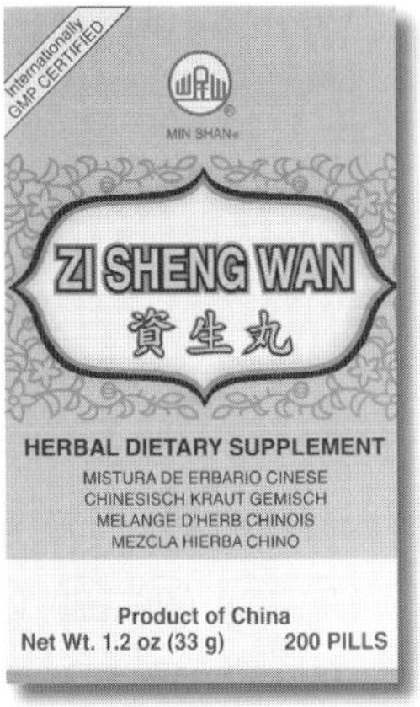

Lanzhou Foci Pharmaceutical Factory (Gansu)
'Aid Life Pills'
Zi Sheng Wan is packaged in bottles of 200 pills
Also available as: Zi Sheng Stomachic Pills

Chinese medical action

Tonifies Spleen qi, moves stagnant qi, dispels damp, alleviates food stagnation, harmonizes the Stomach, stops diarrhea

Biomedical action

Tonic, digestive stimulant, improves digestive function and absorption of nutrients, stomachic

INDICATIONS

- Spleen deficiency and lingering damp heat in the Intestine type relapsing dysenteric disorder. The patient will typically have had an acute gastric infection that has never been completely cleared and flares up when the patient is run down.
- Chronic diarrhea from Spleen deficiency with food stagnation. Also useful for the diarrhea that occurs as a side effect of cold medicines like heat clearing herbs, antibiotics, metformin and some chemotherapy.
- Used for children over 5 years old with Spleen weakness, chronic diarrhea, poor appetite and lack of vitality. *See* **12.1 Bo Ying Compound** or **12.6 Healthy Child Tea** for children under 5.
- Digestive weakness with elements of Spleen deficiency and food stagnation.
- Morning sickness in Spleen qi deficient women with qi stagnation. Also threatened miscarriage from the same etiology.

Composition (each pill contains powdered)

Coix lachryma-jobi (yi yi ren, coix), *Codonopsis pilosula* (dang shen, codonopsis), *Atractylodes macrocephala* (bai zhu, atractylodes), *Citrus reticulata* (chen pi, citrus), *Crategus pinnatifida* (shan zha, crategus), *Dioscorea opposita* (shan yao, dioscorea), *Euryale ferox* (qian shi, euryale seed), *Poria cocos* (fu ling, hoelen), *Glycyrrhiza uralensis* (gan cao, licorice), *Dolichos lablab* (bian dou, hyacinth bean), *Nelumbus nucifera* (lian zi, lotus seed), *Platycodon grandiflorum* (jie geng, platycodon), *Pogostemon cablin* (huo xiang, agastache), *Alisma orientale* (ze xie, alisma), *Alpinia katsumadai* (cao dou kou, katsumadai cardamom), *Coptis chinensis* (huang lian, coptis)

Dosage and method of administration

8-12 pills three times daily on an empty stomach. The dose can be spread out, or taken in two lots of 12-18 pills, morning and evening. In severe cases or during the early stages of treatment (the first few weeks), a 50% increase in dose can be used, then reduced as treatment takes effect.

Pattern identifying features

- **Spleen qi deficiency with lingering damp and food stagnation**
- **morning sickness**
- fatigue
- weakness of the extremities
- weight loss

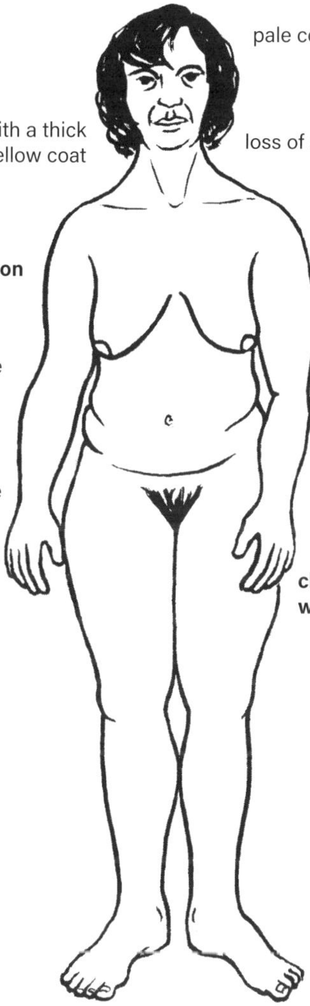

Cautions and contraindications

Contraindicated during the early phase of acute illness such as colds and flu. Not suitable for acute gastroenteritis (*see* **2.1 Xing Jun San** or **2.2 Huo Hsiang Cheng Chi Pien**). The patient should avoid all cold natured or raw foods.

2.17 JIAN PI WAN

健脾丸

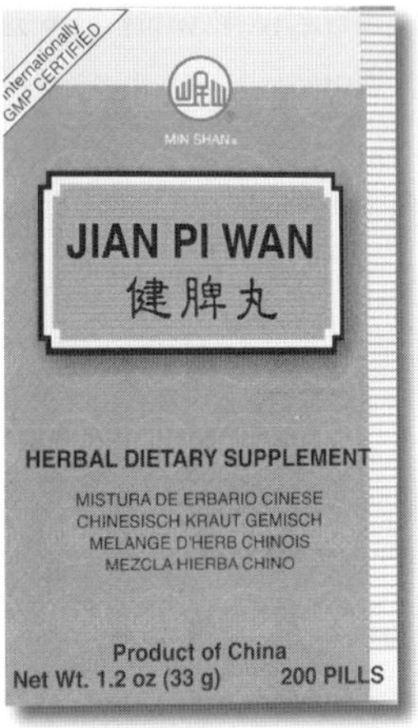

Lanzhou Foci Pharmaceutical Factory (Gansu)
'Strengthen the Spleen Pills'
Jian Pi Wan is packaged in bottles of 200 pills
Also available as: Ginseng Stomachic Pills, Spleen Digest Aid Pill (BE)

Chinese medical action

Alleviates food stagnation, strengthens the Spleen and Stomach

Biomedical action

Enhances digestive functions, digestant, carminative, stomachic

INDICATIONS

- Food stagnation with Spleen and Stomach deficiency. This formula is similar to **2.18 Bao He Wan** in action, with the main focus of this formula equally balanced between strengthening the Spleen and alleviating food stagnation. It is thus more suited to chronic cases of food stagnation complicated by digestive weakness.
- Heartburn and indigestion in late pregnancy.
- With the appropriate identifying features, this formula can be used to treat conditions such as chronic gastritis, peptic ulcer disease, chronic indigestion, dyspepsia, irritable bowel syndrome, autonomic dysfunction of the gastrointestinal tract, chronic colitis and Crohn's disease.

Composition (each pill contains powdered)

Citrus aurantium (zhi shi, aurantium), *Codonopsis pilosula* (dang shen, codonopsis), *Atractylodes macrocephala* (bai zhu, atractylodes), *Crategus pinnatifida* (shan zha, crategus), *Citrus reticulata* (chen pi, citrus). **Note:** Multiple versions of this formula are made, with minor variations in composition. Other herbs that may appear include *Hordeum vulgare* (mai ya, sprouted barley), *Coicis lachryma-jobi* (yi yi ren, coix) and *Amomum cardamomum* (bai dou kou, amomum).

Combine with

- **2.22 Er Chen Wan** for severe rising qi causing nausea and vomiting
- **2.23 Ping Wei San** for patients with more dampness and a very thick tongue coat
- Cloying yin and blood tonic formulas that potentially cause digestive upset

Pattern identifying features

- **Spleen qi deficiency with food stagnation**
- gradual loss of appetite, or decrease in the amount of food that can be consumed before feeling bloated
- fatigue

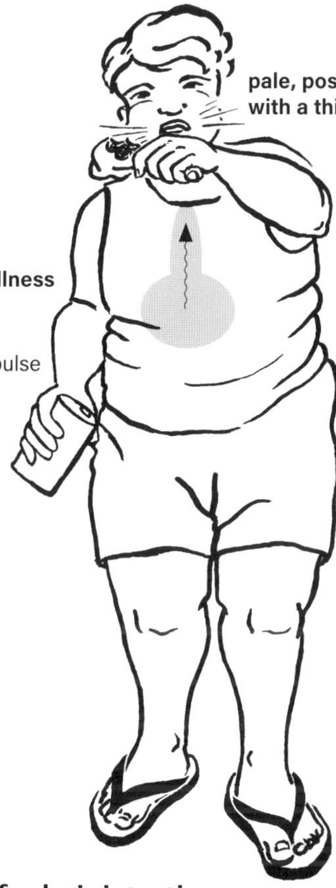

Dosage and method of administration

8-12 pills three times daily on an empty stomach. In severe cases or during the early stages of treatment (the first few weeks), a 50% increase in dose can be used, then reduced to a maintenance dose as the condition settles down and the patient regulates his or her diet.

Cautions and Contraindications

Formulas that contain *Hordeum vulgare* (mai ya, sprouted barley) should be avoided while breast-feeding as this herb can reduce milk production.

2.18 BAO HE WAN

保和丸

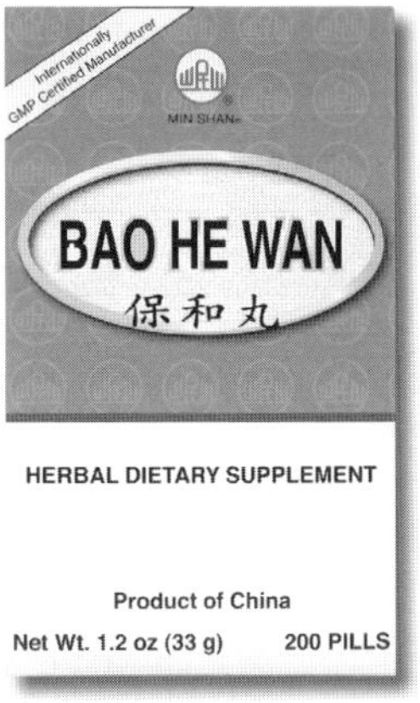

Lanzhou Foci Pharmaceutical Factory (Gansu)
'Preserve Harmony Pills'
Bao He Wan is packaged in bottles of 200 pills
Also available as: Bao He Teapills (PF), Preserve Harmony Pill (BE), Red Tangerine Peel and Crategus Formula (conc. extract)

Chinese medical action

Alleviates food stagnation, harmonizes the Stomach

Biomedical action

Enhances digestive functions, especially absorption of nutrients, digestant, carminative, stomachic

INDICATIONS

- Acute or chronic indigestion, dyspepsia and gastric hyper-acidity. This pattern is primarily related to overindulgence, excess food intake relative to energy output or irregular eating habits, such as eating too late at night, missing meals or eating while working or when stressed. Used for both acute episodes and chronic patterns of food stagnation.
- May be useful as an adjunct therapy for any condition induced by food consumption (often considered to be 'food allergies' or intolerances), such as asthma, skin rashes, sinus congestion, rhinitis and other mucus problems.
- Heartburn and indigestion in late pregnancy.
- For insomnia due to habitual late night snacking (Stomach heat or phlegm heat).
- With the appropriate identifying features, this formula can be used to treat conditions such as chronic indigestion, dyspepsia, acute and chronic gastritis, peptic ulcer disease, autonomic dysfunction of the gastrointestinal tract and chronic cholecystitis.

Composition (each pill contains powdered)

Crategus pinnatifida (shan zha, crategus), *Pinellia ternata* (zhi ban xia, processed pinellia), Massa Fermentata (shen qu), *Poria cocos* (fu ling, hoelen), *Hordeum vulgare* (mai ya, sprouted barley), *Citrus reticulata* (chen pi, citrus), *Forsythia suspensa* (lian qiao, forsythia), *Raphanus sativus* (lai fu zi, radish seed)

Combine with

- **14.2 Huang Lian Su Tablets** for concurrent Stomach heat
- **2.23 Ping Wei San** for severe abdominal distension
- **2.26 Xiang Lian Wan** for severe reflux
- Any 'rich' tonic formula that causes digestive upset

Pattern identifying features

- **food stagnation**
- **indigestion, dyspepsia**
- halitosis

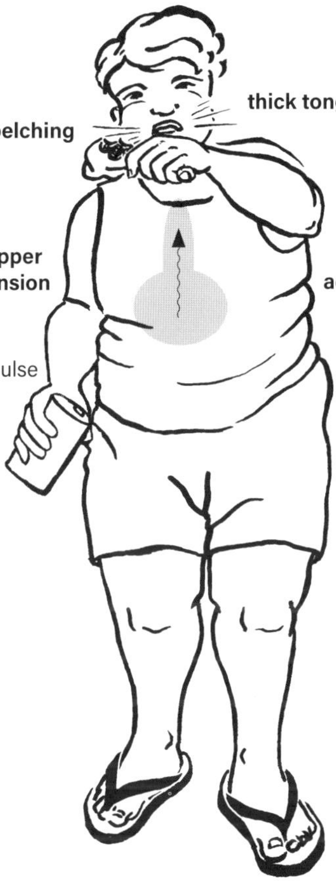

Dosage and method of administration

8-12 pills three times daily before or after a meal. In severe cases a 50% increase in dose may be used, then reduced to a maintenance dose (a few pills before or after a meal) as the condition settles down and the patient regulates their diet.

Cautions and Contraindications

Caution in patients with significant deficiency as this formula is quite dispersing to qi as well as stagnated food (*see* **2.17 Jian Pi Wan**).

1-3/52

2.19 SHEN CHU CHA

神曲茶

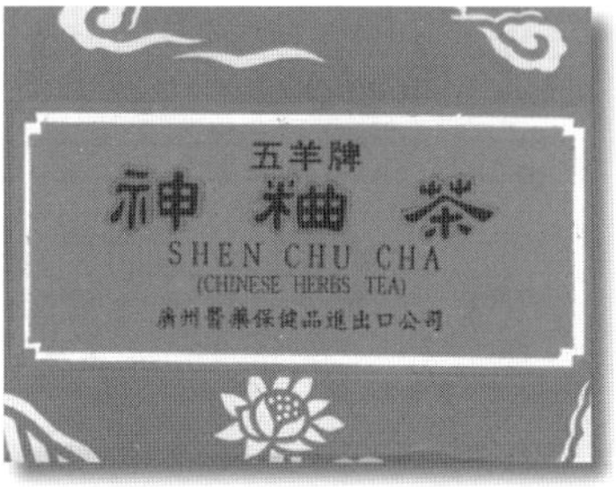

The United Pharmaceutical Manufactory (Guangzhou)
'Medicated Leaven Tea'
Shen Chu Cha is packaged in 38 gram blocks of herbal material wrapped in paper, eight blocks to a box

Chinese medical action

Dispels wind cold and summerdamp, alleviates food stagnation, regulates the Spleen and Stomach

Biomedical action

Diaphoretic, stomachic, alleviates acute gastric conditions

INDICATIONS

- This tea is a mixture of diaphoretic, summerdamp clearing, qi moving and damp draining herbs, designed to treat wind cold common cold during the humid weather of late summer when wind cold exterior symptoms (chills, myalgia, no sweating) are accompanied by digestive symptoms like nausea, vomiting and diarrhea.
- Travelers diarrhea, or digestive upsets that accompany changes in diet. Used for conditions such as stomach flu, food poisoning, acute gastroenteritis, indigestion, dyspepsia, recovery from hangover and the general effects of an extended period of overindulgence.
- Often included in digestive formulas (or used to wash them down), to enhance their resolving and damp clearing action. Can be used to wash down rich tonifying formulas in patients prone to digestive upset (especially the rehmannia formulas).

Composition

Artemesia apiacea (qing hao, artemesia) 4.7%, *Scutellaria baicalensis* (huang qin, scute) 4.7%, *Amomum tsao-ko* (cao guo, tsaoko fruit) 4.7%, *Mosla chinensis* (xiang ru, madder) 4.7%, *Angelica pubescens* (du huo, Tu-huo) 4.7%, *Poria cocos* (fu ling, hoelen) 4.7%, *Glycyrrhiza uralensis* (gan cao, licorice) 5%, *Dioscorea villosa* (shan yao, dioscorea) 5%, *Magnolia officinalis* (hou po, magnolia bark) 4.7%, *Notopterygium incisum* (qiang huo, notopterygium) 4.7%, *Citrus reticulata* (qing pi, blue citrus) 4.7%, *Platycodon grandiflorum* (jie geng, platycodon) 4.7%, *Chaenomeles lagenaria* (mu gua, chinese quince) 4.7%, *Triticum aestivum* (xiao mai, fermented wheat flour) 38%

Combine with

– Cloying yin and blood tonic formulas that potentially cause digestive upset. For this purpose, several blocks can be brewed at one time, the strained liquid stored in a plastic container in the fridge and used to wash down the main formula

Pattern identifying features

- **summerdamp invasion; food stagnation**
- summer colds
- acute gastric upset

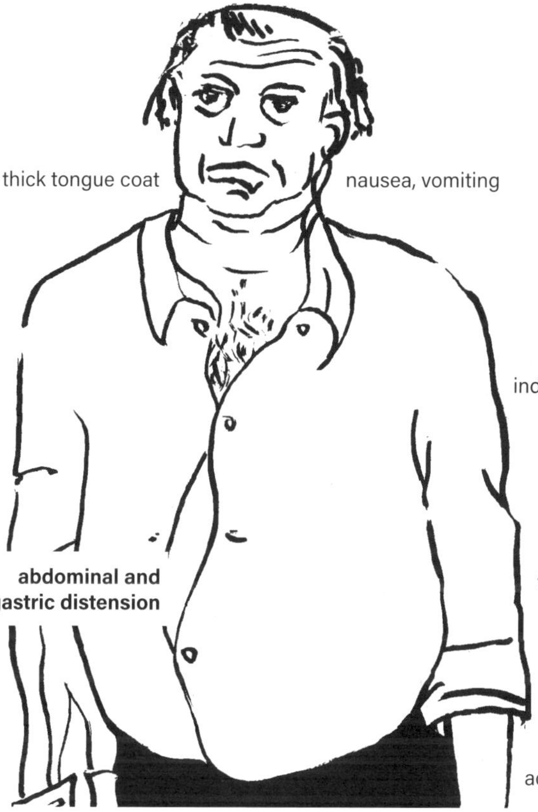

Dosage and method of administration

Simmer one block of **2.19 Shen Chu Cha** in 2 cups of water and reduce by one third. Discard the dregs and take in two doses. With chills or other signs of wind cold, add several thick slices of root ginger before simmering.

Cautions and Contraindications

Not suitable for patients with wheat intolerance or coeliac disease.

2.20 BOJENMI CHINESE TEA

保健美

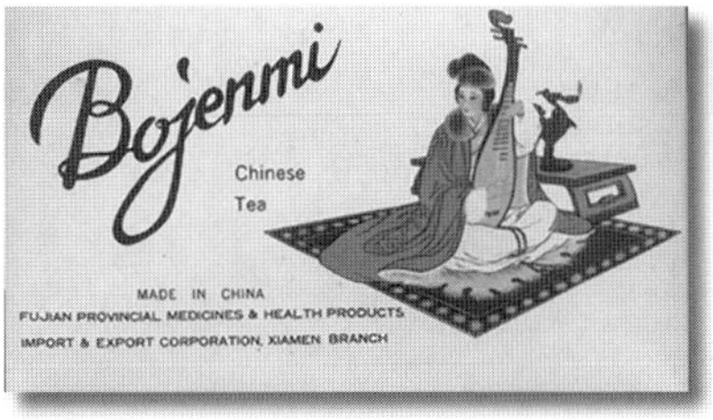

(*Bao Jian Mei*)
Fujian Provincial Medicines and Health Products
'Protect Strength and Beauty Tea'
Bojenmi Chinese Tea is packaged in teabags, twenty bags per box

Chinese medical action

Alleviates food stagnation, harmonizes the Stomach, promotes urination

Biomedical action

Enhances digestive functions, diuretic

INDICATIONS

- Acute or chronic indigestion, dyspepsia and gastric hyper-acidity associated with food stagnation.
- To improve general digestion, fat and fluid metabolism in those with a tendency to being overweight. In conjunction with an appropriate diet and exercise, **2.20 Bojenmi Chinese Tea** may aid in weight loss and improved absorption and metabolism of food. Can assist in lowering blood lipids and cholesterol.
- Fluid retention and edema from Spleen deficiency. May be useful for some patients with hypertension due to its diuretic action.

Composition

Crategus pinnatifida (shan zha, crategus) 9%, *Hordeum vulgare* (mai ya, sprouted barley) 3.5%, *Citrus reticulata* (chen pi, citrus) 3.5%, *Poria cocos* (fu ling, hoelen) 4%, *Alisma orientalis* (ze xie, alisma) 2.5%, Massa Fermentata (shen qu) 3.5%, *Pharbitis nil* (qian niu zi, pharbitis seed) 3%, *Phaseolus angularis* (chi xiao dou, adzuki bean) 4%, *Raphanus sativus* (lai fu zi, radish seed) 2%, *Prunella vulgaris* (xia ku cao, prunella) 8%, *Cassia tora* (jue ming zi, cassia seed) 3%, *Pogostemon cablin* (huo xiang, agastache) 4%, *Camellia sinensis* (cha ye, tea) 50%

Dosage and method of administration

Steep 1-2 teabags in a coffee mug of boiling water for 5 minutes, four times daily.

Cautions and Contraindications

Contraindicated during pregnancy. Avoid while breast-feeding as this product contains *Hordeum vulgare* (mai ya, sprouted barley), a herb that can reduce milk production.

2.21 KEEP FIT CAPSULE

清脂减肥丸

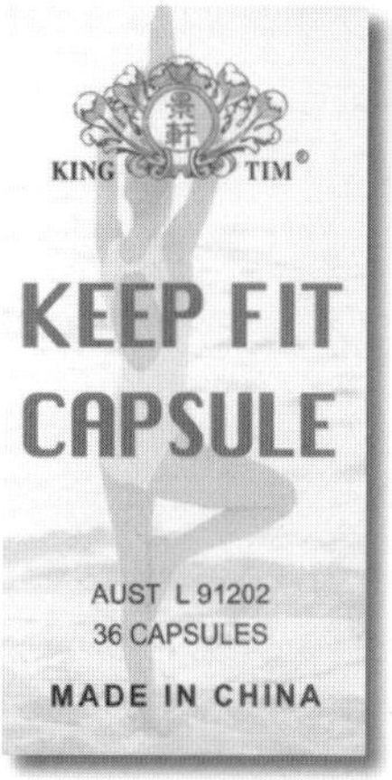

(*Qing Zhi Jian Fei Wan*)
Jing Xian Pharmaceutical Co. (Guangzhou)
'Clear Away Fat and Reduce Obesity Pills'
Keep Fit Capsules are packaged in bottles of 36 capsules

Chinese medical action

Invigorates blood, alleviates food stagnation, transforms phlegm, tonifies qi and blood

Biomedical action

Assists in lowering triglycerides and cholesterol, improves processing of fats, diuretic, strengthens digestive function

INDICATIONS

- In concert with appropriate dietary modifications and a sensible exercise program, this formula may assist in weight loss by improving digestive function and the metabolism of fats.
- High blood cholesterol and triglycerides. This is a modern formulation constructed of herbs with a known action of lowering blood triglycerides and cholesterol.

Composition (each capsule contains herbal extracts equivalent to)

Crategus pinnatifida (shan zha, crategus) 428mg, *Astragalus membranaceous* (huang qi, astragalus) 285mg, *Salvia miltiorrhiza* (dan shen, salvia) 285mg, *Alisma orientalis* (ze xie, alisma) 285mg, *Panax notoginseng* (tian qi, pseudoginseng) 285mg, *Trichosanthes kirilowi* (tian hua fen, trichosanthes root) 285mg, *Polygonum multiflorum* (he shou wu, polygonum root) 285mg, *Raphanus sativus* (lai fu zi, radish seed) 285mg, *Nelumbus speciosum* (he ye, lotus leaf) 142mg, *Panax ginseng* (ren shen, ginseng) 24mg

Dosage and method of administration

2 capsules, three times daily, 20 minutes before meals.

Cautions and contraindications

Contraindicated during pregnancy. Caution in patients who are also taking anticoagulant therapy (aspirin, warfarin, coumarin) as clotting time can be reduced.

2.22 ER CHEN WAN

二陈丸

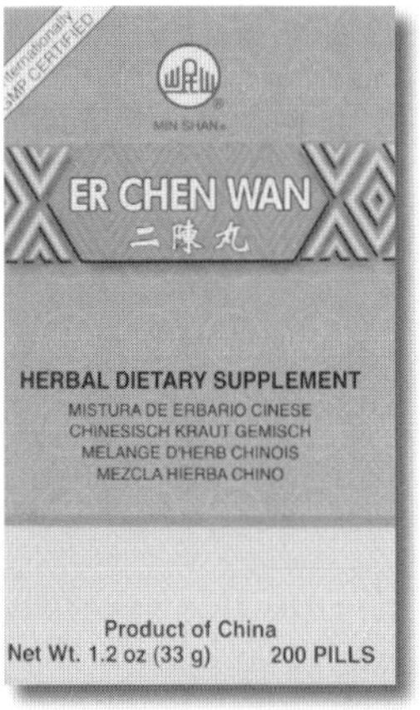

Lanzhou Foci Pharmaceutical Factory (Gansu)
'Two Aged [Ingredient] Pills'
Er Chen Wan is packaged in bottles of 200 pills
Also available as: Pinellia Pachyma Pills, Erh Chen Wan, Citrus and Pinellia Combination (conc. extract)

Chinese medical action

Dries damp and transforms phlegm, regulates qi, harmonizes the middle burner

Biomedical action

Mucolytic, expectorant, anti-emetic

INDICATIONS

- Phlegm damp accumulation. Used primarily for phlegm damp accumulation in the gastrointestinal system and Lungs, but can be used for all chronic mucus problems, regardless of location. **2.22 Er Chen Wan** is the base formula from which all phlegm damp resolving formulas are built. Used when phlegm patterns are not complicated by significant Spleen deficiency (*see* **2.8 Liu Jun Zi Wan** for that problem). Common uses include productive cough with copious white sputum, mucus congestion in the ear ('glue ear'), nose and sinuses, and nausea and vomiting from phlegm damp accumulation in the Stomach, including morning sickness.
- Dizziness, palpitations and insomnia from phlegm accumulation in the head and chest. This pattern may occur following an incompletely resolved upper respiratory tract infection, in which the heat has congealed body fluids into phlegm. May also assist in Meniere's disease of a phlegm damp type.
- Phlegm masses and nodules, such as ovarian and breast cysts, thyroid nodules and swollen lymph glands.
- Can be added to cloying yin and blood tonic formulas to aid digestion and absorption. Frequently combined with other constitutional formulas when enhanced phlegm damp transformation is desired.

Composition (each pill contains powdered)

Pinellia ternata (zhi ban xia, processed pinellia), *Citrus reticulata* (chen pi, citrus), *Poria cocos* (fu ling, hoelen), *Zingiber officinale* (sheng jiang, ginger), *Glycyrrhiza uralensis* (gan cao, licorice)

Combine with

- **2.9 Xiang Sha Liu Jun Wan** to enhance phlegm transformation in patients with Spleen deficiency with copious phlegm damp; as phlegm clears the proportion of **2.22 Er Chen Wan** can be reduced or omitted
- **1.34 Hai Zao Jing Wan** to enhance the phlegm resolving effect when treating phlegm type masses and nodules

Pattern identifying features

- **phlegm damp**
- chronic mucus congestion
- phlegm nodules

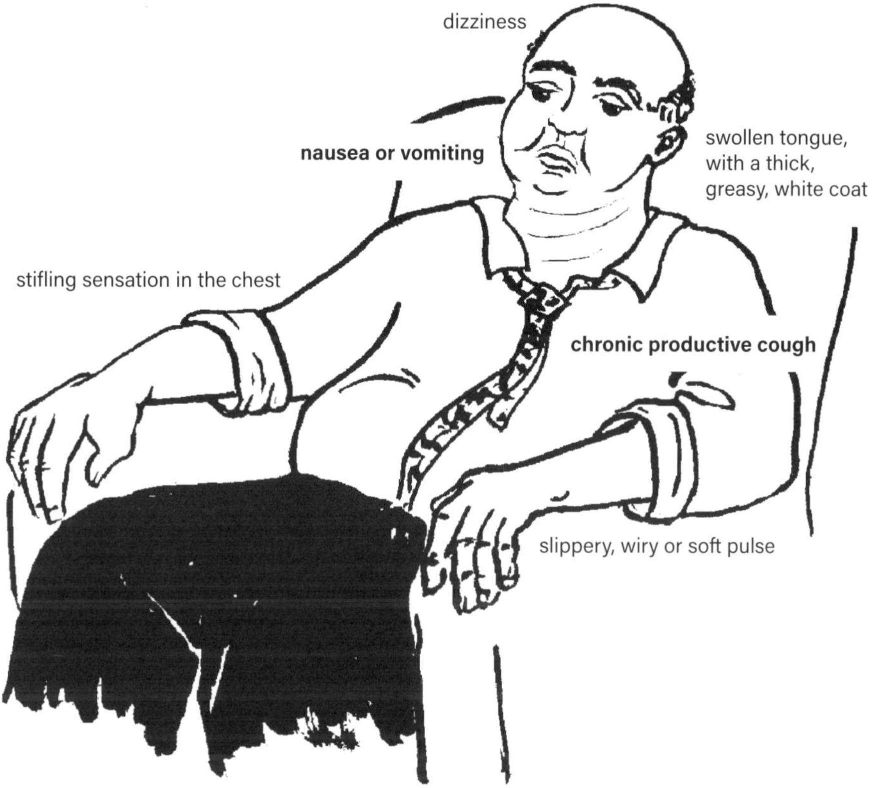

– **6.1 Xiao Chai Hu Wan** for residual productive cough and swollen glands in the aftermath of an upper respiratory tract infection
– **15.4 Tian Ma Gou Teng Wan** for phlegm and ascendant Liver yang type vertigo (as in Ménière's syndrome)
– A small dose to allay the cloying qualities of yin and blood tonic formulas

Dosage and method of administration

8-12 pills three times daily on an empty stomach. The dose can be spread out, or taken in two lots of 12-18 pills, morning and evening. In severe cases or during the early stages of treatment (the first few weeks), a 50% increase in dose can be used, then reduced to a maintenance dose as phlegm clears.

Cautions and Contraindications

Contraindicated (alone) in cough, nausea from dryness or yin deficiency. Not suitable unmodified for constitutionally yin deficient patients with phlegm damp accumulation. **2.22 Er Chen Wan** is parching and can aggravate dryness and thirst in some patients.

2.23 PING WEI SAN

平胃散

Lanzhou Foci Pharmaceutical Factory (Gansu)
'Stomach Calming Powder'.
Ping Wei San is packaged in bottles of 200 pills
Also available as: Calm Stomach Teapills (PF), Magnolia and Ginger Formula (conc. extract)

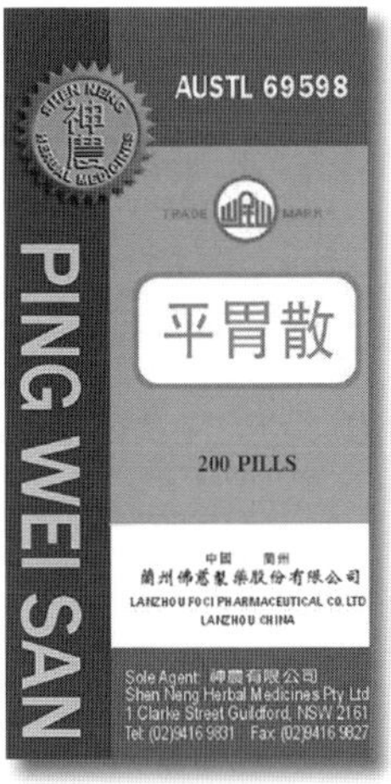

Chinese medical action

Harmonizes the Spleen and Stomach, dries damp, regulates qi in the middle burner

Biomedical action

Enhances digestive functions, digestant, antispasmodic, carminative, stomachic

INDICATIONS

- Damp or cold damp accumulating in the Spleen and Stomach. This can be acute, following invasion of a damp pathogen directly into the digestive system, or a chronic condition due to consumption of an excess of damp producing foods. It can also be the result of poor Spleen function. Damp disrupts the qi dynamic (*see* glossary). Qi and damp accumulate in the middle burner causing pronounced distension. Symptoms often worse first thing in the morning or after periods of inactivity as damp tends to settle and congeal when there is no movement.
- Used to hasten a reluctant labor.
- With the appropriate identifying features, this formula can be used to treat disorders such as acute and chronic gastroenteritis, chronic gastritis, nervous stomach, stomach flu, peptic ulcer disease, narcolepsy and somnolence.

Composition (each pill contains powdered)

Atractylodes lancea (cang zhu, red atractylodes) 48mg, *Magnolia officinalis* (hou po, magnolia bark) 48mg, *Citrus reticulata* (chen pi, citrus) 32mg, *Zingiber officinale* (sheng jiang, ginger) 16mg, *Glycyrrhiza uralensis* (gan cao, licorice) 16mg

Combine with

- **14.1 Huang Lian Jie Du Wan** for marked damp heat in the Stomach
- **2.22 Er Chen Wan** for severe nausea
- **4.2 Wu Ling Wan** for diarrhea with fluid retention and scanty urine
- **6.1 Xiao Chai Hu Wan** for acute infectious illness such as malarial disorder, characterized by alternating fever and chills, muscle aches, heaviness and lethargy, loss of appetite, nausea and vomiting and a soggy pulse

Pattern identifying features

- **cold damp in the middle burner**
- heaviness in the body and limbs
- increased desire to sleep
- fatigue and lethargy
- symptoms worse in the morning
- decreased sense of taste

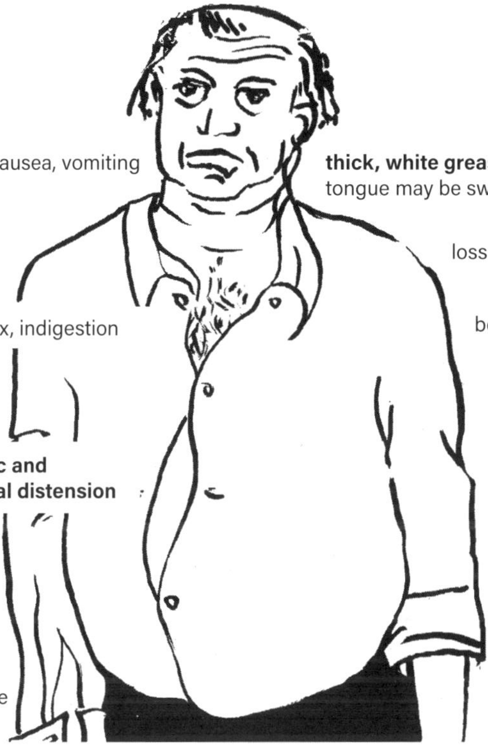

Dosage and method of administration

8-12 pills three times daily on an empty stomach. The dose can be spread out, or taken in two lots of 12-18 pills, morning and evening. In severe cases or during the early stages of treatment (the first 7-10 days), a 50% increase in dosage can be used, then reduced to a maintenance dose as treatment takes effect. To induce labor, double the standard recommended dose is required.

Cautions and Contraindications

Caution during pregnancy (other than when used to induce an overdue labor), and in patients with yin and blood deficiency.

2.24 SHU GAN WAN

舒肝丸

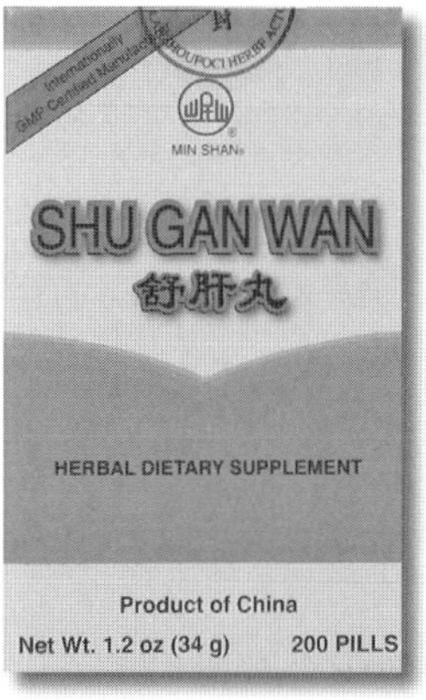

Lanzhou Foci Pharmaceutical Factory (Gansu)
'Soothe the Liver Pills'
Shu Gan Wan is packaged in bottles of 200 pills
Also available as: Soothe Liver Teapills (PF), Bupleurum and Evodia Combination (conc. extract)

Chinese medical action

Invigorates Liver qi and blood, breaks up stagnant qi, stops pain, harmonizes the Liver and Stomach

Biomedical action

Antispasmodic, analgesic, benefits digestion, carminative

INDICATIONS

- Pain and distension from Liver qi constraint and Liver qi invading the Spleen and Stomach. The pain can have elements of both qi and blood stasis – distending, as well as sharp and piercing. Effective for a wide variety of pain conditions, including epigastric, abdominal, chest and hypochondriac pain, intercostal and postherpetic neuralgia, genital pain, qi painful urination, fibromyalgia and chronic muscular pain.
- Indigestion, dyspepsia, acid reflux and indefinable epigastric discomfort from Liver and Stomach disharmony.
- With the appropriate identifying features, this formula can be used to assist in the treatment of conditions such as peptic ulcer disease, chronic gastritis, nervous stomach, chronic cholecystitis, chronic hepatitis, gallstones, chronic pancreatitis, ulcerative colitis, Crohn's disease, irritable bowel syndrome, early hepatic cirrhosis, costochondritis, biliary and esophageal spasm.

Composition (each pill contains powdered)

Cyperus rotundus (xiang fu, cyperus), *Paeonia lactiflora* (bai shao, white peony), *Amomum cardamomum* (bai dou kou, amomum), *Paeonia suffruticosa* (mu dan pi, peony root bark), *Citrus reticulata* (chen pi, citrus), *Bupleurum falcatum* (chai hu, bupleurum), *Citrus aurantium* (zhi shi, aurantium), *Magnolia officinalis* (hou po, magnolia bark), *Corydalis turtschaninovii* (yan hu suo, corydalis), *Saussurea lappa* (mu xiang, saussurea), *Glycyrrhiza uralensis* (gan cao, licorice), *Citrus medica* (xiang yuan, citron), *Curcuma longa* (yu jin, curcuma), *Aquilaria agallocha* (chen xiang, aquilaria), *Santalum album* (tan xiang, sandalwood)

Combine with

- **2.26 Xiang Lian Wan** for epigastric pain and acid reflux. This combination is also used for bleeding and pain associated with ulcerative colitis and Crohn's disease
- **1.12 Shi Xiao Wan** or **5.7 Sunho Multi Ginseng Tablets** for concurrent blood stasis
- **6.11 Li Dan Tablets** or **6.10 Qing Gan Li Dan Tablets** for hypochondriac pain from gallstones
- **10.21 Yan Hu Suo Zhi Tong Wan** for severe pain

Pattern identifying features

- **Liver qi invading the Spleen and Stomach**
- **symptoms worse with emotion or stress**
- **pain syndromes**
- indigestion, nervous stomach
- wiry or paradoxical pulse
- irritability, easily angered

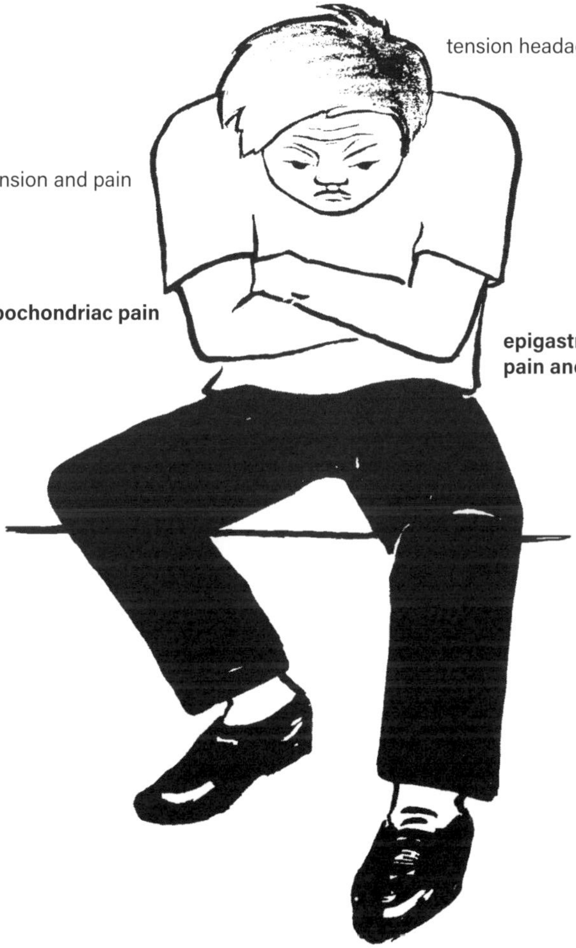

Dosage and method of administration

8-12 pills three times daily on an empty stomach. The dose can be spread out, or taken in two lots of 12-18 pills, morning and evening. In severe cases or during the early stages of treatment, a 50% increase in dosage can be used, then reduced to a maintenance dose as the patient improves.

Cautions and Contraindications

Contraindicated during pregnancy.

GMP

2.25 TONG XIE YAO FANG WAN

痛泻药方丸

3+ 12

Lanzhou Foci Pharmaceutical Factory (Gansu)
'Important Formula [Pills] for Painful Diarrhea'
Tong Xie Yao Wan is packaged in bottles of 200 pills

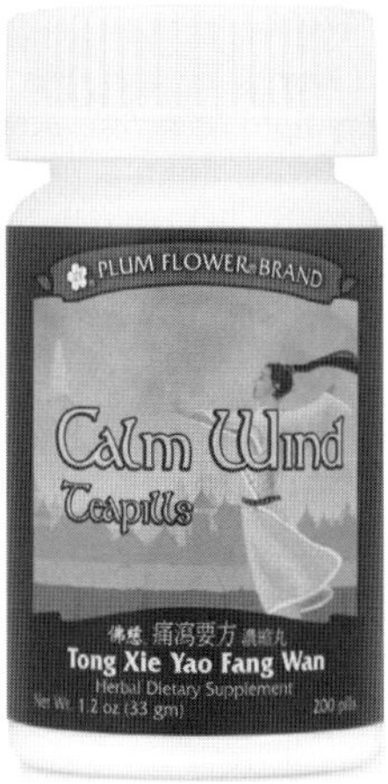

Chinese medical action

Harmonizes the Liver and Spleen, strengthens the Spleen, softens the Liver and regulates Liver qi, eases spasm, stops pain and diarrhea

Biomedical action

Antispasmodic, carminative, benefits digestion

INDICATIONS

- Liver invading the Spleen type diarrhea and abdominal pain. Also known as wood over-controlling earth. The pathology at the basis of this pattern involves the physiological response of the body to prolonged, repeated or severe emotional and psychological stress. Patients prone to this pattern are easily stressed or under significant pressure. The key feature is the relationship of the main symptoms (cramping abdominal pain followed by explosive diarrhea, after which the pain subsides) to the emotional state of the patient. Diarrhea and pain are chronic and recurrent, exacerbating in tandem with the stress levels of the patient.
- Effective for easing smooth muscle spasm in the gastrointestinal tract while gently harmonizing the relationship between the Liver and Spleen. As its focus is primarily at the level of the symptoms, **2.25 Tong Xie Yao Fang Wan** is often combined with an appropriate constitutional formula to enhance the systemic qi regulating treatment.
- With the appropriate identifying features, this formula can be used to treat the diarrhea predominant presentation of irritable bowel syndrome, colitis and the general effects of stress on the gastrointestinal tract.

Composition

Paeonia lactiflora (bai shao, white peony), *Atractylodes macrocephala* (chao bai zhu, dry fried atractylodes), *Citrus reticulata* (chen pi, citrus), *Ledebouriella divaricata* (fang feng, siler)

Combine with

- **6.3 Chai Hu Shu Gan Wan** for Liver invading the Spleen patterns and irritable bowel syndrome in robust patients with little or no deficiency
- **2.18 Bao He Wan** with food stagnation, abdominal distension and indigestion
- **6.4 Xiao Yao Wan** for Liver invading the Spleen patterns and irritable bowel syndrome in patients with blood and qi deficiency

Pattern identifying features

- **Liver qi invading the Spleen**
- symptoms worse with emotional upset and stress
- irritable bowel syndrome

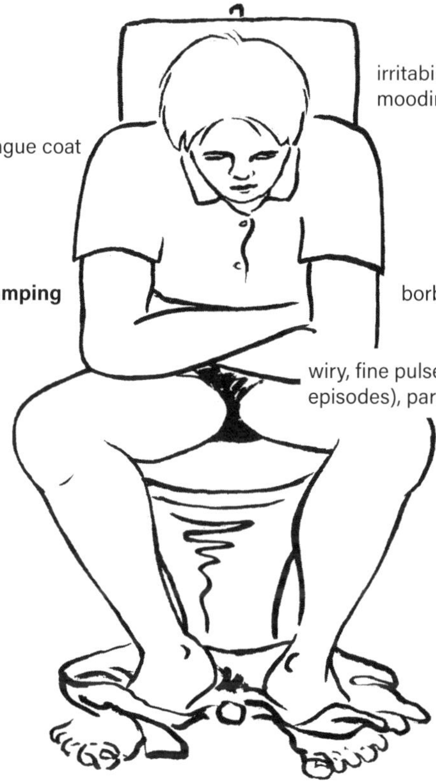

– A small dose of **14.1 Huang Lian Jie Du Wan** or **2.30 Chen Xiang Hua Qi Wan** for damp heat accumulation in the Large Intestine (the Primary Pathological Triad, *see* glossary), manifesting in a greasy yellow coat on the root of the tongue, slippery pulse, tenesmus and burning diarrhea

Dosage and method of administration

8-12 pills three times daily on an empty stomach. The dose can be spread out, or taken in two lots of 12-18 pills, morning and evening. In severe cases or during the early stages of treatment, a 50% increase in dosage can be used, then reduced to a maintenance dose as the patient improves.

Cautions and Contraindications

None noted.

2.26 XIANG LIAN WAN

香连丸

Lanzhou Foci Pharmaceutical Factory (Gansu)
'Saussurea and Coptis Pills'
Xiang Lian Wan is packaged in bottles of 200 pills
Also available as: Aucklandia and Coptis Teapills (PF)

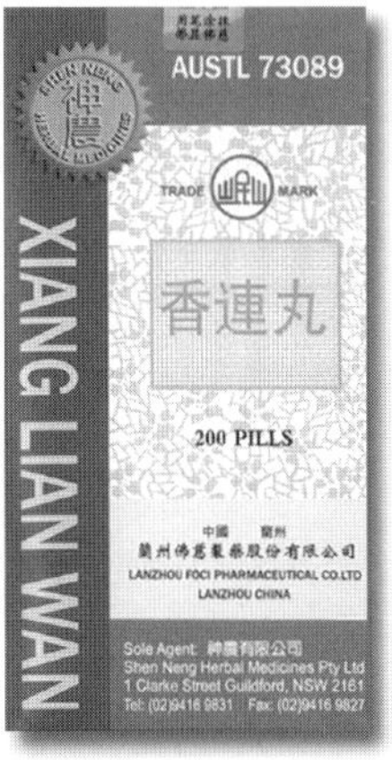

Chinese medical action

Clears toxic heat, transforms damp, directs Stomach qi downwards, regulates qi, harmonizes the Stomach

Biomedical action

Alleviates indigestion, antacid, eases the intestines

INDICATIONS

- Dysenteric disorder (*see* glossary) from accumulation of damp heat in the Large Intestine. This includes true infection (bacterial or amoebic dysentery, Giardia, etc.), and disorders with blood and/or mucus in the stool, such as ulcerative colitis and Crohn's disease.
- Heartburn, acid reflux, gastroesophageal reflux and dyspepsia from Stomach heat or fire. Useful as an addition to a suitable constitutional formula. The coptis utilized in this formula is traditionally prepared with *Evodia rutaecarpae* (wu zhu yu, evodia). When combined, these two herbs are especially effective for heartburn.

Composition (each pill contains powdered)

Coptis japonica (huang lian, coptis) 128mg, *Saussurea lappa* (mu xiang, saussurea) 32mg

Combine with

- **14.1 Huang Lian Jie Du Wan** for tenesmus in dysenteric disorder from lingering damp heat
- **14.5 Chuan Xin Lian Antiphlogistic Tablets** for acute dysenteric disorder or Intestinal abscess
  A large dose of **12.3 Baby Fat Powder** or **14.1 Huang Lian Jie Du Wan** for amoebic dysentery
- **2.10 Xiang Sha Yang Wei Wan** for indigestion arising from Stomach qi stagnation with damp accumulation
- **6.3 Chai Hu Shu Gan Wan** or **2.24 Shu Gan Wan** for indigestion and reflux arising from Liver qi invading the Stomach. These combine with are also useful for some varieties of ulcerative colitis, Crohn's disease and irritable bowel syndrome
- **2.9 Xiang Sha Liu Jun Wan** for indigestion and reflux from Spleen and Stomach qi deficiency

Pattern identifying features

- **damp heat dysenteric disorder**
- Stomach heat, rebellious Stomach qi

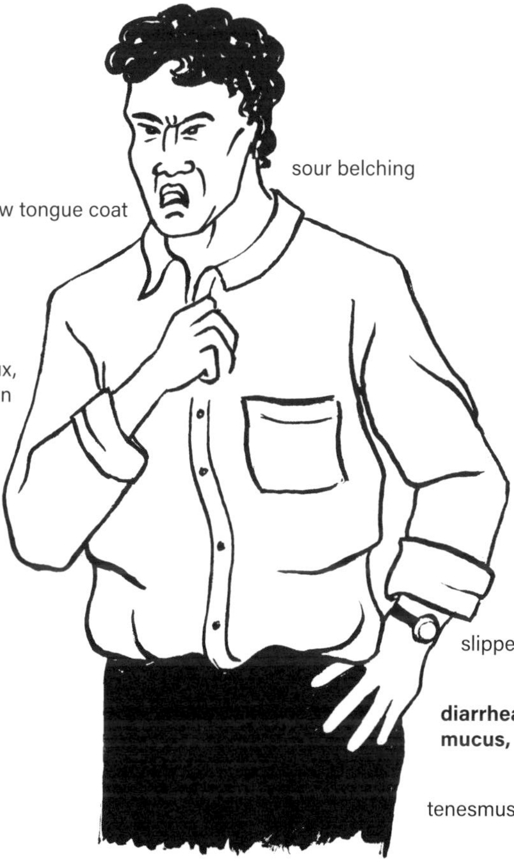

Dosage and method of administration

These pills are usually added to a suitable constitutional formula. The proportion will vary depending on the severity of the symptoms, however a 2:1 ratio of constitutional formula to **2.26 Xiang Lian Wan** is usual. *See also* p.xvii.

Cautions and Contraindications

Caution in patients with Spleen deficiency.

1-3/12

2.27 WEI TE LING

胃特灵

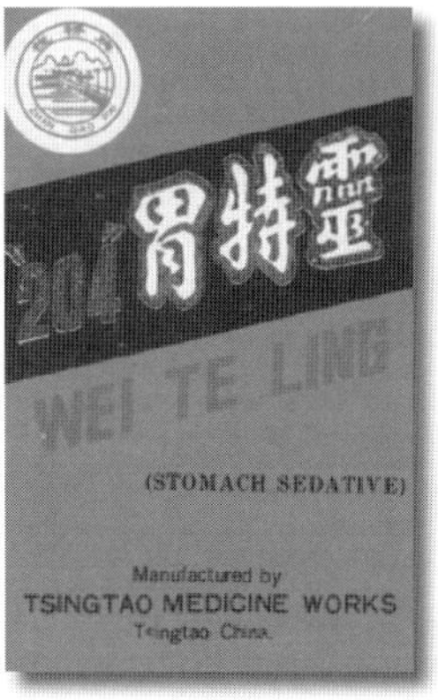

(Wei Te Ling Stomach Sedative)
Qingdao Medicine Works (Shandong)
'Especially Effective (Medicine) for the Stomach'
Wei Te Ling is packaged in bottles of 120 coated tablets

Chinese medical action

Neutralizes gastric acid, regulates qi and invigorates blood in the Stomach, stops pain

Biomedical action

Antacid, analgesic

INDICATIONS

- Gastric hyper-acidity, acid reflux, heartburn, epigastric pain. May be used alone to provide quick relief from reflux, however it is usually combined with a constitutional formula.
- Can be used to assist in the treatment of peptic ulcers, acute and chronic gastritis and gastroesophageal reflux disease (GERD).

Composition

Sepia esculenta (wu zei gu, cuttlefish backbone) 40%, *Corydalis turtschaninovii* (yan hu suo, corydalis) 30%, honey 30%

Combine with

– **6.3 Chai Hu Shu Gan Wan** for hyper-acidity from Liver invading the Stomach
– **2.23 Ping Wei San** for accumulation of phlegm damp in the Stomach
– **2.24 Shu Gan Wan** for acid reflux with marked epigastric pain
– **2.10 Xiang Sha Yang Wei Wan** for Spleen and Stomach qi stagnation with damp accumulation
– **9.8 Qing Wei Wan** for reflux from heat in the Stomach

Pattern identifying features

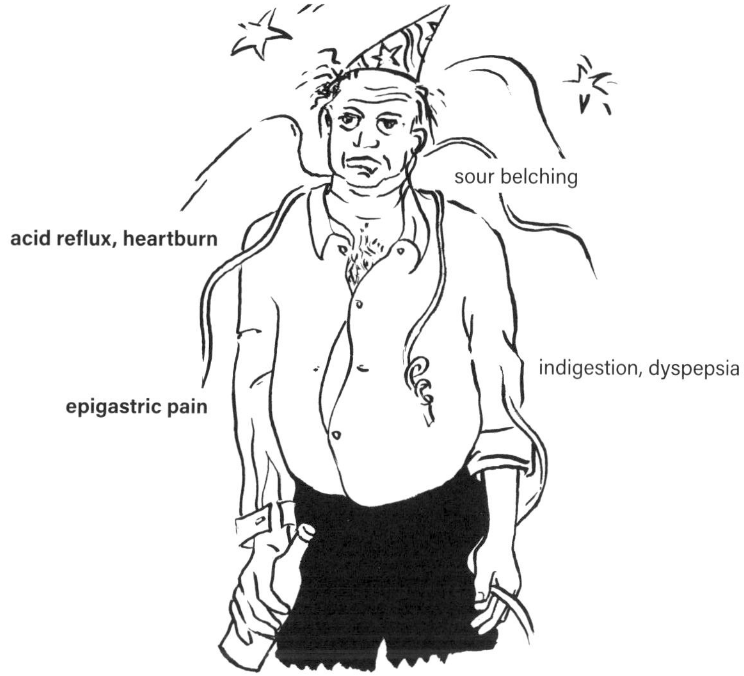

Dosage and method of administration

4-6 pills three times daily on an empty stomach or during an episode of heartburn. In severe cases or the early stages of treatment (the first two weeks), the dose can be increased until the patient experiences relief, then reduced to a maintenance dose (a few pills before or after a meal) as the condition settles down.

Cautions and Contraindications

None noted.

2.28 WEI TONG DING

胃痛定

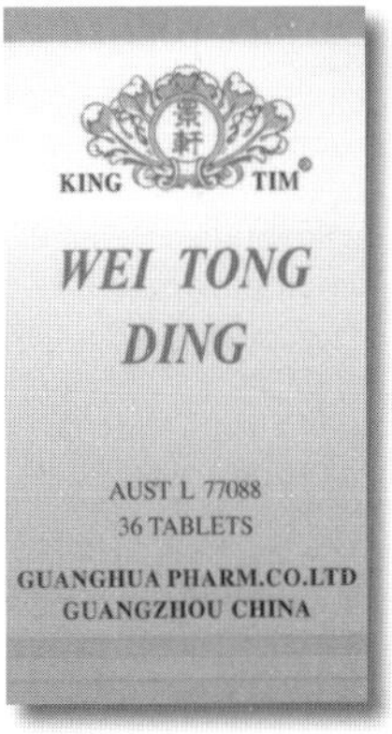

Guanghua Pharmaceutical Co. (Guangzhou)
'Calm Stomach Pain'
Wei Tong Ding is packaged in bottles of 36 tablets

Chinese medical action

Warms the middle burner, dispels cold, regulates qi and restores the qi dynamic, stops pain

Biomedical action

Analgesic, warms the stomach and assists digestion

INDICATIONS

- Epigastric and abdominal pain or discomfort from accumulation of cold, cold and deficiency and/or qi constraint. Pain is typically dull and persistent, improved with the application of warmth from a hot water bottle or warm drink. If cold is abundant, however, the pain may be acute, colicky and relatively severe.
- Persistent hiccup, excessive salivation and drooling, indigestion, epigastric distension, acid reflux, heartburn, nausea, vomiting, from cold accumulation or Spleen qi or yang deficiency.
- With the appropriate identifying features, this formula can assist in the treatment of gastric hyper-acidity, dyspepsia, gastric and duodenal ulcers, chronic gastritis, persistent hiccup and gastroesophageal reflux disease (GERD).

Composition (each pill contains powdered)

Aquilaria sinensis (chen xiang, aquilaria) 60mg, *Cinnamomum cassia* (rou gui, cinnamon bark) 20mg, *Piper nigrum* (hu jiao, black pepper) 20mg, *Syzygium aromaticum* (ding xiang, cloves) 20mg, *Amomum villosum* (sha ren, cardamom) 20mg, *Citrus aurantium* (zhi shi, aurantium) 20mg, *Saussurea lappa* (mu xiang, saussurea) 20mg, *Panax ginseng* (ren shen, ginseng) 20mg,

Combine with

- **2.13 Li Zhong Wan** or **2.15 Xiao Jian Zhong Wan** for abdominal pain or hyper-acidity from Spleen yang deficiency
- **2.10 Xiang Sha Yang Wei Wan** for qi stagnation type abdominal distension, pain or chronic hiccuping
- **2.7 Si Jun Zi Wan** for persistent hiccuping from Spleen and Stomach qi deficiency

Pattern identifying features

- **cold accumulation in the Stomach, Spleen yang qi deficiency**
- vomiting of thin watery fluids
- poor appetite or anorexia
- hiccough
- indigestion, reflux

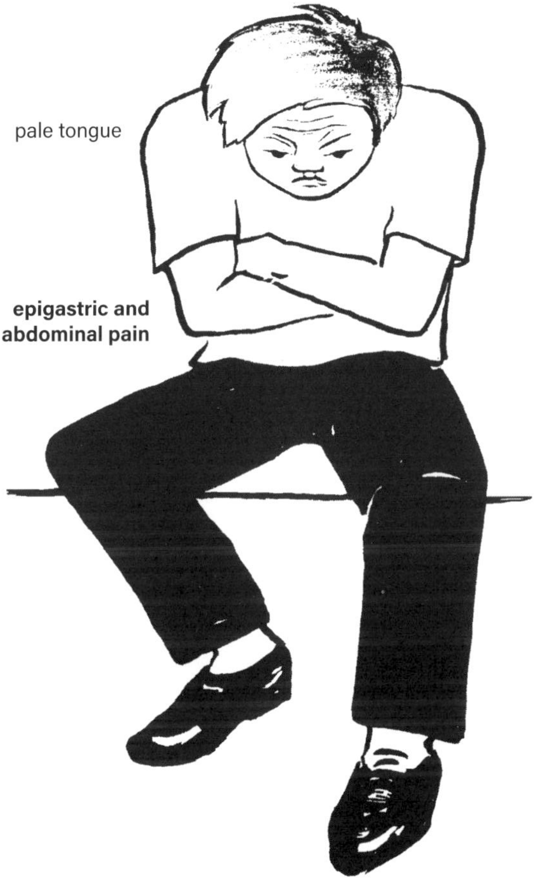

Dosage and method of administration

One tablet, three times daily on an empty stomach.

Cautions and Contraindications

Contraindicated in patients with Stomach heat, fire or yin deficiency.

2.29 MU XIANG SHUN QI WAN

木香顺气丸

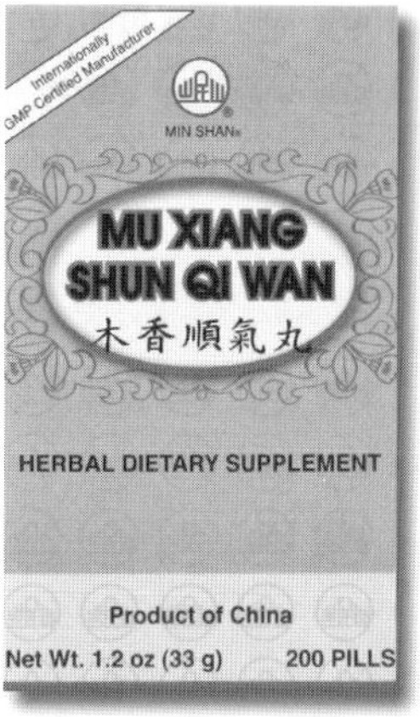

Lanzhou Foci Pharmaceutical Factory (Gansu)
'Saussurea Qi Promoting Pills'
Mu Xiang Shun Qi Wan is packaged in bottles of 200 pills
Also available as: Mu Xiang Shun Qi Teapills (PF), Aplotaxis Carminative Pills, Shun Qi Wan

Chinese medical action

Moves qi in the middle burner, promotes the descent of Stomach qi, relieves food and damp stagnation

Biomedical action

Promotes peristalsis, gentle laxative, antispasmodic

INDICATIONS

- Abdominal pain and bloating, indigestion, flatulence and acid reflux from Liver qi constraint with food and/or damp stagnation in the Intestines. The main strategy of the formula is to drive the qi dynamic with a mix of acrid warm ascending, and bitter descending herbs.
- Sluggish bowel habits or habitual constipation associated with qi stagnation. This typically occurs in stressed and sedentary workers and is usually associated with a slowing down of peristalsis due to hypertonicity in the gastrointestinal system, with secondary weakness of smooth muscle activity.
- Chronic dysenteric disorder from lingering damp heat and qi stagnation, with tenesmus, discomfort preceding a bowel movement and diarrhea with mucus and/or blood.
- With the appropriate identifying features, this formula can be used to treat disorders such as chronic gastritis and colitis, habitual constipation, the constipation predominant presentation of irritable bowel syndrome, dyspepsia, cholecystitis, gallstones, chronic hepatitis and mild ascites.

Composition (each pill contains powdered)

Saussurea lappa (mu xiang, saussurea), *Citrus reticulata* (qing pi, immature citrus), *Citrus reticulata* (chen pi, citrus), *Magnolia officinalis* (hou po, magnolia bark), *Alpinia katsumadai* (cao dou kou, katsumadai cardamom), *Angelica sinensis* (dang gui), *Alpinia oxyphylla* (yi zhi ren, alpinia), *Atractylodes lancea* (cang zhu, red atractylodes), *Zingiber officinalis* (gan jiang, dried ginger), *Pinellia ternata* (zhi ban xia, processed pinellia), *Evodia rutaecarpae* (wu zhu yu, evodia), *Alisma orientalis* (ze xie, alisma), *Poria cocos* (fu ling, hoelen), *Bupleurum falcatum* (chai hu, bupleurum), *Cimicifuga foetida* (sheng ma, cimicifuga)

Pattern identifying features

- **Liver qi constraint with food and damp stagnation**
- indigestion
- flatulence, belching
- acid reflux, heartburn
- borborygmus
- nausea, vomiting

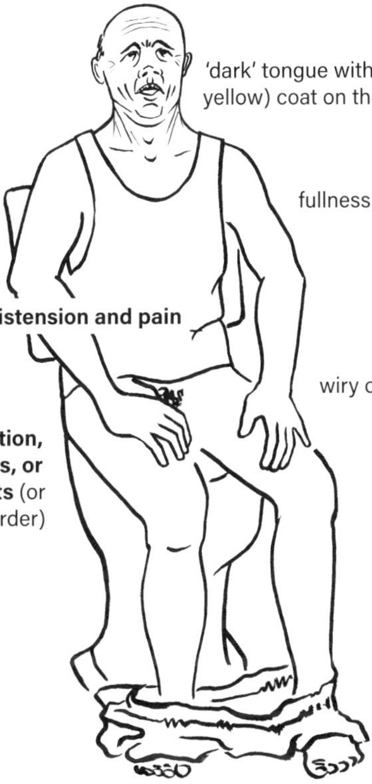

Combine with

– A small dose (2-4 pills each time) of **2.30 Chen Xiang Hua Qi Wan** or **2.33 Da Huang Jiang Zhi Wan** in the early stages of treatment or in resistant cases, until the patient achieves a smooth bowel movement

– **2.26 Xiang Lian Wan** to treat chronic dysenteric disorder from lingering damp heat with severe tenesmus

Dosage and method of administration

Start with 8 pills three times daily on an empty stomach. The dose should be increased until a smooth bowel movement is achieved then reduced to the minimum required to maintain a smooth and regular bowel movement.

Cautions and contraindications

Caution in patients with significant qi or yin deficiency as this formula is quite dispersing.

2.30 CHEN XIANG HUA QI WAN

沉香化气丸

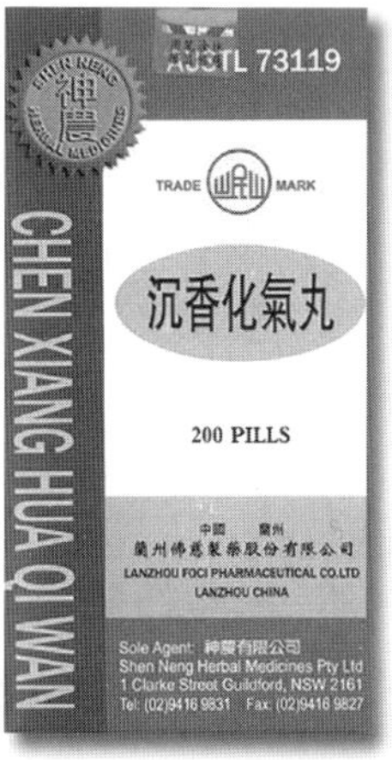

Lanzhou Foci Pharmaceutical Factory (Gansu)
'Aquilaria Qi Transforming Pills'
Chen Xiang Hua Qi Wan is packaged in bottles of 200 pills
Also available as: Aquilaria Pills, Aquilaria Stomachic Pills

Chinese medical action

Regulates and tonifies Spleen qi, restores the qi dynamic, clears damp heat and opens the bowels

Biomedical action

Improves digestive function, laxative

INDICATIONS

- Constipation and indigestion from Spleen qi deficiency with qi dynamic disruption. The deficiency causes failure of Spleen qi to rise and Stomach qi to descend, so qi and incompletely digested food accumulate in the middle and lower burner, with consequent damp heat generation. The formula is composed of qi tonic herbs to encourage the elevation of Spleen qi, and herbs to direct qi downwards and clear damp heat. The combination of these opposing actions drives the qi dynamic, restoring the correct flow and transformation of qi.
- Used for chronic or recurrent diarrhea from lingering damp heat in the Intestines following an incompletely cleared infection. The role of the rhubarb here is to assist the scute in the expulsion of damp heat, while the atractylodes and codonopsis protect the Spleen from further damage.

Composition (each pill contains powdered)

Atractylodes macrocephala (bai zhu, atractylodes), *Codonopsis pilosula* (dang shen, codonopsis), *Scutellaria baicalensis* (huang qin, scute), *Rheum palmatum* (da huang, rhubarb), *Aquilaria agallocha* (chen xiang, aquilaria)

Combine with

- **2.29 Mu Xiang Shun Qi Wan** to enhance the laxative affect of that formula during the early stages of treatment
- **6.4 Xiao Yao Wan**, added a week before menstruation in women prone to premenstrual constipation
- **2.18 Bao He Wan** for severe food stagnation
- **6.3 Chai Hu Shu Gan Wan** for relatively severe qi constraint and Liver invading the Spleen. This combination is also used for constipation predominant irritable bowel syndrome
- **2.25 Tong Xie Yao Fang Wan** for cramping abdominal pain with alternating constipation and occasional explosive diarrhea from Liver invading the Spleen, with damp heat in the Intestines (the Primary Pathological Triad, *see* glossary)

Pattern identifying features

- **Spleen qi deficiency, damp heat in the Intestines, blockage of the qi dynamic**

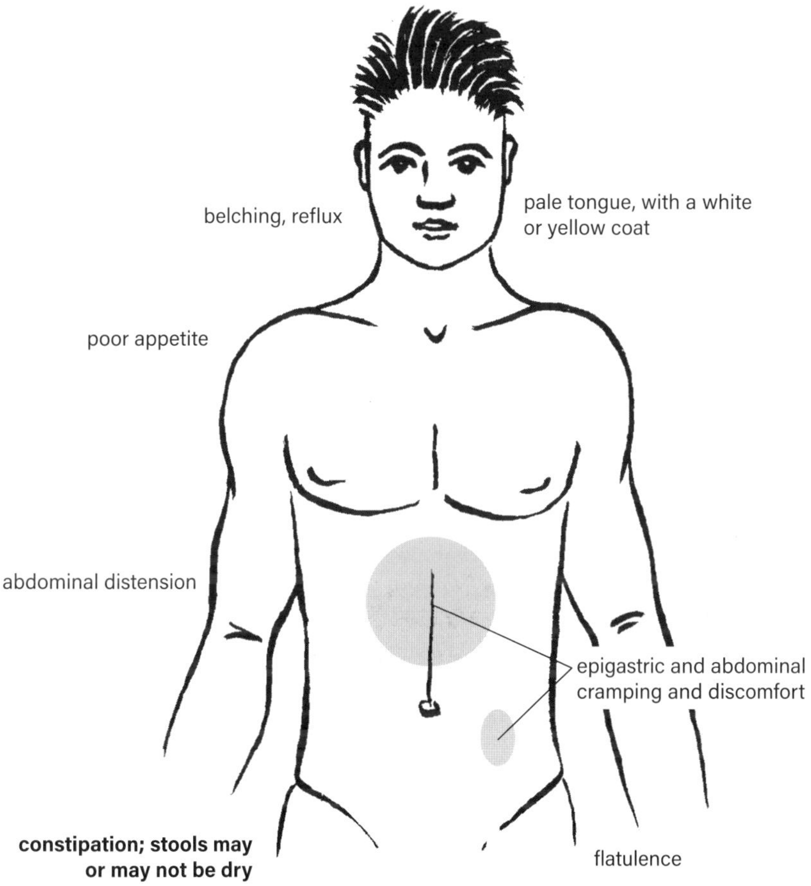

Dosage and method of administration

4-8 pills three times daily on an empty stomach. Best to begin with a small dose and increase it until a smooth bowel movement is achieved. The dose can then be reduced to the minimum required to keep the bowels moving. Usually combined with a constitutional formula and gradually withdrawn as the patient improves. Generally not used for lengthy periods of time as patients can habituate to the rhubarb. When used for recurrent diarrhea, discontinue once the symptoms subside.

Cautions and contraindications

Contraindicated during pregnancy.

2.31 RUN CHANG WAN

润肠丸

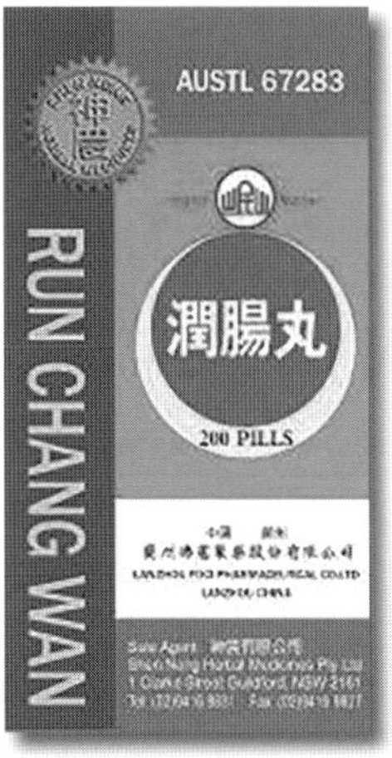

Lanzhou Foci Pharmaceutical Factory (Gansu)
'Lubricate the Intestines Pills'
Run Chang Wan is packaged in bottles of 200 pills
Also available as: Peach Kernel Teapills (PF), Tao Ren Wan, Fructus Persica Pills, Hemp Seed and Rhubarb Formula (conc. extract)

Chinese medical action

Moistens and lubricates the bowel, promotes bowel movement

Biomedical action

Mild moistening laxative

INDICATIONS

- Chronic constipation in blood, fluid or yin deficient patients. Commonly seen in the elderly and postpartum women, or following a febrile disease. Also used for constipation associated with chronic low grade heat in the Intestines.
- This is a relatively gentle laxative formula, commonly added to other primary formulas where a mild laxative action is desired.

Composition (each pill contains powdered)

Prunus persica (tao ren, peach seed) 51.4mg, *Sesamum indicum* (hei zhi ma, black sesame seeds) 51.4mg, *Angelica polymorpha* (dang gui) 25.7mg, *Notopterygium inscisum* (qiang huo, notopterygium) 25.7mg, *Rheum palmatum* (da huang, rhubarb) 25.7mg

Combine with

- **1.2 Si Wu Wan**, **1.9 Gui Pi Wan** or **1.1 Ba Zhen Wan** for postpartum or blood deficiency type constipation
- **1.23 Zhi Bai Di Huang Wan** or **8.1 Tian Wang Bu Xin Dan** for constipation in the elderly with a tendency to heat and dryness

Dosage and method of administration

Usually start with a small dose (4 pills 2-3 times daily) and gradually increase until a smooth bowel movement is achieved. Once a satisfactory dose is found, it can be adjusted from time to time to maintain effectiveness with the aim of gradually reducing the dose. If the patient is taking a constitutional formula to build blood, yin or fluids, **2.31 Run Chang Wan** can be gradually withdrawn as the condition improves. This can take months in some patients.

Pattern identifying features

- **Dry Intestines; blood, yin, fluid deficiency**

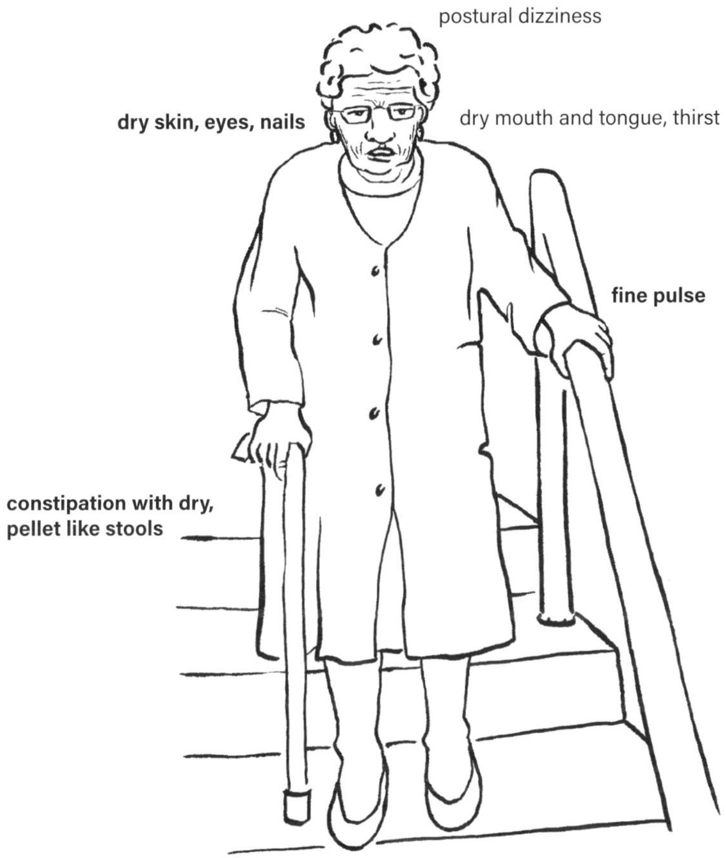

Cautions and contraindications

Contraindicated during pregnancy. Caution in breast-feeding women as rhubarb can pass through the breast milk and affect the child causing colic and diarrhea. Some patients may habituate to the formula when taken alone, so should generally be combined with a constitutional formula. May cause mild abdominal cramping in sensitive patients. Not suitable for constipation from excess heat (*see* **14.10 Liang Ge Wan**)

GMP

2.32 WU REN WAN

五仁丸

Lanzhou Foci Pharmaceutical Factory (Gansu)
'Five Seed Pills'
Wu Ren Wan is packaged in bottles of 200 pills

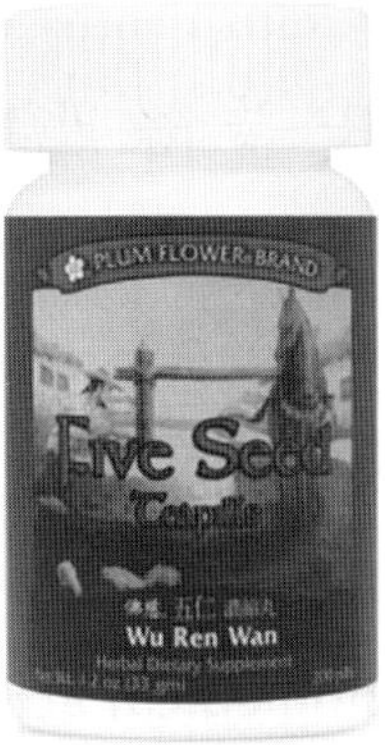

Chinese medical action
Moistens and lubricates the bowel, promotes bowel movement

Biomedical action
Mild moistening laxative

INDICATIONS

- Chronic dry constipation in blood, fluid or yin deficient patients. Commonly seen in the elderly and postpartum women, or following febrile disease.
- A gentle laxative formula, usually added to another primary formula where a mild laxative action is desired. It is somewhat similar in action to **2.31 Run Chang Wan**, but is composed of oily seeds and does not have the purgative action of rhubarb root. Suitable for prolonged use.

Composition
Citrus reticulata (chen pi, citrus), *Prunus armenica* (xing ren, apricot seed), *Prunus persica* (tao ren, peach seed), *Biota orientalis* (bai zi ren, biota seed), *Prunus japonica* (yu li ren, bush cherry seed), *Pinus massoniana* (song zi, pine nut)

Combine with
- **1.2 Si Wu Wan**, **1.9 Gui Pi Wan** or **1.1 Ba Zhen Wan** to enhance blood nourishment and postpartum constipation
- **7.1 Liu Wei Di Huang Wan** or **7.3 Zuo Gui Wan** for constipation in the elderly with dryness and yin deficiency

Dosage and method of administration
4-8 pills, three times daily on an empty stomach. The dose can be gradually increased until a smooth bowel movement is achieved, then adjusted from time to time to maintain effectiveness with the aim of gradually reducing the dose.

Cautions and contraindications
Contraindicated during pregnancy. Caution in patients with phlegm or damp.

2.33 DA HUANG JIANG ZHI WAN

大黄降脂丸

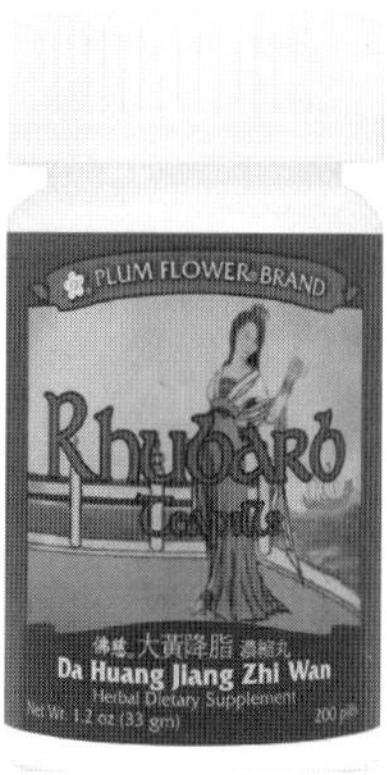

GMP

1-3/12

Lanzhou Foci Pharmaceutical Factory (Gansu)
'Rhubarb Fat Reducing Pills'
Da Huang Jiang Zhi Wan is packaged in bottles of 200 pills

Chinese medical action

Purges the Intestines, promotes bowel movement, clears heat, invigorates blood

Biomedical action

Stimulant laxative, febrifuge, anti-fungal

INDICATIONS

- Constipation. A strong purgative herb, rhubarb is used to stimulate peristalsis and open the bowels in patients with hard or dry impacted stools. It generally works within 6-12 hours following ingestion. Generally combined with a constitutional formula when a purgative action is desired.
- Fungal and bacterial infection of the Intestines. Rhubarb has anti-fungal and antibiotic properties, thus can assist in the treatment of *Candida*, *Shigella* and other infections of the Intestines.
- To reduce blood triglycerides.

Composition

Rheum palmatum (da huang, rhubarb), *Crategus pinnatifida* (jiao shan zha, baked crategus), *Hordeum vulgare* (chao mai ya, dry fried sprouted barley)

Dosage and method of administration

2-4 pills, twice daily. When used as an anti-fungal agent, purgation is not desired, so 1-2 pills per day may be sufficient.

Cautions and contraindications

Contraindicated during pregnancy. Caution in breast-feeding women as rhubarb can pass through the breast milk and affect the child causing colic and diarrhea. Not suitable for prolonged use as patients may habituate to it and its bitter coldness can damage Spleen yang. Best combined with a constitutional formula. May cause mild abdominal cramping in sensitive patients.

2.34 CONG RONG BU SHEN WAN

苁蓉补肾丸

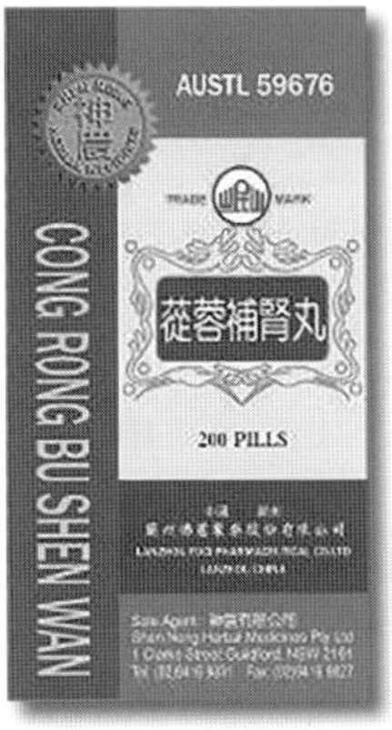

Lanzhou Foci Pharmaceutical Factory (Gansu)
'Cistanches Kidney Tonic Pills'
Cong Rong Bu Shen Wan is packaged in bottles of 200 pills

Chinese medical action

Tonifies Kidney yang, improves transformation of qi and bowel function

Biomedical action

Lubricates the bowel and enhances peristalsis

INDICATIONS

- Chronic atonic constipation from qi or yang deficiency. The main feature is a lack of desire to defecate and stools that are not dry when voided. This type of constipation is usually seen in elderly or post surgical patients.
- Yang deficiency type infertility, impotence, cold pains and weakness in the low back and knees, urinary frequency and uterine bleeding.

Composition

Cistanches deserticola (rou cong rong, cistanches) 66.3mg, *Rehmannia glutinosa* (shu di, processed rehmannia) 66.3mg, *Cuscuta chinensis* (tu su zi, cuscuta) 66.3mg, *Schizandra chinensis* (wu wei zi, schizandra) 1.1mg

Combine with

- A warming and yang strengthening formula such as **7.9 Jin Gui Shen Qi Wan**, **7.10 You Gui Wan**, **2.14 Li Chung Yuen Medical Pills**, or **2.13 Li Zhong Wan** to address the constitutional components of the problem
- **1.2 Si Wu Wan** or **1.1 Ba Zhen Wan** for postpartum constipation with blood and Kidney deficiency symptoms. This combination is also used for infertility from blood and yang deficiency
- **1.20 Cu Yun Yu Tai Capsule** or **1.21 Tiao Jing Cu Yun Wan** for infertility in a patient with marked yang deficiency, cold intolerance and copious vaginal discharge
- **1.9 Gui Pi Wan** for recurrent uterine bleeding from deficiency and cold in the Uterus

Pattern identifying features

- **Kidney qi and/or yang deficiency lack of stool propulsion**
- no urge to move bowels
- nocturia, frequent clear urination
- impotence, infertility

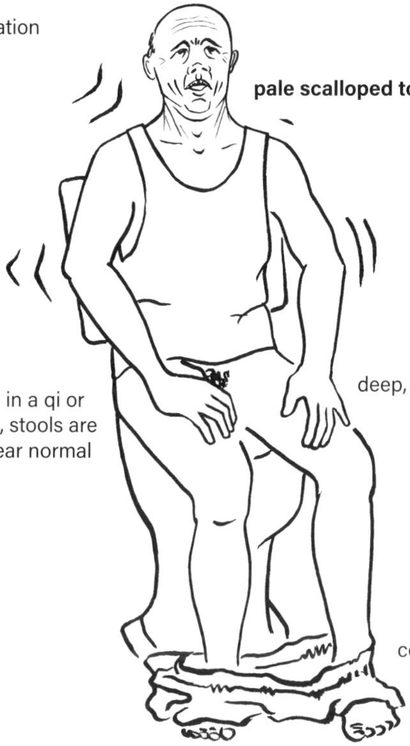

Dosage and method of administration

8-12 pills three times daily, before meals. The dose can be spread out, or taken in two lots of 12-18 pills, morning and evening. In severe cases or during the early stages of treatment (the first few weeks), a 50% increase in dose can be used, then reduced as the treatment takes effect. **2.34 Cong Rong Bu Shen Wan** needs to be used for prolonged periods for a sustained result. When combined with a constitutional yang tonic formula, a half dose may be sufficient.

Cautions and contraindications

Contraindicated during the early phase of acute illness such as colds and flu and in patients with diarrhea from Spleen deficiency.

GMP

2.35 YU QUAN WAN

玉泉丸

3+/12

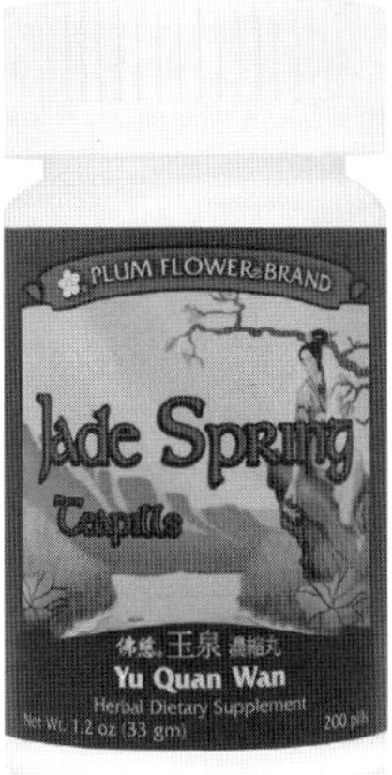

Lanzhou Foci Pharmaceutical Factory (Gansu)
'Jade Spring Pills'
Yu Quan Wan is packaged in bottles of 200 pills
Also available as: Jade Source Combination (conc. extract)

Chinese medical action

Nourishes yin, generates fluids, moistens dryness, stops thirst, strengthens the Spleen and tonifies qi

Biomedical action

Hypoglycemic, demulcent, energy stimulant

INDICATIONS

- Diabetes mellitus type 2 and prediabetes associated with Kidney, Spleen and Stomach qi and yin deficiency. The herbs in this formula are selected on the basis of their action in tonifying qi and enriching yin, as well as their known effects on reducing blood sugar levels. Traditionally considered a type of wasting and thirsting disorder (*xiāo kě* 消渴).
- Many patients with diabetes or hyperglycemia are medicated and the classical features, thirst, frequent copious urination, weight loss and hunger, absent. In fact, many patients with adult onset diabetes are overweight and overfed, with elements or phlegm damp (*see* **2.23 Ping Wei San**) or phlegm heat (*see* **8.8 Wen Dan Wan**), so care must be taken to differentiate patterns carefully and avoid tonifying when a reducing method is more appropriate.

Composition

Trichosanthes kirilowi (tian hua fen, trichosanthes root), *Pueraria lobata* (ge gen, kudzu), *Codonopsis pilosula* (dang shen, codonopsis), *Astragalus membranaceous* (huang qi, astragalus), *Poria cocos* (fu ling, hoelen), *Rehmannia glutinosa* (sheng di, raw rehmannia), *Ophiopogon japonicus* (mai dong, ophiopogon), *Prunus mume* (wu mei, black plum), *Glycyrrhiza uralensis* (gan cao, licorice), *Schizandra chinensis* (wu wei zi, schizandra)

Combine with

- **2.36 Sugarid** to assist in reducing blood sugar
- **2.12 Shen Ling Bai Zhu Wan** for patients tending to more qi deficiency

Pattern identifying features

- **Kidney, Spleen, Stomach qi and yin deficiency**
- thirst
- hunger
- frequent urination

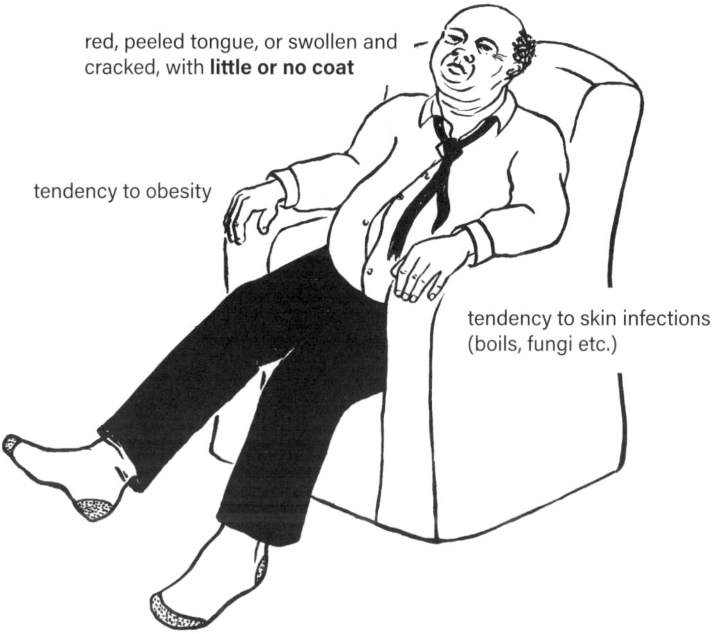

Dosage and method of administration

8-15 pills three times daily on an empty stomach. In severe cases or during the early stages of treatment, a 50% increase in dose can be used, then reduced to a maintenance dose (~8-12 pills three times daily) as treatment takes effect.

Cautions and contraindications

Contraindicated in patients with phlegm damp, phlegm heat, or any other excess heat pattern. Medication alone is insufficient to control type 2 diabetes. Prepared medicines are one part of a comprehensive treatment plan involving diet and exercise. Over time, requirements for hypoglycemic medications may decrease, however this must be allowed to occur naturally.

2.36 SUGARID

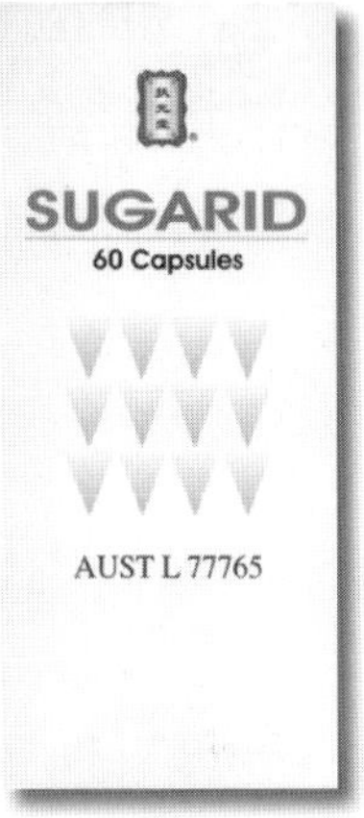

扶糖平胶囊

(*Fu Tang Ping Jiao Nang*)
Fu Yuan Tang Industrial Co. (Guangzhou)
'Assist [Blood] Glucose Capsules'
Sugarid is packaged in bottles of 60 capsules

Chinese medical action

Dries damp and transforms phlegm, clears heat, strengthens the Spleen

Biomedical action

Hypoglycemic, assists in lowering triglycerides and cholesterol, antioxidant, assists blood circulation

INDICATIONS

- Hyperglycemia, prediabetes, type 2 diabetes mellitus. This formula is based on modern pharmacological studies. Bitter buckwheat has been shown to be effective at reducing blood glucose and lipids, and to have antioxidant effects. Andrographis reduces blood glucose and its extreme bitterness stimulates the digestive process, in particular the digestion of fats, when used in relatively small doses.

Composition (each capsule contains herbal extracts equivalent to)

Fagopyrum esculentum (ku ji, bitter buckwheat) 11g, *Andrographis paniculata* (chuan xin lian, andrographis) 383mg, propolis 89mg

Combine with

- **2.35 Yu Quan Wan** for type 2 diabetes of a qi and yin deficient type
- **7.1 Liu Wei Di Huang Wan** for patients with Kidney yin deficiency
- **2.12 Shen Ling Bai Zhu Wan** for patients tending to more qi deficiency

Dosage and method of administration

3-5 capsules, three times daily, 20 minutes before meals.

Cautions and contraindications

Contraindicated during pregnancy. Propolis may cause allergic reactions in some people. Contraindicated in patients with allergy to bee stings, an atopic constitution and asthma.

2.37 HUAI JIAO DI YU WAN

槐角地榆丸

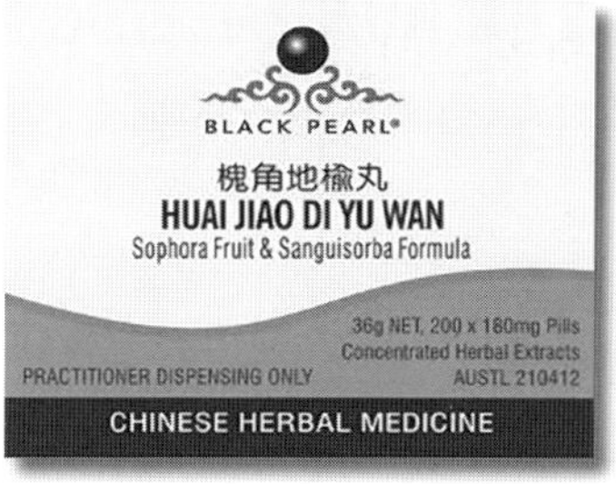

Sunherbal (Australia)
'Sophora and Sanguisorba Pills'
Huai Jiao Di Yu Wan is packaged in bottles of 200 pills
A formula with similar action is available as: Sophora Flower Formula (conc. extract)

Chinese medical action

Clears damp heat from the Large Intestine, stops bleeding, dispels wind, nourishes the blood

Biomedical action

Anti-inflammatory, analgesic, hemostatic

INDICATIONS

- Rectal bleeding of fresh blood prior to or following defecation, with blood on the stool or toilet paper. Often without pain, itch, distension or swelling. Technically known as 'Intestinal wind', this generally corresponds to the early stages of hemorrhoids.
- To alleviate discomfort and bleeding from for anal fissures and fistulas.

Composition

Sophora japonica (huai jiao, styphnolobioum fruit), *Sophora japonica* (huai hua mi, styphnolobioum flower bud), *Sanguisorba officinalis* (di yu, poterium), *Scutellaria baicalensis* (huang qin, scute), *Citrus aurantium* (zhi ke, aurantium), *Ledebouriella divaricata* (fang feng, siler), *Angelica polymorpha* (dang gui, chinese angelica), *Rehmannia glutinosa* (sheng di, rehmannia), *Panax notoginseng* (tian qi, tian qi ginseng)

Combine with

– **2.11 Bu Zhong Yi Qi Wan** for bleeding hemorrhoids from qi deficiency

Dosage and method of administration

8-12 pills three times daily on an empty stomach. The dose can be spread out, or taken in two lots of 12-18 pills, morning and evening. In severe cases, a 50% increase in dosage can be used until, bleeding stops, then reduced to a maintenance dose until fully resolved.

Cautions and contraindications

Contraindicated during pregnancy and in bleeding from yin deficiency.

2.38 HUA ZHI LING TABLET

强力化痔灵

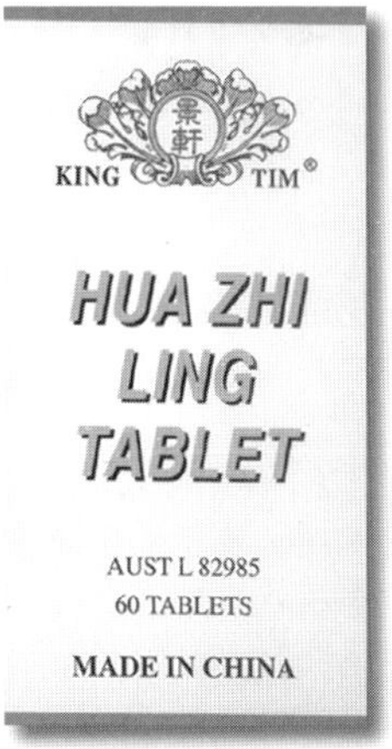

(*Qiang Li Hua Zhi Ling*)
Jing Xian Pharmaceutical Co. (Guangzhou)
'Extra Strength Miraculous Hemorrhoid Transforming Tablets'
Hua Zhi Ling Tablets are packaged in bottles of 60 sugar coated tablets

Chinese medical action

Clears damp heat from the Large Intestine, cools the blood and stops bleeding, invigorates blood and stops pain

Biomedical action

Anti-inflammatory, analgesic, hemostatic

INDICATIONS

- Hemorrhoids. For internal, external, thrombosed, inflamed, painful or bleeding hemorrhoids arising from damp heat accumulation in the Large Intestine with blood stasis. The inclusion of blood invigorating frankincense and myrrh increase the analgesic qualities of the formula, effectively alleviating pain associated with thrombosed hemorrhoids. There may or may not be systemic signs and symptoms of damp heat.
- Rectal bleeding associated with damp heat and/or blood stasis. This occurs in some inflammatory disorders of the Large Intestine.
- With the appropriate identifying features, this formula can be used to treat some conditions in addition to hemorrhoids, such as anal fissure, anal fistula, Crohn's disease and ulcerative colitis.

Composition (each tablet contains extracts equivalent to dry)

Angelica polymorpha (dang gui, chinese angelica) 390mg, *Sophora japonica* (huai hua, sophora flower bud) 300mg, *Agrimonia pilosa* (xian he cao, agrimony) 300mg, *Panax notoginseng* (tian qi, tian qi ginseng) 300mg, *Sanguisorba officinalis* (di yu, sanguisorba) 390mg, *Lonicera japonica* (jin yin hua, honeysuckle flower) 625mg, *Boswellia carteri* (ru xiang, frankincense) 12mg, *Commiphora myrrha* (mo yao, myrrh) 12mg

Combine with

- **13.14 Ching Wan Hung** or **2.40 Hemorrhoids Ointment** topically for inflamed or thrombosed hemorrhoids
- **14.1 Huang Lian Jie Du Wan** for severe damp heat
- **14.5 Chuan Xin Lian Antiphlogistic Tablets** or **14.6 Fu Fang Nan Ban Lan Gen** with severe inflammation
- **10.2 Raw Tienchi Tablets** for severe bleeding
- **10.21 Yan Hu Suo Zhi Tong Wan** for severe pain
- **10.5 Huo Luo Xiao Ling Dan** for severe blood stasis
- **6.3 Chai Hu Shu Gan Wan** for colitis, rectal bleeding and pain associated with Liver qi invading the Spleen and Intestines

Pattern identifying features

- **damp heat in the Large Intestine**
- tenesmus
- abdominal distension
- thirst
- concentrated urine
- tendency to constipation or sluggish loose stools

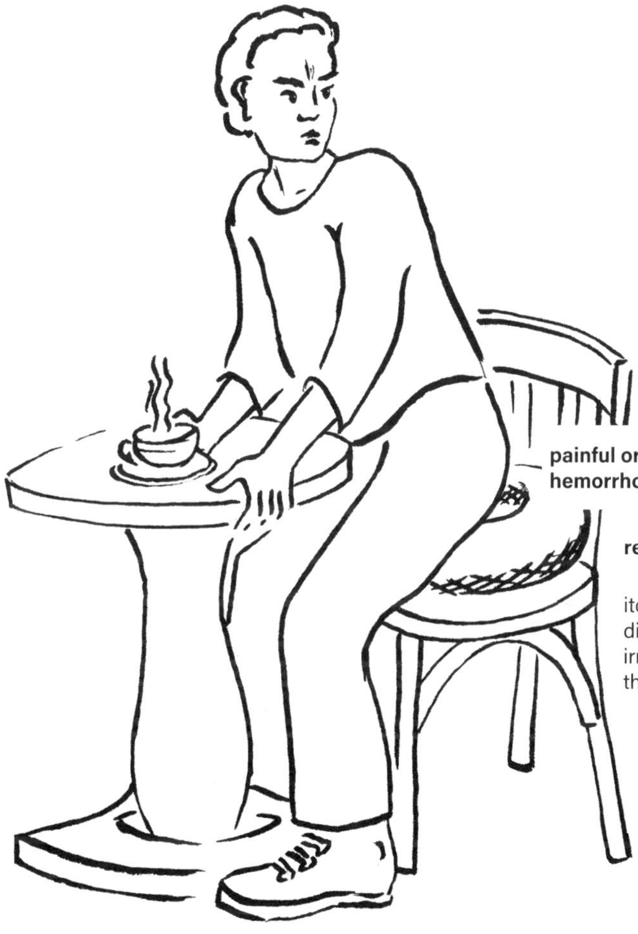

Dosage and method of administration

3-4 tablets three times daily on an empty stomach. One or two bottles is often enough to get a result, however in severe or very chronic cases, five or six bottles may be needed before a result is seen.

Cautions and contraindications

Contraindicated during pregnancy and in bleeding from yin deficiency.

2.39 FARGELIN FOR PILES

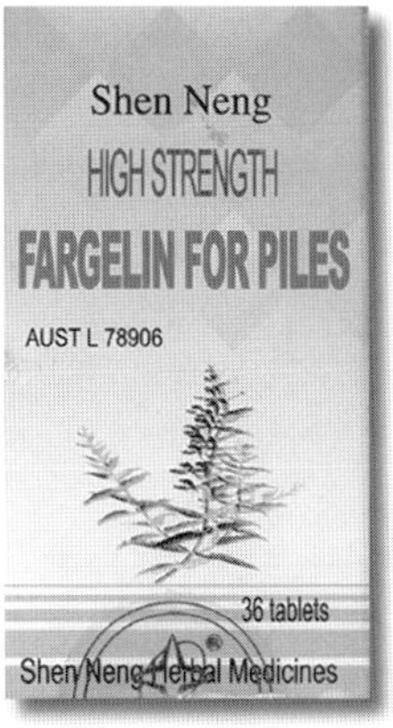

强力化痔灵

(*Qiang Li Hua Zhi Ling*)
Guangzhou Qixing Pharmaceutical Factory (Guangzhou)
'Extra Strength Miraculous Hemorrhoid Transforming Tablets'
Fargelin for Piles is packaged in bottles of 36 sugar coated tablets
A formula with similar action is available as: Fargelin Pills (PF)

Chinese medical action

Clears damp heat from the Large Intestine, cools the blood and stops bleeding, invigorates blood and stops pain

Biomedical action

Anti-inflammatory, analgesic, hemostatic

INDICATIONS

- As for **2.38 Hua Zhi Ling Tablet**. This formula is similar in overall action to **2.38 Hua Zhi Ling Tablet**, although it has slightly less blood invigorating activity and is slightly cooler.

Composition (each tablet contains extracts equivalent to dry)

Panax notoginseng (tian qi, tian qi ginseng) 400mg, *Scutellaria baicalensis* (huang qin, scute) 300mg, *Sanguisorba officinalis* (di yu, sanguisorba) 200mg, *Sophora japonica* (huai hua, sophora flower bud) 300mg, *Callicarpa pedunculata* (zi zhu cao, callicarpa) 300mg, *Corydalis turtschaninovii* (yan hu suo, corydalis) 100mg

Dosage and method of administration

3-4 tablets three times daily on an empty stomach. One or two bottles is often enough to get a result, however in severe or very chronic cases, five or six bottles may be needed before a result is seen.

Cautions and contraindications

Contraindicated during pregnancy and in bleeding from yin deficiency.

2.40 HEMORRHOIDS OINTMENT

特效痔疮膏

TGA

1-3/52

E

(*Te Xiao Zhi Chuang Gao*)
Jing Xian Pharmaceutical Co. (Guangzhou)
'Especially Effective Hemorrhoid Ointment'
Hemorrhoids Ointment is packaged in tubes of 20 grams

Chinese medical action

Clears damp heat from the Large Intestine, invigorates blood, stops bleeding, itch and pain

Biomedical action

Anti-inflammatory, analgesic, hemostatic

INDICATIONS

- Applied topically for relief of the discomfort, pain and itching of internal or external, thrombosed, inflamed, painful or bleeding hemorrhoids arising from damp heat accumulation in the Large Intestine.
- To relieve the discomfort and itching of anal lesions such as fissures and fistulas.

Composition (each 1 gram ointment contains extracts equivalent to dry)

Dryobalanops camphora (bing pian, borneol) 200mg, *Pinus massoniana* (hu po, amber) 840mg, *Sanguisorba officinalis* (di yu, sanguisorba) 840mg, *Sophora japonica* (huai jiao sophora fruit) 240mg, *Ostrea gigas* (mu li, oyster shell powder) 32mg

Dosage and method of administration

For external use only. Apply to the affected area, 3-4 times daily.

Cautions and contraindications

None noted.

肺病 3

Respiratory

3.1.1 YIN CHIAO CHIEH TU PIEN

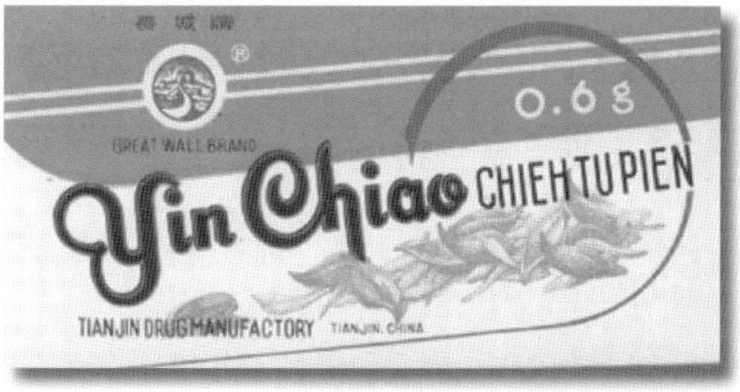

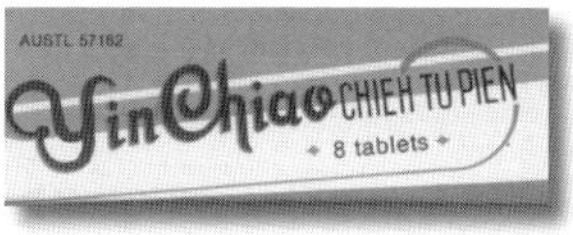

1-3/52

银翘解毒片

(*Yin Qiao Jie Du Pian*)
Tianjin Drug Manufactory (Shandong)
'Lonicera and Forsythia Antitoxic Pills'
Yin Chiao Chieh Tu Pien is packaged in vials of eight uncoated tablets, ten vials to a box
Also available as: Lonicera and Forsythia Formula (conc. powder)

Chinese medical action
Dispels wind heat, clears toxic heat

Biomedical action
Antipyretic, diaphoretic, anti-inflammatory, antiviral

INDICATIONS

- Wind heat common cold. The most important formula for the acute phase (the first few days) of a wind heat invasion or warm disease (*see* glossary). Conditions classified as wind heat or warm disease include acute upper respiratory tract infections, (viral or bacterial), the common cold, the early stage of influenza, tonsillitis, conjunctivitis, the acute phase of disorders such as otitis media and mumps, and the viral rash diseases of childhood, such as measles and chicken pox.
- Acute itchy red skin diseases such as urticaria, eczema and dermatitis. The rashes that may be treated by this formula usually affect the upper body and are characterized by redness, heat and itch which start suddenly and may move quickly from place to place.

Composition **(each tablet contains extracts equivalent to dry)**
Lonicera japonica (jin yin hua, lonicera) 1.33g, *Forsythia suspensa* (lian qiao, forsythia) 1.33g, *Arctium lappa* (niu bang zi, burdock seeds) 813mg, *Mentha haplocalyx* (bo he, mint) 739mg, *Lophatherum gracile* (dan zhu ye, bamboo leaves) 517mg, *Schizonepeta tenuifolia* (jing jie, schizonepeta) 517mg, *Glycine max* (dou chi, prepared soybean) 66mg, *Platycodon grandiflorum* (jie geng, platycodon) 65mg, *Glycyrrhiza uralensis* (gan cao, licorice) 53mg

Combine with
- **9.9 Superior Sore Throat Powder** topically for acute sore throat
- **14.5 Chuan Xin Lian Antiphlogistic Tablets** for itchy chicken pox
- **2.2 Huo Hsiang Cheng Chi Pien** for wind heat sinus congestion or hay fever
- **13.2 Xiao Feng Wan** for very acute itchy urticaria or nettle rash

Pattern identifying features

- **wind heat common cold**
- fever, mild (or absent) chills

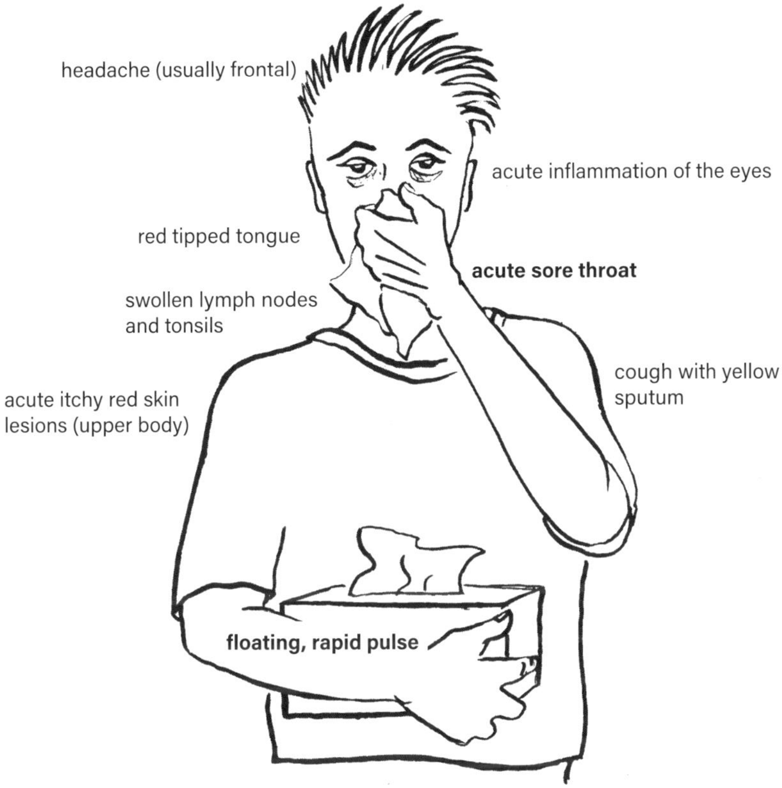

Dosage and method of administration

The adult dose of **3.1.1 Yin Chiao Chieh Tu Pien** is eight tablets (one vial) 3-4 times daily, or in severe cases, every 2 hours. Not suitable for younger children due to the dimensions of the tablet. For wind heat common cold in small children, see **12.7 Xiao Er Gan Mao Chong Ji**.

Cautions and contraindications

Not suitable for wind cold type colds or flu characterized by dominant chills, muscle aches and an absence of sweating (*see* **3.5 Ma Huang Tang** or **3.9 Chuan Xiong Cha Tiao Wan** for that problem)

3.1.2 YIN CHIAO JIE DU PIAN

银翘解毒片

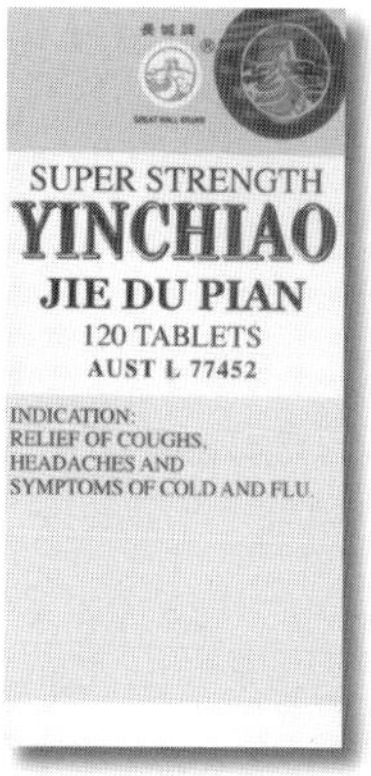

Tianjin Drug Manufactory (Shandong)
'Tianjin Lonicera and Forsythia Antitoxic Pills'
Yin Chiao Jie Du Pian is packaged in bottles of 120 coated pills
Also available as: Tianjin Yin Chiao Plus

Chinese medical action

Dispels wind heat, clears toxic heat

Biomedical action

Antipyretic, diaphoretic, anti-inflammatory, antiviral

INDICATIONS

- Same indications as for **3.1.1 Yin Chiao Chieh Tu Pien**. This formula includes the heat clearing *Procaprea gutterosa pallas* (goat horn). This addition makes this version, **3.1.2 Yin Chiao Jie Du Pian**, slightly more cooling, even though the total amount of herb per dose is smaller.

Composition (each tablet contains)

Lonicera japonica (jin yin hua, lonicera) 1.04g, *Forsythia suspensa* (lian qiao, forsythia) 1.04g, *Mentha haplocalyx* (bo he, mint) 626mg, *Glycine max* (dou chi, prepared soybean) 520mg, *Schizonepeta tenuifolia* (jing jie, schizonepeta) 416mg, *Lophatherum gracile* (dan zhu ye, bamboo leaves) 416mg, *Platycodon grandiflorum* (jie geng, platycodon) 63mg, *Glycyrrhiza uralensis* (gan cao, licorice) 52mg, *Procaprea gutterosa pallas* (goat horn) 3.24mg

Combine with

– As for **3.1.1 Yin Chiao Chieh Tu Pien**

Dosage and method of administration

The adult dose of **3.1.2 Yin Chiao Jie Du Pian** is 2-4 tablets 3-4 times daily; in severe cases take a dose every 2 hours. Take on an empty stomach. Half dose for children 8-12 years old. Not suitable for younger children due to the dimensions of the tablet. For wind heat patterns in small children, see **12.7 Xiao Er Gan Mao Chong Ji**.

Cautions and contraindications

– As for **3.1.1 Yin Chiao Chieh Tu Pien**.

3.1.3 YIN CHIAO JIE DU WAN

银翘解毒丸

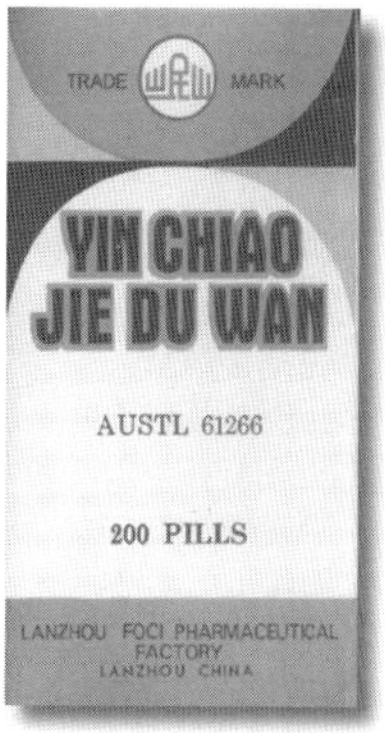

Lanzhou Foci Pharmaceutical Factory (Gansu)
'Lonicera and Forsythia Antitoxic Pills'
Yin Chiao Jie Du Wan is packaged in bottles of 200 pills

Chinese medical action
Dispels wind heat, clears toxic heat

Biomedical action
Antipyretic, diaphoretic, anti-inflammatory, antiviral

INDICATIONS
- As for **3.1.1 Yin Chiao Chieh Tu Pien**.

Composition (each pill contains powdered)
Lonicera japonica (jin yin hua, lonicera) 28.5mg, *Forsythia suspensa* (lian qiao, forsythia) 28.5mg, *Arctium lappa* (niu bang zi, burdock seeds) 17.3mg, *Mentha haplocalyx* (bo he, mint) 17.3mg, *Platycodon grandiflorum* (jie geng, platycodon) 14.2mg, *Glycyrrhiza uralensis* (gan cao, licorice) 14.2mg, *Schizonepeta tenuifolia* (jing jie, schizonepeta) 11.4mg, *Lophatherum gracile* (dan zhu ye, bamboo leaves) 11.4mg

Combine with
– As for **3.1.1 Yin Chiao Chieh Tu Pien**

Dosage and method of administration
8-12 pills three to five times daily on an empty stomach. Not suitable for younger children due to the number of pills required. For wind heat patterns in small children, see **12.7 Xiao Er Gan Mao Chong Ji**.

Cautions and contraindications
– As for **3.1.1 Yin Chiao Chieh Tu Pien**.

3.1.4 PEKING YIN CHIAO JIE DU PIAN

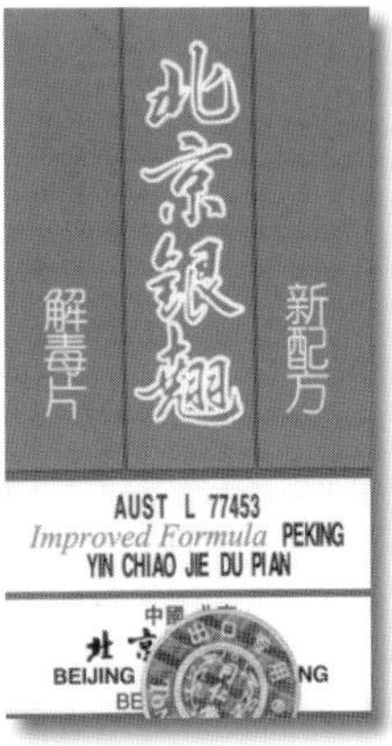

北京银翘

(*Bei Jing Yin Qiao*)
Tong Ren Tang (Beijing)
'Beijing Lonicera and Forsythia Antitoxic Pills'
Peking Yin Chiao Jie Du Pian is packaged in bottles of 50 tablets

Chinese medical action
Dispels wind heat, clears toxic heat

Biomedical action
Antipyretic, diaphoretic, anti-inflammatory, antiviral

INDICATIONS
- As for **3.1.1 Yin Chiao Chieh Tu Pien.**

Composition (each tablet contains)
Lonicera japonica (jin yin hua, lonicera) 1.33g, *Forsythia suspensa* (lian qiao, forsythia) 1.2g, *Mentha haplocalycis* (bo he, mint) 600mg, *Schizonepeta tenuifolia* (jing jie, schizonepeta) 600mg, *Platycodon grandiflorum* (jie geng, platycodon) 600mg, *Procaprea gutterosa pallas* (goat horn) 1.2mg,

Combine with
– As for **3.1.1 Yin Chiao Chieh Tu Pien.**

Dosage and method of administration
2-4 tablets, twice daily. In severe cases, 2-4 tablets may be taken every 2-3 hours. Half dose for children 8-12 years old. Not suitable for younger children due to the dimensions of the tablet. For wind heat patterns in small children, see **12.7 Xiao Er Gan Mao Chong Ji.**

Cautions and contraindications
– As for **3.1.1 Yin Chiao Chieh Tu Pien.**

3.1.5 INFLUENZA AND COLD RELIEVER

银翘解毒片

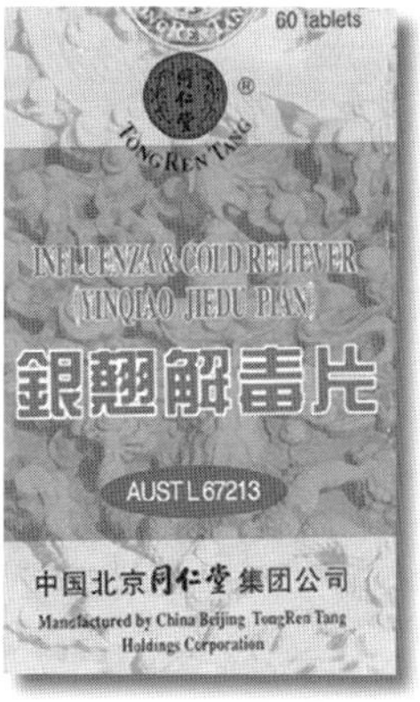

(*Yin Qiao Jie Du Pian*)
Tong Ren Tang (Beijing)
'Lonicera and Forsythia Antitoxic Pills'
Influenza and Cold Reliever is packaged in bottles of 60 tablets

Chinese medical action

Dispels wind heat, clears toxic heat

Biomedical action

Antipyretic, diaphoretic, anti-inflammatory, antiviral

INDICATIONS

- As for **3.1.1 Yin Chiao Chieh Tu Pien**.

Composition (each tablet contains)

Lonicera japonica (jin yin hua, lonicera) 200g, *Forsythia suspensa* (lian qiao, forsythia) 200g, *Platycodon grandiflorum* (jie geng, platycodon) 120mg, *Arctium lappa* (niu bang zi, burdock seeds) 120mg, *Glycine max* (dou chi, prepared soybean) 100mg, *Lophatherum gracile* (dan zhu ye, bamboo leaves) 80.7mg, *Mentha haplocalyx* (bo he, mint essential oil) 1.1mg, *Schizonepeta tenuifolia* (jing jie, schizonepeta essential oil) 762mcg

Combine with

– As for **3.1.1 Yin Chiao Chieh Tu Pien**.

Dosage and method of administration

4 tablets, 2-3 times daily. In severe cases, a dose may be taken every 2-3 hours. Half dose for children 8-12 years old. Not suitable for younger children due to the dimensions of the tablet. For wind heat patterns in small children, see **12.7 Xiao Er Gan Mao Chong Ji**.

Cautions and contraindications

– As for **3.1.1 Yin Chiao Chieh Tu Pien**.

GMP

3.2 GAN MAO ZHI KE CHONG JI

感冒止咳冲剂

1/52

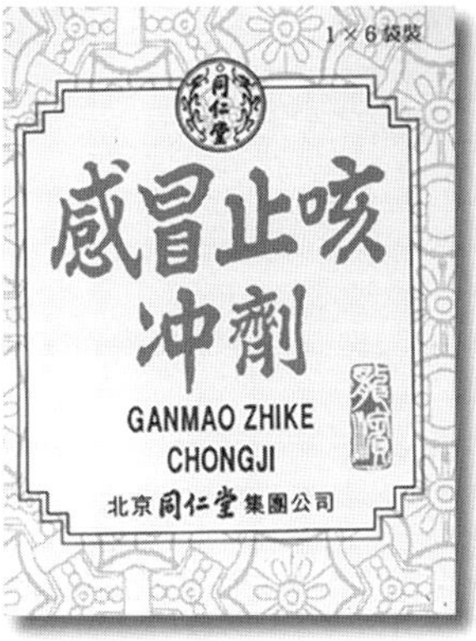

Tong Ren Tang (Beijing)
'Cough and Cold Granules'
Gan Mao Zhi Ke Chong Ji is packaged in 10 gram sachets of soluble granules, six sachets per box

Chinese medical action

Dispels wind heat, stops cough, harmonizes *shào yáng*

Biomedical action

Antipyretic, expectorant, diaphoretic

INDICATIONS

- Acute wind heat common cold with cough.
- *Shào yáng* syndrome, or *tài yáng/shào yáng* overlap patterns. This type of disorder occurs in the post acute phase (around 3-7 days after onset) of an exterior syndrome as the pathogen begins to penetrate further into the body. The speed of change depends on the strength of the pathogen and the vitality of the patient. The symptoms in the *tài yáng/shào yáng* overlap pattern display a mixture of both levels.
- As an adjunct formula, combined with a constitutional formula, for any acute heat disorder that exhibits alternating fever and chills. This may include conditions such as acute urinary tract infection, mastitis and pelvic inflammatory disease.

Composition

Bupleurum sinensis (chai hu, bupleurum) 19.99%, *Pueraria lobata* (ge gen, pueraria) 19.99%, *Scutellaria baicalensis* (huang qin, scute) 15%, *Forsythia suspensa* (lian qiao, forsythia) 15%, *Artemesia annua* (qing hao, artemesia) 10%, *Platycodon grandiflorum* (jie geng, platycodon) 10%, *Lonicera japonica* (jin yin hua, lonicera) 10%, Menthol 0.02%

Combine with

- **9.9 Superior Sore Throat Powder** topically for severe sore throat
- **3.25 Nin Jiom Pei Pa Kao** for dry irritating cough
- **14.5 Chuan Xin Lian Antiphlogistic Tablets** for acute mastitis with alternating fever and chills
- **4.6 Ba Zheng San Wan** for acute urinary tract infection with alternating fever and chills
- **1.36 Fu Yan Qing Tablet** for acute pelvic infection with alternating fever and chills

Pattern identifying features

- **wind heat common cold; *tài yáng-shào yáng* overlap patterns**
- mild fever, or **alternating fever and chills**
- acute or post acute phase of wind heat invasion
- fatigue

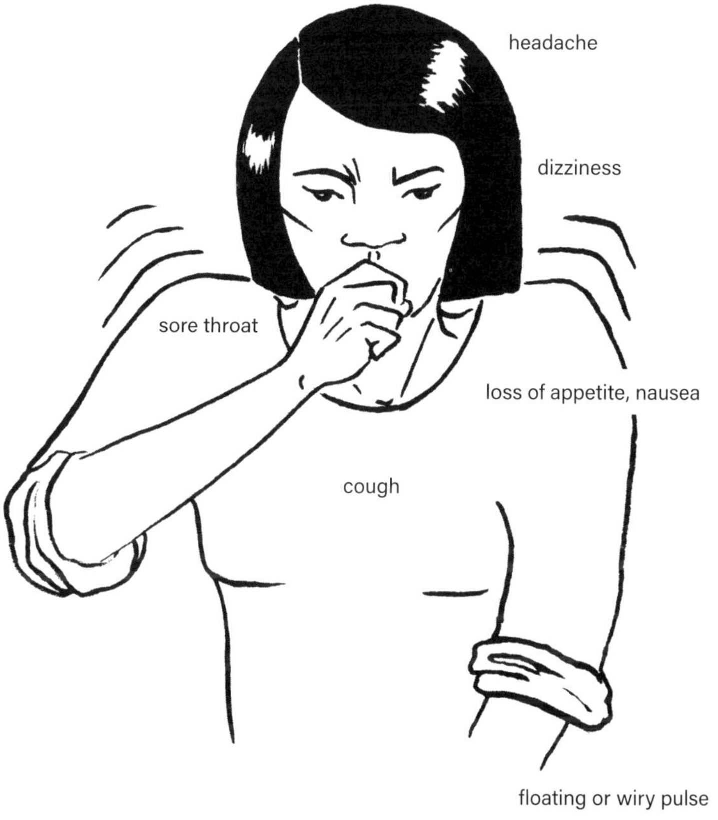

Dosage and method of administration

The recommended dose is one sachet dissolved in hot water 3-6 times daily depending on the severity of the symptoms. Half dose for children.

Cautions and contraindications

Not suitable for acute wind cold patterns (*see* **3.5 Ma Huang Tang**, **3.8 Xiao Qing Long Wan**, **3.9 Chuan Xiong Cha Tiao Wan** or **3.7 Su Zi Jiang Qi Wan**).

3.3 SANG JU WAN

桑菊丸

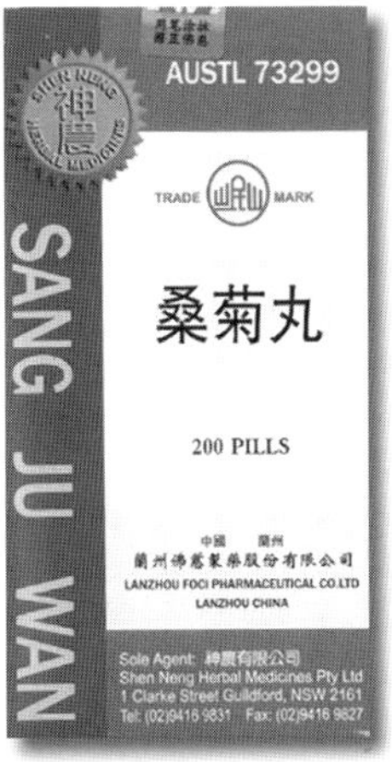

Lanzhou Foci Pharmaceutical Factory (Gansu)
'Mulberry Leaf and Chrysanthemum Pills'
Sang Ju Wan is packaged in bottles of 200 pills
Also available as: Clear Wind Heat Teapills (PF), Sang Ju Yin Wan–Early Defence Formula (JD), Mulberry and Chrysanthemum Combination (conc. extract)

Chinese medical action

Dispels wind heat, cools and moistens the Lungs, stops cough

Biomedical action

Antipyretic, antitussive, diaphoretic

INDICATIONS

- Acute cough from mild to moderate wind heat common cold. The main features are dry cough, slight fever, thirst, a white tongue coat and a floating, rapid pulse. Similar in action to **3.1.1 Yin Chiao Chieh Tu Pien** but with less diaphoretic and heat clearing action and more emphasis on stopping the cough. Also used to moisten the Lungs for cough associated with external dryness.
- Wind heat eye disorders, with redness and pain.

Composition (each pill contains powdered)

Phragmites communis (lu gen, reed rhizome) 32.7mg, *Morus alba* (sang ye, mulberry leaf) 22.9mg, *Chrysanthemum sinense* (ju hua, chrysanthemum flower) 22.9mg, *Platycodon grandiflorum* (jie geng, platycodon) 22.9mg, *Forsythia suspensa* (lian qiao, forsythia) 22.9mg, *Prunus armeniaca* (xing ren, apricot seed) 19.6mg, *Glycyrrhiza uralensis* (gan cao, licorice) 8.2mg, *Mentha haplocalycis* (bo he, mint) 8.2mg

Dosage and method of administration

8-12 pills three to five times daily, on an empty stomach.

Cautions and contraindications

Not suitable for wind cold type colds or flu characterized by dominant chills, muscle aches and absence of sweating.

3.4 GAN MAO LING

感冒灵

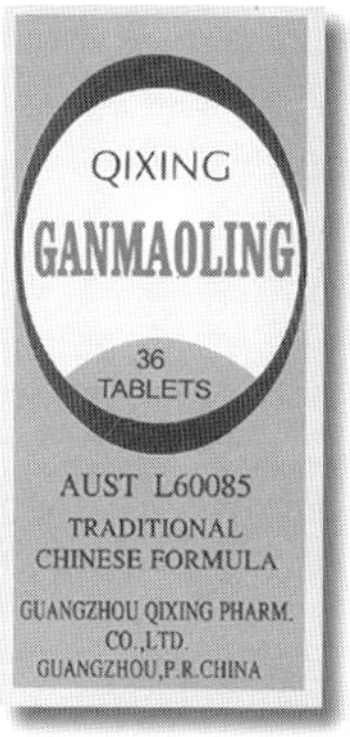

Guangzhou Qixing Pharmaceutical Co. (Guangzhou)
'Miraculous Common Cold Pills'
Gan Mao Ling is packaged in bottles of 36 tablets

Chinese medical action

Dispels wind, clears toxic heat

Biomedical action

Antipyretic, antiviral

INDICATIONS

- Acute external wind (and either heat or mild cold, but best for heat, mixed or unclear) common cold patterns. The herbs in this unusual formula are all toxic heat clearing and, in biomedical terms, antiviral.
- Used for the common cold, influenza, acute upper respiratory tract infections, mild bronchitis, tracheitis and tonsillitis.

Composition (each pill contains extracts equivalent to dry)

Ilex aquifolium (english holly) 1.2g, *Evodia lepta* (san jiao bie) 765mg, *Chrysanthemum indicum* (ye ju hua, wild chrysanthemum) 450.7mg, *Vitex negrundo* (mu jing ye, chinese vitex) 450.7mg, *Isatis tinctora* (ban lan gen, isatis) 450.7mg, *Lonicera japonica* (jin yin hua, lonicera) 166mg

Dosage and method of administration

The recommended dose is four tablets, three times daily, however in most cases the dose can be doubled or tripled for a swift effect. Take on an empty stomach.

Cautions and contraindications

Not suitable for severe wind cold patterns (*see* **3.5 Ma Huang Tang**, **3.8 Xiao Qing Long Wan**, **3.9 Chuan Xiong Cha Tiao Wan** or **3.7 Su Zi Jiang Qi Wan**).

GMP

3.5 MA HUANG TANG

麻黄汤

1/52

Vitapharm USA
'Ephedra Decoction'
Ma Huang Tang is packaged in bottles of 90 capsules
Also available as: Ephedra Combination (conc. extract)

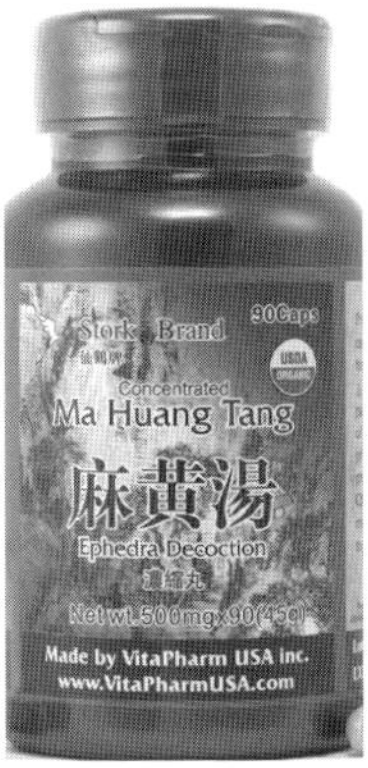

Chinese medical action

Dispels wind cold, directs Lung qi downwards, stops wheezing

Biomedical action

Diaphoretic, anti-asthmatic, diuretic

INDICATIONS

- Wind cold common cold with wheezing and cough. A strong diaphoretic formula, **3.5 Ma Huang Tang** is indicated for wind cold common cold with the cold firmly lodged in the *tài yáng* superficial layers of the body. This is described as 'wind cold with exterior excess' (*shāng hán biǎo shí* 伤寒表实). The cold, by 'freezing and constricting' shuts and locks the pores behind it, hence the key features of mild fever with prominent chills and no sweating, muscle and joint aches, occipital headache, cough and wheezing and a floating tight pulse.
- Wind cold acute edema. Edema of this type occurs because normal distribution of fluids is retarded by obstruction to Lung qi descent and diffusion, and closure of the pores by a wind cold pathogen. Edema begins abruptly, first affecting the orbits and face, accompanied by scanty urination and wind cold pattern identifying features opposite.
- Cold induced urticaria. This occurs on parts of the body exposed to cold, such as the hands and forearms of those frequently in and out of fridges and freezers.
- Acute wind cold painful obstruction.
- With the appropriate identifying features this formula can assist in the treatment of conditions such as acute asthma, asthmatic bronchitis, the common cold, influenza, acute glomerulonephritis and urticaria.

Composition

Ephedra sinica (ma huang*, ephedra), *Cinnamomum cassia* (gui zhi, cinnamon twigs), *Prunus armenica* (xing ren, apricot seed), *Glycyrrhiza uralensis* (zhi gan cao, honey fried licorice) [**Restricted use in some jurisdictions; may be subject to substitution*]

Dosage and method of administration

For acute wind cold patterns the dose is 8-12 pills every two hours or so, on an empty stomach. The pills can be taken with hot soup or rice and ginger porridge to encourage sweat. Following a dose with a hot bath to encourage sweat is beneficial.

Pattern identifying features

- **wind cold common cold (exterior excess); cold dominant**
- **no sweating**
- simultaneous fever and chills; chills more prominent than fever

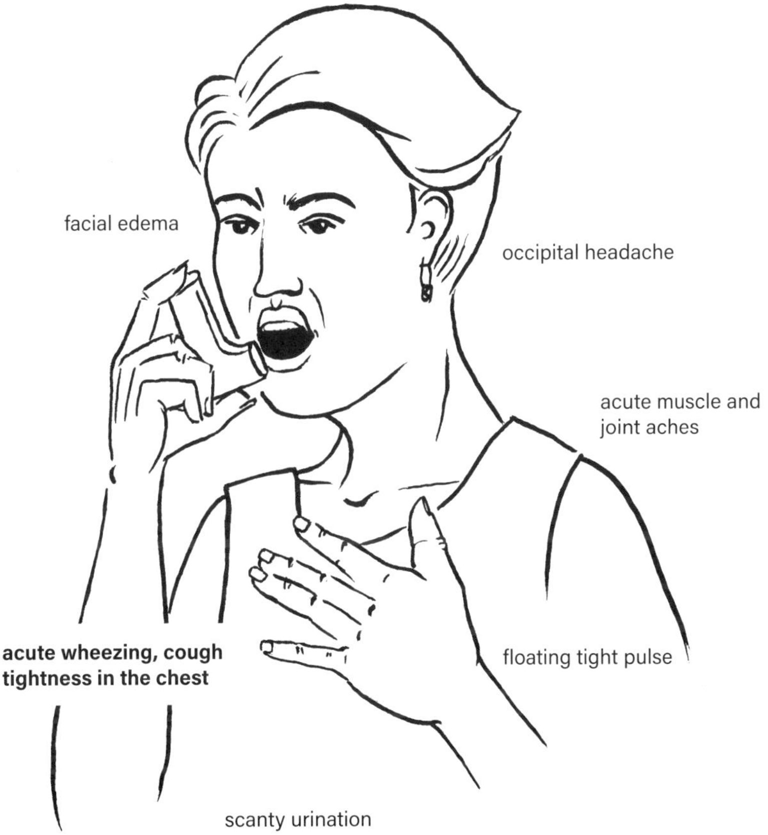

Cautions and contraindications

Contraindicated in wind cold patterns with sweating (*see* **3.6 Gui Zhi Wan**), wind heat induced wheezing and in patients with frequent urination and general debility. Caution in patients with hypertension. May cause or aggravate insomnia in some patients due to presence of ephedra. Suitable for short term use only.

GMP

3.6 GUI ZHI WAN

1-3/12

桂枝丸

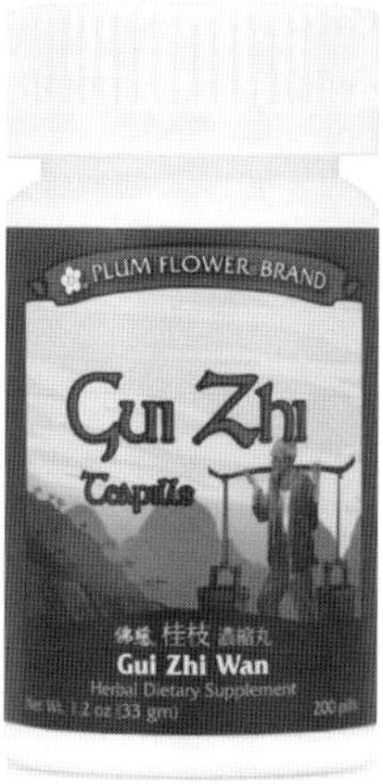

Lanzhou Foci Pharmaceutical Factory (Gansu)
'Cinnamon Twig Pills'
Gui Zhi Wan is packaged in bottles of 200 pills
Available as: Cinnamon Combination (conc. extract)

Chinese medical action

Dispels wind from the exterior, balances nutritive and defensive qi, harmonizes the Spleen and Stomach

Biomedical action

Mild diaphoretic, antispasmodic

INDICATIONS

- Wind cold common cold with wind predominant. Also used for wind cold in patients with preexisting weak defensive qi that is unable to keep the pores closed. In contrast to **3.5 Ma Huang Tang**, which is preferred for a *tài yáng* invasion with exterior excess, this formula is for *tài yáng* invasion with exterior deficiency (*zhòng fēng biǎo xū* 中风表虚). This manifests in mild or lingering upper respiratory tract disorders that are unrelieved by diaphoresis, characterized by sweating or clamminess, aversion to wind, mild fever and chills, fatigue, nasal congestion, loss of appetite, dry retching and a floating moderate or weak pulse. Patients prone to this type of pattern are typically run down, convalescing or debilitated in some way.
- Itchy dry skin diseases initiated or aggravated by cold weather, exposure to cold water, that recur each Winter and that are not red or inflamed. Also indicated for the sensation of 'worms or insects crawling under the skin'.
- Cold type pain in the joints, extremities, epigastrium and abdomen; numbness in the extremities and skin.
- With the appropriate identifying features, this formula can assist in the treatment of conditions such as the common cold, the common cold in the debilitated, postpartum fever, postpartum colds, morning sickness, allergic rhinitis, eczema, urticaria, idiopathic pruritus, frostbite, neuralgia, sciatica and rheumatism.

Composition

Cinnamomum cassia (gui zhi, cinnamon twigs), *Paeonia lactiflora* (bai shao, white peony), *Zingiber officinale* (sheng jiang, ginger), *Zizyphus jujuba* (da zao, chinese dates), *Glycyrrhiza uralensis* (zhi gan cao, honey fried licorice)

Pattern identifying features

- **wind cold common cold (exterior deficiency); wind dominant**
- mild fever and chills
- aversion to wind
- no thirst

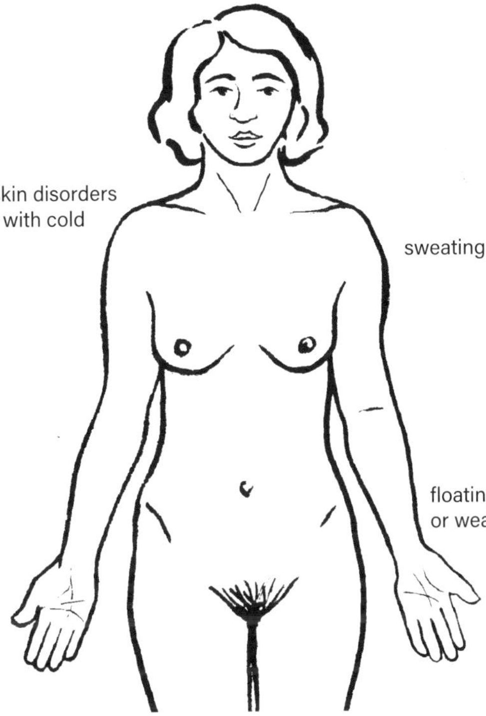

Combine with

- **10.22 Shao Yao Gan Cao Wan** for wind invasion with more severe abdominal pain
- **6.1 Xiao Chai Hu Wan** for *tài yáng – shào yáng* overlap syndrome, abdominal pain due to Liver and Spleen disharmony, wind damp joint pain or creaking in the joints

Dosage and method of administration

8-12 pills, three times daily on an empty stomach. The pills can be taken with hot soup or rice and ginger porridge to encourage mild sweating.

Cautions and contraindications

Contraindicated in exterior excess patterns (*see* **3.5 Ma Huang Tang**, **3.8 Xiao Qing Long Wan**, or **3.9 Chuan Xiong Cha Tiao Wan**), external cold with internal heat patterns, wind heat, acute warm or damp heat patterns, internal heat and yin deficiency.

3.7 SU ZI JIANG QI WAN

苏子降气丸

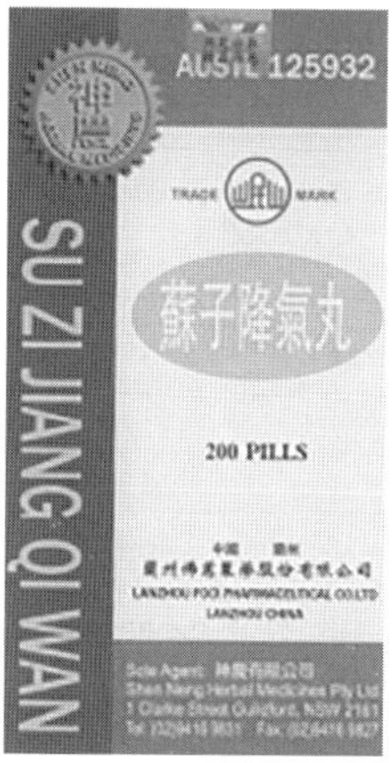

Lanzhou Foci Pharmaceutical Factory (Gansu)
'Perilla Seed Pills to Redirect Qi Downwards'
Su Zi Jiang Qi Wan is packaged in bottles of 200 pills
Also available as: Perilla Seed Combination (conc. extract)

Chinese medical action

Redirects Lung qi downwards, stops cough and wheezing, warms and transforms thin phlegm

Biomedical action

Anti-asthmatic, antitussive, mucolytic, expectorant

INDICATIONS

- Acute and chronic coughing and wheeze from wind cold with accumulation of phlegm damp or cold phlegm in the Lungs. Used for acute patterns with clear signs of exterior wind cold, and chronic patterns where the phlegm damp accumulation is primary. In either case, the sputum is copious and thin or watery. The formula is warming and drying in nature and its main focus is on transforming and expelling phlegm, and encouraging the downward movement of Lung qi.
- With the appropriate identifying features, this formula can be used to treat disorders such as acute and chronic asthma, chronic bronchitis and emphysema.

Composition (each pill contains powdered)

Perilla frutescens (su zi, perilla seed) 24.24mg, *Pinellia ternata* (zhi ban xia, processed pinellia) 24.24mg, *Prunus armenica* (xing ren, apricot seed) 21mg, *Peucedanum decursivum* (qian hu, peucedanum) 19.4mg, *Magnolia officinalis* (hou po, magnolia bark) 19.4mg, *Angelica polymorpha* (dang gui, chinese angelica) 16.2mg, *Ephedra sinica* (ma huang*, ephedra) 12.9mg, *Aquilaria agallocha* (chen xiang, aquilaria) 12.9mg, *Glycyrrhiza uralensis* (gan cao, licorice) 9.7mg [**Restricted use in some jurisdictions; may be subject to substitution*]

Combine with

- **3.30 Tong Xuan Li Fei Kou Fu Ye** for marked dyspnea with copious sputum or obvious rattles and rales, used until sputum starts to break up
- **2.22 Er Chen Wan** for very thick or hard to expectorate sputum

Pattern identifying features

- **wind cold with phlegm damp/cold accumulation in the Lungs**
- **wheezing, dyspnea**
- breathlessness

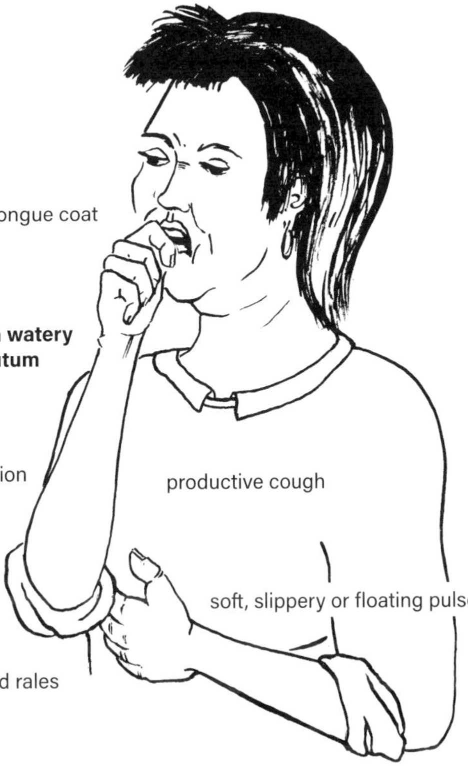

Dosage and method of administration

8-12 pills three times daily on an empty stomach. Half dose for children. In severe cases or during the early stages of treatment (the first 7-10 days), a 50% increase in dose can be used, then reduced to a maintenance dose as treatment takes effect.

Cautions and contraindications

Contraindicated in cases of wheezing, breathlessness and asthma from heat in the Lungs or Lung yin deficiency. Caution in patients with hypertension. May cause or aggravate insomnia in some patients due to presence of ephedra.

3.8 XIAO QING LONG WAN

小青龙丸

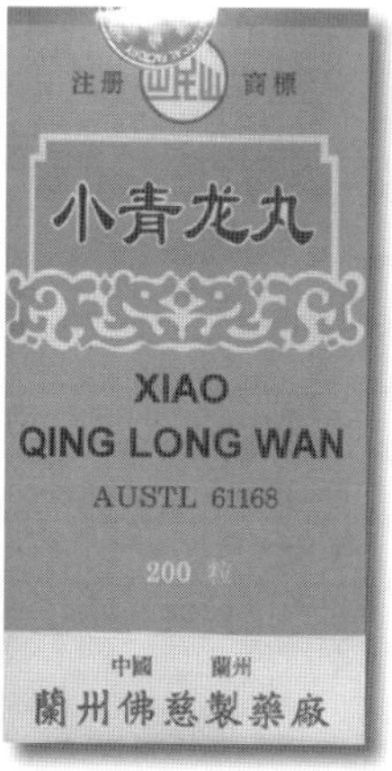

Lanzhou Foci Pharmaceutical Factory (Gansu)
'Minor Blue Green Dragon Pills'
Xiao Qing Long Wan is packaged in bottles of 200 pills
Also available as: Minor Blue Dragon Combination (conc. extract)

Chinese medical action

Dispels wind cold, warms the Lungs and transforms phlegm and thin mucus, directs qi downward, stops wheezing

Biomedical action

Diaphoretic, anti-asthmatic, antitussive, expectorant

INDICATIONS

- Wind cold type common cold with congested thin fluids. The main feature of this formula is its ability to warm, dry and transform fluids, and improve fluid metabolism. Preexisting fluids from Lung and Spleen deficiency are stirred up by the wind cold, or fluids accumulate as descent of Lung qi is blocked by the pathogen.
- Acute episodes of hay fever and other atopic conditions characterized by copious discharge of thin watery fluids from the nasal sinuses, eyes or lungs.
- With the appropriate identifying features, this formula can be used to treat conditions such as the common cold, influenza, asthma, asthmatic bronchitis, acute exacerbation of chronic bronchitis, emphysema and hay fever.

Composition

Paeonia lactiflora (bai shao, white peony), *Pinellia ternata* (zhi ban xia, processed pinellia), *Cinnamomum cassia* (gui zhi, cinnamon twigs), *Schizandra chinensis* (wu wei zi, schizandra), *Ephedra sinica* (ma huang*, ephedra), *Zingiber officinale* (gan jiang, dry ginger), *Asarum seiboldi* (xi xin*, asarum), *Glycyrrhiza uralensis* (gan cao, licorice) [**Restricted use in some jurisdictions; may be subject to substitution*]

Combine with

- **3.30 Tong Xuan Li Fei Kou Fu Ye** for marked dyspnea with copious sputum and obvious rattles and rales, used until sputum starts to break up
- **2.22 Er Chen Wan** for copious sputum and difficulty lying flat (orthopnea)

Dosage and method of administration

8-15 pills three times daily on an empty stomach. For acute wind cold common cold patterns the pills can be taken with hot soup or rice and ginger porridge to encourage sweating. It is also of benefit to follow a dose with a hot bath. In severe cases or during the early stages of treatment, a 50% increase in dose can be used, then reduced to a maintenance dose (~8-12 pills three times daily) as treatment takes effect.

Pattern identifying features

- **wind cold common cold with copious thin phlegm**
- **no sweating**
- simultaneous fever and chills; chills more prominent than fever

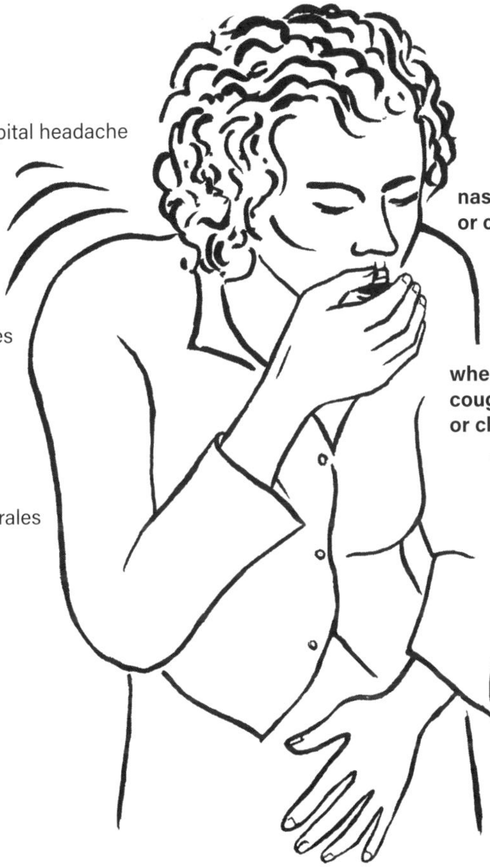

Cautions and contraindications

Not suitable for long term use. Contraindicated in cases of wheezing, breathlessness, asthma and hay fever arising from qi and yin deficiency, or heat in the Lungs.

Contraindicated in wind cold exterior deficiency patterns with sweating (*see* **3.6 Gui Zhi Wan**). Caution in patients with hypertension. May cause or aggravate insomnia in some patients due to presence of ephedra.

3.9 CHUAN XIONG CHA TIAO WAN

川芎茶调丸

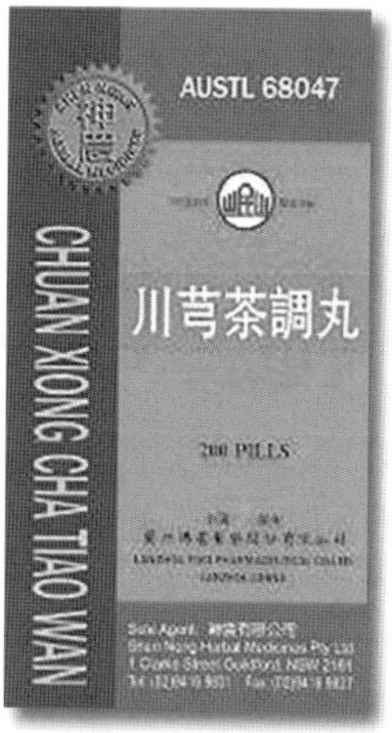

1-3/52

Lanzhou Foci Pharmaceutical Factory (Gansu)
'Ligusticum and Tea Regulating Pills'
Chuan Xiong Cha Tiao Wan is packaged in bottles of 200 pills
Also available as: Chuan Xiong Wan (PF), Ligusticum and Tea Formula (conc. extract)

Chinese medical action

Dispels wind cold, stops pain, invigorates the circulation of qi and blood in the face and head

Biomedical action

Antipyretic, diaphoretic, analgesic

INDICATIONS

- Headache and neck stiffness from acute external wind invasion. While considered best for wind cold patterns, this formula is quite well balanced and can be used for wind heat or wind damp patterns with headache, especially when combined with a specific wind heat or damp formula.
- Headache (either acute, chronic or recurrent, including migraines) or facial pain triggered by sudden exposure to cold, changes in weather or by going from a warm to a cold environment. Acute frontal headaches associated with sinus congestion, sinusitis and rhinitis, as long as the nasal discharge is watery or white.
- With the appropriate identifying features, this formula can be used to treat conditions such as acute upper respiratory tract infection, the common cold, influenza, acute rhinitis, trigeminal neuralgia, migraine headaches, tension headaches, neurogenic headaches, acute torticollis and Bell's palsy.

Composition (each pill contains powdered)

Ligusticum wallici (chuan xiong, ligusticum), *Mentha haplocalycis* (bo he, mint), *Schizonepeta tenuifolia* (jing jie, schizonepeta), *Notopterygium incisum* (qiang huo, notopterygium), *Angelica dahurica* (bai zhi, angelica), *Glycyrrhiza uralensis* (gan cao, licorice), *Ledebouriella divaricata* (fang feng, siler), *Cinnamomum cassia* (gui zhi, cinnamon twigs)

Combine with

- **15.9 Headache and Dizziness Reliever** for severe occipital headache
- **9.18 Xin Yi San** for acute frontal headache, rhinitis or sinus congestion from wind cold invasion
- **3.4 Gan Mao Ling** or **3.3 Sang Ju Wan** for wind heat patterns
- **3.10 Jing Fang Bai Du Wan** for wind damp patterns

Pattern identifying features

- **external wind invasion common cold with headache**
- pain initiated or aggravated by exposure to cold or sudden changes of temperature
- chills, mild fever
- no sweating

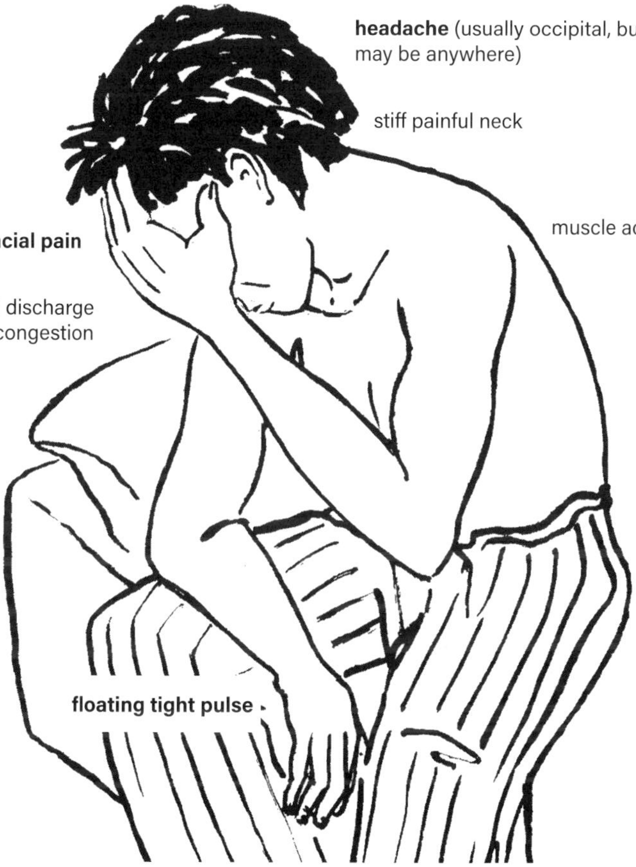

Dosage and method of administration

For acute wind cold patterns the dose is 8-12 pills every two hours or so, on an empty stomach. The pills can be taken with hot soup or rice and ginger porridge to encourage sweating. When used for acute wind cold patterns, one week or less is usually sufficient. When used for recurrent headaches the formula can be used continually for several months at a lower dose (8-12 pills three times daily).

Cautions and contraindications

Not suitable for headaches due to deficiency.

GMP

3.10 JING FANG BAI DU WAN

荆防败毒丸

1/52

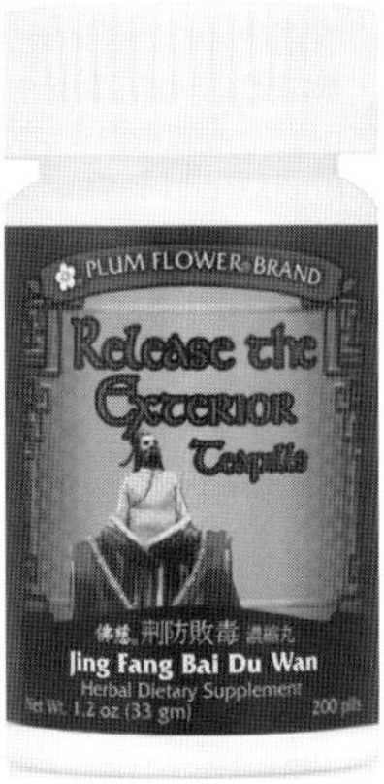

Lanzhou Foci Pharmaceutical Factory (Gansu)
'Schizonepeta and Siler Pills to Overcome Toxin'
Jing Fang Bai Du Wan is packaged in bottles of 200 pills
Also available as: Schizonepeta and Siler Formula (conc. extract)

Chinese medical action

Dispels wind cold damp, stops pain, expels phlegm

Biomedical action

Antipyretic, diaphoretic, analgesic, expectorant

INDICATIONS

- Acute wind cold damp type common cold. A broad acting and relatively strong formula for dispelling strong pathogens from the surface. Particularly useful when wind cold damp pathogens are on the edge of transforming into heat, usually observed in a sore throat amidst clear wind cold signs and symptoms. Initial signs and symptoms are generally marked reflecting the intensity of the battle between the strong pathogen and robust normal qi.
- With the appropriate identifying features, this formula can be used to treat conditions such as the common cold, the early stage of superficial suppurative lesions, acute rheumatic joint pain, epidemic influenza, bronchitis, and epidemic parotitis (mumps).

Composition

Schizonepeta tenuifolia (jing jie, schizonepeta), *Ledebouriella divaricata* (fang feng, siler), *Bupleurum falcatum* (chai hu, bupleurum), *Peucedanum praeruptorum* (qian hu, peucedanum), *Ligusticum wallici* (chuan xiong, ligusticum), *Notopterygium incisum* (qiang huo, notopterygium), *Angelica pubescens* (du huo, Tu-huo), *Poria cocos* (fu ling, hoelen), *Platycodon grandiflorum* (jie geng, platycodon), *Citrus aurantium* (zhi ke, aurantium), *Glycyrrhiza uralensis* (gan cao, licorice), *Zingiber officinale* (sheng jiang, ginger)

Combine with

- **9.7 Jie Geng Wan** for the beginnings of a sore throat from heat transformation
- **15.9 Headache and Dizziness Reliever** for severe occipital headache
- **9.18 Xin Yi San** for acute frontal headache, rhinitis or sinus congestion from wind cold invasion
- **3.30 Tong Xuan Li Fei Kou Fu Ye** for wind cold with copious watery sputum

Pattern identifying features

- **wind cold damp common cold**
- **acute simultaneous fever and chills, chills > fever**
- maybe high fever with shivering or rigors
- no sweating

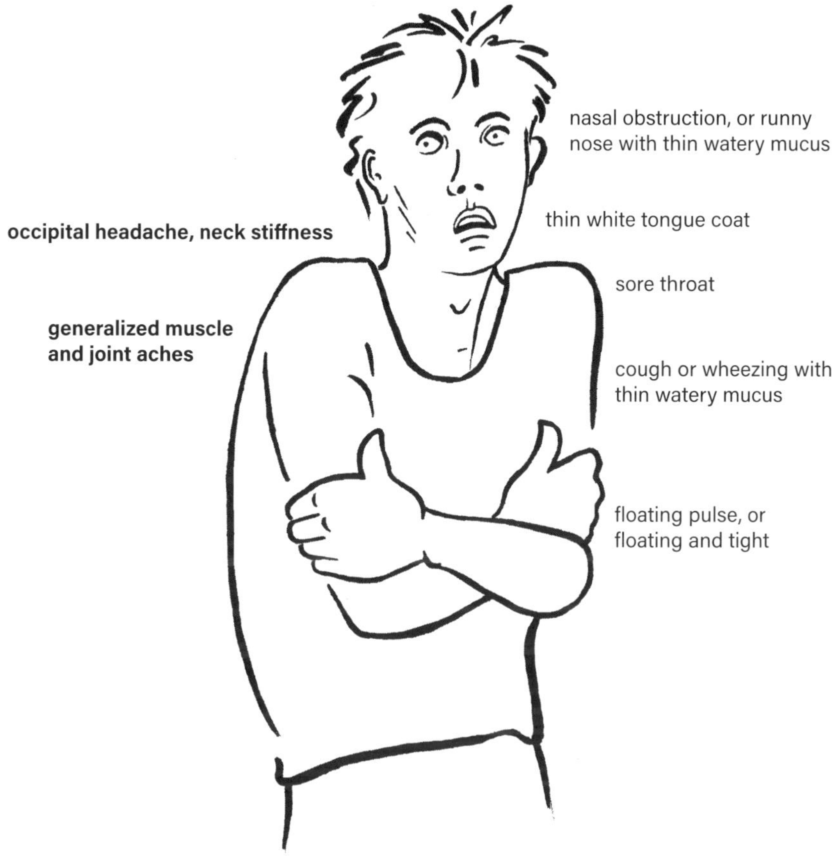

Dosage and method of administration

For acute wind cold damp patterns the dose is 8-12 pills every two hours or so, on an empty stomach. The pills can be taken with hot soup or rice and ginger porridge to encourage sweating. Following a dose with a hot bath to encourage sweat is beneficial. Used for acute wind cold patterns, one week or less is usually sufficient.

Cautions and contraindications

Not suitable for full blown wind heat patterns or warm diseases.

GMP

3.11 GE GEN WAN

葛根丸

1-3 / 52

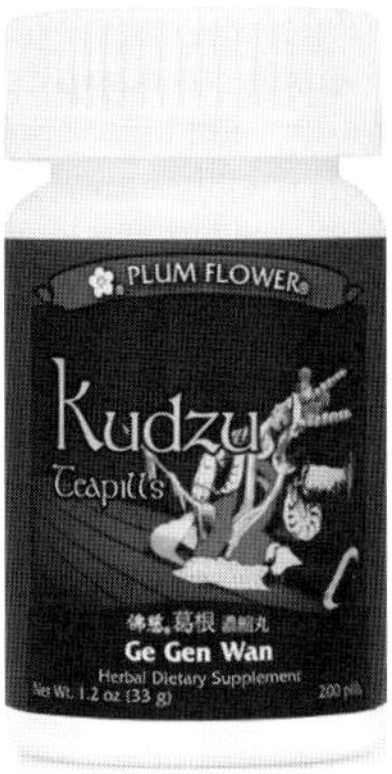

Lanzhou Foci Pharmaceutical Factory (Gansu)
'Pueraria Pills'
Ge Gen Wan is packaged in bottles of 200 pills
Also available as: Pueraria Combination (conc. extract)

Chinese medical action

Dispels wind cold, eases muscles, alleviates spasm, stops pain

Biomedical action

Diaphoretic, analgesic, muscle relaxant, calmative

INDICATIONS

- Neck, upper back and shoulder stiffness and pain from wind cold invasion into the *tài yáng* channels of the upper back. Although designed for wind cold patterns, its use has been expanded to include stiff and painful neck, upper back and shoulders from a variety of causes as long as there is no significant heat.
- Acute *tài yáng* syndrome with diarrhea. Cold (when strong or in a weakened host) can swiftly penetrate the surface layers into the deeper recesses of the body, inhabiting multiple levels. In such cases there are symptoms of both *tài yáng* syndrome–chills, fever, myalgia, and *yáng míng* (Stomach and Intestines) or *tài yīn* (Spleen) involvement. With *yáng míng* involvement, cold usually transforms into heat, diarrhea is urgent and signs of internal heat are appearing (yellow tongue coat on the root of the tongue). With *tài yīn* involvement, the cold damages Spleen yang and diarrhea is watery, the appetite poor and fatigue increasing.
- Wind cold type nasal and skin conditions – allergic rhinitis, sinus congestion and urticaria aggravated or initiated by exposure to cold or cold weather.
- With the appropriate identifying features, this formula can assist in the treatment of conditions such as the common cold, influenza, early stage of meningitis or encephalitis, acute torticollis, wry neck, cervical spondylosis, chronic pediatric diarrhea, early stage of dysenteric disorder, early stage of measles, eczema and urticaria.

Composition

Pueraria lobata (ge gen, kudzu), *Ephedra sinica* (ma huang*, ephedra), *Zingiber officinale* (sheng jiang, ginger), *Cinnamomum cassia* (gui zhi, cinnamon twigs), *Paeonia lactiflora* (bai shao, white peony), *Glycyrrhiza uralensis* (gan cao, licorice), *Zizyphus jujuba* (da zao, chinese dates) [**Restricted use in some jurisdictions; may be subject to substitution*]

Combine with

- **15.9 Headache and Dizziness Reliever** for severe occipital headache, stiff neck and upper back pain
- **10.30 Po Sum On Medicated Oil** topically for neck and upper back stiffness and pain

Pattern identifying features

- **wind cold common cold with neck and upper back pain**
- chills, mild fever
- no sweating
- generalized myalgia
- maybe diarrhea and nausea

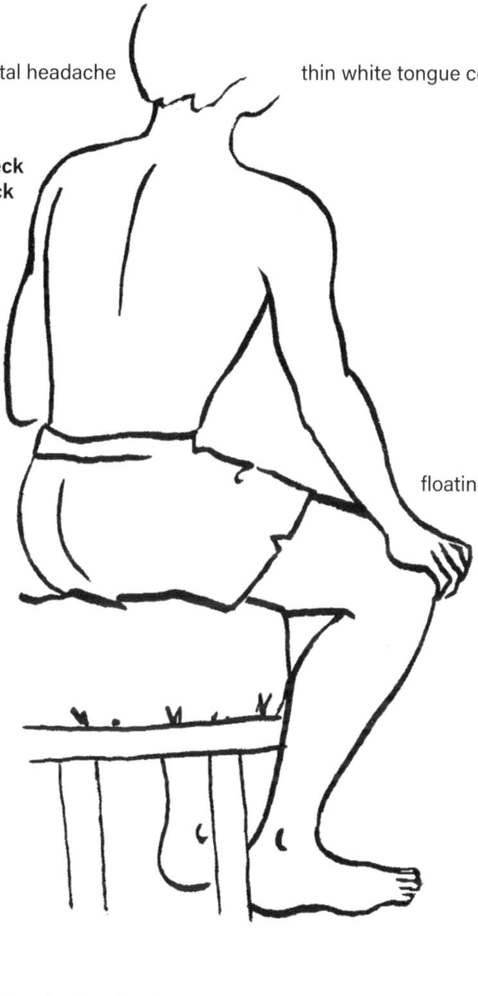

Dosage and method of administration

For acute wind cold common cold patterns the dose is 8-12 pills every two hours or so, on an empty stomach. The pills can be taken with hot soup or rice and ginger porridge to encourage sweating. Following a dose with a hot bath to encourage sweat is beneficial. Used for acute wind cold patterns, one week or less is usually sufficient.

Cautions and contraindications

Contraindicated in wind cold exterior deficiency patterns with sweating (*see* **3.6 Gui Zhi Wan**). Caution in patients with hypertension. May cause or aggravate insomnia in some patients due to presence of ephedra.

3.12 GAN MAO QING RE CHONG JI

感冒清热冲剂

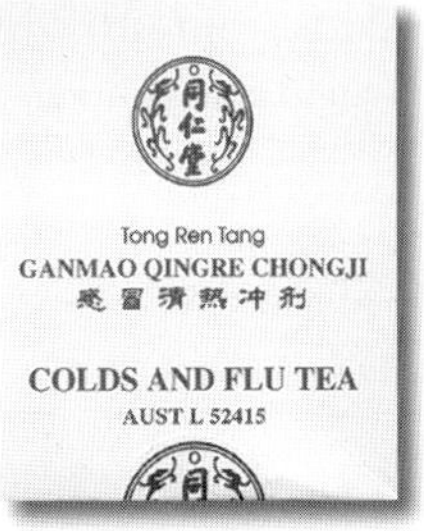

(Colds and Flu Tea)
Tong Ren Tang (Beijing)
'Cold and Fever Clearing Granules'
Gan Mao Qing Re Chong Ji is packaged as dissolving granules in single dose sachets, 10 sachets per box

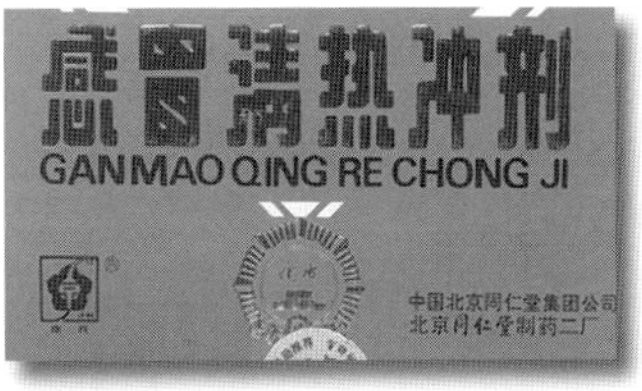

Chinese medical action

Dispels wind cold, directs Lung qi downward, eases muscle aches

Biomedical action

Diaphoretic, antipyretic, analgesic

INDICATIONS

- Wind cold type common cold, especially good when muscle aches and headaches are a prominent feature.
- Two varieties are manufactured, with and without sugar. The sugarless variety is quite bitter; the sweet version well tolerated by children.
- With the appropriate identifying features, this formula can treat conditions such as influenza and the common cold.

Composition (each sachet contains decoctions equivalent to fresh)

Corydalis turtschaninovii (yan hu suo, corydalis) 2.95g, *Phragmites communis* (lu gen, reed rhizome) 2.36g, *Bupleurum falcatum* (chai hu, bupleurum) 1.47g, *Ledebouriella divaricata* (fang feng, siler) 1.47g, *Pueraria lobata* (ge gen, pueraria) 1.47g, *Prunus armenica* (xing ren, apricot seed) 1.18g, *Angelica dahurica* (bai zhi, angelica) 880mg, *Platycodon grandiflorum* (jie geng, platycodon) 880mg, *Schizonepeta tenuifolia* (jing jie, schizonepeta essential oil) 17.6mcl, *Perilla frutescens* (zi su ye, perilla leaf essential oil) 0.09mcl, *Mentha haplocalycis* (bo he, mint oil) 3.5mcl

Dosage and method of administration

The recommended dose is one sachet dissolved in hot water twice daily, however to get the best therapeutic effect the dose should be doubled or trebled. Take one sachet every hour or two. Half dose for children.

Cautions and contraindications

Contraindicated during pregnancy.

3.13 GAN MAO QING RE KE LI

感冒清热颗粒

GMP

1-3/7

Tong Ren Tang (Beijing)
'Cold and Fever Clearing Granules'
Gan Mao Qing Re Ke Li is packaged as dissolving granules in single dose sachets, 10 sachets per box

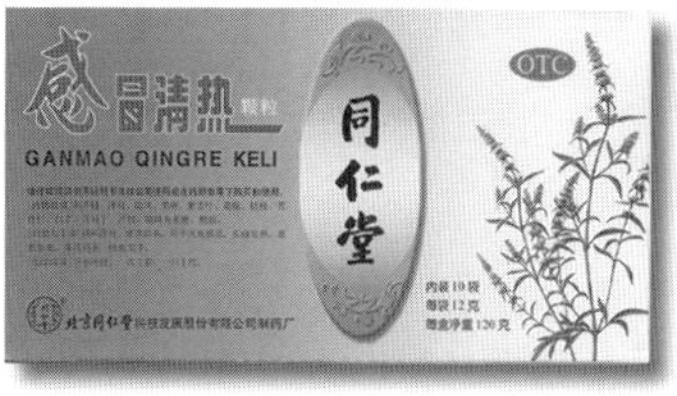

Chinese medical action

Dispels wind cold, clears heat from the throat

Biomedical action

Diaphoretic, antipyretic, antiviral

INDICATIONS

- Wind cold type common cold. Also used for mild wind heat patterns or wind cold patterns that are beginning to transform into heat. Similar to **3.12 Gan Mao Qing Re Chong Ji**, with the addition of *Viola yedoensis* (zi hua di ding, viola) to clear toxic heat.
- With the appropriate identifying features, this formula can treat conditions such as influenza, the common cold, laryngitis and early tonsillitis.

Composition

Schizonepeta tenuifolia (jing jie sui, schizonepeta), *Mentha haplocalycis* (bo he, mint), *Ledebouriella divaricata* (fang feng, siler), *Bupleurum falcatum* (chai hu, bupleurum), *Perilla frutescens* (zi su ye, perilla leaf), *Pueraria lobata* (ge gen, pueraria), *Platycodon grandiflorum* (jie geng, platycodon), *Prunus armenica* (xing ren, apricot seed), *Angelica dahurica* (bai zhi, angelica), *Phragmites communis* (lu gen, reed rhizome), *Viola yedoensis* (zi hua di ding, viola)

Dosage and method of administration

The recommended dose is one sachet dissolved in hot water twice daily, however to get the best therapeutic effect the dose should be doubled or trebled. Take one sachet every hour or two. Half dose for children.

Cautions and contraindications

None noted.

GMP

3.14 REN SHEN BAI DU WAN

人参败毒丸

1-3/52

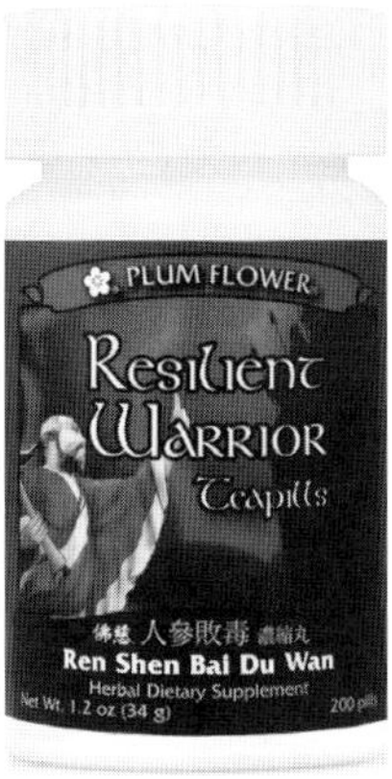

Lanzhou Foci Pharmaceutical Factory (Gansu)
'Ginseng Pills to Overcome Toxin'
Ren Shen Bai Du Wan is packaged in bottles of 200 pills
Also available as: Ginseng and Mint Formula (conc. extract)

Chinese medical action

Dispels wind cold damp, tonifies qi, expels phlegm

Biomedical action

Antipyretic, diaphoretic, analgesic, expectorant

INDICATIONS

- Wind cold damp type common cold in patients with qi deficiency. Mostly seen in patients convalescing from illness, in children and postpartum women, the elderly and debilitated. Wind cold patterns such as this tend to drag on as normal qi is unable to expel the pathogen.
- The difference between this formula and **3.10 Jing Fang Bai Du Wan** is relatively small – replacement of two wind expelling herbs, schizonepeta and siler, with mint and ginseng. This alteration subtly shifts the focus of the formula to expelling wind cold while supporting normal qi. The overall pattern is the similar to that in **3.10 Jing Fang Bai Du Wan**. The preexisting qi deficiency does, however, result in two phenomena that help differentiate between the two formulas – the patient gets colds more easily, and when a cold occurs symptoms are more subdued due to the relative weakness of the battle between the pathogen and the deficient normal qi.

Composition

Notopterygium incisum (qiang huo, notopterygium), *Angelica pubescens* (du huo, Tu-huo), *Ligusticum wallici* (chuan xiong, ligusticum), *Bupleurum falcatum* (chai hu, bupleurum), *Peucedanum praeruptorum* (qian hu, peucedanum), *Poria cocos* (fu ling, hoelen), *Platycodon grandiflorum* (jie geng, platycodon), *Citrus aurantium* (zhi ke, aurantium), *Mentha haplocalycis* (bo he, mint), *Panax ginseng* (ren shen, ginseng), *Glycyrrhiza uralensis* (gan cao, licorice), *Zingiber officinale* (sheng jiang, ginger)

Pattern identifying features

- **wind cold damp common cold with qi deficiency**
- chills > fever
- no sweating

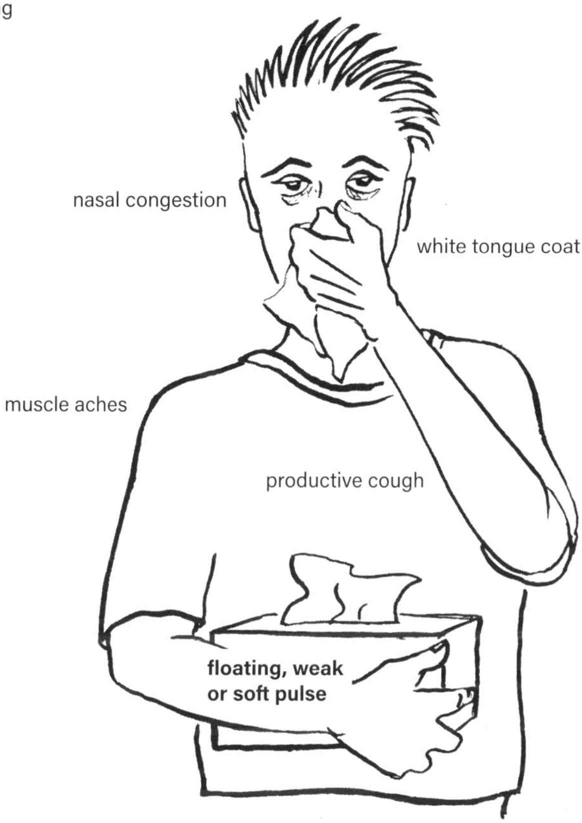

Dosage and method of administration

8-12 pills every two hours or so, on an empty stomach. The pills can be taken with hot soup or rice and ginger porridge to encourage mild sweating. Following a dose with a hot bath to encourage sweat is beneficial.

Cautions and contraindications

Not suitable for wind heat patterns or warm diseases.

3.15 QING QI HUA TAN WAN

清气化痰丸

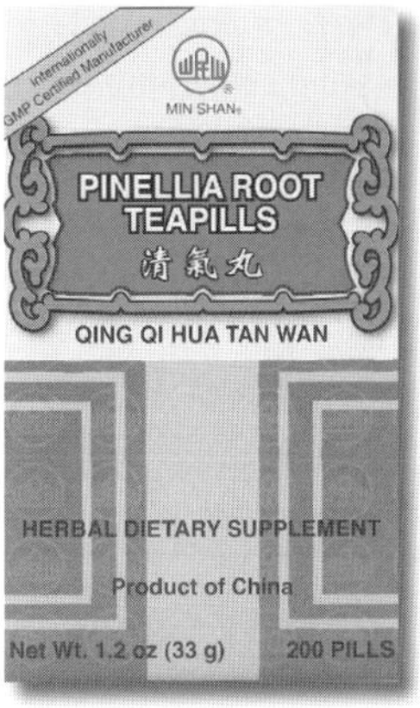

Lanzhou Foci Pharmaceutical Factory (Gansu)
'Clear the Qi and Transform Phlegm Pills'
Qing Qi Hua Tan Wan is packaged in bottles of 200 pills
Also available as: Clean Air Teapills (PF), Pinellia Expectorant Pills, Clear Damp and Transform Phlegm Pill (BE), Pinellia and Scute Formula (conc. extract)

Chinese medical action
Clears phlegm heat from the Lungs, stops cough

Biomedical action
Expectorant, decongestant, febrifuge, antitussive

INDICATIONS

- Acute and chronic phlegm heat in the Lungs. The main feature is the nature and quantity of the sputum – copious, thick, sticky, yellow or green. The patient has difficulty breathing or wheezes, with audible rattles and rales. Cough is loud and productive, although sometimes the sputum is so sticky that it can be hard to expectorate and may not be immediately apparent; this is usually the case during the early stage and when the heat component is relatively strong.
- Lingering or low grade phlegm heat patterns of the Lungs with chronic cough and sticky yellow or green sputum.
- Chronic phlegm heat congestion in the sinuses.
- With the appropriate identifying features, this formula can be used to treat conditions such as acute and chronic bronchitis, bronchiectasis, pneumonia, whooping cough, bronchial asthma and chronic sinusitis.

Composition (each pill contains powdered)
Scutellaria baicalensis (huang qin, scute), *Poria cocos* (fu ling, hoelen), *Trichosanthes kirilowi* (gua lou, trichosanthes), *Pinellia ternata* (zhi ban xia, processed pinellia), *Prunus armenica* (xing ren, apricot seed), *Arisaema cosanguinium* (dan nan xing, pig bile treated arisaema), *Citrus aurantium* (zhi shi, aurantium), *Citrus nobilis* (chen pi, citrus peel)

Combine with
- **14.5 Chuan Xin Lian Antiphlogistic Tablets** or **3.16 Ching Fei Yi Huo Pien** for severe cases (the latter when there is constipation)
- **3.21 She Dan Chuan Bei Ye** for chronic phlegm heat in the Lungs with very sticky sputum
- **2.22 Er Chen Wan** for milder chronic cases with mixtures of yellow and white sticky sputum

Pattern identifying features

- **phlegm heat in the Lungs**
- cough worse at night and early in the morning
- dry mouth, thirst, or an unpleasant sticky sensation in the mouth
- maybe fever and night sweats

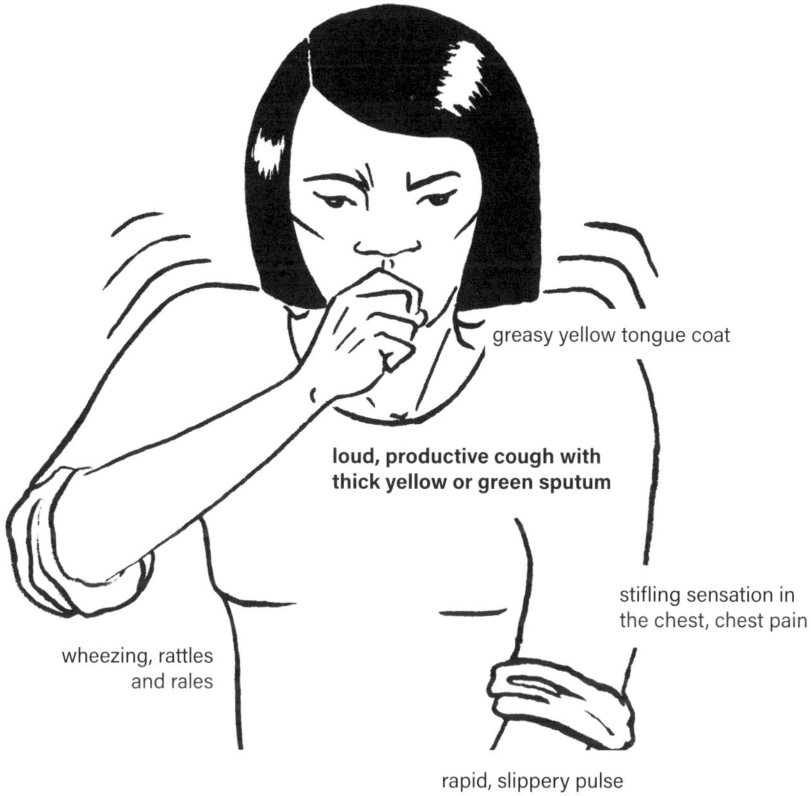

Dosage and method of administration

The recommended dose is 8 pills three times daily, however to get a good result in acute cases a larger dose is generally required, 12-18 pills every 2 hours, to a maximum of around 80-100 pills per day. Therefore in acute cases one jar (200 pills) should only last 2-3 days. In chronic cases of lingering phlegm heat, 8-16 pills three times daily is usually sufficient. Take on an empty stomach.

Cautions and contraindications

Not suitable for hot dry cough, cough with thin watery sputum or cough from yin deficiency.

3.16 CHING FEI YI HUO PIEN

清肺抑火片

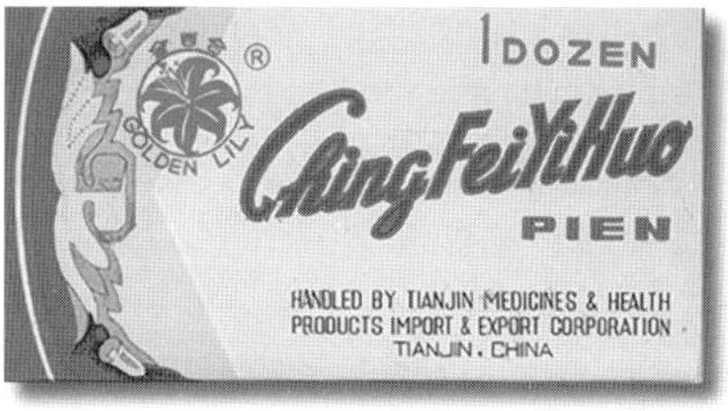

(*Qing Fei Yi Huo Pian*)
Tianjin Drug Manufactory (Shandong)
'Clear the Lungs and Restrain fire Pills'
Ching Fei Yi Huo Pien is packaged in vials of eight pills, twelve vials per box

Chinese medical action

Clears heat and fire from the Lungs, stops cough, promotes descent of Lung and Large Intestine qi

Biomedical action

Antipyretic, anti-inflammatory, antibiotic, laxative

INDICATIONS

- Lung heat or Lung fire, characterized by acute onset of loud, painful, barking cough, or wheezing, with or without yellow sputum. Coughing typically begins a few days after an unresolved or severe wind cold or wind heat invasion. Patients tend to be prone to recurrent episodes, with the illness repeatedly lodging in the same part of the upper respiratory tract, the lungs, throat or sinuses.
- Acute sore throat (toxic heat in the throat) and acute sinusitis (phlegm heat or fire in the sinuses).
- *Yáng míng* organ syndrome with acute constipation, abdominal pain, fever and thirst. Because it can clear heat (and damp) from the Intestines, it can also be used for the early stages of dysenteric disorder.
- With the appropriate identifying features, this formula can be used to treat conditions such as acute upper respiratory tract infection, bronchitis, pneumonia, whooping cough, pleurisy, tonsillitis, pharyngitis, tracheitis, sinusitis, uncomplicated appendicitis, acute cholecystitis and acute pancreatitis.

Composition (each tablet contains extracts equivalent to dry)

Scutellaria baicalensis (huang qin, scute) 955mg, *Gardenia florida* (shan zhi zi, gardenia) 887mg, *Anemarrhena aspheloides* (zhi mu, anemarrhena) 665mg, *Sophora flavescentis* (ku shen, sophora root) 409mg, *Rheum palmatum* (da huang, rhubarb root) 106mg, *Trichosanthes kirilowi* (tian hua fen, trichosanthes root) 71mg, *Peucedanum praeruptorum* (qian hu, peucedanum) 318mg, *Platycodon grandiflorum* (jie geng, platycodon) 71mg

Combine with

- **14.5 Chuan Xin Lian Antiphlogistic Tablets** for severe heat in the Lungs, or the early stages of dysenteric disorder
- **10.2 Raw Tienchi Tablets** for hemoptysis
- **3.15 Qing Qi Hua Tan Wan** for copious colored sputum
- **9.9 Superior Sore Throat Powder** for sore throat
- **9.13 Pe Min Kan Wan** or **9.19 Cang Er Zi Wan** for acute sinus infection

Pattern identifying features

- **Lung heat or fire**
- sore red throat
- fever
- focal chest pain with cough

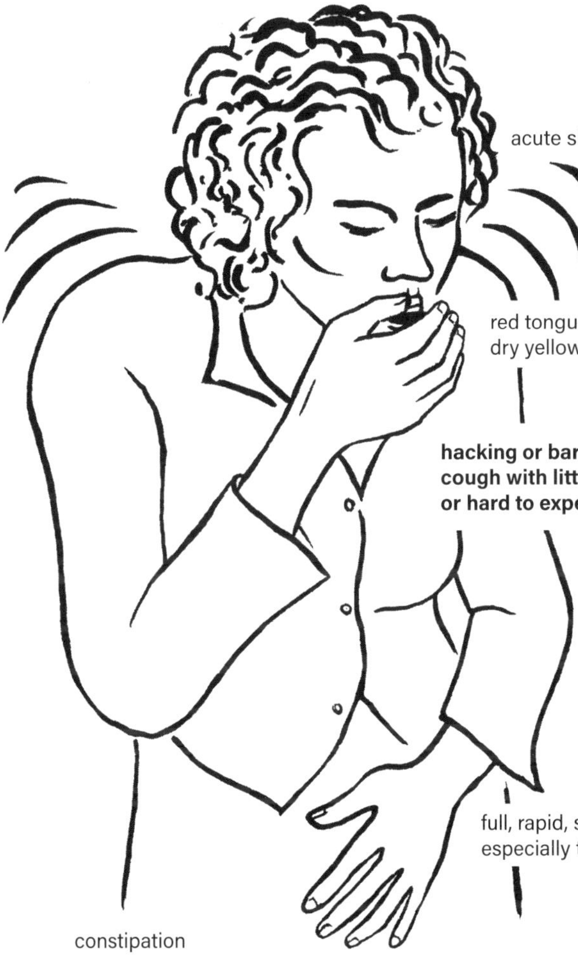

Dosage and method of administration

The recommended dose is 4 pills twice daily, but to be effective in strong acute Lung fire patterns, one vial can be taken every 2 hours. Take on an empty stomach. Usually not necessary for more than 4-7 days. Patients should be advised they may experience diarrhea.

Cautions and contraindications

Contraindicated during pregnancy and for acute cough from wind cold or cough due to Lung yin deficiency.

3.17 PI PA COUGH TEA

止咳川贝枇杷冲剂

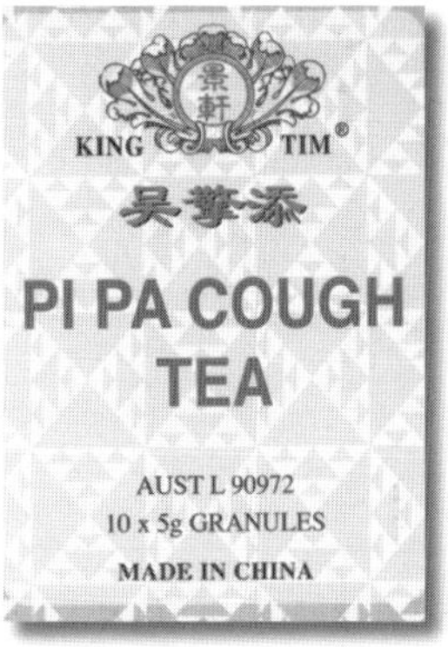

(*Zhi Ke Chuan Bei Pi Pa Chong Ji*)
Jing Xian Pharmaceutical Co. (Guangzhou)
'Antitussive Fritillaria and Loquat Leaf Soluble Granules'
Pi Pa Cough Tea is packaged in 5 gram sachets, 10 sachets per box

Chinese medical action

Clears heat from the Lungs, moistens the Lungs, expels phlegm, stops cough

Biomedical action

Antitussive, expectorant, febrifuge

INDICATIONS

- Cough from wind heat, Lung heat or phlegm heat. The heat may follow an acute wind heat or wind cold common cold, or be the result of hot dry weather, or smoking. The main features are hacking dry or productive cough, with or without sticky yellow sputum. Coughing produces chest pain, a dry, sore throat, hoarse voice and fever. In some cases there will be constipation.
- With the appropriate identifying features, this formula can assist in the treatment of conditions such as upper respiratory tract infection, acute bronchitis, tonsillitis and pleurisy.

Composition (each sachet contains extracts equivalent to dry)

Fritillaria cirrhosa (chuan bei mu, fritillaria) 1.8g, *Eriobotria japonica* (pi pa ye, loquat leaf) 1.8g, *Glycyrrhiza uralensis* (gan cao, licorice) 1.8g, *Lonicera japonica* (jin yin hua, honeysuckle) 1.8g, *Platycodon grandiflorum* (jie geng, platycodon) 1.4g, *Scutellaria baicalensis* (huang qin, scute) 900mg, *Morus alba* (sang bai pi, mulberry root bark) 900mg, *Mentha haplocalyx* (bo he, mint) 900mg, *Perilla frutescens* (su zi, perilla seed) 900mg, *Lepidium apetalum* (ting li zi, lepidium seed) 900mg, *Trichosanthis kirilowii* (gua luo ren, trichosanthes seed) 900mg, *Peucedanum praeruptorum* (qian hu, peucedanum) 750mg, *Aster tataricus* (zi wan, aster) 750mg, *Stemona sessifolia* (bai bu, stemona) 750mg, *Lilium lancifolium* (bai he, lily), *Cynanchum stauntonii* (bai qian, cynanchum) 540mg

Pattern identifying features

- **heat type cough**

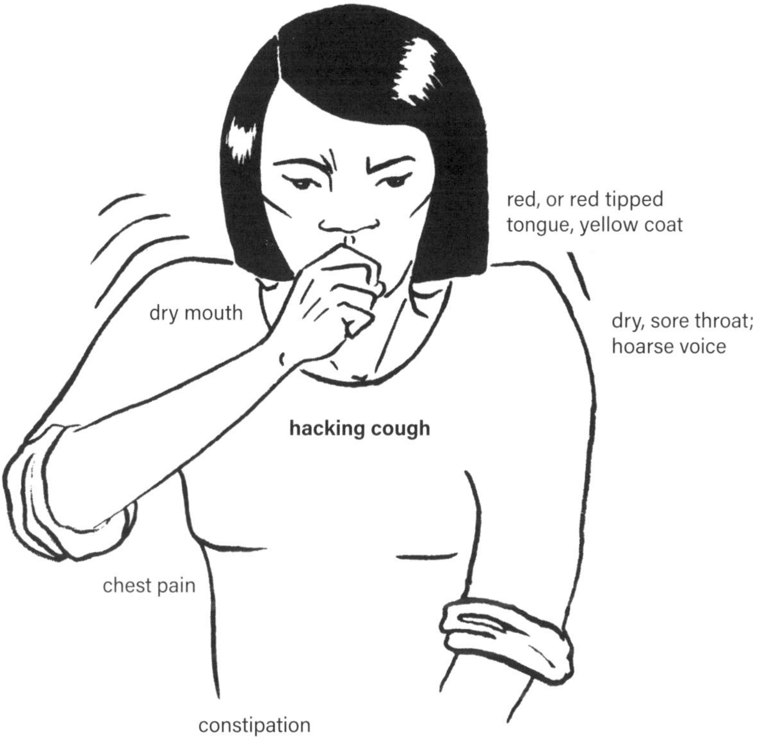

Dosage and method of administration

Adults: 1-2 sachets dissolved in hot water, three times daily.
Children over 4 years: 1 sachet dissolved in hot water, two or three times daily.
Children under 4 years *see* **12.1 Bo Ying Compound**.

Cautions and contraindications

Contains aspartame and phenylalanine. Not suitable for phenylketonurics.

3.18 TUNG HSUAN LI FEI PIEN

通宣理肺片

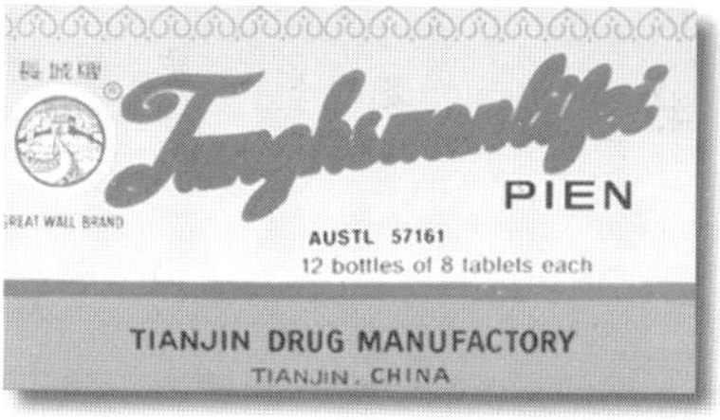

(*Tong Xuan Li Fei Pian*)
Tianjin Drug Manufactory (Shandong)
'Open, Diffuse and Regulate Lung Pills'
Tung Hsuan Li Fei Pien is packaged in vials of eight pills, twelve vials per box

Chinese medical action

Stops cough, benefits the throat, detoxifies and promotes healing

Biomedical action

Antitussive, antispasmodic, demulcent, anti-inflammatory

INDICATIONS

- Cough from various etiologies. Used for acute and chronic coughs, from external or internal causes, with heat or cold, with or without phlegm congestion. Good for smokers cough, and especially good for dryness and mild heat patterns.
- Sore throat from various etiologies, including acute and chronic sore throat, dry sore throat and sore throat with phlegm congestion.
- To assist in healing of gastric ulcers and treatment of chronic upper gastrointestinal disorders, such as gastritis, with elements of qi and yin deficiency. Disorders such as these are characterized by indefinable epigastric discomfort (*see* glossary), morning nausea, belching, epigastric fullness and pain and perhaps a peeled patch in the center of the tongue (the Stomach area).

Composition (each pill contains extracts equivalent to dry)

Glycyrrhiza uralensis (gan cao, licorice) 2.07g, *Perilla frutescens* (zi su ye, perilla leaf) 1.18g, *Platycodon grandiflorum* (jie geng, platycodon) 665mg, *Peucedanum praeruptorum* (qian hu, peucedanum) 636mg, *Citrus aurantium* (zhi shi, aurantium) 591mg, *Citrus reticulata* (chen pi, citrus) 369mg, *Polygonatum odoratum* (yu zhu, polygonatum) 318mg, *Pueraria lobata* (ge gen, pueraria) 318mg, *Lilium lancifolium* (bai he, lily) 240mg

Combine with

- **3.4 Gan Mao Ling** for acute cough from severe wind heat
- **2.27 Wei Te Ling** for epigastric pain and hyper-acidity associated with peptic ulcer disease
- **9.9 Superior Sore Throat Powder** for sore throat from acute or chronic tonsillitis
- **3.33 Yang Yin Qing Fei Wan** or **3.35 Mai Wei Di Huang Wan** for recurrent sore throat from Lung yin deficiency
- **3.29 African Sea Coconut Cough Syrup** for persistent irritating tickle in the throat

Pattern identifying features

- **Lung dryness and heat**

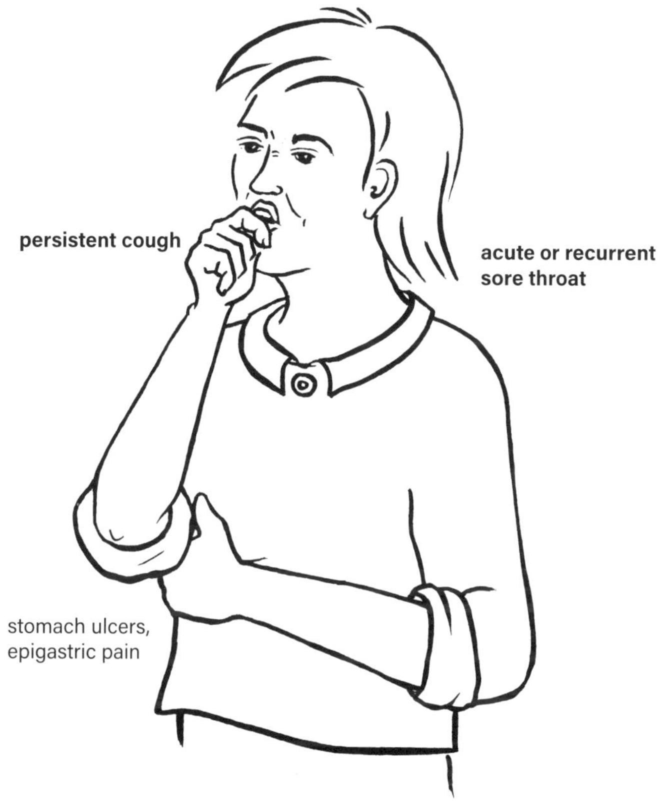

Dosage and method of administration

4 pills twice daily on an empty stomach. In severe cases, or during the early stages of treatment (the first week or so), the dose can be increased by 50%, then reduced as treatment takes effect.

Cautions and contraindications

Can aggravate digestive damp and abdominal distension and nausea in some patients. This can usually be relieved by reducing the dose. Licorice root has a sodium sparing and potassium leaching effect and when used in large doses can cause edema. Caution in patients with hypertension and fluid problems. May counteract spironolactone (Aldactone) and potentiate potassium depleting loop diuretics (like Lasix) leading to hypokalemia.

3.19 DING CHUAN WAN

定喘丸

Lanzhou Foci Pharmaceutical Factory (Gansu)
'Calm Wheezing Pills'
Ding Chuan Wan is packaged in bottles of 200 pills
Also available as: Clear Mountain Air Teapills (PF), Ephedra and Ginkgo Combination (conc. extract)

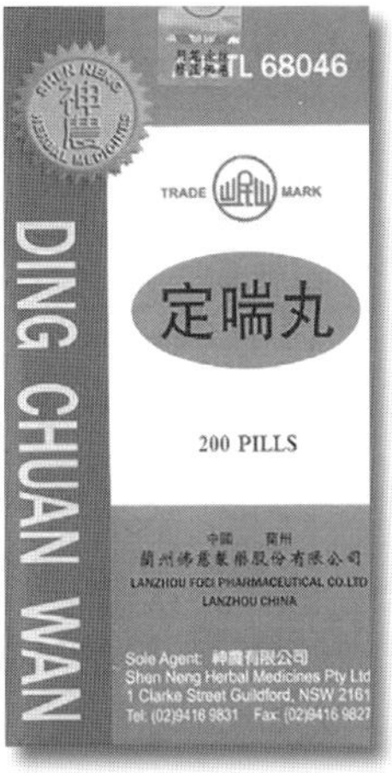

Chinese medical action

Stops wheezing and cough, redirects Lung qi downwards, transforms phlegm, clears heat from the Lungs

Biomedical action

Anti-asthmatic, antitussive, expectorant

INDICATIONS

- Acute and chronic wheezing and asthma associated with phlegm or phlegm heat congestion in the Lungs. The phlegm is usually preexisting, stirred up and mobilized by some trigger. Once mobilized, phlegm obstructs the bronchi causing difficulty in breathing. The trigger for wheezing can be a wind invasion, sudden change in temperature or exposure to an allergen. The main focus of this formula is in transforming and expelling phlegm, with directing Lung qi downward and alleviating wheezing secondary.
- With the appropriate identifying features, this formula can be used to treat conditions such as asthma, asthmatic bronchitis, chronic bronchitis and emphysema.

Composition (each pill contains powdered)

Ginko biloba (yin xing, ginko seed) 22mg, *Morus alba* (sang bai pi, mulberry bark) 22mg, *Platycodon grandiflorum* (jie geng, platycodon) 18.4mg, *Perilla frutescens* (zi su ye, perilla leaf) 18.4mg, *Prunus armenica* (xing ren, apricot seed) 18.4mg, *Scutellaria baicalensis* (huang qin, scute) 18.4mg, *Pinellia ternata* (zhi ban xia, processed pinellia) 18.4mg, *Stemona sessifolia* (bai bu, stemona) 14.7mg, *Glycyrrhiza uralensis* (gan cao, licorice) 14.7mg, *Aster tataricus* (zi wan, aster) 14.7mg

Combine with

- **3.21 She Dan Chuan Bei Ye** for patients with copious sputum or obvious rattles and rales, until the sputum starts to break up
- **2.22 Er Chen Wan** for very thick or hard to expectorate sputum
- **3.15 Qing Qi Hua Tan Wan** for wheezing from deep rooted phlegm heat

Pattern identifying features

- **phlegm heat accumulation in the Lungs**
- **dyspnea, wheezing**

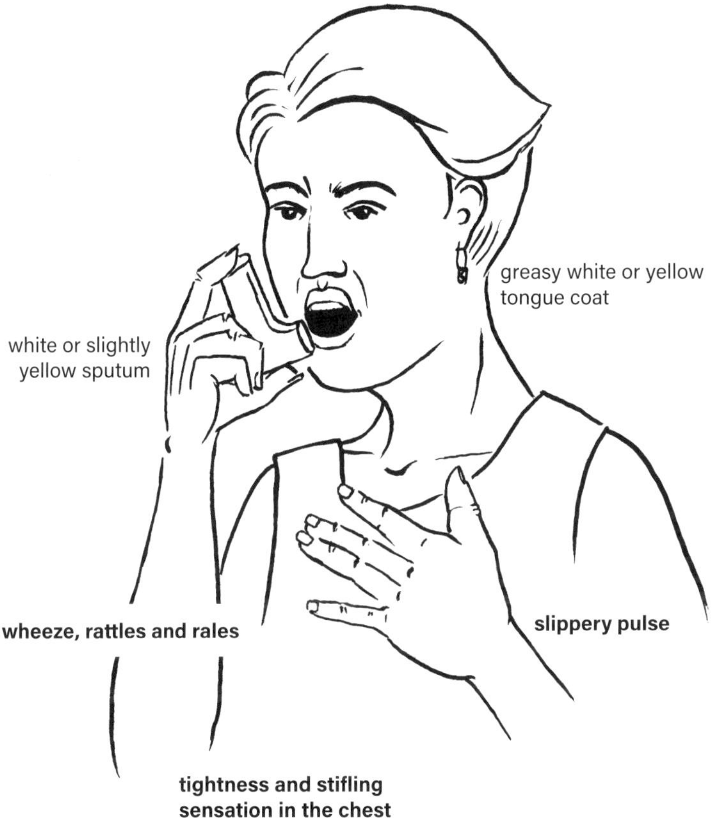

Dosage and method of administration

15 pills three times daily on an empty stomach. In severe cases or during the early stages of treatment (the first 7-10 days), a 50% increase in dose can be used, then reduced to a maintenance dose (~8-12 pills three times daily) as treatment takes effect.

Cautions and contraindications

Contraindicated in cases of wheezing, breathlessness and asthma from qi or yin deficiency.

3.20 QI GUAN YAN KE SOU TAN CHUAN WAN

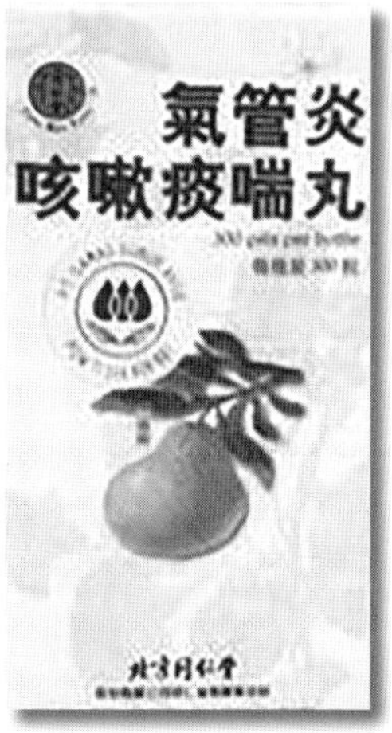

气管炎咳嗽痰喘丸

Tong Ren Tang (Beijing)
'Bronchitis, Cough, Phlegm and Wheezing Pills'
Qi Guan Yan Ke Sou Tan Chuan Wan is packaged in bottles of 300 pills

Chinese medical action

Stops cough, redirects Lung qi downwards, transforms phlegm

Biomedical action

Anti-asthmatic, antitussive, expectorant

INDICATIONS

- Chronic cough from phlegm congestion in the Lungs. Most suitable for chronic bronchitis with underlying Spleen deficiency.
- With the appropriate identifying features, this formula can be used to assist in treatment of conditions such as chronic bronchitis, emphysema, asthmatic bronchitis and bronchiectasis.

Composition (30 pills contains powdered)

Codonopsis pilosula (dang shen, codonopsis) 570mg, *Platycodon grandiflorum* (jie geng, platycodon) 300mg, *Morus alba* (sang ye, mulberry leaf) 270mg, *Zingiber officinalis* (sheng jiang, ginger) 270mg, *Peucedanum praeruptorium* (qian hu, peucedanum) 180mg, *Cynanchum stauntonii* (bai qian, cynanchum) 180mg, *Pinellia ternata* (zhi ban xia, processed pinellia) 180mg, *Fritillaria thunbergii* (zhe bei mu, fritillaria) 180mg, *Perilla frutescens* (zi su ye, perilla leaf) 180mg, *Aster tataricus* (zi wan, aster) 180mg, *Poria cocos* (fu ling, hoelen) 180mg, *Glycyrrhiza uralensis* (gan cao, licorice) 180mg, *Polygala sibiricum* (yuan zhi, polygala) 180mg, *Paeonia lactiflora* (bai shao, white peony) 180mg, *Stemona sessifolia* (bai bu, stemona) 180mg, *Belamcanda chinensis* (she gan, belamcanda) 180mg, *Allium macrostemon* (xie bai, allium bulb) 180mg, *Prunus armenica* (xing ren, apricot seed) 150mg, *Citrus reticulata* (chen pi, citrus) 120mg, *Schizandra chinensis* (wu wei zi, schizandra) 120mg, *Fritillaria cirrhosa* (chuan bei mu, Sichuan fritillaria) 90mg, *Scutellaria baicalensis* (huang qin, scute) 90mg, *Baphicacanthus cusia* (da qing ye) 90mg, *Cinnamomum cassia* (gui zhi, cinnamon twigs) 60mg, *Asarum seiboldi* (xi xin*, wild ginger) 30mg, *Eriobotrya japonica* (pi pa ye, loquat leaf) 2.4mg [**Restricted use in some jurisdictions; may be subject to substitution*]

Pattern identifying features

- **phlegm damp accumulation in the Lungs**
- dyspnea, orthopnea
- breathlessness
- white or slightly yellow sputum

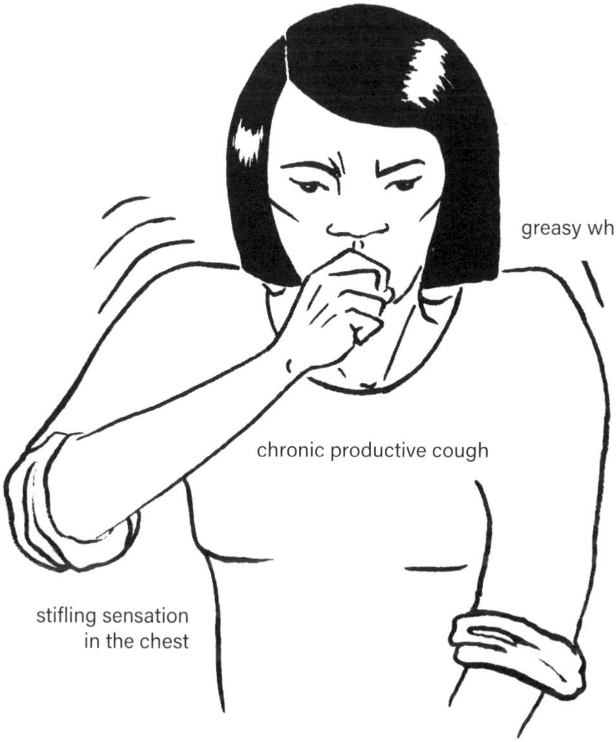

Combine with

– **3.21 She Dan Chuan Bei Ye** or **3.30 Tong Xuan Li Fei Kou Fu Ye** for copious sputum with obvious rattles and rales, until sputum starts to break up
– **2.22 Er Chen Wan** for very thick or hard to expectorate sputum.

Dosage and method of administration

The recommended dose for adults is 30 pills twice daily, before meals. Not suitable for children due to the number of pills required.

Cautions and contraindications

Contraindicated in cases of cough, wheezing, breathlessness and asthma arising from yin deficiency or Lung dryness.

3.21 SHE DAN CHUAN BEI YE

蛇胆川贝液

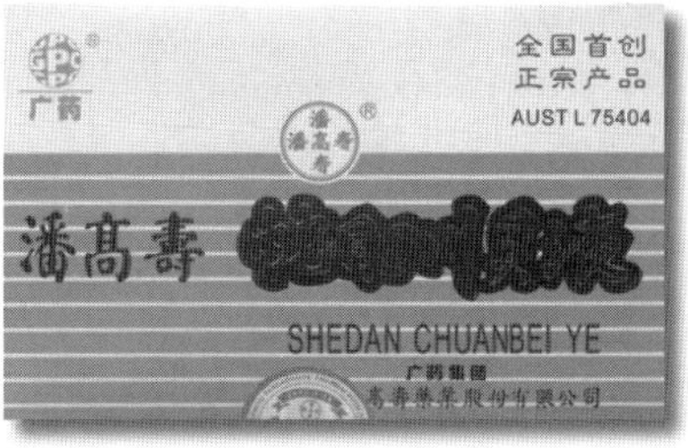

Guangzhou Pangaoshou Pharmaceutical Company (Guangzhou)
'Snake Bile and Fritillaria Liquid'
She Dan Chuan Bei Ye is packaged in vials of liquid extract, six vials to a box. The vials are pierced with a sharpened straw (supplied)

Chinese medical action

Breaks up, transforms and expels phlegm, stops cough

Biomedical action

Mucolytic, expectorant, antitussive

INDICATIONS

- Phlegm damp congestion in the Lungs. For relief of persistent productive cough, or cough with deep lying and hard to expectorate sputum, especially continuing sputum in the convalescent phase of an upper respiratory tract infection.
- With the appropriate identifying features, this formula can be used to treat persistent sputum in the convalescent phase of acute bronchitis or pneumonia, the tenacious sputum of whooping cough, bronchiectasis or chronic bronchitis.

Composition (each vial contains by volume)

Snake bile (she dan) 2.7%, *Fritillaria cirrhosa* (chuan bei mu, fritillaria) 10.13%, *Prunus armenica* (xing ren, apricot seed) 4.05%, menthol 0.01%, honey 0.5%, water, sucrose, benzoate as preservative

Combine with

- **3.15 Qing Qi Hua Tan Wan** for chronic or residual phlegm heat in the Lungs in the post acute phase of an upper respiratory tract infection
- **3.19 Ding Chuan Wan** for wheezing from phlegm heat congestion
- **2.9 Xiang Sha Liu Jun Wan** for persistent productive cough in a patient with Spleen deficiency (often following repeated antibiotic treatment)

Dosage and method of administration

In adults with severe cough and copious sputum, 4-6 vials per day may be used. For maintenance treatment, 1-3 vials per day is sufficient. For children over 4 years old 1-2 vials per day (for children below 4 years *see* **12.1 Bo Ying Compound**).

Pattern identifying features

- **phlegm damp in the Lungs**
- **persistent productive cough with either green or white, hard to expectorate or tenacious sputum**

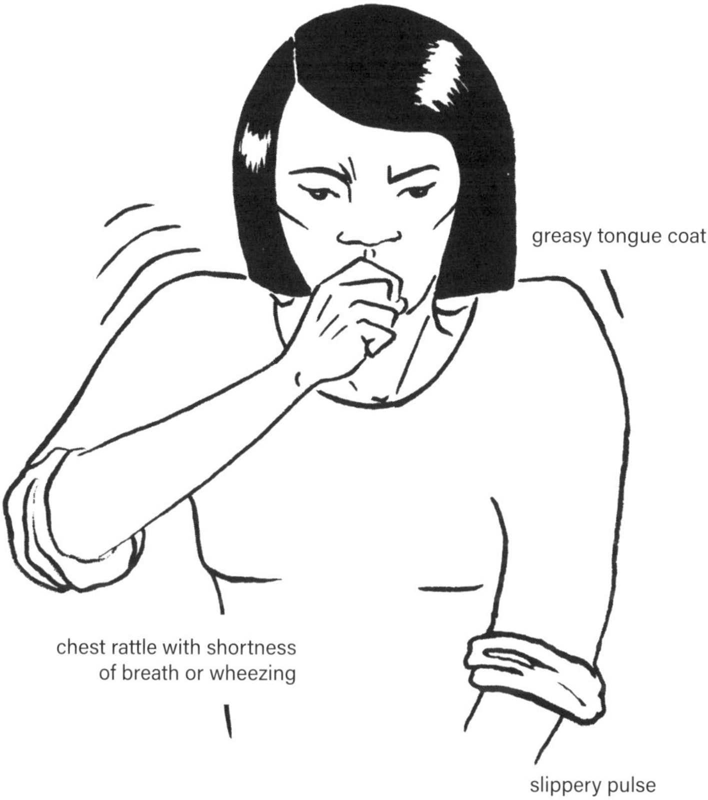

Cautions and contraindications

Not suitable during the acute stages of Lung heat (with fever and purulent sputum, *see* **3.15 Qing Qi Hua Tan Wan** or **3.16 Ching Fei Yi Huo Pien**), or for persistent unproductive cough (*see* **3.33 Yang Yin Qing Fei Wan**, **3.34 Bai He Gu Jin Wan**, **3.35 Mai Wei Di Huang Wan** or **3.31.1 Zhi Sou Wan**).

3.22 ORANGE PEEL POWDER

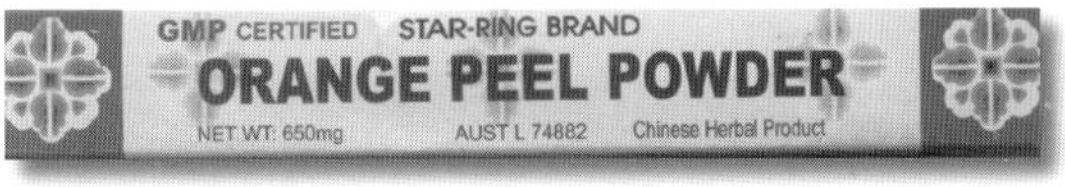

三蛇胆陈皮末

(*San She Dan Chen Pi Mo*)
Guangzhou Qixing Pharmaceutical Co. (Guangzhou)
'Three Snakes Bile and Orange Peel Powder'
Orange Peel Powder is packaged as a single dose powder in a plastic tube of 650mg

Chinese medical action

Transforms and expels phlegm, regulates qi, stops cough

Biomedical action

Expectorant, mucolytic

INDICATIONS

- Phlegm damp congestion in the Lungs. For relief of persistent productive cough or cough with deep lying and hard to expectorate sputum. Especially good for continuing sputum in the convalescent phase of an upper respiratory tract infection. The citrus assists in breaking up and transforming copious thick sputum. In contrast to **3.23 Tendrilleaf Fritillary Powder**, this formula is better when the cough is more productive.
- With the appropriate identifying features, this formula may assist in the treatment of disorders such as persistent sputum in the convalescent phase of acute bronchitis or pneumonia, the tenacious sputum of whooping cough, bronchiectasis or chronic bronchitis.

Composition (each vial contains by volume)

Citrus reticulata (chen pi, citrus) 600mg, Snake bile (she dan) 50mg

Dosage and method of administration

The adult dose is 1 vial mixed in warm water two or three times daily. In severe cases, the dose can be safely doubled for a few days. For children over 4 years old reduce the dose by half. For children below 4 years *see* **12.1 Bo Ying Compound**).

Cautions and contraindications

Not suitable for long term use. Caution during pregnancy.

3.23 TENDRILLEAF FRITILLARY POWDER

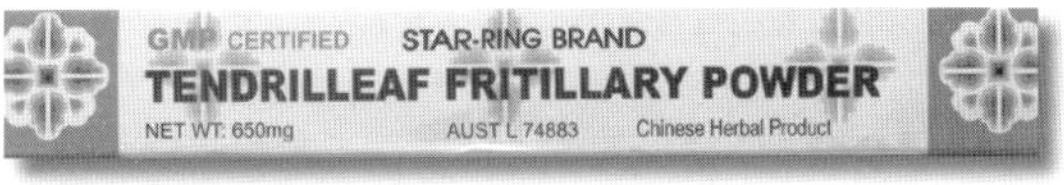

三蛇胆川贝末

(*San She Dan Chuan Bei Mo*)
Guangzhou Qixing Pharmaceutical Co. (Guangzhou)
'Three Snakes Bile and Fritillaria Powder'
Tendrilleaf Fritillary Powder is packaged as a single dose powder in a plastic tube of 650mg

Chinese medical action

Transforms and expels phlegm, moistens the Lungs, stops cough

Biomedical action

Expectorant, mucolytic

INDICATIONS

- Phlegm damp or residual phlegm heat congestion in the Lungs. For relief of persistent productive cough or cough with deep lying and hard to expectorate sputum, especially continuing sputum in the convalescent phase of an upper respiratory tract infection. Fritillaria excels at moistening and expelling dry or hard to expectorate sputum. In contrast to **3.22 Orange Peel Powder** this formula is better when there is a degree of heat and the sputum is dryer and harder to shift.
- With the appropriate identifying features, this formula may be used to treat disorders such as persistent sputum in the convalescent phase of acute bronchitis or pneumonia, the tenacious sputum of whooping cough, bronchiectasis or chronic bronchitis.

Composition (each vial contains)

Fritillaria cirrhosa (chuan bei mu, fritillaria) 600mg, Snake bile (she dan) 50mg

Dosage and method of administration

The adult dose is 1 vial mixed in warm water two or three times daily. In severe cases, the dose can be safely doubled for a few days. For children over 4 years old reduce the dose by half. For children below 4 years *see* **12.1 Bo Ying Compound**).

Cautions and contraindications

Not suitable for long term use. Caution during pregnancy.

3.24 SHE DAN CHUAN BEI PI PA GAO

蛇胆川贝枇杷膏

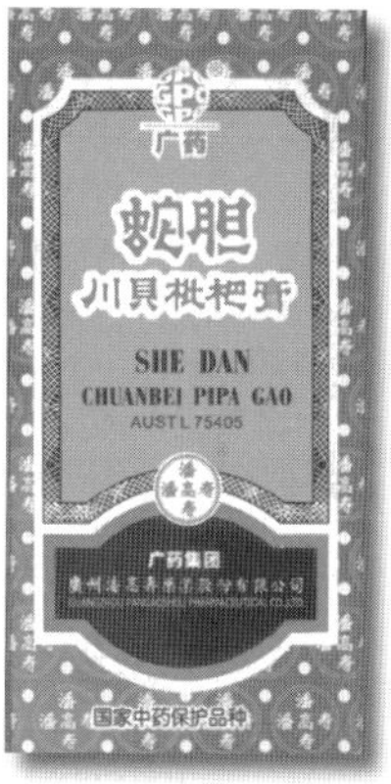

Guangzhou Pangaoshou Pharmaceutical Company (Guangzhou)
'Snake Bile, Fritillaria and Loquat Syrup'
She Dan Chuan Bei Pi Pa Gao is packaged as a sweet syrup in 100ml bottles

Chinese medical action

Breaks up, transforms and expels phlegm, stops cough

Biomedical action

Antitussive, expectorant, mucolytic

INDICATIONS

- Phlegm damp in the Lungs. Relief of persistent productive cough or cough with deep lying and hard to expectorate sputum. Similar in composition and action to **3.21 She Dan Chuan Bei Ye**, although slightly stronger and more focused on alleviating the cough that accompanies persistent phlegm congestion in the Lungs. Much used for persistent sputum in the convalescent phase of an upper respiratory tract infection.
- With the appropriate identifying features, this formula may be used to assist in the treatment of persistent sputum in the convalescent phase of acute bronchitis or pneumonia, and the tenacious sputum of whooping cough, bronchiectasis or chronic bronchitis.

Composition

Snake bile (she dan), *Fritillaria cirrhosa* (chuan bei mu, fritillaria), *Eriobotrya japonica* (pi pa ye, loquat leaf), *Platycodon grandiflorum* (jie geng, platycodon), *Pinellia ternata* (zhi ban xia, processed pinellia), menthol, honey, sucrose, benzoate as preservative

Dosage and method of administration

The recommended adult dose is one tablespoon (~ 15ml) three times daily, although many people swig straight from the bottle every now and then, with no untoward effects. For children, reduce the dose by half to a third (for children below 4 years *see* **12.1 Bo Ying Compound**).

Pattern identifying features

- **phlegm damp in the Lungs**

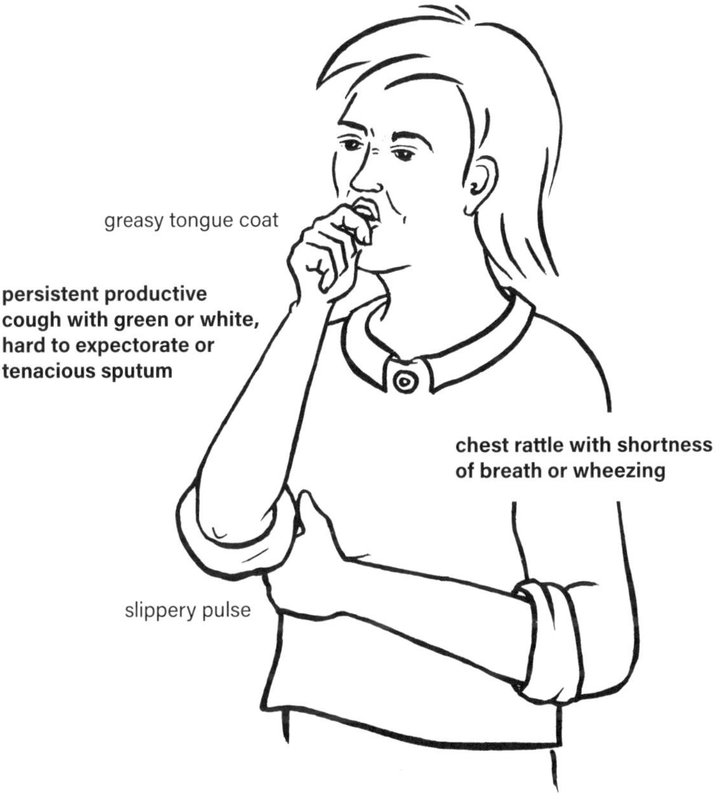

Cautions and contraindications

Not suitable during the acute stages of a lung infection (with fever and purulent sputum, *see* **3.15 Qing Qi Hua Tan Wan** or **3.16 Ching Fei Yi Huo Pien**), or for persistent unproductive cough (*see* **3.33 Yang Yin Qing Fei Wan**, **3.34 Bai He Gu Jin Wan**, **3.35 Mai Wei Di Huang Wan** or **3.31.1 Zhi Sou Wan**).

TGA

3.25 NIN JIOM PEI PA KAO

川贝枇杷膏

1-3/52

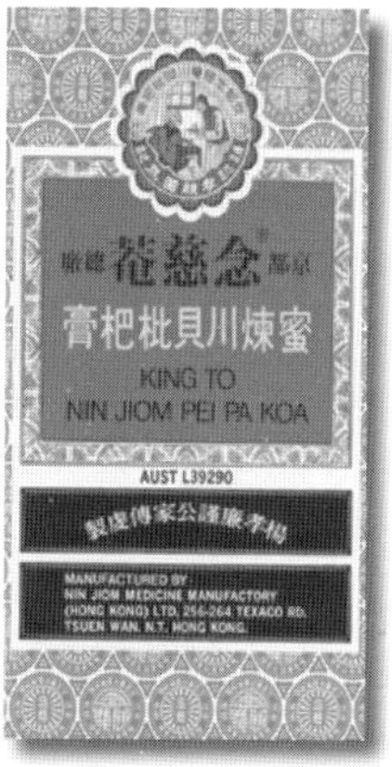

(*Chuan Bei Pi Pa Gao*)
Nin Jiom Manufactory (Hong Kong)
'Fritillaria and Loquat Leaf Syrup'
Nin Jiom Pei Pa Kao is packaged as a thick sweet syrup

Chinese medical action

Transforms and expels phlegm, clears heat, moistens Lung yin, stops cough

Biomedical action

Antitussive, expectorant, mucolytic.

INDICATIONS

- Phlegm, phlegm heat, or phlegm heat in the Lungs, with mild damage to yin and Lung fluids. Particularly useful for persistent phlegm heat cough that has begun to damage yin fluids in the Lungs. Sputum is sticky and hard to expectorate. Also for persistent cough following an upper respiratory tract infection and smokers cough. Good for children as they like the sweet taste. **3.25 Nin Jiom Pei Pa Kao** can be used for long periods for people who persist in smoking, perhaps acting to prevent some of the potential damage smoking can cause by helping break up phlegm and by moistening and cooling the Lungs. Although tending to be cooling in general, this formula is mild enough to be used for phlegm congestion without heat.
- For hoarse voice, aphonia or sore throat from phlegm, dryness or overuse. Helps soothe recurrent sore throat from phlegm heat congestion and mild dryness. This formula is particularly good for throat problems of this type as its viscosity helps it adheres to and soothe the throat.

Composition (each 15ml contains)

Eriobotria japonica (pi pa ye, loquat leaf) 600mg, *Fritillaria cirrhosa* (chuan bei mu, fritillaria) 300mg, *Prunus armenica* (xing ren, apricot seed) 300mg, *Platycodon grandiflorum* (jie geng, platycodon) 300mg, *Polygala tenuifolia* (yuan zhi, polygala) 300mg, *Glycyrrhiza uralensis* (gan cao, licorice) 300mg, *Trichosanthis kirilowii* (gua luo ren, trichosanthes seed) 300mg, *Glehnia littoralis* (sha shen, glehnia) 150mg, *Citrus reticulata* (chen pi, citrus) 150mg, *Zingiber officinale* (sheng jiang, ginger) 150mg, *Mentha arvensis* (bo he, mint) 30mg, honey

Combine with

- **3.1.1 Yin Chiao Chieh Tu Pien** for acute cough from wind heat
- **3.15 Qing Qi Hua Tan Wan** for acute cough from phlegm heat
- **3.35 Mai Wei Di Huang Wan**, **3.33 Yang Yin Qing Fei Wan** or **3.34 Bai He Gu Jin Wan** for yin deficiency or dry cough with residual sticky sputum
- **9.11 Qing Yin Wan** for dry throat problems associated with overuse or strain

Pattern identifying features

- **phlegm or phlegm heat in the Lungs with mild damage to yin fluids**

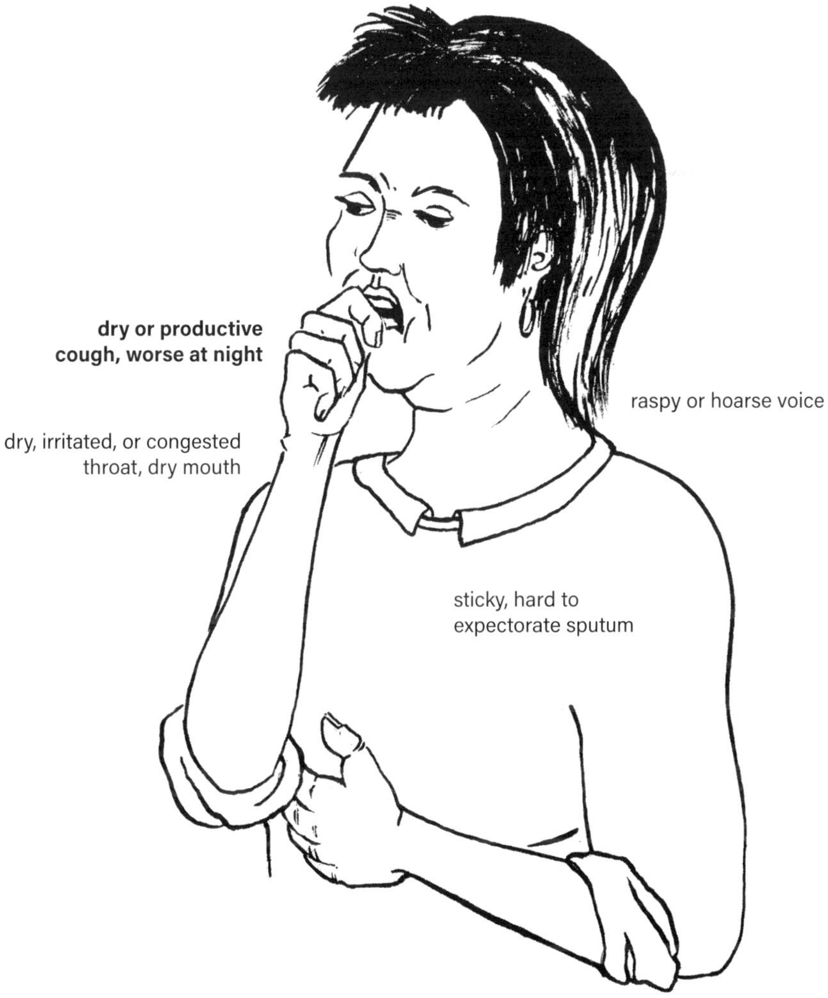

Dosage and method of administration

In chronic cases the dose for adults is one tablespoon (~15ml) three times daily (half dose for children). In general, this dose can be doubled for acute or severe cases.

Cautions and contraindications

Contraindicated in diabetic patients (due to sugar content).

3.26 MI LIAN CHUAN BEI PI PA GAO

蜜炼川贝枇杷膏

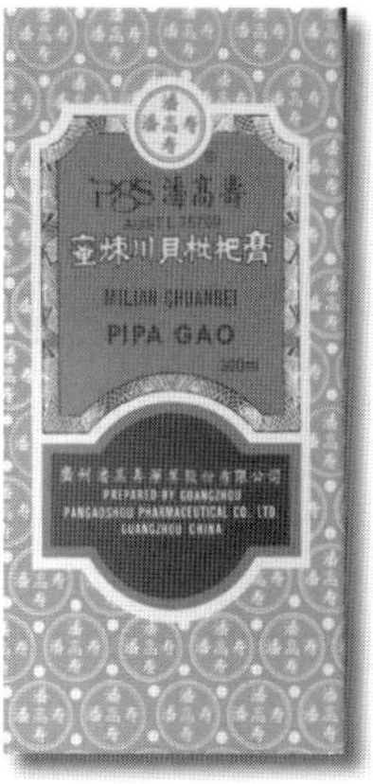

Guangzhou Pangaoshou Pharmaceutical Company (Guangzhou)
'Fritillaria and Loquat Leaf Honey Syrup'
Mi Lian Chuan Bei Pi Pa Gao is packaged as a thick sweet syrup

Chinese medical action

Transforms and expels phlegm, clears heat, moistens Lung yin, stops cough

Biomedical action

Antitussive, expectorant, mucolytic

INDICATIONS

- As for **3.25 Nin Jiom Pei Pa Kao**

Composition (w/v)

Eriobotria japonica (pi pa ye, loquat leaf) 10%, *Platycodon grandiflorum* (jie geng, platycodon) 3%, *Prunus armenica* (xing ren, apricot seed) 2%, *Adenophora tetraphylla* (nan sha shen, adenophora) 2%, *Citrus reticulata* (chen pi, citrus) 2%, *Pinellia ternata* (zhi ban xia, processed pinellia) 2%, *Schizandra chinensis* (wu wei zi, schizandra) 0.5% *Mentha arvensis* (bo he, mint oil) 0.02%, *Fritillaria cirrhosa* (chuan bei mu, fritillaria) 0.8%, honey, sucrose, benzoate as preservative.

Dosage and method of administration

In chronic cases the dose for adults is one tablespoon (~15ml) three times daily (half dose for children). In general, this dose can be doubled for acute or severe cases.

Cautions and contraindications

Caution in diabetic patients due to sugar content.

3.27 FRITILLARY AND LOQUAT LEAF MIXTURE

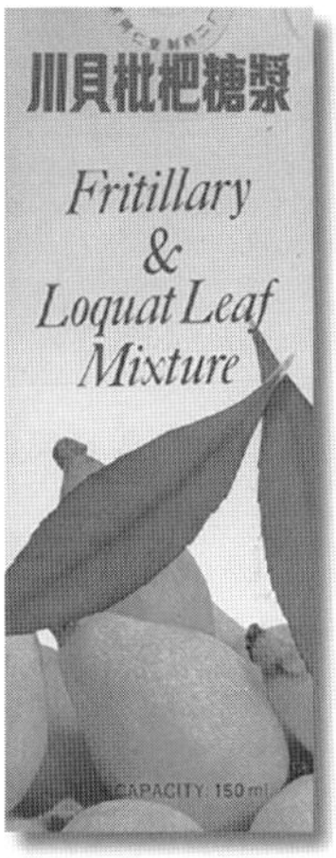

川贝枇杷糖浆

(*Chuan Bei Pi Pa Tang Jiang*)
Tong Ren Tang (Beijing)
Fritillary and Loquat Leaf Mixture is packaged in bottles of 150ml

Chinese medical action

Transforms and expels phlegm, clears heat, moistens Lung yin, stops cough

Biomedical action

Antitussive, expectorant, mucolytic

INDICATIONS

- Acute and chronic cough from phlegm or phlegm heat in the Lungs.
- Also used for cough from acute wind heat and Lung heat patterns, as well as more persistent coughs. This formula is rather thin in consistency and does not adhere to the throat on the way down, and is best suited for cough without sore throat.

Composition (each 10ml contains extracts equivalent to dry)

Eriobotria japonica (pi pa ye, loquat leaf) 3g, *Fritillaria cirrhosa* (chuan bei mu, fritillaria) 450mg, *Platycodon grandiflorum* (jie geng, platycodon) 450mg

Dosage and method of administration

Shake well before use. In chronic cases the dose for adults is one tablespoon (~15ml) three times daily (half dose for children). In general, this dose can be doubled for acute cases.

Cautions and contraindications

None noted.

3.28 LOQUAT LEAF COUGH SYRUP

止咳川贝枇杷露

1-3 / 52

(*Zhi Ke Chuan Bei Pi Pa Lu*)
Guangzhou Pangaoshou Pharmaceutical Company (Guangzhou)
Loquat Leaf Cough Syrup is packaged in bottles of 150ml

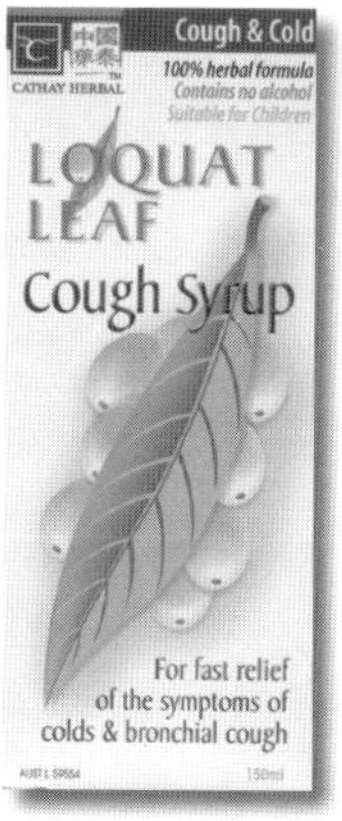

Chinese medical action

Transforms and expels phlegm, clears heat, moistens Lung yin, stops cough

Biomedical action

Antitussive, expectorant, mucolytic

INDICATIONS

- Acute and chronic cough from phlegm or phlegm heat accumulation in the Lungs. Similar to **3.27 Fritillary and Loquat Leaf Mixture**, with the addition of *Pinellia ternata* (zhi ban xia, processed pinellia) to strengthen the mucolytic action. Can be used for productive coughs associated with acute wind heat and Lung heat patterns, as well as more persistent coughs.

Composition (each 10ml contains extracts equivalent to dry)

Eriobotria japonica (pi pa ye, loquat leaf) 6.74g, *Pinellia ternata* (zhi ban xia, processed pinellia) 1.98g, *Fritillaria cirrhosa* (chuan bei mu, fritillaria) 690mg, *Platycodon grandiflorum* (jie geng, platycodon) 590mg, sucrose, benzoic acid and ethyl hydroxybenzoate (as preservatives)

Dosage and method of administration

Shake well before use. Take the appropriate dose 3-5 times daily.
2-5 years.............................. 4ml
6-12 years............................ 8ml
12+ years............................. 10-20ml

Cautions and contraindications

Not suitable for children under 2 years of age without medical advice.

3.29 AFRICAN SEA COCONUT COUGH SYRUP

非洲海底椰

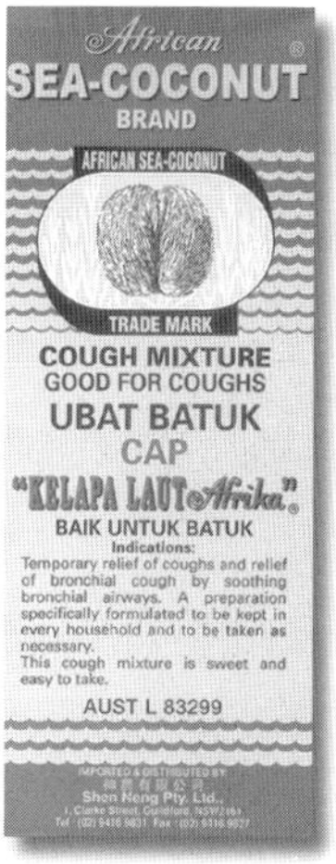

(*Fei Zhou Hai Di Ye*)
Luen Fook Medicine Co. (Malaysia)
'African Sea Coconut'
African Sea Coconut Cough Syrup is packaged in 177ml bottles of flavored syrup

Chinese medical action
Transforms phlegm and stops cough

Biomedical action
Antitussive, expectorant, mucolytic

INDICATIONS
- Cough with phlegm congestion. Good for loosening phlegm and easing persistent cough and wheezing associated with colds and flu, chronic bronchitis, asthma, bronchiectasis and general mucus congestion.
- Soothes sore throat, dry throat and throat irritation from infection, overuse, strain or smoking.

Composition (each 10ml contains)
Cephaelis ipecacuanha (tincture of ipecac) 0.224ml, *Drinia indica* (squill extract) 0.224ml, Wild Cherry Syrup 0.224ml, *Glycyrrhiza uralensis* (gan cao, licorice extract) 0.224ml, *Myroxylon balsamum* (tolu syrup) 0.448ml, sucrose, benzoate as preservative

Dosage and method of administration
Shake well before use. Take the appropriate dose 4-5 times daily mixed with an equal volume of hot water.
Infants under one year old......... ½-1 teaspoon
Children one to two years.......... 1-2 teaspoons
Children 2-16 years .... 2-3 teaspoons
Adults....................................... 4 teaspoons

Cautions and contraindications
Not suitable for children under 2 years of age without medical advice.

3.30 TONG XUAN LI FEI KOU FU YE

通宣理肺口服液

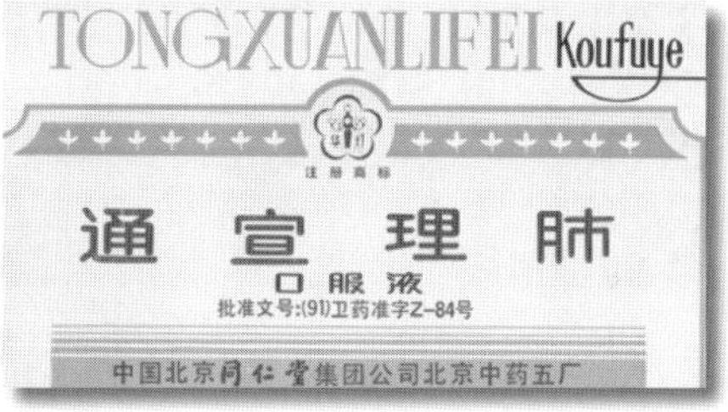

Tong Ren Tang (Beijing)
'Open, Diffuse and Regulate Lung Drink'
Tong Xuan Li Fei Kou Fu Ye is packaged in 10ml vials of liquid extract, ten vials to a box. The vials are pierced with a sharpened straw (supplied)

Chinese medical action

Stops cough and wheezing, redirects Lung qi downwards, transforms phlegm damp

Biomedical action

Antitussive, expectorant

INDICATIONS

- Phlegm damp in the Lungs causing productive cough with sticky or frothy white or slightly yellow sputum. This formula is suitable for both acute and chronic patterns, as long as phlegm damp is present.
- Wind cold common cold with productive cough or wheezing, headache and stuffy nose.

Composition (each 10ml vial contains extracts equivalent to dry)

Peucedanum praeruptorum (qian hu, peucedanum) 192mg, *Perilla frutescens* (zi su ye, perilla leaf) 164.8mg, *Platycodon grandiflorum* (jie geng, platycodon) 110.7mg, *Citrus aurantium* (zhi shi, aurantium) 110.7mg, *Citrus reticulata* (chen pi, citrus) 110.7mg, *Scutellaria baicalensis* (huang qin, scute) 110.7mg, *Poria cocos* (fu ling, hoelen) 110.7mg, *Glycyrrhiza uralensis* (gan cao, licorice) 83.6mg, *Pinellia ternata* (zhi ban xia, processed pinellia) 83.6mg, *Ephedra sinica* (ma huang*, ephedra) 44mg, *Prunus armenica* (xing ren, apricot seed) 2.5mg [**Restricted use in some jurisdictions; may be subject to substitution*]

Combine with

- **3.9 Chuan Xiong Cha Tiao Wan** for wind cold patterns with productive cough
- **3.20 Qi Guan Yan Ke Sou Tan Chuan Wan** for chronic phlegm damp in the Lungs

Dosage and method of administration

2 vials three times daily on an empty stomach (half dose for children).

Pattern identifying features

- **phlegm damp accumulation in the Lungs**
- wind cold common cold

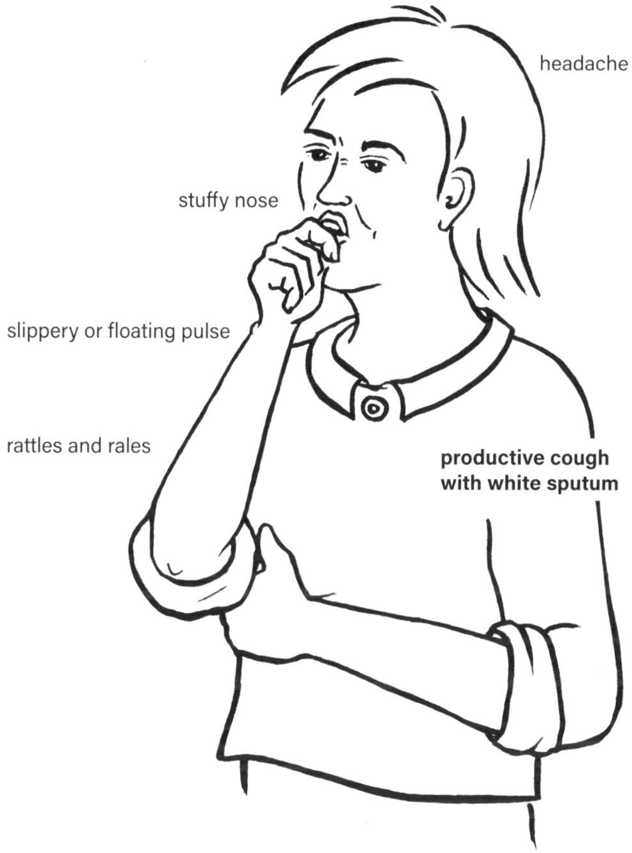

Cautions and contraindications

Contraindicated in cases with little or no sputum, or with cough, wheezing, breathlessness and asthma from yin or qi deficiency, or dryness in the Lungs. Caution in patients with hypertension. May cause or aggravate insomnia in some patients due to presence of ephedra.

3.31.1 ZHI SOU WAN

止嗽散

1-3/52

Lanzhou Foci Pharmaceutical Factory (Gansu)
'Antitussive Pills'
Zhi Sou Wan is packaged in bottles of 200 pills
Also available as: Citrus and Aster Formula (conc. extract)

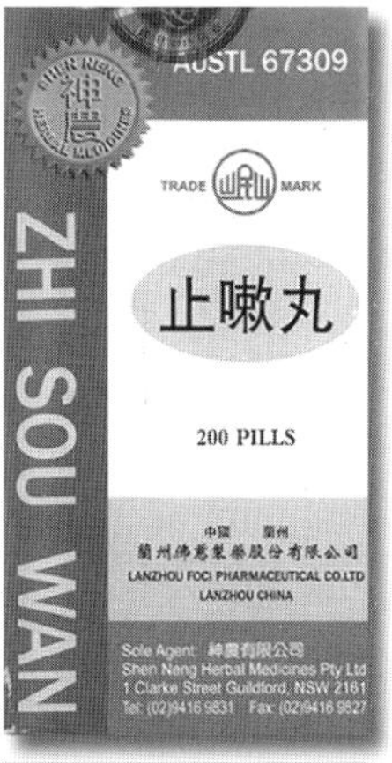

Chinese medical action

Stops cough, expels wind from the Lungs, transforms phlegm, aids the descent of Lung qi

Biomedical action

Antitussive, mildly mucolytic

INDICATIONS

- Persistent cough in the aftermath of an upper respiratory tract infection. This usually follows a wind cold or wind heat attack that was not completely cleared from the Lungs. This is a useful and broad acting antitussive formula for a range of persistent coughs in both adults and children. It can be combined with other formulas to deal with any complicating pathology (other than those noted under contraindications).

Composition (each pill contains powdered)

Schizonepeta tenuifolia (jing jie, schizonepeta) 30.6mg, *Aster tartaricus* (zi wan, aster) 30.6mg, *Stemona sessilifolia* (bai bu, stemona) 30.6mg, *Cynanchum stauntonii* (bai qian, cynanchum) 30.6mg, *Glycyrrhiza uralensis* (gan cao, licorice) 25.6mg, *Platycodon grandiflorum* (jie geng, platycodon) 20.9mg, *Citrus reticulata* (chen pi, citrus) 11.2mg

Combine with

- **2.22 Er Chen Wan** for white sputum
- **3.25 Nin Jiom Pei Pa Kao** for a dry, irritated, ticklish throat
- **3.21 She Dan Chuan Bei Ye** for sticky, yellow, residual sputum

Dosage and method of administration

15 pills three times daily on an empty stomach (one third to one half dose for children over 8 years; for small children *see* **12.5 Gan Mao Tea**). In severe cases the dose can be increased by 50%. The dose should be spread out evenly, and can be taken every two hours. If the cough persists longer than 7-10 days, or at least shows no signs of improvement in that time, the patient should be reassessed.

Pattern identifying features

- **Residual cough unresolved following wind invasion**

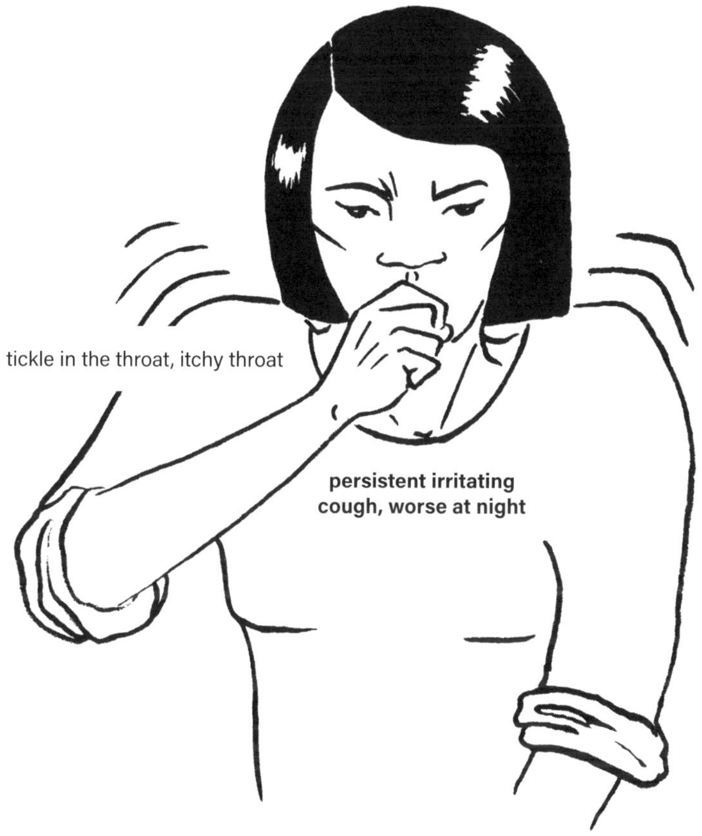

Cautions and contraindications

Not suitable for acute cough from wind cold or cough due to Lung yin deficiency.

3.31.2 ZHI SOU SAN

止嗽散

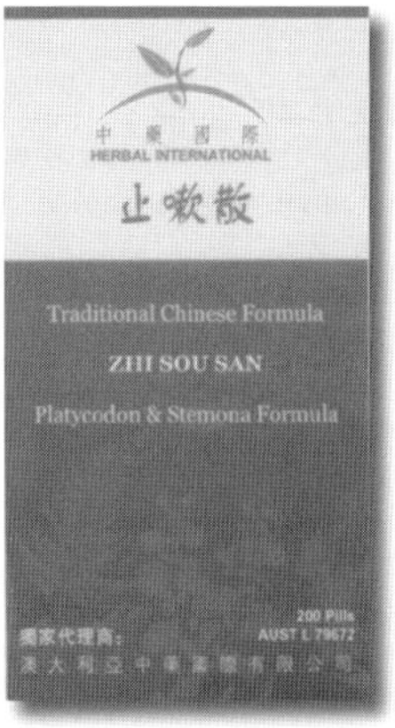

Guandong Yifang Pharmaceutical Factory (Guandong)
'Antitussive Powder'
Zhi Sou San is packaged in bottles of 200 pills

Chinese medical action

Stops cough, expels wind from the Lungs, transforms phlegm, clears heat, aids the descent of Lung qi

Biomedical action

Antitussive, mucolytic

INDICATIONS

- As for **3.31.1 Zhi Sou Wan**. This formulation is slightly stronger than **3.31.1 Zhi Sou Wan**, and includes herbs to clear heat and phlegm heat from the Lungs, making it more suitable for residual cough with sticky yellow, or hard to expectorate, sputum.

Composition (each pill contains extracts equivalent to dry)

Platycodon grandiflorum (jie geng, platycodon) 127.5mg, *Peucedanum praeruptorum* (qian hu, peucedanum) 127.5mg, *Stemona sessilifolia* (bai bu, stemona) 127.5mg, *Aster tartaricus* (zi wan, aster) 102mg, *Trichosanthes kirilowi* (gua lou, trichosanthes) 102mg, *Glycyrrhiza uralensis* (gan cao, licorice) 76.5mg, *Citrus reticulata* (chen pi, citrus) 68mg, *Schizonepeta tenuifolia* (jing jie, schizonepeta) 68mg, *Eriobotrya japonica* (pi pa ye, loquat leaf) 51mg

Combine with

– **3.25 Nin Jiom Pei Pa Kao** for a dry, irritated, ticklish throat
– **3.21 She Dan Chuan Bei Ye** for sticky, yellow, residual sputum

Dosage and method of administration

8 pills three times daily on an empty stomach. In severe cases the dose can be increased by 50%. The dose should be spread out evenly, or can be taken every two hours. If the cough persists longer than 7-10 days, or at least shows no signs of improvement in that time, the patient should be reassessed.

Cautions and contraindications

Not suitable for acute cough from wind cold or coughs due to Lung yin deficiency.

GMP

1-3/52

3.32 NING SOU WAN

宁嗽丸

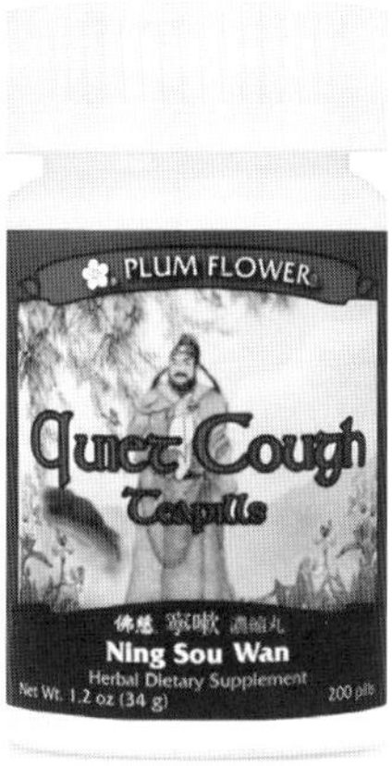

Lanzhou Foci Pharmaceutical Factory (Gansu)
'Calm Cough Pills'
Ning Sou Wan is packaged in bottles of 200 pills.
Also available as: Fritillaria and Platycodon Formula (conc. extract)

Chinese medical action

Transforms phlegm, stops cough, moistens Lung yin

Biomedical action

Antitussive, mucolytic

INDICATIONS

- Post acute or chronic cough associated with Lung heat, dryness or mild yin deficiency. Best for lingering cough following an upper respiratory tract infection or wind heat common cold that has not been cleared completely, and that has left a residue of heat and dryness. The cough is dry and hacking, worse at night, with small amounts of sticky or hard to expectorate sputum.

Composition

Fritillaria cirrhosa (chuan bei mu, fritillaria), *Pinellia ternata* (jiang ban xia, ginger processed pinellia), *Perilla frutescens* (su zi, perilla seed), *Platycodon grandiflorum* (jie geng, platycodon), *Glehnia littoralis* (bei sha shen, glehnia), *Poria cocos* (fu ling, hoelen), *Morus alba* (sang bai pi, mulberry root bark), *Mentha arvensis* (bo he, mint), *Prunus armenica* (xing ren, apricot seed), *Citrus erythrocarpae* (ju hong, tangerine peel), *Oryza sativa* (gu ya, sprouted rice), *Glycyrrhiza uralensis* (gan cao, licorice)

Combine with

– **3.21 She Dan Chuan Bei Ye** for sticky, yellow sputum

Dosage and method of administration

8-12 pills three times daily on an empty stomach. In severe cases or the early stages a 50% increase in dose can be used, then reduced to a maintenance dose as treatment takes effect.

Cautions and contraindications

Not suitable for acute cough from wind cold (*see* **3.5 Ma Huang Tang**), cough due to severe phlegm heat (*see* **3.15 Qing Qi Hua Tan Wan**) or Lung yin deficiency (*see* **3.33 Yang Yin Qing Fei Wan** or **3.34 Bai He Gu Jin Wan**).

3.33 YANG YIN QING FEI WAN

养阴清肺丸

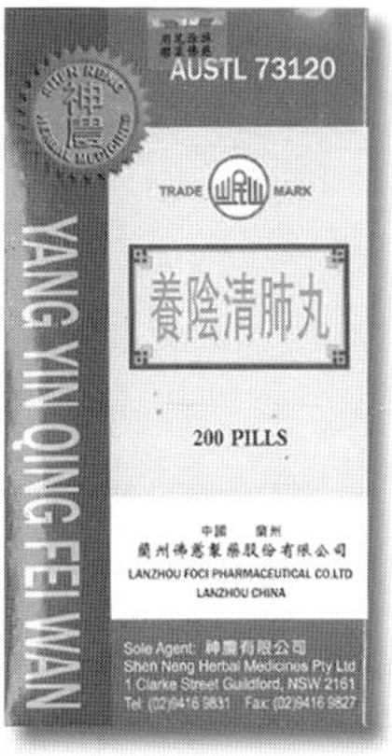

Lanzhou Foci Pharmaceutical Factory (Gansu)
'Pills to Nourish Yin and Clear (Heat from) the Lungs'
Yang Yin Qing Fei Wan is packaged in bottles of 200 pills

Chinese medical action

Nourishes and moistens Lung yin, cools the Lungs, benefits the throat, moistens the Intestines

Biomedical action

Demulcent febrifuge, antitussive, mild laxative

INDICATIONS

- Dry cough and wheezing from Lung yin deficiency. For all chronic respiratory illness resulting in Lung yin deficiency, or yin damage following an acute episode of heat or fire in the Lungs.
- Recurrent dry, sore or irritated throat.
- Dryness of the gastrointestinal system. This includes constipation following a febrile illness that has damaged yin and fluids, and dryness of the oral cavity, either from local pathology, the after effects of radiation treatment, or systemic pathology like diabetes and Sjögren's syndrome.
- Useful for smokers of tobacco and other substances that introduce heat into the Lungs, damaging Lung yin. This formula can aid in repair and cooling of the Lungs, while clearing stubborn phlegm accumulation.
- With the appropriate identifying features, this formula may be used to treat disorders such as the chronic dry cough of patients with lung cancer, tuberculosis and other chronic respiratory diseases, chronic tonsillitis, pharyngitis and smokers cough.
- Originally created to treat epidemic 'white throat disorder' (*bái hóu* 白喉), analogous to diptheria, with a white curd like membrane on the respiratory mucosa, swollen throat and fever. Diptheria is life threatening and should be managed in hospital.

Composition (each pill contains powdered)

Rehmannia glutinosa (sheng di, rehmannia) 25.6mg, *Ophiopogon japonicus* (mai dong, ophiopogon) 25.6mg, *Scrophularia ningpoensis* (xuan shen, scrophularia) 25.6mg, *Paeonia suffruticosa* (mu dan pi, moutan) 25.6mg, *Paeonia lactiflora* (bai shao, white peony) 25.6mg, *Mentha haplocalycis* (bo he, mint) 11.2mg, *Glycyrrhiza uralensis* (gan cao, licorice) 11.2mg, *Fritillaria cirrhosa* (chuan bei mu, fritillaria) 9.6mg

Combine with

- **10.2 Raw Tienchi Tablets** for blood streaked sputum or coughing blood
- **9.9 Superior Sore Throat Powder** for sore throat
- **1.34 Hai Zao Jing Wan** for the swollen rubbery cervical lymph nodes that sometimes occur in chronic Lung yin deficiency
- **7.1.1 Liu Wei Di Huang Wan** for chronic constipation from yin deficiency

Pattern identifying features

- **Lung yin deficiency**
- low grade, afternoon or tidal fever

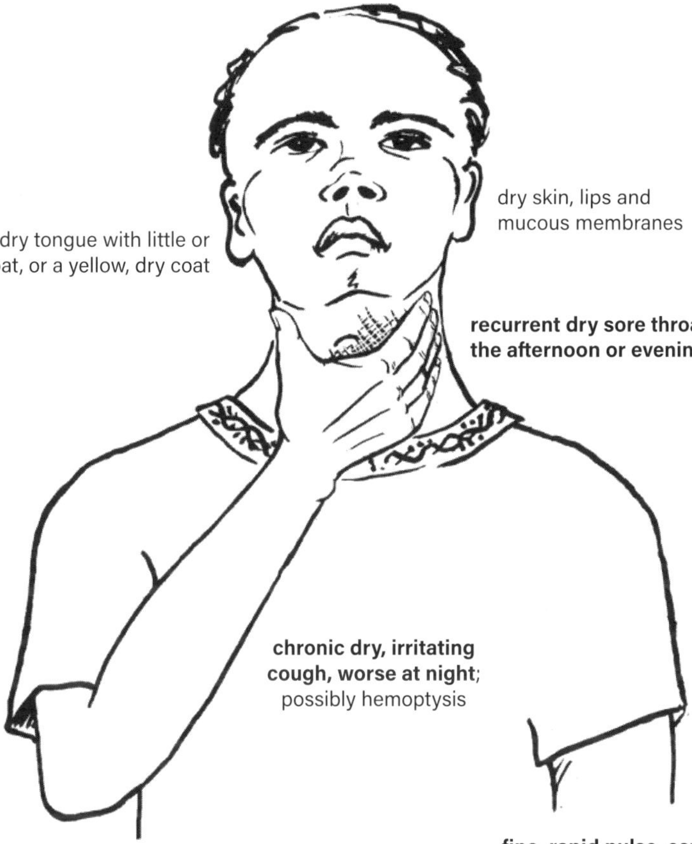

Dosage and method of administration

8-12 pills three times daily on an empty stomach. In severe cases or during the early stages of treatment (the first few weeks), a 50% increase in dose can be used, then reduced to a maintenance dose as treatment takes effect.

Cautions and contraindications

Contraindicated during pregnancy. Not suitable for acute cough from an external pathogenic invasion. This formula can be cloying, and can aggravate damp and Spleen deficiency in some patients. This can usually be alleviated by taking the pills with a small dose (3-6 pills at the same time) of **2.18 Bao He Wan**.

3.34 BAI HE GU JIN WAN

百合固金丸

T G A

3+ 12

Lanzhou Foci Pharmaceutical Factory (Gansu)
'Lily Pills to Strengthen Metal (Lungs)'
Bai He Gu Jin Wan is packaged in bottles of 200 pills
Also available as: Lilium Teapills (PF), Lily Combination (conc. extract)

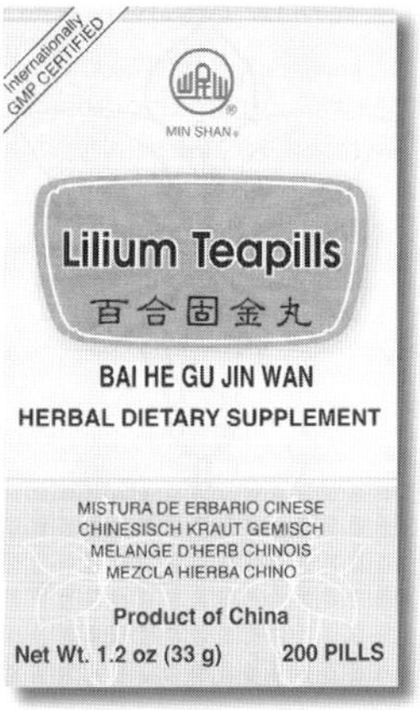

Chinese medical action

Nourishes and moistens Lung and Kidney yin, cools the Lungs, transforms phlegm and stops cough, moistens the Intestines

Biomedical action

Demulcent febrifuge, antitussive, mild laxative

INDICATIONS

- Lung and Kidney yin deficiency. Similar in action to **3.33 Yang Yin Qing Fei Wan**, but more enriching to yin. Used for chronic Lung and Kidney yin deficiency with dry cough, wheezing and persitent dry, sore throat. Cough is worse at night with sporadic hemoptysis or blood streaked sputum. Throat soreness is worse in the afternoon and towards the evening; the throat is usually not especially red or inflamed.
- Dryness of the gastrointestinal system, post febrile constipation, oral effects of radiation treatment, Sjögren's syndrome.
- Useful for patients with chronic respiratory disorders being treated by oral steroids. Rehmannia formulas have a steroid sparing effect.
- With the appropriate identifying features, this formula may be used to treat disorders such as the chronic dry cough of patients with lung cancer, tuberculosis, silicosis and other chronic respiratory diseases, chronic tonsillitis, pharyngitis and smokers cough.

Composition (each pill contains powdered)

Rehmannia glutinosa (shu di, cooked rehmannia), *Rehmannia glutinosa* (sheng di, raw rehmannia), *Scrophularia ningpoensis* (xuan shen, scrophularia), *Ophiopogon japonicus* (mai dong, ophiopogon), *Paeonia lactiflora* (bai shao, white peony), *Lilium brownii* (bai he, lily), *Fritillaria cirrhosa* (chuan bei mu, fritillaria), *Glycyrrhiza uralensis* (gan cao, licorice), *Angelica polymorpha* (dang gui, chinese angelica), *Platycodon grandiflorum* (jie geng, platycodon)

Dosage and method of administration

8-12 pills three times daily on an empty stomach. The dose can be spread out, or taken in two lots of 12-18 pills, morning and evening. In severe cases or during the early stages of treatment (the first few weeks), a 50% increase in dose can be used, then reduced as treatment takes effect.

Pattern identifying features

- **Lung and Kidney yin deficiency**
- dry skin, lips and mucous membranes
- thirst, dry mouth and throat
- low grade, afternoon or tidal fever
- night sweats
- heat in the palms and soles

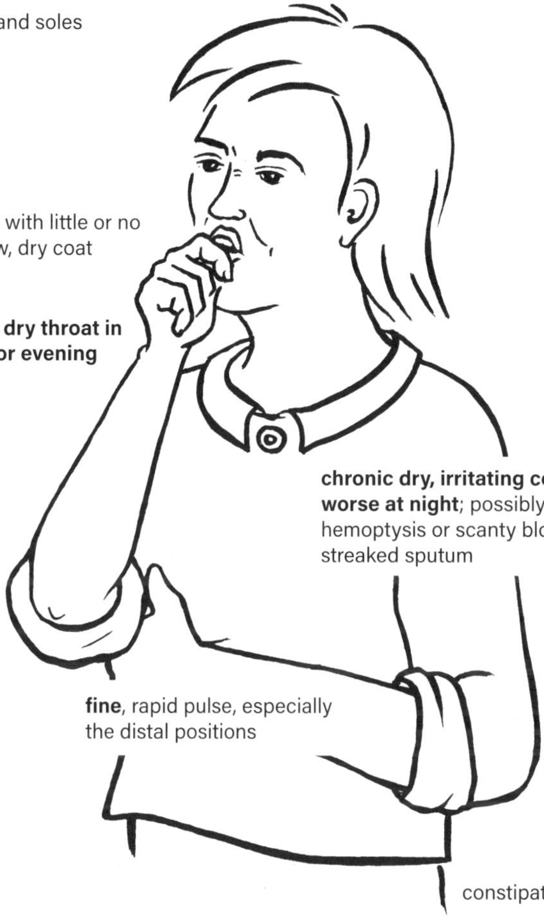

Cautions and contraindications

Not suitable for acute cough from an external pathogenic invasion or phlegm accumulation. This formula is quite rich and cloying, and can aggravate dampness and Spleen deficiency in some patients. This can usually be alleviated by taking the pills with a small dose (3-6 pills at the same time) of **2.18 Bao He Wan**.

3.35 MAI WEI DI HUANG WAN
麦味地黄丸

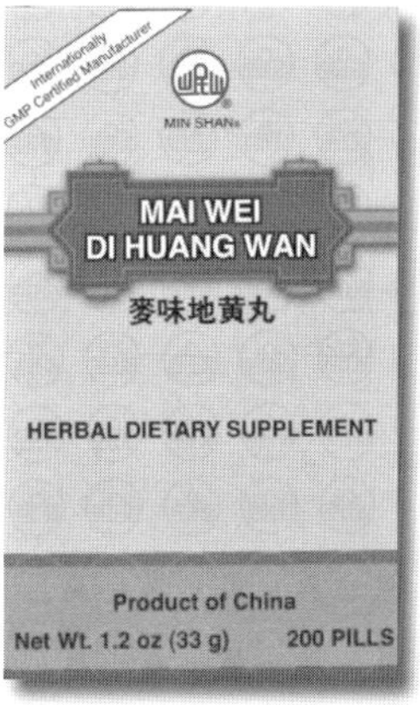

Lanzhou Foci Pharmaceutical Factory (Gansu)
'Eight Immortal Pill for Longevity'
Mai Wei Di Huang Wan is packaged in bottles of 200 pills
Also available as: Ba Xian Chang Shou Wan, Eight Immortals Teapills (PF)

Chinese medical action
Nourishes and moistens Lung and Kidney yin

Biomedical action
Antitussive, hypoglycemic, anti-hypertensive, improves kidney function

INDICATIONS
- Lung and Kidney yin deficiency respiratory disorders. A variation of **7.1.1 Liu Wei Di Huang Wan**, the main indications are dry consumptive coughing, asthma, wheezing and recurrent sore throat. Cough worse at night, with sporadic hemoptysis or blood streaked sputum. Throat soreness worse in the afternoon and towards evening, with the throat usually not especially red or inflamed.
- Useful for patients with chronic respiratory disorders being treated by oral steroids. Rehmannia formulas have a steroid sparing effect and can moderate the negative effects of steroids.
- With the appropriate identifying features, this formula may be used to assist in treatment of disorders such as the chronic dry cough of patients with lung cancer, tuberculosis, silicosis and other chronic respiratory diseases, chronic tonsillitis, pharyngitis and smokers cough.

Composition (each pill contains powdered)
Rehmannia glutinosa (shu di, processed rehmannia), *Cornus officinalis* (shan zhu yu, cornus), *Dioscorea opposita* (shan yao, dioscorea), *Poria cocos* (fu ling, hoelen), *Alisma orientalis* (ze xie, alisma), *Paeonia suffruticosa* (mu dan pi, moutan), *Ophiopogon japonicus* (mai dong, ophiopogon), *Schizandra chinensis* (wu wei zi, schizandra)

Combine with
– **9.11 Qing Yin Wan** or **3.36 Luo Han Kuo Beverage** for chronic sore dry throat and hoarseness

Dosage and method of administration
8-12 pills three times daily on an empty stomach. The dose can be spread out, or taken in two lots of 12-18 pills, morning and evening. In severe cases or during the early stages of treatment (the first few weeks), a 50% increase in dose can be used, then reduced as treatment takes effect.

Pattern identifying features

- **Kidney and Lung yin deficiency**
- dry skin, lips and mucous membranes
- thirst, dry mouth and throat
- low grade, afternoon or tidal fever
- night sweats
- heat in the palms and soles
- weight loss

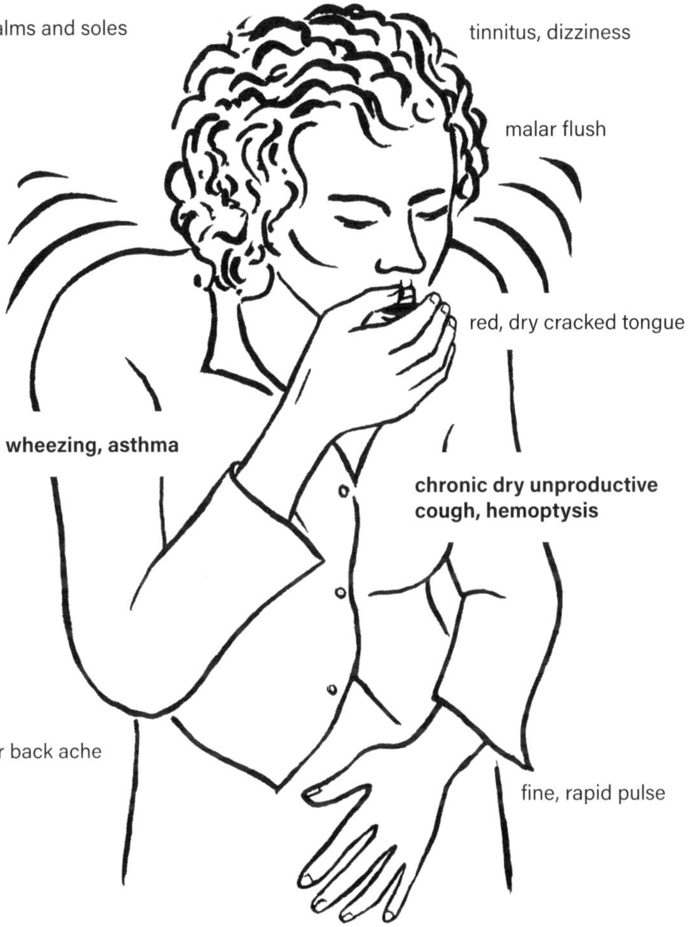

Cautions and contraindications

Not suitable for acute cough from an external pathogenic invasion. This formula is rich and cloying, and can aggravate damp and Spleen deficiency in some patients. This can usually be alleviated by adding a small dose (3–6 pills at the same time) of **2.18 Bao He Wan**.

1-3/12

3.36 LO HAN KUO BEVERAGE

罗汉果冲剂

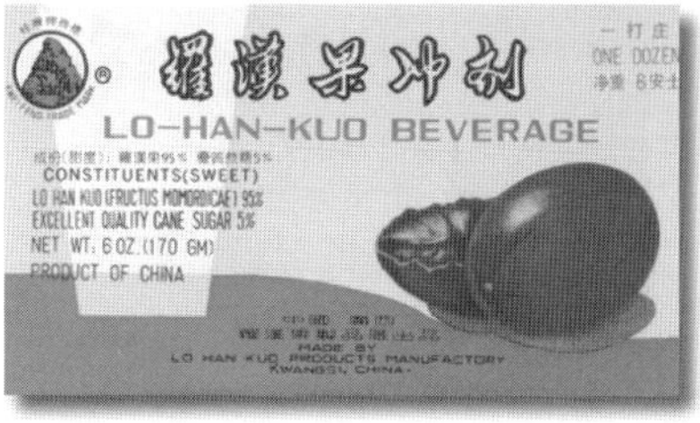

(*Luo Han Guo Chong Ji*)
Luo Han Kuo Products Manufactory (Guangxi)
'Momordica Soluble Granules'
Lo Han Guo Beverage is packaged in blocks of soluble compressed granules, twelve blocks per box

Chinese medical action

Nourishes and moistens Lung yin, cools the Lungs, stops cough, moistens the Intestines

Biomedical action

Antitussive, demulcent

INDICATIONS

- Dry cough and generalized dryness of the respiratory system (lips, mucous membranes) from Lung heat. Used for stubborn, chronic dry cough following an upper respiratory tract infection and smoking, and recurrent sore throat from Lung dryness.
- Hoarse voice or loss of voice from overuse, smoking, environmental dryness or following an upper respiratory tract infection.
- Constipation from dryness of the Intestines or following a febrile illness that damages Intestinal yin and fluids.
- With the appropriate identifying features, this medicine may assist in the treatment of disorders such as acute and chronic bronchitis, acute and chronic tonsillitis and pharyngitis, whooping cough and smoker's cough.

Composition

Momordica grosvenori (luo han guo, momordica fruit) 95%, sugar 5%

Dosage and method of administration

One block dissolved in a cup of boiling water 2-3 times daily.

Cautions and contraindications

Caution in patients with Spleen deficiency or diarrhea.

GMP

1-3/12

3.37 SHA SHEN MAI MEN DONG WAN

沙参麦门冬丸

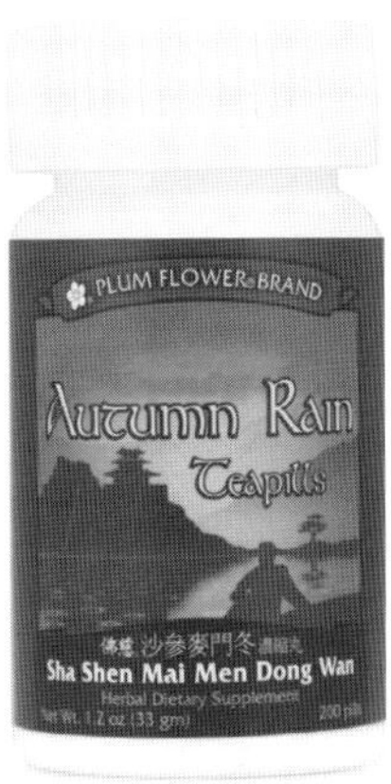

Lanzhou Foci Pharmaceutical Factory (Gansu)
'Adenophora and Ophiopogon Pills'
Sha Shen Mai Men Dong Wan is packaged in bottles of 200 pills
Also available as: Glehnia and Ophiopogon Combination (conc. extract)

Chinese medical action
Moistens dryness, nourishes Lung and Stomach yin

Biomedical action
Demulcent, antitussive

INDICATIONS

- Dryness patterns of the Lungs and Stomach. Both these organs are sensitive to dryness and are easily affected by the pathogenic heat patterns, weather, habits such as smoking and diet. This formula assists in replenishing healthy moist linings on dry or damaged tissues, and improves function and health of mucus membranes. Typical features are dry cough, dry mouth and throat, thirst, a dry tongue with little or no coat and a fine, rapid pulse. Helpful in alleviating the adverse effects of very dry climates.
- With the appropriate identifying features, this medicine may assist in the treatment of biomedical disorders such as residual dry cough following an upper respiratory tract infection, smokers cough, pharyngitis and gastritis.

Composition
Adenophora tetraphylla (nan sha shen, adenophora), *Glehnia littoralis* (bei sha shen, glehnia), *Ophiopogon japonicus* (mai dong, ophiopogon), *Polygonatum odoratum* (yu zhu, polygonatum), *Morus alba* (sang ye, mulberry leaf), *Trichosanthes kirilowi* (tian hua fen, trichosanthes root), *Dolichos lablab* (bian dou, hyacinth bean), *Glycyrrhiza uralensis* (gan cao, licorice)

Dosage and method of administration
8-12 pills three times daily on an empty stomach. The dose can be spread out, or taken in two lots of 12-18 pills, morning and evening. In severe cases or during the early stages of treatment, a 50% increase in dose can be used, then reduced as treatment takes effect.

Cautions and contraindications
Contraindicated in phlegm damp patterns.

3.38 SHENG MAI SAN WAN

生脉散丸

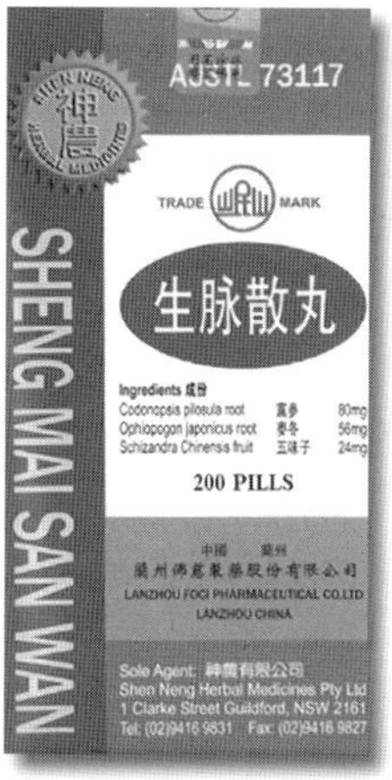

Lanzhou Foci Pharmaceutical Factory (Gansu)
'Generate the Pulse Pills'
Sheng Mai San Wan is packaged in bottles of 200 pills
Also available as: Great Pulse Teapills (PF), Ginseng and Ophiopogon Formula (conc. extract)

Chinese medical action

Tonifies qi and yin (especially of the Lungs, Heart and Stomach), moistens dryness, stops sweating

Biomedical action

Demulcent, energy stimulant, anhidrotic

INDICATIONS

- Chronic respiratory disorders, in particular coughing, wheezing and breathlessness, from Lung qi and yin deficiency.
- Convalescence following febrile illness. A high fever, especially when the Lungs and/or Stomach are affected, often damages qi and yin, with patients suffering night sweats and easy sweating, persistent fatigue, insomnia and restlessness in the post-acute phase of the infection.
- Cardiac disorders such as cardiac weakness, palpitations, cardiac arrhythmias (irregularity, tachycardia and bradycardia), and *shén* disturbances from Heart qi and yin deficiency.
- An elegant formula with wide application, and as long as the basic pattern is one of qi and yin deficiency, it can be used to treat a variety of cardiac and respiratory disorders such as chronic asthma and persistent cough, cardiac arrhythmia, tachycardia, chronic obstructive airways disease (COAD), chronic bronchitis, post febrile weakness, debility following sunstroke, post coronary artery bypass debility, coronary artery disease and gastritis.

Composition (each pill contains powdered)

Codonopsis pilosula (dang shen, codonopsis) 80mg, *Ophiopogon japonicus* (mai dong, ophiopogon) 56mg, *Schizandra chinensis* (wu wei zi, schizandra) 24mg

Combine with

- **7.23 Yu Ping Feng Wan** for spontaneous sweating and low immunity from defensive qi deficiency
- **7.1.1 Liu Wei Di Huang Wan** for chronic Lung and Kidney qi and yin deficiency respiratory weakness and wheezing

Pattern identifying features

- **Lung, Heart and Stomach qi and yin deficiency**
- post febrile yin damage
- spontaneous sweating, night sweats
- breathlessness
- dry mouth and throat
- insomnia

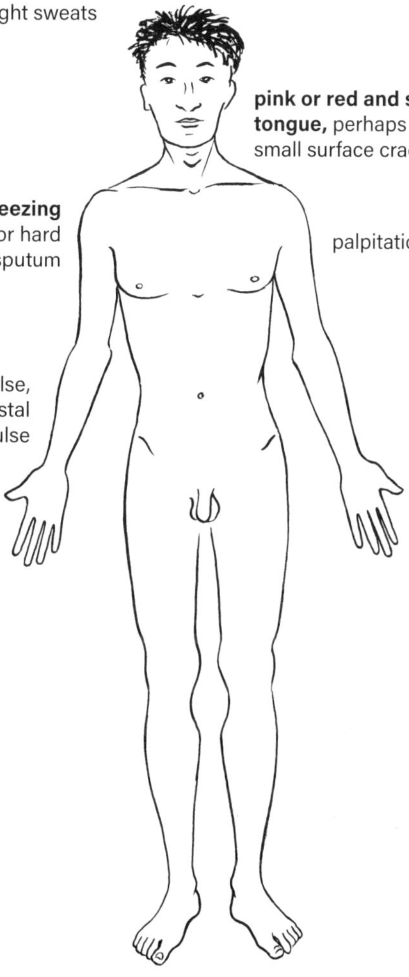

Dosage and method of administration

15-20 pills three times daily on an empty stomach, or two lots of 22-30 pills twice daily, morning and evening. Once the patient notices an effect, reduce the dose to a maintenance level (around 24-36 pills daily).

Cautions and contraindications

Contraindicated in the early stages of a febrile illness, or when there is residual pathogenic influence remaining in the Lungs.

3.39 YULIN BU SHEN WAN

玉林补肾丸

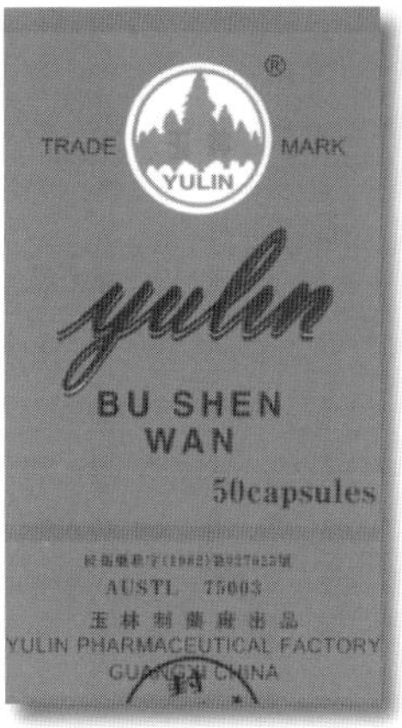

Yulin Pharmaceutical Factory (Guangxi)
'Tonify Kidney Pills from Yulin'
Yulin Bu Shen Wan is packaged in bottles of 50 capsules.
A similar formula is available as: Gecko Tonic Teapills (PF)

Chinese medical action

Strengthens, warms and supports Kidney yang, tonifies source qi and essence, strengthens the Spleen

Biomedical action

Stimulant and tonic, adaptogenic, warms the body, improves respiratory function

INDICATIONS

- Chronic wheezing, asthma and breathlessness from Lung and Kidney yang qi deficiency. Used to strengthen the Kidneys and their action of assisting inspiration for patients with a long history of respiratory weakness, asthma and emphysema.
- Urinary disorders associated with deficiency Kidney yang, including frequent urination, nocturia, incontinence of urine, broken stream or difficulty getting started.
- Useful for supporting essence. Used for all essence disorders in children and adults, including failure to thrive, slow development, learning problems, congenital disorders, loss of memory, weakening of the bones and teeth.
- Loss of libido, impotence, infertility.
- Generalized debility, convalescence from a debilitating, prolonged or serious illness or surgery. A good general tonic for the elderly and excellent to build immunity in weak and immunocompromised patients with a tendency to yang deficiency.

Composition (each capsule contains powdered)

Gecko gecko (ge jie, gecko) 100mg, *Cervus japonicus* (lu rong, deer velvet) 25mg, *Panax ginseng* (ren shen, ginseng) 25mg, *Astragalus membranaceous* (huang qi, astragalus) 50mg, *Eucommia ulmoides* (du zhong, eucommia) 50mg, *Lycium chinensis* (gou qi zi, lycium) 50mg, *Cordyceps sinensis* (dong chong xia cao, cordyceps stroma) 25mg, *Poria cocos* (fu ling, hoelen) 85mg, *Atractylodes macrocephala* (bai zhu, atractylodes) 65mg

Combine with

– **7.23 Yu Ping Feng Wan** or **2.11 Bu Zhong Yi Qi Wan** for severe spontaneous sweating and immune deficiency

Dosage and method of administration

3-4 capsules, two or three times daily on an empty stomach. Half dose for children 8-12 years old. For infants and small children, one or two capsules per day can be opened and mixed in with a suitable soft and disguising food.

Pattern identifying features

- **Kidney failing to grasp Lung qi; Lung and Kidney yang deficiency**
- urinary dysfunction
- fatigue, increased desire to sleep
- spontaneous sweating

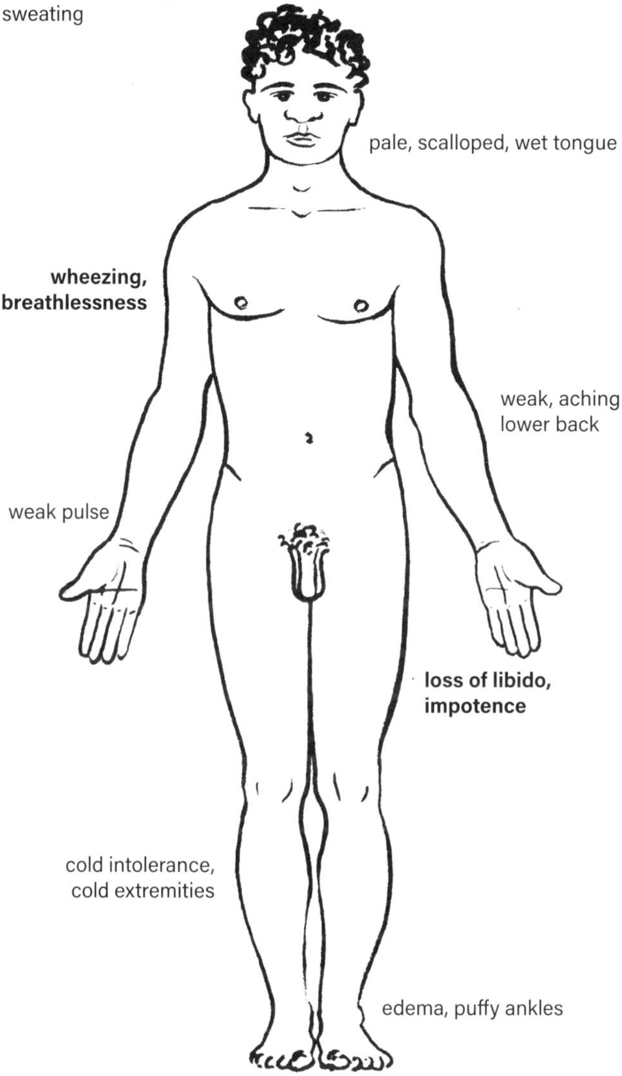

Cautions and contraindications

Contraindicated during the early phase of acute illness such as colds and flu. This formula is quite warming, and may overheat some patients, especially if they are taking other warming medications, such as steroids. Best to start with a smaller than standard dose for a week or two and gradually increase it until the desired dose level is achieved. If overheating occurs, reduction in dose will alleviate it.

GMP

3.40 BU FEI WAN

3+/12

补肺丸

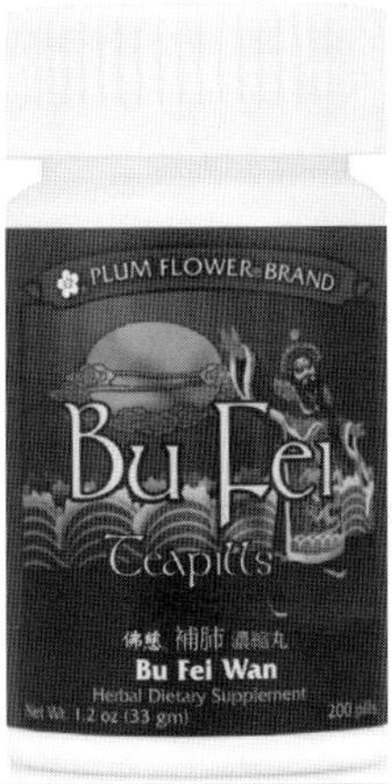

Lanzhou Foci Pharmaceutical Factory (Gansu)
'Pills to Tonify the Lungs'
Bu Fei Wan is packaged in bottles of 200 pills
Also available as: Ginseng and Aster Combination (conc. extract)

Chinese medical action

Tonifies Lung qi and defensive qi, nourishes yin, stops cough and sweating

Biomedical action

Antitussive, energy stimulant, anhidrotic

INDICATIONS

- Chronic cough, wheezing, breathlessness, sweating and fatigue from Lung qi deficiency causing. The cough is weak and persistent, tires the patient out, and is aggravated or initiated by exertion, fatigue or exposure to wind. Sputum, if present, is thin and mostly clear, frothy or white.
- With the appropriate identifying features this formula can assist in the treatment of conditions such as chronic asthma, persistent cough, chronic obstructive airways disease (COAD) and chronic bronchitis.

Composition

Astragalus membranaceous (huang qi, astragalus), *Rehmannia glutinosa* (shu di, processed rehmannia), *Morus alba* (sang bai pi, mulberry root bark), *Aster tataricus* (zi wan, aster), *Changium smyrnioides* (ming dang shen, changium), *Schizandra chinensis* (wu wei zi, schizandra), *Panax ginseng* (ren shen, ginseng)

Combine with

- **7.23 Yu Ping Feng Wan** or **3.41 Xu Han Ting** for severe spontaneous sweating and low immunity from defensive qi deficiency
- **2.8 Liu Jun Zi Wan** or **7.22 Shen Qi Da Bu Wan** for more severe Spleen qi deficiency
- **7.15 Yulin Da Bu Wan** if Kidney weakness is contributing to wheezing
- **3.22 Orange Peel Powder** for copious white sputum

Dosage and method of administration

8-12 pills three times daily on an empty stomach. The dose can be spread out, or taken in two lots of 12-18 pills, morning and evening. In severe cases or during the early stages of treatment (the first few weeks), a 50% increase in dose can be used, then reduced as treatment takes effect.

Pattern identifying features

- **Lung qi deficiency**
- weak low voice or a reluctance to speak
- frequent colds
- aversion to wind

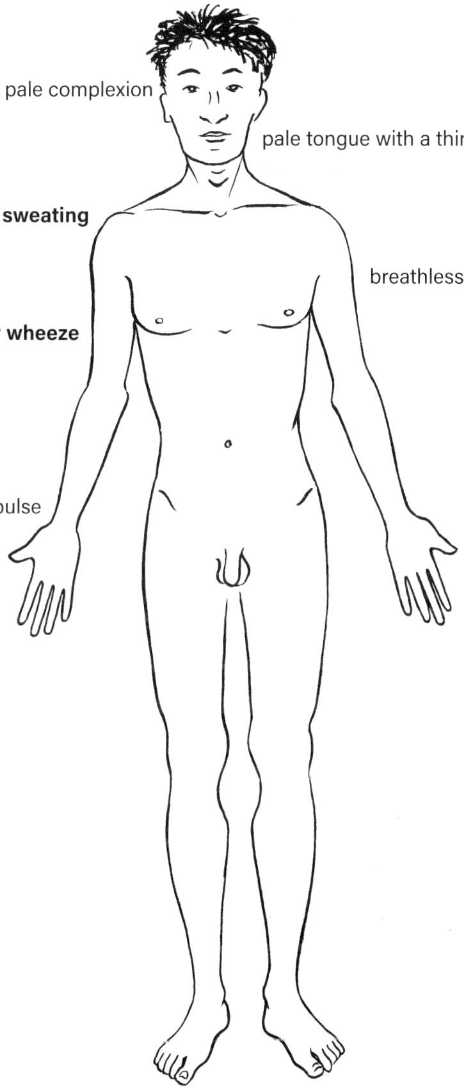

Cautions and contraindications

Contraindicated in the early stages of a febrile illness, or when there is residual pathogenic influence remaining in the Lungs.

3.41 XU HAN TING

虛汗停

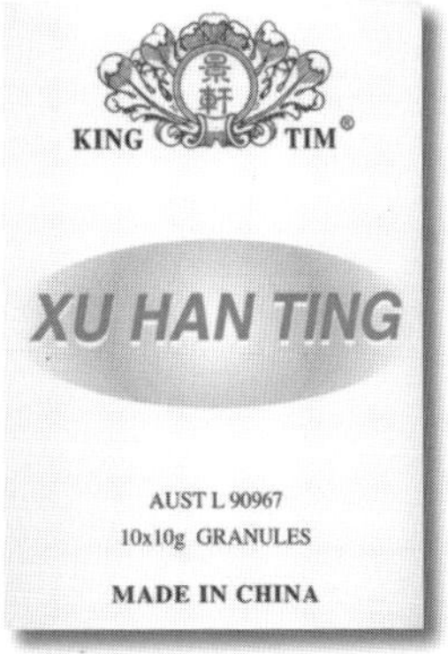

Jing Xian Pharmaceutical Co. (Guangzhou)
'Stop Sweating from Deficiency'
Xu Han Ting is packaged in 10 gram sachets of soluble granules, ten sachets per box

Chinese medical action

Tonifies Spleen and Lung qi, fortifies defensive qi, stops sweating

Biomedical action

Astringent, anhidrotic, stimulates immunity

INDICATIONS

- Sweating associated with defensive qi deficiency. The focus of this astringent formula is on controlling the symptom of sweating, while secondarily strengthening the source of defensive qi, the Spleen. Although it is targeted at defensive qi, it can be used for any type of excessive sweating disorder when combined with the appropriate constitutional formula.
- Weakened immunity. Can be used alone for weak immunity, especially good for children. Can be used preventively for those at risk of increased exposure to pathogens, such as children starting daycare or during influenza epidemics.
- Allergies. May be useful in hay fever, asthma and other atopic respiratory conditions, as these are often associated with defensive qi deficiency and chronic retention of wind in the nasal and respiratory mucous membranes.

Composition (each sachet contains extracts equivalent to dry)

Astragalus membranaceous (huang qi, astragalus) 2.97g, *Zizyphus jujuba* (da zao, chinese dates) 2.97g, *Oryza sativa* (nuo dao gen, glutinous rice root) 3.96g, *Triticum aestivum* (fu xiao mai, wheat) 3.96g, *Dioscorea opposita* (shan yao, dioscorea) 1.98g, *Atractylodes macrocephala* (bai zhu, atractylodes) 1.32g, *Pseudostellaria heterophylla* (tai zi shen, pseudostellaria) 1.32g, *Ostrea gigas* (mu li, oyster shell powder) 600mg

Combine with

- **1.25 Er Xian Wan** or **1.23 Zhi Bai Di Huang Wan** for frequent night sweats from yin deficiency
- **2.11 Bu Zhong Yi Qi Wan** or **7.23 Yu Ping Feng Wan** for spontaneous sweating and frequent colds from defensive qi deficiency
- **3.38 Sheng Mai San Wan** for sweating from qi and yin deficiency in the aftermath of a febrile illness
- **7.9 Jin Gui Shen Qi Wan** for copious sweating associated with yang deficiency

Pattern identifying features

- **Defensive qi deficiency**
- frequent colds

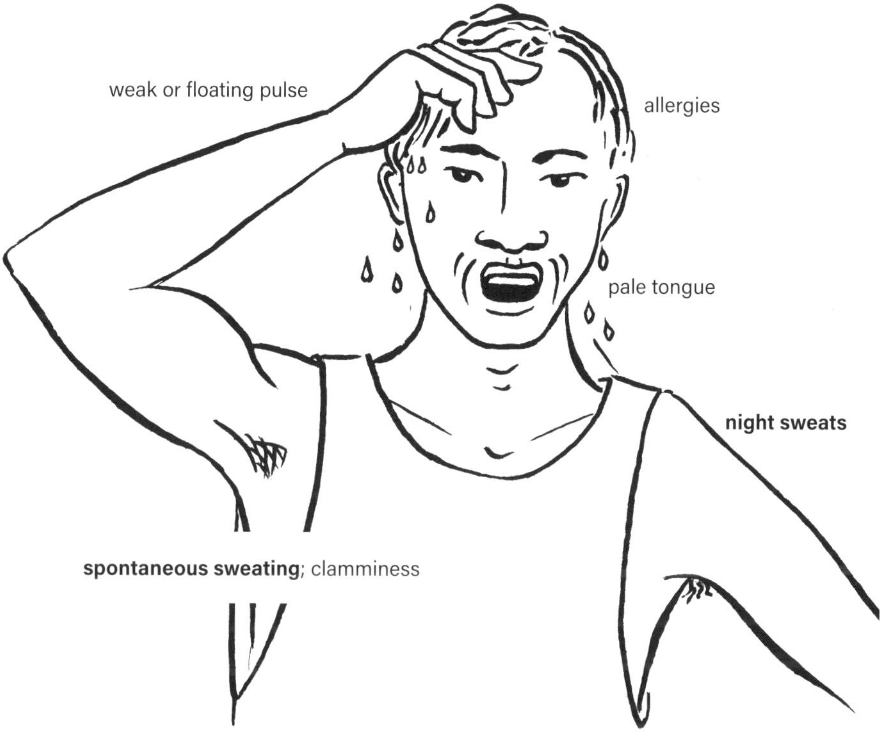

Dosage and method of administration

Adults.............. 1-2 sachets dissolved in hot water, three times daily.
Children.......... ½-1 sachet, dissolved in hot water, once or twice daily.

Cautions and contraindications

Contraindicated in the early stages of a febrile or other acute upper respiratory tract illness (wind heat or wind cold common cold), such as the common cold or flu.

肾膀胱病 4

Genitourinary

GMP

4.1 ZHEN WU WAN

真武丸

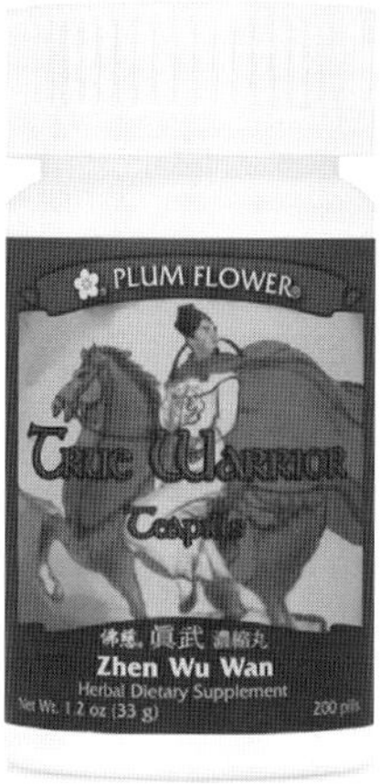

1-3/12

Lanzhou Foci Pharmaceutical Factory (Gansu)
'True Warrior Pills'
Zhen Wu Wan is packaged in bottles of 200 pills
Also available as: Zhen Wu Tang (HT), Ginger, Aconite, Poria and Peony Combination (conc. extract)

Chinese medical action

Warms the Kidney, Heart and Spleen, mobilizes yang and activates fluid metabolism, promotes urination

Biomedical action

Diuretic, cardiac stimulant

INDICATIONS

- Edema and fluid metabolism problems from Kidney and Heart yang deficiency. This is a type of cold transformation *shào yīn* syndrome (cf. heat transformation type **8.1 Tian Wang Bu Xin Dan**). Edema is worse in the lower body and ankles and usually pitting. In addition to edema, weakness of fluid metabolism can lead to pathological collection of fluids in body cavities (ascites, pleural effusion, prostatic hypertrophy, fluid in the middle ear) and organs such as the Lungs resulting in wet productive cough, dyspnea or orthopnea.
- Abdominal pain, chronic diarrhea, weak digestion, poor fluid metabolism and dizziness from Spleen and Kidney yang deficiency.
- Cold damp in the joints and tissues of the extremities with localized pain that is significantly improved by heat.
- With the appropriate identifying features, this formula can assist in the treatment of conditions such as congestive cardiac failure, cardiac edema, cor pulmonale, chronic nephritis, nephrotic syndrome, chronic hepatic disease resulting in ascites, Ménière's disease, hypothyroidism, chronic colitis and chronic arthritic pain.

Composition

Poria cocos (fu ling, hoelen), *Atractylodes macrocephala* (bai zhu, atractylodes), *Paeonia lactiflora* (bai shao, white peony), *Aconite carmichaeli* (zhi fu zi, processed aconite), *Zingiber officinale* (sheng jiang, ginger)

Combine with

– **4.2 Wu Ling Wan** for severe edema
– **3.38 Sheng Mai San Wan** for cough or orthopnea with copious watery sputum
– **7.1.1 Liu Wei Di Huang Wan** for nephrotic syndrome of a yang deficient type

Pattern identifying features

- **Kidney and Heart yang deficiency edema and fluid metabolism disorder**
- cold intolerance
- increased desire to sleep
- fatigue, exhaustion
- cough with watery sputum
- joint pain, especially finger and toes

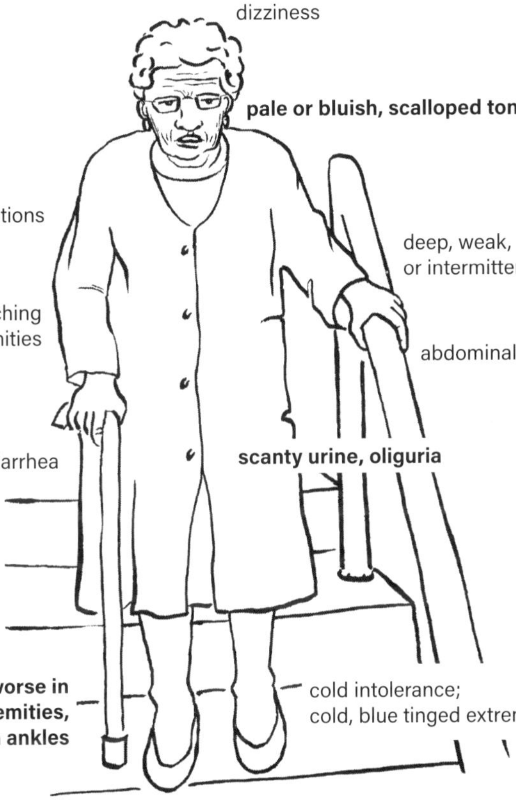

Dosage and method of administration

8-12 pills three times daily on an empty stomach. The dose can be spread out, or taken in two lots of 12-18 pills, morning and evening. In severe cases or during the early stages of treatment (the first few weeks), a 50% increase in dose can be used, then reduced as treatment takes effect.

Cautions and contraindications

Contraindicated during pregnancy. A very warming formula, not suitable for patients with swelling associated with heat or damp heat patterns.

GMP
4.2 WU LING WAN

五苓丸

1-3/12

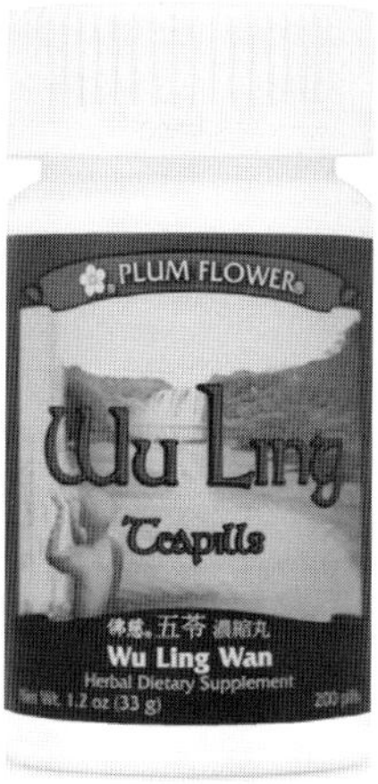

Lanzhou Foci Pharmaceutical Factory (Gansu)
'Five Ingredient Pills with Poria'
Wu Ling Wan is packaged in bottles of 200 pills
Available as: Poria Five Herb Formula (conc. extract)

Chinese medical action
Promotes fluid metabolism and urination, strengthens the Spleen

Biomedical action
Diuretic

INDICATIONS

- Mild edema from Spleen qi deficiency with accumulation of pathological fluids. **4.2 Wu Ling Wan** can be used alone or combined with other constitutional formulas. Edema is more noticeable in the upper body, in particular around the eyes and fingers.
- Edema associated with an acute pathogenic invasion. Acute onset of edema and oliguria accompanied by fever and chills, headache, thirst, vomiting immediately after drinking , with a floating pulse. This is a type of *tài yáng* syndrome, in which the pathogen (usually wind cold) obstructs the *tài yáng* organ system (channel pathway and Bladder organ), disrupting the transformation of Bladder qi and blocking the passage of urine, which rebels upward through the Triple Burner.
- Summerdamp invasion or sudden turmoil disorder with acute vomiting and diarrhea. In this case, promoting urination provides an alternative outlet for the pathogen.
- With the appropriate identifying features, this formula can assist in treatment of conditions such as edema, nephritic edema, acute gastroenteritis, post surgical urinary inhibition or difficulty, paralysis of the bladder sphincter, mild ascites and neurogenic bladder syndrome.

Composition
Alisma orientalis (ze xie, alisma), *Poria cocos* (fu ling, hoelen), *Polyporus umbellatus* (zhu ling, polyporus), *Atractylodes macrocephala* (bai zhu, atractylodes), *Cinnamomum cassia* (gui zhi, cinnamon twigs)

Combine with
- **2.7 Si Jun Zi Wan** for edema associated with Spleen qi deficiency
- **6.4 Xiao Yao Wan** for premenstrual fluid retention
- **2.23 Ping Wei San** for accumulation of pathological fluids and dampness in the Spleen and Stomach
- **4.1 Zhen Wu Wan** for relatively severe edema associated with Spleen and Kidney yang deficiency
- **1.2 Si Wu Wan** for edema during pregnancy

Pattern identifying features

- **Spleen qi deficiency with mild generalized edema**
- **Edema from *tài yáng* organ syndrome** (with external symptoms such as fever and chills, oliguria, headache and thirst with vomiting after drinking)

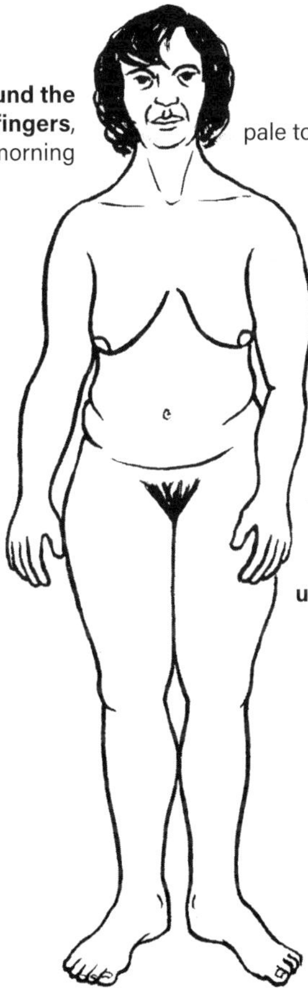

Dosage and method of administration

8-12 pills three times daily on an empty stomach. The dose can be spread out, or taken in two lots of 12-18 pills, morning and evening. As a mild formula, the dose required to effect a result may be higher than recommended, so patients can increase the dose until urinary output increases.

Cautions and contraindications

Contraindicated in difficult urination associated with yin deficiency. Although generally mild and well tolerated, overuse of the diuretic herbs in this formula can damage qi and yin, so prolonged use is not recommended. If overused, dizziness and loss of appetite may occur.

GMP

4.3 WU PI YIN WAN

五皮饮丸

1-3/12

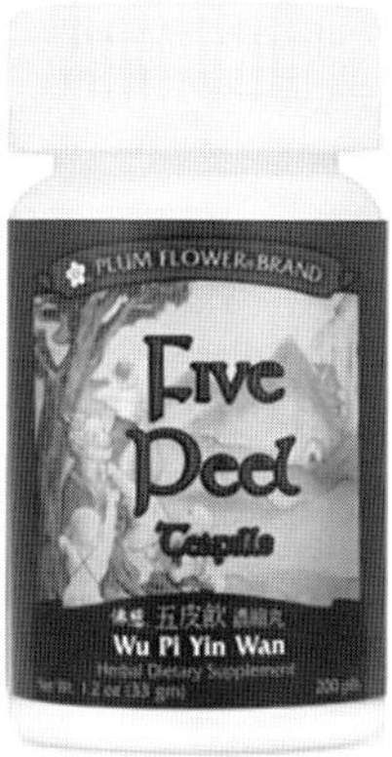

Lanzhou Foci Pharmaceutical Factory (Gansu)
'Five Peel Drink Pills'
Wu Pi Yin Wan is packaged in bottles of 200 pills
A similar formula available as: Poria and Areca Combination (conc. extract)

Chinese medical action

Promotes urination

Biomedical action

Diuretic

INDICATIONS

- Mild superficial or interstitial edema. Suitable for edema from dysfunction of any of the organs of fluid metabolism – Lungs, Spleen and Kidney. Typically combined with a constitutional formula aimed at correcting the underlying cause of the edema.
- With the appropriate identifying features, this formula can be used to treat conditions such as edema of pregnancy, premenstrual and menopausal edema and chronic nephritis.

Composition (each pill contains powdered)

Poria cocos (fu ling pi, hoelen skin), *Alisma orientalis* (ze xie, alisma), *Morus alba* (sang bai pi, mulberry root bark), *Citrus reticulata* (chen pi, citrus), *Zingiber officinale* (sheng jiang pi, ginger skin), *Dolichos lablab* (bai bian dou, hyacinth bean)

Combine with

- **1.2 Si Wu Wan** for edema during pregnancy
- **4.2 Wu Ling Wan** for marked generalized edema
- **2.7 Si Jun Zi Wan** for edema associated with Spleen qi deficiency
- **6.4 Xiao Yao Wan** for premenstrual fluid retention
- **2.23 Ping Wei San** for accumulation of pathological fluids and damp in the Spleen and Stomach
- **4.1 Zhen Wu Wan** for relatively severe edema associated with Spleen and Kidney yang deficiency

Dosage and method of administration

8-12 pills three times daily on an empty stomach. The dose can be spread out, or taken in two lots of 12-18 pills, morning and evening. In severe cases or during the early stages of treatment (the first few weeks), a 50% increase in dose can be used, then reduced as treatment takes effect.

Pattern identifying features

- **mild edema from various causes**

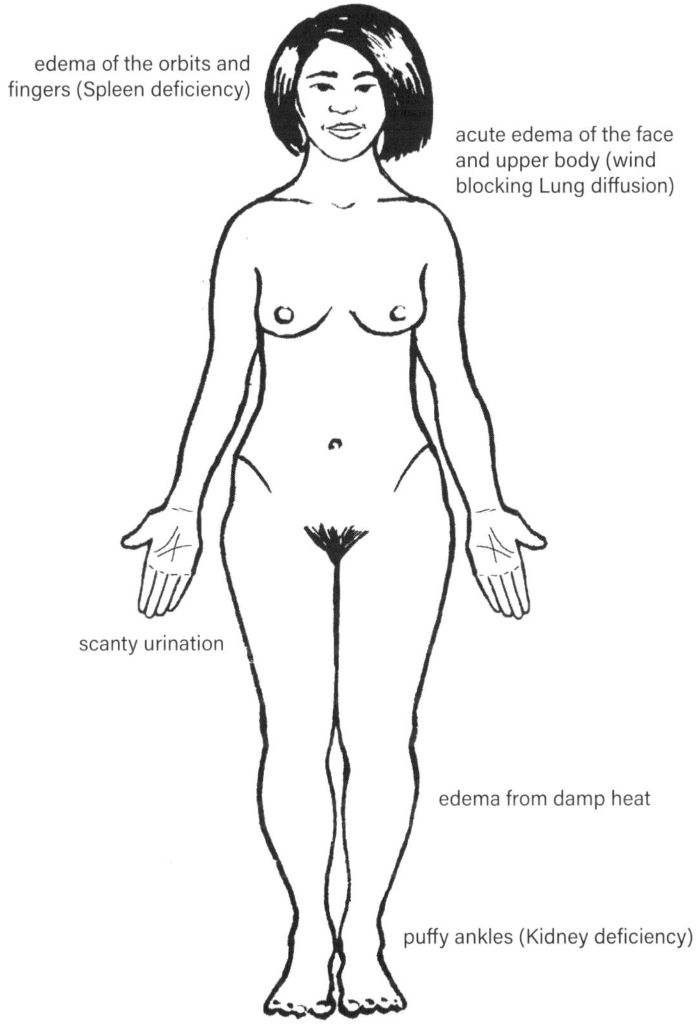

Cautions and contraindications

Although a mild formula, overuse of diuretic herbs can damage qi and yin. Prolonged use of this formula alone is not recommended.

GMP

4.4 FANG JI HUANG QI WAN

防己黄芪丸

1-3/12

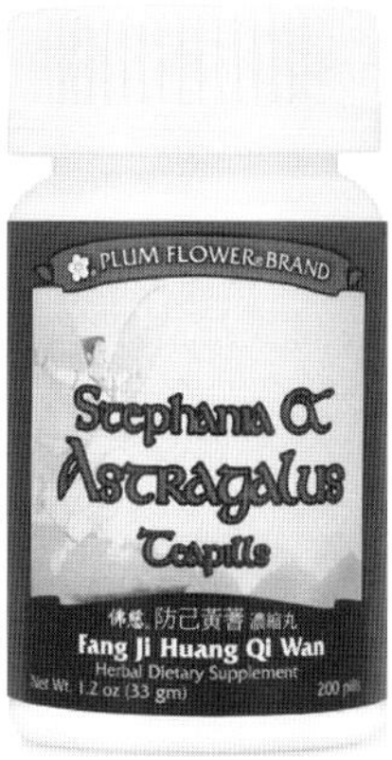

Lanzhou Foci Pharmaceutical Factory (Gansu)
'Stephania and Astragalus Pills'
Fang Ji Huang Qi Wan is packaged in bottles of 200 pills
Also available as: Stephania and Astragalus Combination (conc. extract)

Chinese medical action

Strengthens the Spleen and tonifies qi, promotes urination, dispels wind damp, stops pain

Biomedical action

Diuretic, analgesic

INDICATIONS

- Wind edema (*see* glossary). An acute condition characterized by sudden onset of edema and oliguria, due to invasion of superficial tissues by wind damp in patients with qi deficiency.
- Wind damp painful obstruction, mostly affecting the lower limbs, especially knees, in patients with qi deficiency. Commonly used for swelling and pain in the knees in clammy, overweight, fatigued individuals.
- With the appropriate identifying features, this formula can be used to treat conditions such as osteoarthritis or rheumatoid arthritis of the knees, chronic nephritis, post streptococcal glomerulonephritis, and edema associated with malnutrition and protein deficiency. Can assist in alleviating lymphedema following mastectomy.

Composition

Astragalus membranaceous (huang qi, astragalus), *Stephania tetrandra* (fang ji, stephania), *Atractylodes macrocephala* (bai zhu, atractylodes), *Zizyphus jujuba* (da zao, chinese dates), *Zingiber officinale* (sheng jiang, ginger), *Glycyrrhiza uralensis* (gan cao, licorice)

Combine with

- **4.2 Wu Ling Wan** for severe swelling in the knees or chronic nephritis
- **10.22 Shao Yao Gan Cao Wan** for wind edema with abdominal pain
- **3.5 Ma Huang Tang** for wheezing or breathlessness and edema
- **1.17 Gui Zhi Fu Ling Wan** for edema, joint pain and palpitations following rheumatic heart disease
- **7.22 Shen Qi Da Bu Wan** for relatively severe qi deficiency

Dosage and method of administration

8-12 pills three times daily on an empty stomach. The dose can be spread out, or taken in two lots of 12-18 pills, morning and evening. In severe cases or during the early stages of treatment (the first few weeks), a 50% increase in dose can be used, then reduced as treatment takes effect.

Pattern identifying features

- **qi deficiency with wind damp and edema**
- general sensation of heaviness and fatigue
- frequent colds and flu
- poor appetite, loose stools
- patients often overweight
- females more affected than males

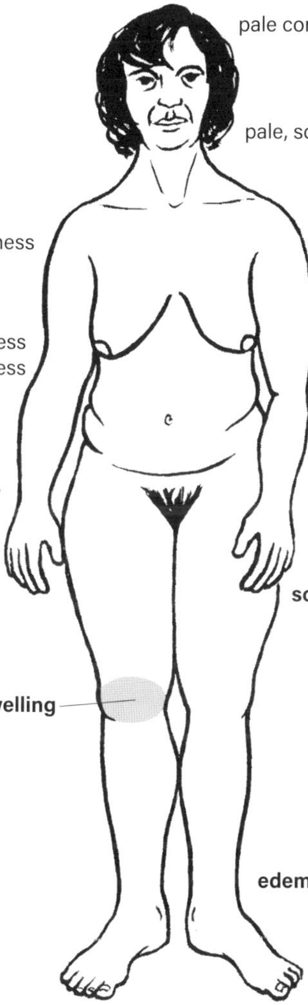

Cautions and contraindications

Contraindicated in edema or pain pathology from excess without underlying deficiency, such as damp heat or blood stasis.

4.5 BI XIE FEN QING WAN

TGA

萆薢分清丸

1-3/12

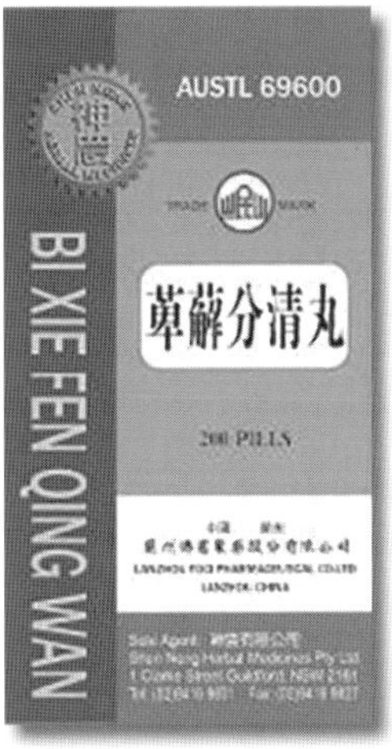

Lanzhou Foci Pharmaceutical Factory (Gansu)
'Fish Poison Yam Pills to Separate and Clear'
Bi Xie Fen Qing Wan is packaged in bottles of 200 pills
Also available as: Bi Xie Fen Qing Teapills (PF), Tokoro Combination (conc. extract)

Chinese medical action

Promotes urination and leaches damp, warms the Kidneys, separates the turbid from the clear

Biomedical action

Diuretic

INDICATIONS

- Kidney yang qi deficiency with accumulation of damp in the lower burner causing cloudy or turbid painful urination (see glossary), copious watery or white leukorrhea and white or mucoid discharges.
- With the appropriate identifying features, this formula can be used to treat conditions such as vaginal thrush (candidiasis), leukorrhea, chronic or recurrent urinary tract infections, chronic cystitis, chronic prostatitis or urinary discomfort with chyluria, albuminuria or urinary sediment, chronic nephritis and nephrotic syndrome.

Composition (each pill contains powdered)

Dioscorea hypoglauca (bei xie, fish poison yam) 35mg, *Alpinia oxyphylla* (yi zhi ren, alpinia) 35mg, *Lindera strychnifolia* (wu yao, lindera) 35mg, *Poria cocos* (fu ling, hoelen) 32mg, *Glycyrrhiza uralensis* (gan cao, licorice) 20.4mg

Combine with

- **7.9 Jin Gui Shen Qi Wan** for prostate swelling with marked yang deficiency
- **2.23 Ping Wei San** for severe damp
- **2.13 Li Zhong Wan** for Spleen yang deficiency with damp sinking downward
- **2.12 Shen Ling Bai Zhu Wan** for copious cold damp leukorrhea from Spleen qi deficiency
- **11.1 Qian Lie Xian Capsule** or **11.2 Prostate Gland Pills** for damp accumulation in the prostate causing chronic swelling, perineal discomfort and discharge

Dosage and method of administration

8-12 pills three times daily on an empty stomach. The dose can be spread out, or taken in two lots of 12-18 pills, morning and evening. In severe cases or during the early stages of treatment (the first few weeks), a 50% increase in dose can be used, then reduced as treatment takes effect.

Pattern identifying features

- **Cloudy urine from Kidney yang qi deficiency with damp accumulation**
- frequent urination, nocturia

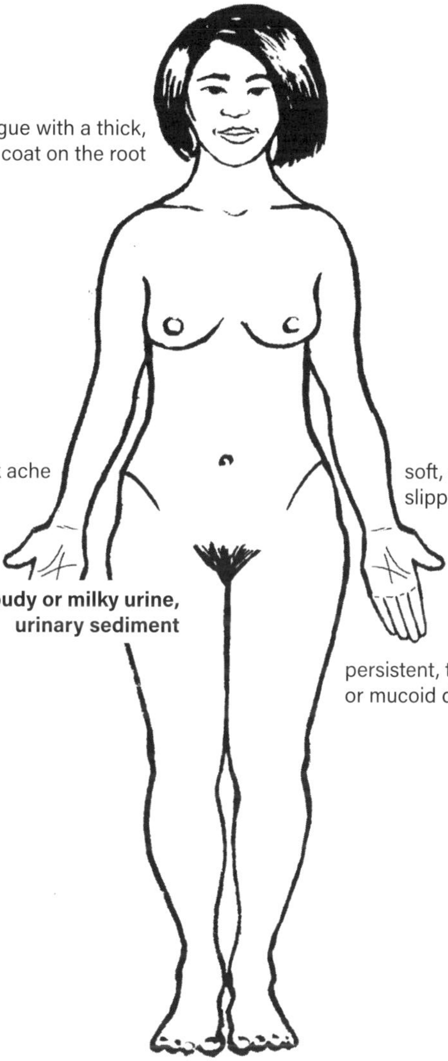

Cautions and contraindications

Not suitable unmodified for patients with lingering damp heat.

4.6 BA ZHENG SAN WAN

八正散丸

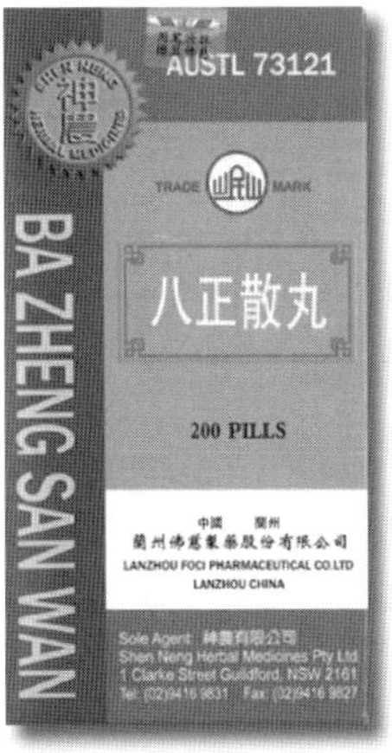

Lanzhou Foci Pharmaceutical Factory (Gansu)
'Eight (Herbs to) Correct Pills'
Ba Zheng San Wan is packaged in bottles of 200 pills
Also available as: Eight Righteous Teapills (PF), Dianthus Formula (conc. extract)

Chinese medical action

Clears damp heat from the Bladder

Biomedical action

Diuretic, anti-inflammatory, urinary antiseptic

INDICATIONS

- Acute pain and burning with urination from damp heat in the Bladder. The damp heat may be from an external invasion, or generated internally. This is the classical formula for damp heat painful urination. Used for a variety of acute presentations with dysuria, including those associated with urinary tract stones or sand, hematuria or cloudy urine.
- With the appropriate identifying features, this formula can be used to treat such conditions as acute urinary tract infection, nephritis, cystitis and urethritis, prostatitis, urinary calculi, pyelonephritis and glomerulonephritis.

Composition (each tablet contains powdered)

Lysimachia christina (jin qian cao, golden coin grass) 28.8mg, *Clematis armandii* (mu tong, akebia) 22.4mg, *Gardenia florida* (shan zhi zi, gardenia fruit) 22.4mg, *Plantago asiatica* (che qian zi, plantago) 19.2mg, *Polygonum aviculare* (bian xu, knotweed) 19.2mg, *Lopatherum gracile* (dan zhu ye, bamboo leaf) 16mg, *Juncus effusus* (deng xin cao, juncus) 12.8mg, *Rheum palmatum* (da huang, rhubarb root) 9.6mg, *Glycyrrhiza uralensis* (gan cao, licorice) 9.6mg

Combine with

- **14.1 Huang Lian Jie Du Wan** for severe pain with urination
- **6.1 Xiao Chai Hu Wan** for acute cystitis with alternating fever and chills
- **10.2 Raw Tienchi Tablets** for dysuria with bleeding
- **4.10 Shi Lin Tong** for stone painful urination with damp heat

Pattern identifying features

- **damp heat in the Bladder**
- may be fever, or alternating fever and chills

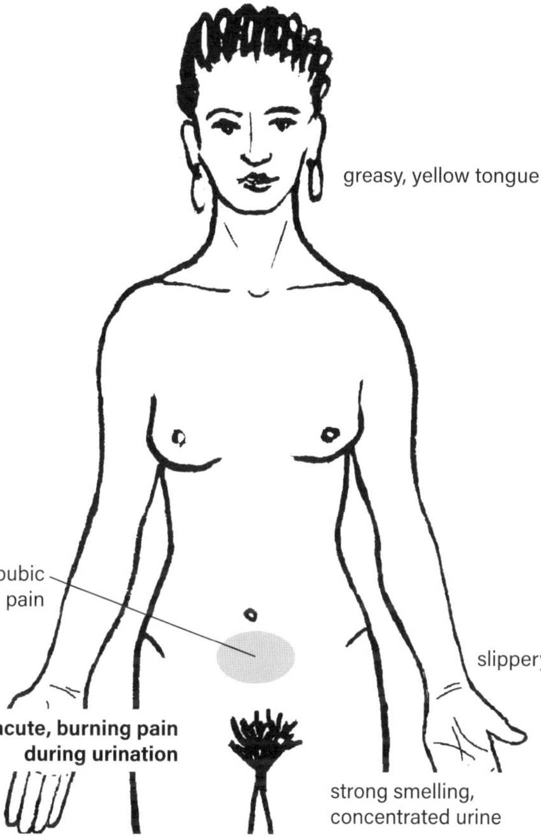

Dosage and method of administration

The recommended dose is 8-12 pills three times daily, however to be effective in acute and severe cases a higher dose is usually required, in the order of 16-24 pills three times daily (or about 12 pills every two hours), on an empty stomach.

Cautions and contraindications

Contraindicated during pregnancy.

4.7 QING RE QU SHI TEA

清热祛湿冲剂

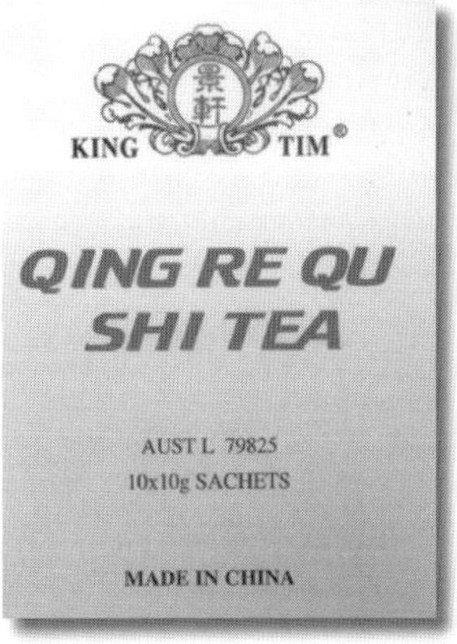

(*Qing Re Qu Shi Chong Ji*)
Jing Xian Pharmaceutical Co. (Guangzhou)
'Heat Clearing, Damp Dispelling Granules'
Qing Re Qu Shi Tea is packaged in 10 gram sachets of soluble granules, ten sachets per box

Chinese medical action

Clears damp heat and toxic heat, promotes urination

Biomedical action

Diuretic, anti-inflammatory, urinary antiseptic

INDICATIONS

- Damp heat and/or toxic heat in the genitourinary system. A strong formula for acute infection and inflammation of the reproductive system, urinary bladder and kidneys. The main focus of the formula is on clearing toxic heat, with diuresis secondary. Suitable for acute and relatively severe patterns.
- Damp heat lodged in the skin with red, itchy vesicular rashes, especially in the lower body.
- With the appropriate identifying features, this formula can assist in the treatment of conditions such as acute urinary tract infection, acute cystitis and urethritis, acute prostatitis, pyelonephritis, glomerulonephritis, pelvic inflammatory disease, salpingitis, vaginitis, shingles, eczema, genital eczema, Bartholin's cyst and acute genital herpes.

Composition (each sachet contains extracts equivalent to dry)

Chrysanthemum indicum (ye ju hua, wild chrysanthemum) 7.2g, *Coix lachryma-jobi* (yi yi ren, coix) 4.8g, *Lonicera japonica* (jin yin hua, lonicera) 4.3g, *Plantago asiatica* (che qian zi, plantago) 3.8g, *Lysimachia christina* (jin qian cao, golden coin grass) 3.2g, *Taraxacum mongolicum* (pu gong ying, dandelion) 3g, *Gardenia florida* (shan zhi zi, gardenia fruit) 3g, *Atractylodes lancea* (cang zhu, red atractylodes) 2.6g

Combine with

- **14.1 Huang Lian Jie Du Wan** for severe pain with urination
- **6.1 Xiao Chai Hu Wan** for acute cystitis with alternating fever and chills
- **10.1 Yunnan Paiyao** for dysuria with bleeding
- **4.10 Shi Lin Tong** for stone painful urination with damp heat
- **14.5 Chuan Xin Lian Antiphlogistic Tablets** for pelvic infection
- **6.6 Long Dan Xie Gan Wan** for genitourinary infections, eczema or herpes associated with Liver fire or damp heat in the Liver channel

Pattern identifying features

- **damp heat and/or toxic heat in the genitourinary system**
- infection of the genitourinary system
- fever, or fever and chills
- colored discharges

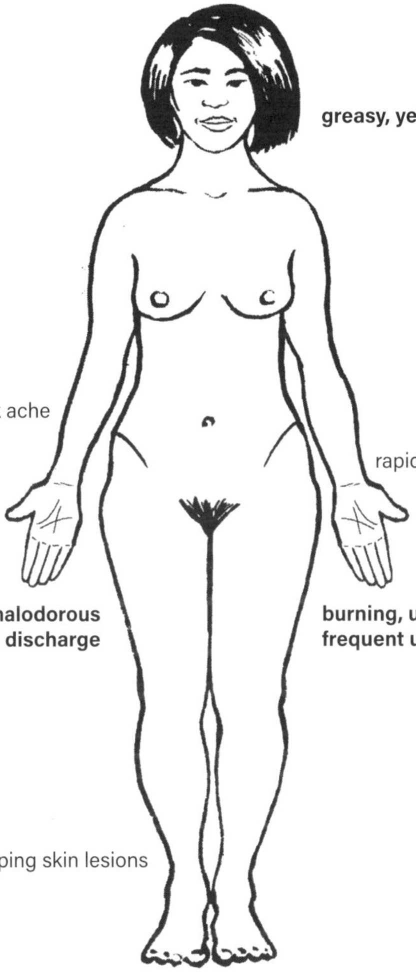

Dosage and method of administration

1-2 sachets dissolved in hot water, three times daily. In severe cases, the dose may be safely doubled.

Cautions and contraindications

Not suitable in the absence of damp or toxic heat, for cold damp discharges, or for prolonged use.

4.8 TAO CHIH PIEN

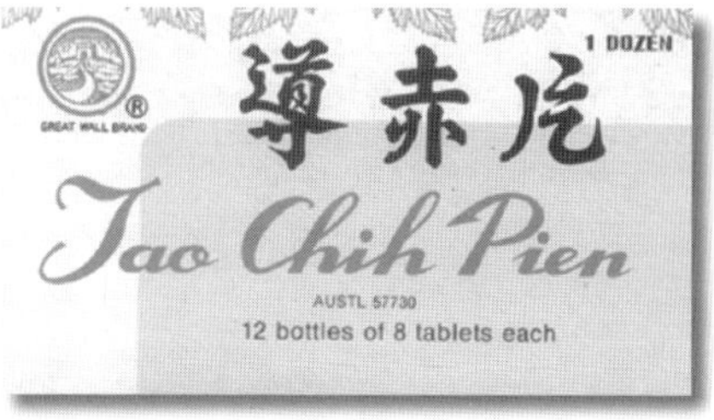

导赤片

(*Dao Chi Pian*)
Tianjin Drug Manufactory (Shandong)
'Guide [out the] Red Pills'
Tao Chih Pien is packaged in vials of eight small tablets, twelve vials per box
Also available as: Red Door Teapills (PF), Rehmannia and Clematis Armandi Formula (conc. extract)

Chinese medical action

Clears heat, promotes urination, eases painful urination

Biomedical action

Diuretic, anti-inflammatory, urinary antiseptic

INDICATIONS

- Heat/fire affecting the Heart and allied systems – Heart fire flaring upwards to the mouth and tongue, and Heart fire invading the Small Intestine. Typically associated with emotional turmoil, symptoms are triggered by sudden, significant or prolonged emotional trauma. Good for acute mouth ulcers, particularly in children. Also helpful for sleep disturbances, disturbing dreams or nightmares, irritability or anxiety from heat affecting the Heart.
- Heart fire invading the Small Intestine, a type of urinary tract irritation, infection or inflammation with a pronounced emotional component. The Small Intestine plays a role in urinary function in Chinese medicine, and it is paired in a yin yang relationship with the Heart. The distinctive feature of this pattern is the onset of urinary symptoms following emotional upheaval, anxiety, period of sleep deprivation or post traumatic stress.
- With the appropriate identifying features, this formula can treat conditions such as acute mouth and tongue ulcers, urinary tract infection, cystitis, pyelonephritis, nightmares and the mental and physical effects of emotional trauma or shock.

Composition **(each tablet contains extracts equivalent to dry)**

Gardenia florida (shan zhi zi, gardenia) 1.16g, *Rehmannia glutinosa* (sheng di, rehmannia) 773mg, *Glycyrrhiza uralensis* (gan cao, licorice) 394mg, Calcium sulphate 163mg, *Rheum palmatum* (da huang, rhubarb root) 87mg, *Poria cocos* (fu ling, hoelen) 23mg, *Alsima orientale* (ze xie, alisma) 23mg

Dosage and method of administration

The adult dose is 4-8 tablets every 2-3 hours.

For children 1-2 years ....one tablet 2-3 times daily
3-5 years........one tablet 3-4 times daily
6-10 years......one to two tablets 4 times daily

Pattern identifying features

- **Heart fire, Heart fire transmitted the Small Intestine**
- **urinary tract infection**, cystitis, urethritis
- irritability, **agitation**, anxiety
- **insomnia**, dream disturbed sleep

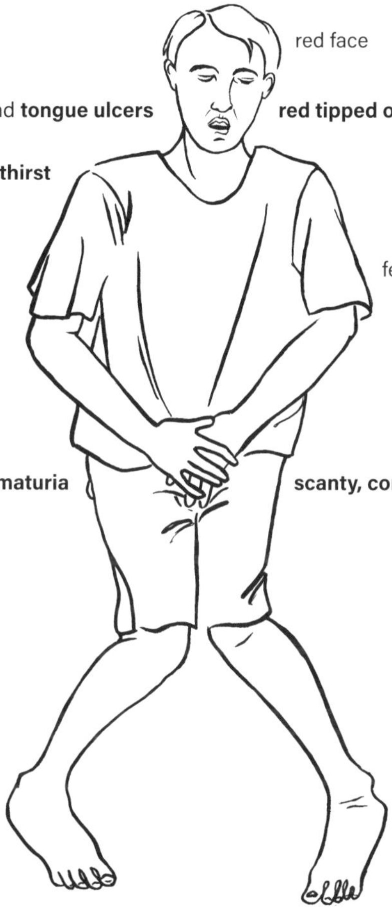

Note: This product is noted on the packaging 'for babies', but the tablet size is too large for children under 6 years old. Tablets can be ground up and mixed with hot water or other liquid to create a suspension that can be delivered to a small child in an eye-dropper. For infants and small children *see also* **12.9 Xiao Er Qi Xing Cha Chong Ji**.

Cautions and contraindications

Contraindicated during pregnancy. Tablets must be crushed before giving to children to avoid choking. May cause diarrhea.

GMP

4.9 DBD CAPSULE

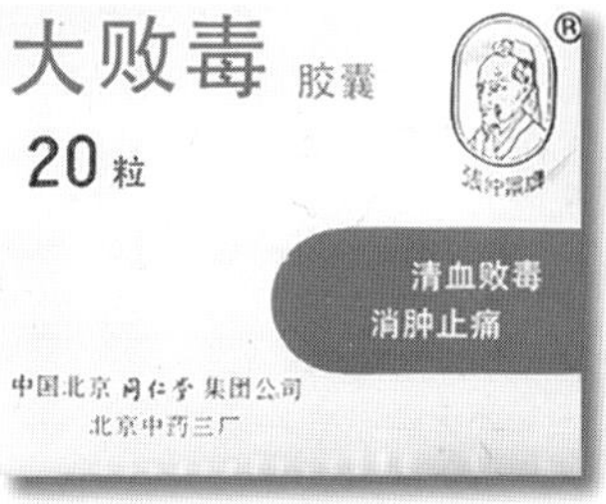

大败毒胶囊

1-3/7

(Da Bai Du Jiao Nang)
Tong Ren Tang (Beijing)
'Great Toxin Relieving Capsules'
DBD Capsule is packaged in gelatine capsules on blister sheets, twenty capsules per box

Chinese medical action
Clears toxic heat, cools the blood, reduces swelling, stops pain

Biomedical action
Antibiotic, anti-inflammatory, detoxicant

INDICATIONS

- Internal excess heat and toxic heat patterns, especially of the genitourinary system.
- Suppurative swellings and superficial sores, ulcers and carbuncles.
- With the appropriate identifying features, this formula can be used to treat disorders such as urinary tract infection, cystitis, hematuria, pyelonephritis, syphilis, abscesses, carbuncles and furuncles.

Composition
Taraxacum mongolicum (pu gong ying, dandelion), *Lonicera japonica* (jin yin hua, lonicera), *Rheum palmatum* (da huang, rhubarb root), *Bufo bufo* (chan su, cane toad venom), *Angelica sinensis* (dang gui), Snake skin slough (she tui)

Combine with
– **10.2 Raw Tienchi Tablets** for hematuria

Dosage and method of administration
For acute disorders, the recommended dose is five capsules, 4 times daily and the length of treatment is usually no more than a few days. For syphilis, the length of treatment is longer, with the dose reduced by 50-75%.

Cautions and contraindications
Contraindicated during pregnancy.

4.10 SHI LIN TONG

石淋通

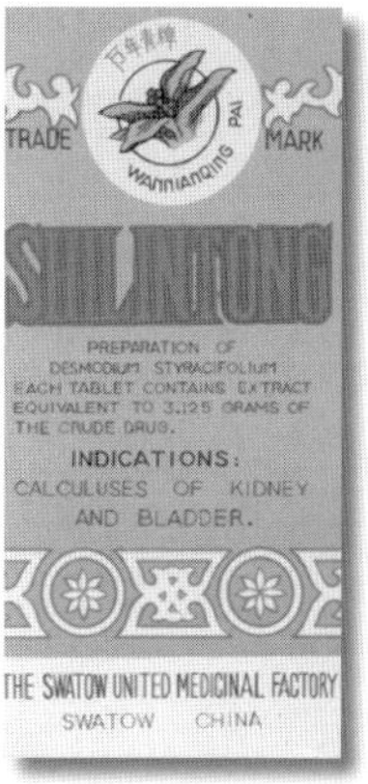

Swatow United Medicinal Factory
'Open (and Clear) Stone Painful Urination'
Shi Lin Tong is packaged in bottles of 200 pills
A formula with similar action is available as: *Jie Shi Ling* (Stone Formula PF)

Chinese medical action

Clears damp heat, promotes urination, dissolves stones and small calculi

Biomedical action

Diuretic

INDICATIONS

- Kidney and Bladder calculi. Composed of the main herb in the Chinese materia medica for urinary stones, it is effective in dissolving and easing the passage of small stones. Generally not effective for large or staghorn calculi. Usually needs to be taken for at least 3-6 months for an effect to be felt. The patient must increase water intake during therapy.
- Also used for Gallstones associated with damp, damp heat or qi constraint.
- May also be useful for sialolith.

Composition (each tablet contains extracts equivalent to)

Desmodium styracifolium (guang jin qian cao, desmodium) 3.125g

Combine with

- **1.23 Zhi Bai Di Huang Wan** for Kidney yin deficiency
- **4.6 Ba Zheng San Wan** for damp heat in the Bladder
- **1.15 Tong Jing Wan** for stones with blood stasis causing back pain
- **6.11 Li Dan Tablets** for gallstones from damp heat
- **6.3 Chai Hu Shu Gan Wan** for gallstones associated with constrained qi

Dosage and method of administration

6-10 tablets two or three times daily on an empty stomach.

Cautions and contraindications

Desmodium can leach potassium from the body when used long term, potentially causing palpitations and dizziness. This can be remedied by increasing potassium intake in the form of bananas or potassium replacement pills. Caution in patients with large stones.

4.11 BA JI YIN YANG WAN

巴戟阴阳丸

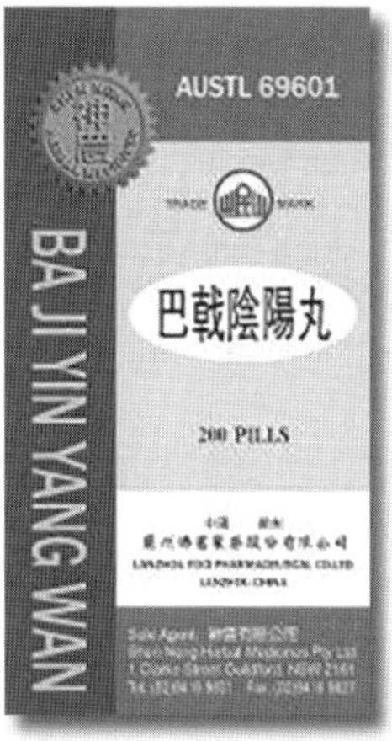

Lanzhou Foci Pharmaceutical Factory (Gansu)
'Morinda Pills to Balance Yin and Yang'
Ba Ji Yin Yang Wan is packaged in bottles of 200 pills
Also available as: Ba Ji Yin Yang Teapills (PF)

Chinese medical action

Tonifies Kidney yang, strengthens the Spleen, benefits fluid metabolism, secures essence and restrains leakage of fluids

Biomedical action

Stimulant, improves fluid metabolism

INDICATIONS

- Kidney yang deficiency. Focuses on strengthening the Kidneys' role of governing fluid metabolism and control of the lower yin (urethra and anus). Used for leakage of fluids such as urinary frequency, nocturia and incontinence, as well as chronic cockcrow diarrhea and copious watery leukorrhea.
- Strengthens the Lung Kidney axis to alleviate chronic or congenital respiratory weakness and hypersensitivity. This manifests as conditions such as allergic rhinitis, atopic asthma and atopic eczema.
- Impotence, erectile dysfunction, low libido, sperm disorders, premature ejaculation, infertility, luteal phase defect and long menstrual cycles
- Chronic mild to moderate lower back and leg pain and weakness from Kidney deficiency with wind cold damp in the channels.
- With the appropriate identifying features, this formula can assist in the treatment of conditions such as benign prostatic hypertrophy, chronic nephritis, infertility, impotence, allergies, chronic colitis, chronic cystitis and chronic pelvic inflammatory disease.

Composition (each pill contains powdered)

Morinda officinalis (ba ji tian, morinda) 19.7mg, *Epimedium brevicornu* (xian ling pi, epimedium) 19.7mg, *Rehmannia glutinosa* (shu di, processed rehmannia) 19.7mg, *Dioscorea opposita* (shan yao, dioscorea) 13.6mg, *Paeonia lactiflora* (bai shao, white peony root) 13.6mg, *Nelumbium speciosum* (lian zi, lotus seed) 10.7mg, *Cornus officinalis* (shan zhu yu, cornus) 10.7mg, *Rosa laevigata* (jin ying zi, chinese rose fruit) 9.1mg, *Dipsacus asper* (xu duan, dipsacus) 9.1mg, *Cibotium barometz* (gou ji, cibotium fern) 9.1mg, *Eucommia ulmoides* (du zhong, eucommia) 9.1mg, *Lycium barbarum* (gou qi zi, lycium fruit) 9.1mg, *Angelica sinensis* (dang gui, chinese angelica) 6.9mg

Combine with

- **4.14 Chin So Ku Ching Wan** or **4.15 Sang Piao Xiao Wan** for severe urinary frequency or nocturia

Pattern identifying features

- **Kidney yang deficiency with weakness of fluid metabolism, leakage of fluids and reproductive function**
- **impotence, low libido**
- chronic allergies and atopy
- fatigue, lassitude
- cold intolerance

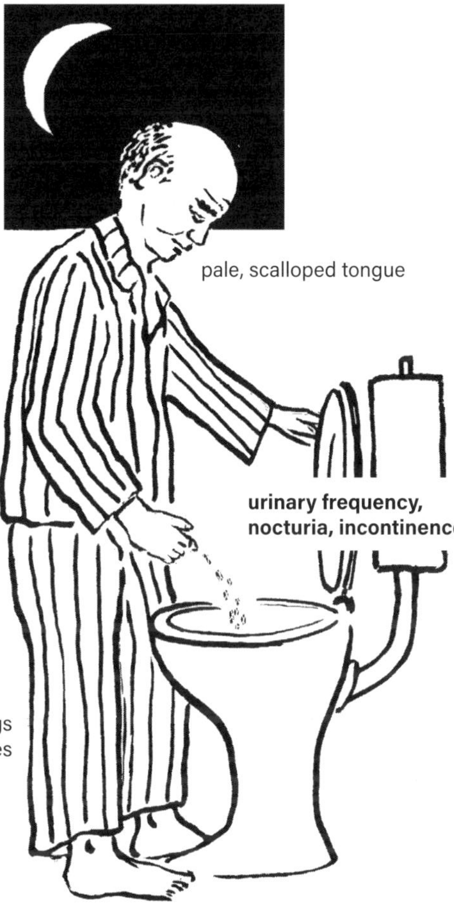

- **2.13 Li Zhong Wan** for cockcrow diarrhea, or persistent Spleen and Kidney yang deficient diarrhea
- **11.8 Kang Wei Ling Wan** for impotence from yang deficiency with blood stasis
- **9.18 Xin Yi San** for congenital Lung and Kidney deficiency allergy and hay fever

Dosage and method of administration

8-12 pills three times daily on an empty stomach. The dose can be spread out, or taken in two lots of 12-18 pills, morning and evening. In severe cases or during the early stages of treatment (the first two weeks), a 50% increase in dose can be used, then reduced as treatment takes effect.

Cautions and contraindications

Contraindicated during the early phase of acute illness such as colds and flu. This formula is well tolerated and rarely causes digestive problems.

GMP

4.12 SAN YUEN MEDICAL PILLS

宁心补肾丸

1-3/12

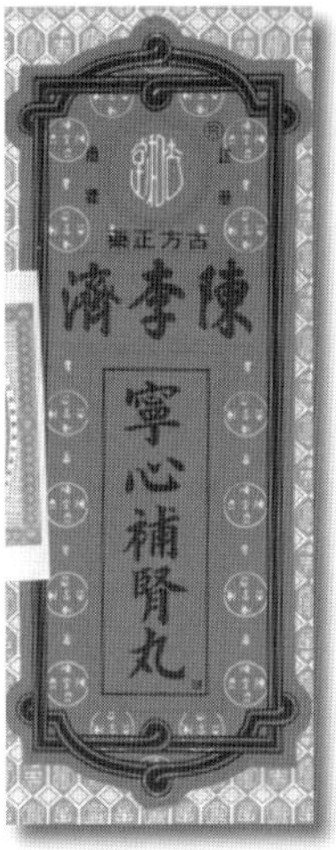

(*Ning Xin Bu Shen Wan*)
Chan Li Chai Medical Factory (Hong Kong)
'Pills to Calm the Heart and Tonify the Kidneys'
San Yuen Medical Pills are packaged as large honey pills sealed in yellow wax balls

Chinese medical action

Tonifies and warms Kidney yang, strengthens the Spleen and benefits qi, secures essence and restrains leakage of fluids

Biomedical action

Astringent

INDICATIONS

- Frequent urination, enuresis and nocturia from Kidney yang qi deficiency. Also used for leakage of other fluids that rely on a degree of Kidney control for restraint, such as premature ejaculation and copious watery leukorrhea.
- Recurrent miscarriage, impotence or infertility. Can be used for a variety of sperm problems, including poor motility, low sperm count and high proportion of abnormal forms. In this respect the formula is somewhat similar to **11.5 Wu Zi Yan Zong Wan**.
- Fearfulness, anxiety, easy fright or emotional timidity associated with loss of communication between the Heart and Kidneys. This is a type of *shào yīn* syndrome associated with disruption to the Heart Kidney axis from a sudden shock, trauma or prolonged emotional distress.
- Weakness of the eyes from Liver and Kidney deficiency.

Composition

Codonopsis pilosula (dang shen, codonopsis) 25.6%, *Psoralea corylifolia* (bu gu zhi, psoralea) 12.8%, *Polygonum multiflorum* (he shou wu, polygonum root) 10.24%, *Euryale ferox* (qian shi, euryale) 10.24%, *Eucommia ulmoides* (du zhong, eucommia bark) 10.24%, *Rosa laevigata* (jin ying zi, chinese rose fruit) 7.82%, *Cuscuta japonica* (tu si zi, cuscuta) 7.7%, *Rubus coreanus* (fu pen zi, rubus) 5.12%, *Poria cocos* (fu shen, hoelen) 5.12%, *Allium odorum* (jiu zi, chinese chive seed) 5.12%

Combine with

- **7.9 Jin Gui Shen Qi Wan** for severe cold
- **7.1.1 Liu Wei Di Huang Wan** for yin deficient urinary disorders
- **8.1 Tian Wang Bu Xin Dan** for Heart and Kidney yin and yang deficiency anxiety states, premature ejaculation and insomnia
- **10.41 Gou Pi Gao** plaster topically on key acupuncture points of the lower abdomen (such as CV-6 (*qì hǎi*) and CV-4 (*guān yuán*) to warm the Kidneys and invigorate lower burner qi

Pattern identifying features

- **Kidney yang qi deficiency**
- **infertility, sperm disorders**

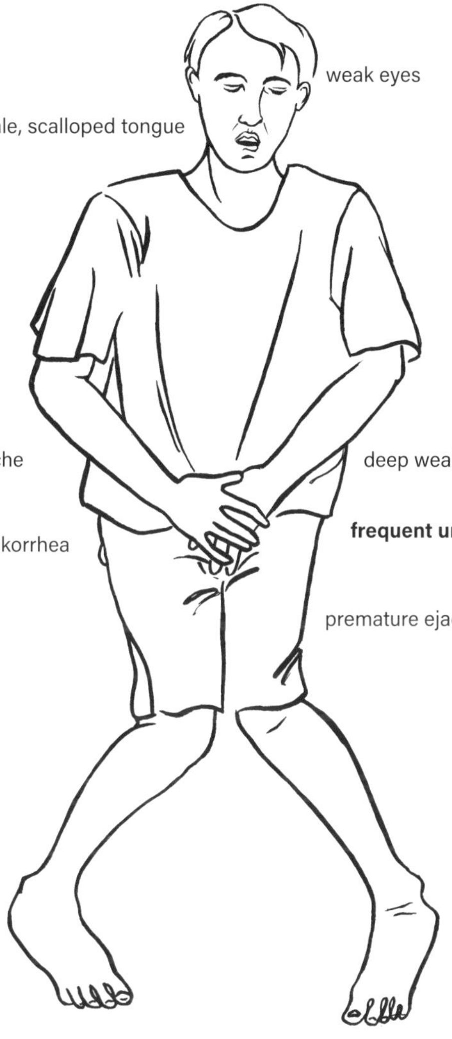

Dosage and method of administration

The recommended dose is one pill twice daily before meals. The pills are often hard and need to be softened by soaking in hot water for ten minutes or so before ingestion.

Cautions and contraindications

Not suitable for Kidney deficiency patterns with oliguria and edema.

4.13 ZI SHEN DA BU CAPSULE

滋肾大补丸

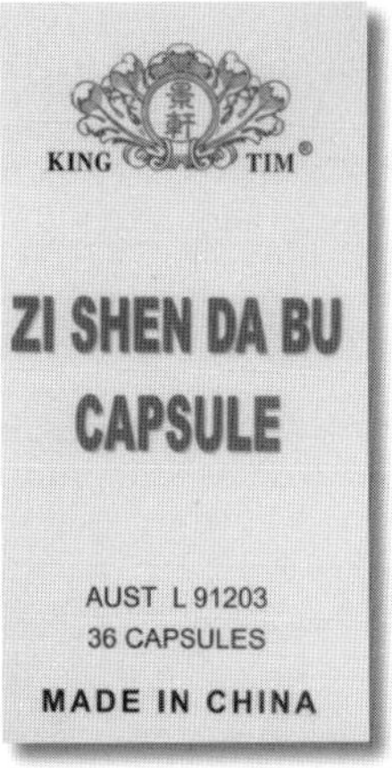

(Zi Shen Da Bu Wan)
Jing Xian Pharmaceutical Co. (Guangzhou)
'Pills to Nourish and Powerfully Tonify the Kidneys'
Zi Shen Da Bu Capsule is packaged in bottles of 36 capsules

Chinese medical action

Warms and tonifies Kidney yang, strengthens the Spleen, benefits fluid metabolism, secures essence and restrains leakage of fluids

Biomedical action

Astringent

INDICATIONS

- Kidney yang qi deficiency. Effective for leakage or loss of fluids, in particular urine. Used to treat urinary frequency, nocturia, incontinence and enuresis. Also treats loss or leakage of other fluids that should be secured by Kidney yang, such as premature ejaculation and copious watery leukorrhea.
- Male infertility, impotence and sperm disorders such as low sperm count, poor quality sperm or a high proportion of abnormal forms.
- With the appropriate identifying features, this formula can be used to treat conditions such as benign prostatic hypertrophy, chronic nephritis, prolapsed bladder, infertility and impotence.

Composition (each capsule contains extracts equivalent to dry)

Epimedium brevicornu (xian ling pi, epimedium) 500mg, *Dioscorea opposita* (shan yao, dioscorea) 240mg, *Rosa laevigata* (jin ying zi, chinese rose) 175mg, *Cuscuta hygrophila* (tu su zi, cuscuta) 150mg, *Nelumbium speciosum* (lian zi, lotus seed) 140mg, *Alpinia oxyphylla* (yi zhi ren, alpinia) 140mg, *Rehmannia glutinosa* (shu di, processed rehmannia) 140mg, *Paeonia lactiflora* (bai shao, white peony) 125mg, *Curculigo orchioides* (xian mao, curculigo) 125mg, *Euryale ferox* (qian shi, euryale seed) 100mg

Combine with

- **2.11 Bu Zhong Yi Qi Wan** for urinary frequency from Spleen and Kidney deficiency with urinary bladder prolapse, or uterine prolapse that presses on the Bladder
- **4.14 Chin So Ku Ching Wan** for persistent incontinence of urine

Dosage and method of administration

3-4 capsules, three times daily on an empty stomach.

Pattern identifying features

- **Kidney yang qi deficiency**
- **clear copious urine**
- fatigue, lack of vitality
- cold intolerance
- easy sweating

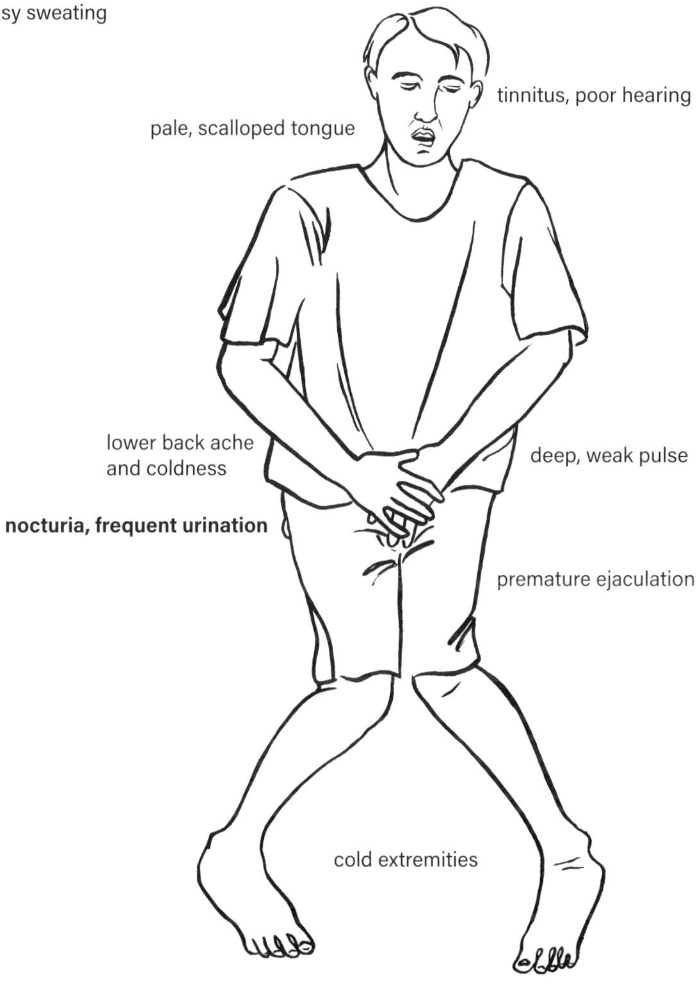

Cautions and contraindications

Contraindicated during the early phase of acute illness such as colds and flu, and in urinary dysfunction or other patterns associated with lingering damp heat or other pathogen that requires expulsion.

4.14 CHIN SO KU CHING WAN

金锁固精丸

(Jin Suo Gu Jing Wan)
Lanzhou Foci Pharmaceutical Factory (Gansu)
'Golden Lock Pills to Contain Essence'
Chin So Ku Ching Wan is packaged in bottles of 200 pills
Also available as: Lotus Stamen Formula (conc. extract)

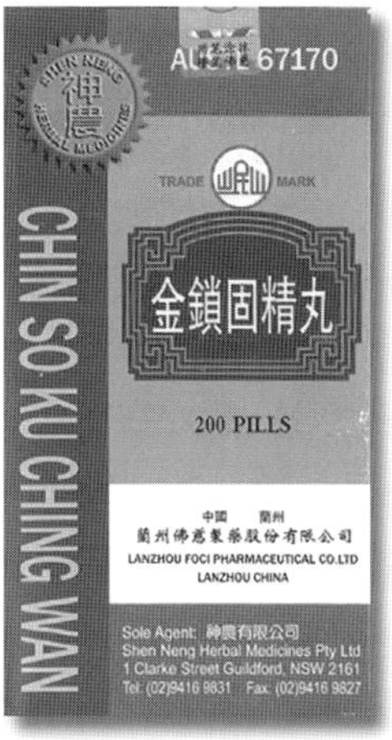

Chinese medical action

Consolidates the Kidney, secures essence and prevents leakage of fluids

Biomedical action

Astringent

INDICATIONS

- Chronic leakage of fluids associated with Kidney deficiency. An astringent and thermally neutral formula that simply restrains fluids, it is usually combined with an appropriate constitutional formula that deals with the underlying cause of the fluid leakage. Most commonly used for urinary frequency, nocturia, enuresis, incontinence of urine, premature ejaculation or copious watery or white mucoid leukorrhea.
- Can assist in alleviating excessive sweating and chronic diarrhea.
- With the appropriate identifying features, this formula may be used to treat conditions such as benign prostatic hypertrophy, childhood enuresis, bladder prolapse, chronic nephritis, chronic nephritic albuminuria, chyluria and chronic pelvic inflammatory disease.

Composition (each pill contains powdered)

Nelumbium speciosum (lian zi, lotus seed) 60mg, *Nelumbium speciosum* (lian xu, lotus stamen) 30mg, *Euryale ferox* (qian shi, euryale seed) 30mg, *Astragalus complanatus* (sha yuan ji li, astragalus seed) 30mg, *Ostrea gigas* (mu li, oyster shell) 15mg, Calcium sulphate 15mg

Combine with

- **7.9 Jin Gui Shen Qi Wan**, **4.11 Ba Ji Yin Yang Wan** or **4.13 Zi Shen Da Bu Capsule** for nocturia, urinary frequency or incontinence arising from Kidney yang deficiency
- **7.1.1 Liu Wei Di Huang Wan** for nocturia, urinary frequency or incontinence in patients with a tendency to Kidney yin deficiency
- **2.11 Bu Zhong Yi Qi Wan** for prolapsed Bladder causing incontinence and defensive qi deficiency type excessive sweating
- **4.5 Bi Xie Fen Qing Wan** for chyluria and copious leukorrhea

Pattern identifying features

- **Kidney qi deficiency**
- leakage of fluids
- diarrhea, sweating

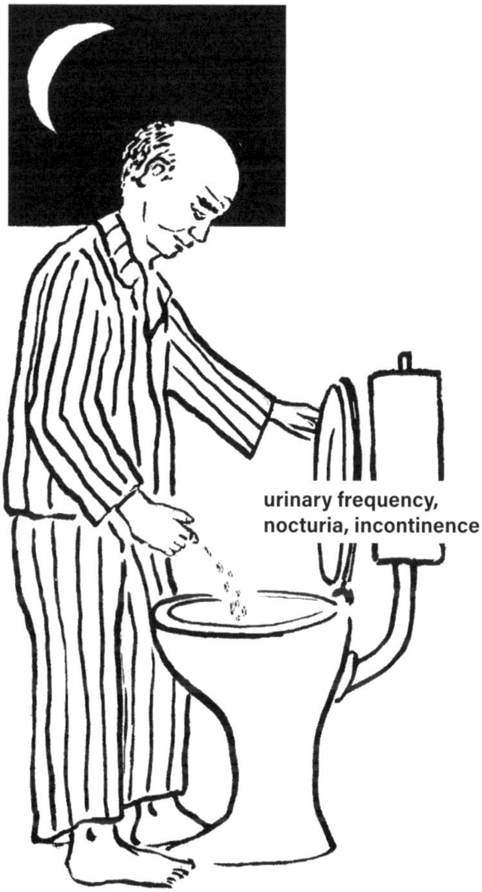

Dosage and method of administration

The recommended dose if used alone is 12 pills three times daily before meals, however, as it is usually combined with a constitutional formula, the dose can be reduced by 25-50%.

Cautions and contraindications

Contraindicated during the early phase of acute illness such as colds and flu, and in urinary dysfunction or other patterns associated with lingering damp heat or other pathogens that require expulsion.

GMP

4.15 SANG PIAO XIAO WAN

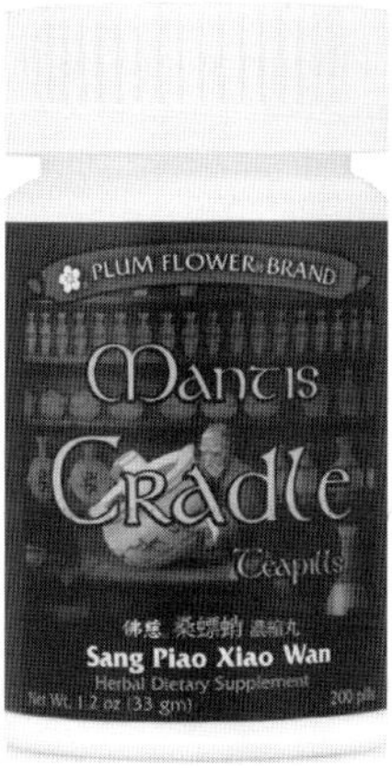

桑螵蛸丸

1-3/12

Lanzhou Foci Pharmaceutical Factory (Gansu)
'Mantis Egg Case Pills'
Sang Piao Xiao Wan is packaged in bottles of 200 pills
Also available as: Mantis Cocoon Formula (conc. extract)

Chinese medical action

Regulates and tonifies Heart and Kidney qi, restrains leakage of urine and secures essence

Biomedical action

Astringent

INDICATIONS

- Urinary frequency, incontinence of urine, nocturia and enuresis associated with Heart and Kidney qi deficiency. Urinary frequency and enuresis fluctuate with the patient's anxiety levels, and, in children especially, bed-wetting is often associated with night-time fearfulness and fear of the dark. The pathology is common in feeble or timid children with weak Kidney energy unable to support and anchor the *shén*. The focus of this formula is primarily on restraining leakage of fluids while secondarily tonifying the deficiency, so it combines well with more tonic formulas for long term results.
- With the appropriate identifying features, this formula can be used to assist in the treatment of conditions such as bed wetting, diabetes mellitus and insipidus, and neurogenic bladder dysfunction.

Composition

Ootheca Mantidis (sang piao xiao, mantis egg case), *Os draconis* (long gu, dragon bone), *Chinemys reevesii* (gui ban, turtle shell), *Panax ginseng* (ren shen, ginseng), *Poria cocos* (fu ling, hoelen), *Angelica sinensis* (dang gui, chinese angelica), *Acorus gramineus* (shi chang pu, acorus), *Polygala sibirica* (yuan zhi, polygala)

Combine with

- **7.1.1 Liu Wei Di Huang Wan** for diabetes associated with Kidney yin deficiency
- **2.15 Xiao Jian Zhong Wan** for qi deficiency urinary problems in children
- **2.35 Yu Quan Wan** for diabetes
- **7.9 Jin Gui Shen Qi Wan**, **4.11 Ba Ji Yin Yang Wan** or **4.13 Zi Shen Da Bu Capsule** for nocturia, urinary frequency or incontinence from Kidney yang deficiency

Pattern identifying features

- **Heart and Kidney qi deficiency**
- nocturia, incontinence of urine
- cloudy urine
- anxiety, dream disturbed sleep, insomnia
- tendency to timidity or fearfulness
- memory problems

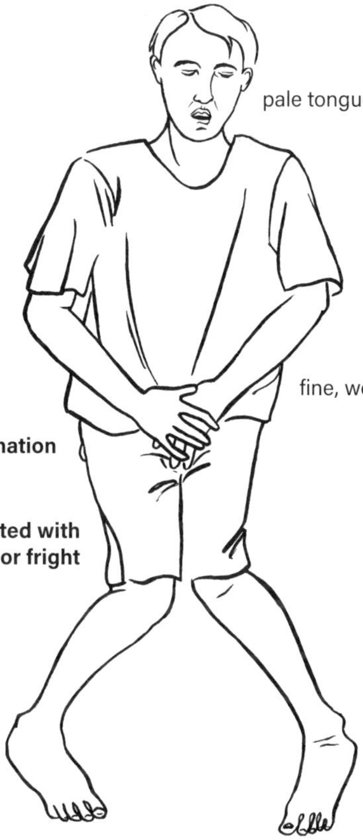

Dosage and method of administration

In adults, the dose is 8-12 pills three times daily on an empty stomach. The dose can be spread out, or taken in two lots of 12-18 pills, morning and evening. In severe cases or during the early stages of treatment (the first few weeks), a 50% increase in dose can be used, then reduced as treatment takes effect. Reduce the dose by 50-75% for children depending on their age and weight. Not suitable in pill form for children under 5 years.

Cautions and contraindications

Contraindicated in frequent urination patterns associated with heat or damp heat.

心脏血管病 5

Cardiovascular

5.1 XUE FU ZHU YU WAN

血府逐瘀丸

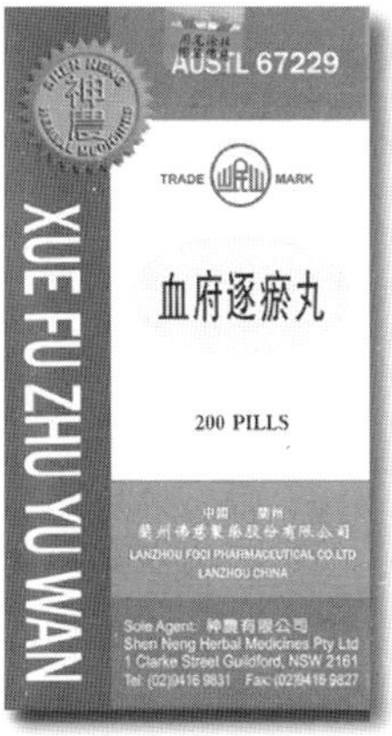

Lanzhou Foci Pharmaceutical Factory (Gansu)
'Pills to Dispel Static Blood from the Palace of Blood'
Xue Fu Zhu Yu Wan is packaged in bottles of 200 pills
Also available as: Stasis in the Mansion of Blood Teapills (PF), Persica and Carthamus Combination (conc. extract)

Chinese medical action

Invigorates qi and blood, dispels static blood

Biomedical action

Vasodilator, antispasmodic, anti-platelet action

INDICATIONS

- Qi and blood stasis. An important and effective blood stasis dispelling formula, with significant qi regulating capacity as well. Especially good for chronic Liver qi constraint complicated by blood stasis.
- Mostly used for chronic blood stasis patterns of the upper body, head, chest and Liver organ system (including reproductive system and channel pathway), but can be effective for all systemic blood stasis problems.
- Being such a broad acting formula, it can assist in the treatment of a wide variety of conditions, as long as the appropriate identifying features are present.
  - Cardiovascular: coronary artery disease, angina, sequelae of rheumatic fever, peripheral vascular insufficiency, varicose veins, Raynaud's syndrome, Buerger's disease, vasculitis, hypertension, thrombocytemia, hemochromatosis
  - Liver: chronic hepatitis, early stage hepatic cirrhosis
  - Head: post-concussion or head trauma syndrome, migraine headaches, trigeminal neuralgia, cerebrovascular insufficiency
  - Chest: post herpetic neuralgia, intercostal neuralgia, post traumatic chest wall pain, costochondritis
  - Gastrointestinal: peptic ulcer disease, diverticulosis, abdominal masses
  - Gynecological: dysmenorrhea, endometriosis, painful fibroids, ovarian cysts, uterine bleeding with dark clotted blood, infertility, interstitial cystitis
  - Psychiatric: chronic depression, bipolar mood disorder, schizophrenia, chronic recalcitrant insomnia, memory problems
  - Connective tissue: lupus, scleroderma, mixed connective tissue disease

Composition (each pill contains powdered)

Prunus persica (tao ren, peach seed), *Angelica sinensis* (dang gui, chinese angelica), *Rehmannia glutinosa* (sheng di, raw rehmannia), *Carthamus tinctorius* (hong hua, carthamus), *Achyranthes bidentata* (niu xi, achyranthes), *Citrus aurantium* (zhi ke, aurantium), *Paeonia lactiflora* (bai shao, white peony), *Ligusticum wallici* (chuan xiong, ligusticum), *Bupleurun falcatum* (chai hu, bupleurum), *Glycyrrhiza uralensis* (gan cao, licorice), *Platycodon grandiflorum* (jie geng, platycodon)

Pattern identifying features

- **qi and blood stasis**
- **fixed sharp pain anywhere in the body**
- **purple discoloration; vascular congestion; purple lips; dark circles around eyes**
- **masses**
- low grade hectic fevers
- dry, scaly skin
- recalcitrant insomnia

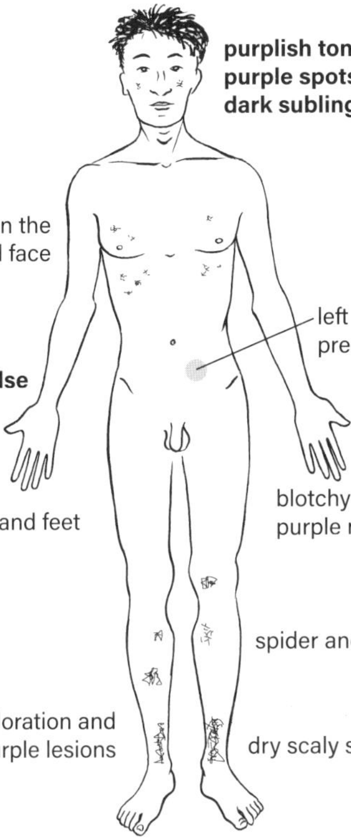

Combine with

- **6.9 Jigucao Wan** for chronic hepatitis or early cirrhosis
- **5.7 Sunho Multi Ginseng Tablets** for chronic depression and insomnia. This combination is also used for fixed headaches and migraine
- **15.8 Fu Fang Jiang Ya Capsule** for chronic essential hypertension associated with blood stasis

Dosage and method of administration

8-12 pills three times daily on an empty stomach. The dose can be spread out, or taken in two lots of 12-18 pills, morning and evening. In severe cases or during the early stages of treatment, a 50% increase in dose can be used, then reduced as treatment takes effect.

Cautions and contraindications

Contraindicated during pregnancy, in women with menorrhagia, and in patients with bleeding disorders. Caution in patients taking anticoagulants. Watch for bruising or increased tendency to bleeding. Prolonged use can disperse normal qi and blood, so a break every 2-3 months with a change to a simple qi and blood tonic formula for a few weeks, is recommended.

5.2 DAN SHEN PILL

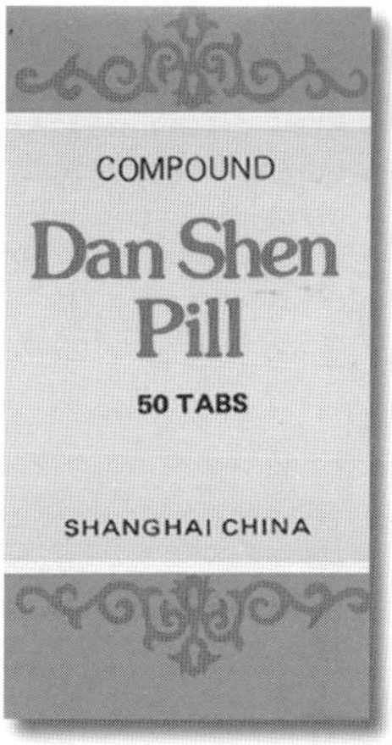

复方丹参片

(*Fu Fang Dan Shen Pian*)
China National Chemicals Corp. (Shanghai)
'Salvia Compound Pills'
Dan Shen Pills are packaged in bottles of 50 pills

Chinese medical action

Invigorates blood flow in the chest, dispels static blood and phlegm, opens the vessels, regulates qi, stops pain

Biomedical action

Anti-platelet action, vasodilator, lowers cholesterol and triglycerides, improves coronary circulation

INDICATIONS

- Blood stasis affecting the Heart and chest, giving rise to angina pectoris, cardiovascular disease, atherosclerosis and arteriosclerotic heart disease.
- Used to lower blood cholesterol and triglycerides.
- With the appropriate identifying features, this formula can assist in the treatment of conditions such as the early stage of coronary heart disease, angina pectoris, hypercholesterolemia, cerebrovascular insufficiency, transient ischaemic attacks, carotid stenosis, peripheral vascular disease, Raynaud's syndrome and Buerger's disease.

Composition

Salvia miltiorrhiza (dan shen, salvia) 59%, *Panax notoginseng* (tian qi, tianqi ginseng) 39%, Borneol (bing pian) 2%

Combine with

- **5.1 Xue Fu Zhu Yu Wan** for cardiac disease and cerebrovascular insufficiency
- **7.16 Shi Quan Da Bu Wan** and **13.14 Ching Wan Hung** topically for chronic non-healing ulcers and sores on the legs associated with qi and blood deficiency
- **2.18 Bao He Wan** for hypercholesterolemia in an overweight, damp patient

Dosage and method of administration

3 pills, three times daily on an empty stomach. Patients should expect to see some improvement within 1-3 months.

Pattern identifying features

- **blood stasis in the chest**
- **stifling sensation in the chest, chest oppression**
- palpitations, arrhythmia
- cardiovascular disease
- angina

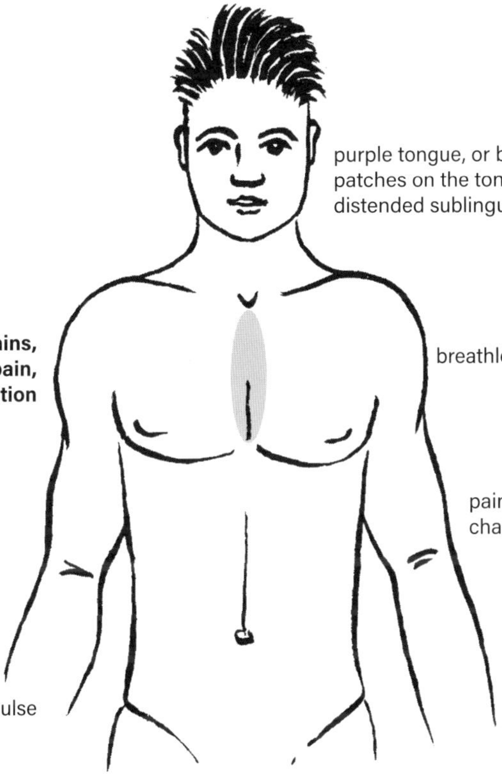

Cautions and contraindications

Contraindicated during pregnancy. Caution in patients taking mild anticoagulant therapy such as aspirin and fish oil as clotting time can be reduced. Contraindicated in patients taking warfarin (coumarin).

GMP

5.3 DAN SHEN YIN WAN

丹参饮丸

3+/12

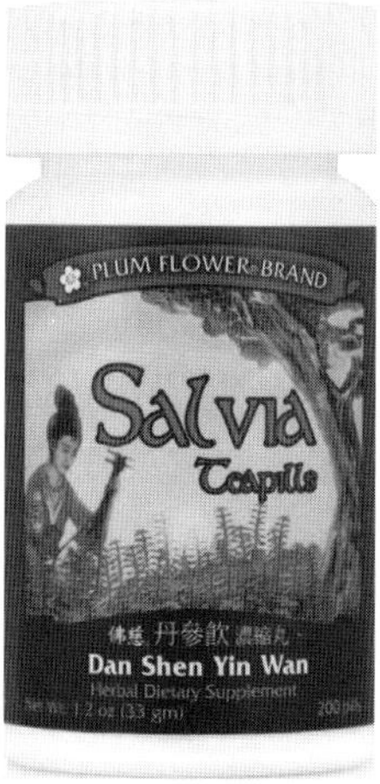

Lanzhou Foci Pharmaceutical Factory (Gansu)
'Salvia Pills'
Dan Shen Yin Wan is packaged in bottles of 200 pills
Also available as: Dan Shen Wan (HT)

Chinese medical action

Invigorates the circulation of qi and blood circulation in the chest and Stomach, invigorates blood, dispels static blood and stops pain

Biomedical action

Anti-platelet action, vasodilator, lowers cholesterol and triglycerides, improves coronary circulation

INDICATIONS

- Blood and qi stagnation patterns of the Heart and Stomach. A simple formula that utilizes a high proportion of salvia to invigorate blood and disperse blood stasis, it is best used in chronic, mild to moderate patterns with focal pain, but without severe systemic signs and symptoms of static blood.
- For mild to moderate qi and blood stasis patterns affecting the Liver causing hypochondriac pain.
- With the appropriate identifying features, this formula can assist in the treatment of conditions such as the early stage of coronary heart disease, angina pectoris, atherosclerosis, arteriosclerosis, chronic gastritis, peptic ulcer disease, chronic hepatitis, early hepatic cirrhosis and dysmenorrhea.

Composition

Salvia miltiorrhiza (dan shen, salvia), *Santalum album* (tan xiang, sandalwood), *Amomum villosum* (sha ren, cardamon), *Glycyrrhiza uralensis* (gan cao, licorice)

Combine with

- **5.1 Xue Fu Zhu Yu Wan** for cardiac disease and cerebrovascular insufficiency
- **10.21 Yan Huo Suo Zhi Tong Wan** for relatively severe pain

Dosage and method of administration

8-12 pills three times daily on an empty stomach. The dose can be spread out, or taken in two lots of 12-18 pills, morning and evening. In severe cases or during the early stages of treatment, a 50% increase in dose can be used, then reduced as treatment takes effect.

Pattern identifying features

- **mild blood stasis in the Heart or Stomach**

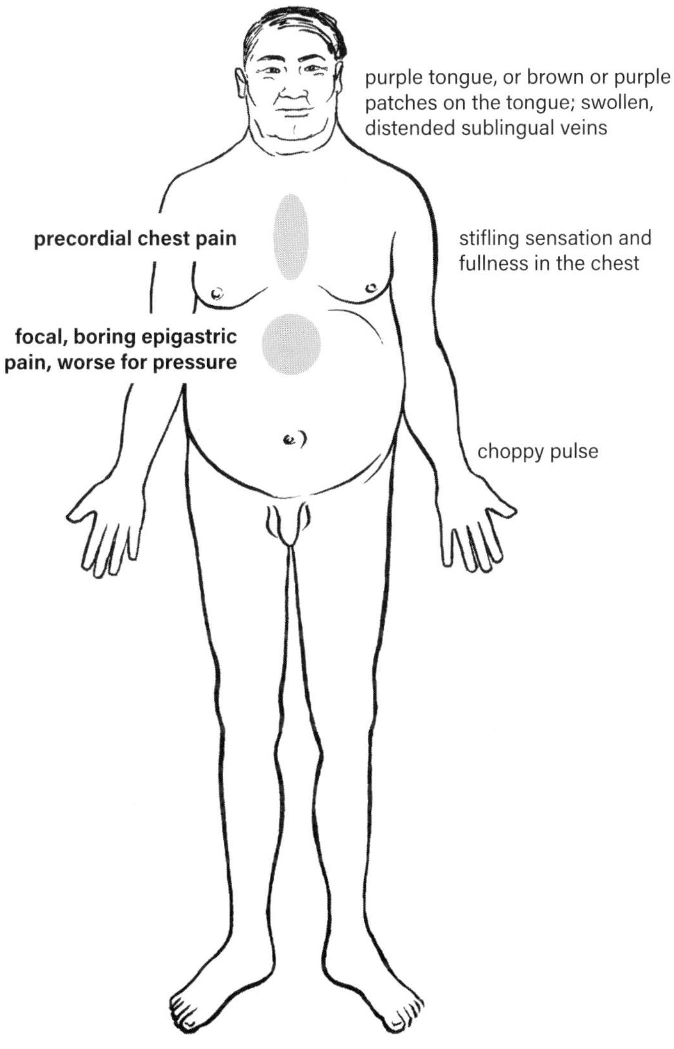

Cautions and contraindications

Contraindicated during pregnancy, in patients with bleeding disorders and patients taking warfarin (coumarin). Caution in patients taking mild anticoagulant therapy such as aspirin and fish oil as clotting time can be reduced.

5.4 XIN MAI LING

心脉灵

Guanghua Pharmaceutical Co. (Guangzhou)
'Miraculously Effective Pills for Coronary Circulation'
Xin Mai Ling is packaged in bottles of 36 capsules

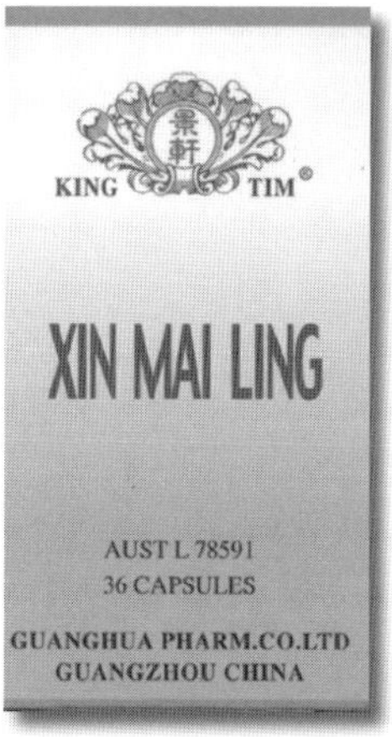

Chinese medical action
Invigorates blood circulation in the chest and periphery, dispels static blood, opens the vessels, clears toxic heat

Biomedical action
Anti-platelet action, vasodilator, lowers cholesterol and triglycerides, improves coronary circulation

INDICATIONS

- Blood stasis patterns of the heart, chest and periphery. The main herb, Ilex, is widely used in China to treat cardiac and peripheral blood stasis problems. Used to help restore circulation in those with peripheral vascular disease and hemiplegia. Especially good when peripheral blood stasis is complicated by heat.
- Used to lower blood cholesterol and triglycerides. Also useful as a preventative against cardiovascular and cerebrovascular disease for those at risk.
- With the appropriate identifying features, this formula can be used to assist in the treatment of conditions such as the early stage of coronary heart disease, angina pectoris, hypercholesterolemia, cerebrovascular insufficiency, transient ischaemic attacks (TIA's), hemiplegia, carotid stenosis, thrombophlebitis, peripheral vascular disease, diabetic vascular disease and ulcers, Raynaud's syndrome, Buerger's disease and central retinitis.

Composition (each capsule contains extracts equivalent to dry)
Ilex pubescens (mao dong qing, ilex) 3.75g, *Salvia miltiorrhiza* (dan shen, salvia) 315mg, *Panax notoginseng* (tian qi, tianqi ginseng) 50mg

Combine with
- **5.1 Xue Fu Zhu Yu Wan** for cardiac disease, cerebrovascular insufficiency and peripheral vascular disease associated with stagnation of qi and blood
- **7.16 Shi Quan Da Bu Wan** and **13.14 Ching Wan Hung** topically for chronic non-healing ulcers and sores on the legs

Dosage and method of administration
3 capsules three times daily on an empty stomach. In severe cases the dose can be increase to 4-5 capsules three times daily. In general, quite a large dose of Ilex is required for a satisfactory therapeutic effect.

Pattern identifying features

- **blood stasis with heat in the chest and extremities**

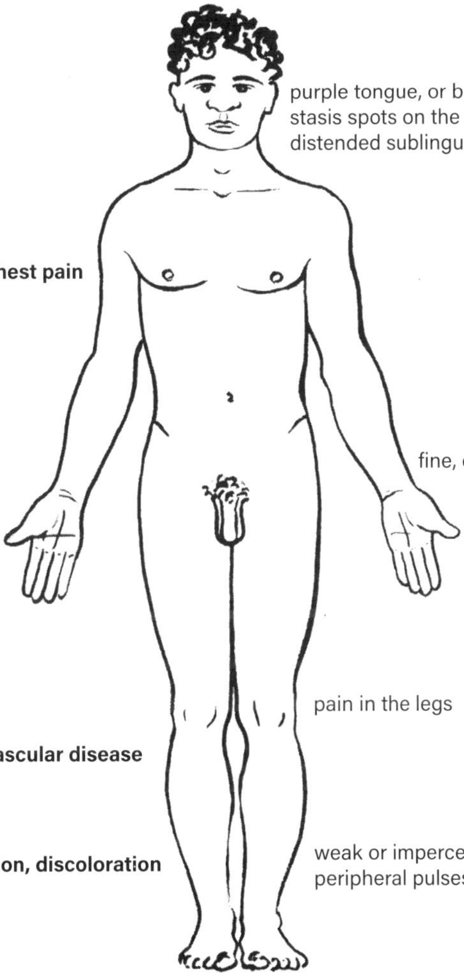

Cautions and contraindications

Contraindicated during pregnancy and in patients taking warfarin (coumarin). Caution in patients taking mild anticoagulant therapy such as aspirin and fish oil as clotting time can be reduced. This formula is quite cooling and not recommended alone for patients with deficient cold patterns with blood stasis. Although Ilex is considered safe and well tolerated, occasional side effects like nausea, dizziness and abdominal pain can occur. These can be alleviated by reducing the dose.

GMP

5.5 ZHI GAN CAO WAN

炙甘草丸

3+/12

Lanzhou Foci Pharmaceutical Factory (Gansu)
'Honey Fried Licorice Pills'
Zhi Gan Cao Wan is packaged in bottles of 200 pills
Also available as: Licorice Combination (conc. extract)

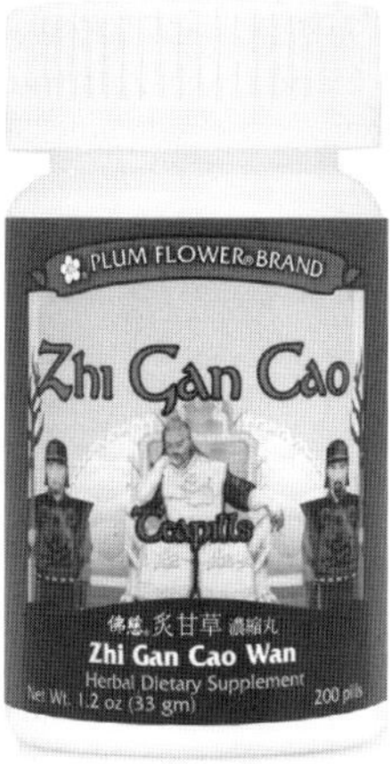

Chinese medical action

Tonifies Heart qi, blood and yin, promotes circulation of Heart yang, restores the pulse, calms the *shén*

Biomedical action

Anti-arrhythmic, improves cardiac function, sedative and tranquillizer

INDICATIONS

- Palpitations and cardiac arrhythmia associated with Heart qi, blood and/or yin deficiency. Palpitations or arrhythmias are initiated or aggravated by exertion and when fatigued. The specific arrhythmia referred to here is an irregularly irregular beat, that is, beats are dropped at irregular intervals. The formula can, however, also be used for heart beats dropped at regular intervals, as well as tachycardia and bradycardia.
- Consumptive Lung disease (*fèi láo* 肺痨 or *fèi wěi* 肺痿), characterized by chronic dry cough, or cough with blood streaked sputum, weight loss, breathlessness, low grade fever, night sweats and spontaneous sweating and generalized dryness.
- With the appropriate identifying features, this formula can assist in the treatment of conditions such as supraventricular arrhythmia, sick sinus syndrome, premature ectopic asystole, bradycardia, hyperthyroidism, cardiomyopathy, viral myocarditis, sequelae of rheumatic heart disease, coronary artery disease, and pulmonary tuberculosis.

Composition

Rehmannia glutinosa (sheng di, raw rehmannia), *Glycyrrhiza uralensis* (zhi gan cao, honey fried licorice), *Ophiopogon japonicus* (mai dong, ophiopogon), *Cannabis sativa* (huo ma ren, cannabis seeds), *Cinnamomum cassia* (gui zhi, cinnamon twigs), *Zingiber officinale* (sheng jiang, ginger), *Zizyphus jujuba* (da zao, chinese dates), *Panax ginseng* (ren shen, ginseng), *Equus asinus* (e jiao, donkey skin gelatin)

Combine with

- **2.7 Si Jun Zi Wan** for patients with a greater degree of qi deficiency
- **1.2 Si Wu Wan** for patients with a greater degree of blood deficiency
- **1.16 Tao Hong Si Wu Wan** with mild blood stasis

Pattern identifying features

- **Heart qi, blood and/or yin deficiency**
- insomnia, difficulty falling asleep (and switching off the mind), dream disturbed sleep
- symptoms exacerbated by exertion and when fatigued
- forgetfulness, poor memory, poor concentration
- fatigue and weakness
- breathlessness

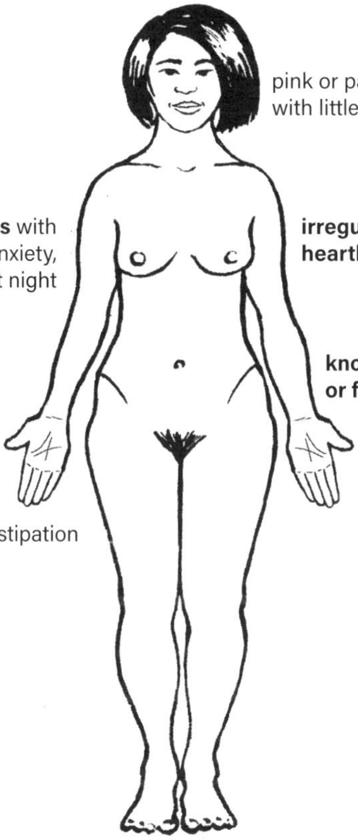

Dosage and method of administration

8-12 pills three times daily on an empty stomach. The dose can be spread out, or taken in two lots of 12-18 pills, morning and evening. In severe cases or during the early stages of treatment, a 50% increase in dose can be used, then reduced as treatment takes effect.

Cautions and contraindications

Caution in patients with loose bowels or diarrhea, and where prescribed alone for patients with significant heat generated by deficiency. Caution in patients with hypertension and fluid problems due to the large proportion of licorice. May counteract spironolactone (Aldactone) and potentiate potassium depleting loop diuretics, such as Lasix, leading to hypokalemia.

5.6 GUAN XIN AN KOU FU YE

冠心安口服液

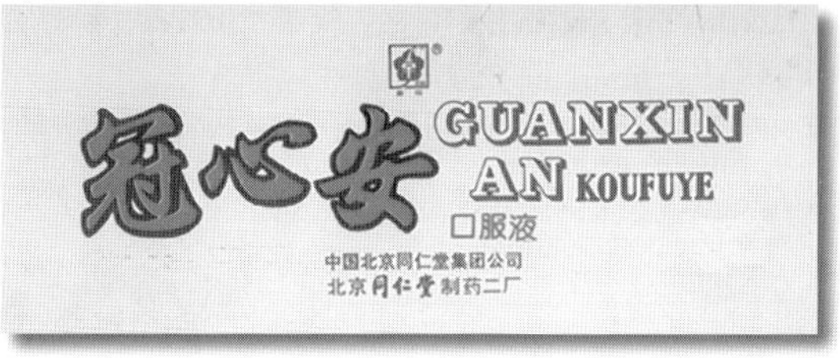

Tong Ren Tang (Beijing)
'Calm Coronary Artery Drink'
Guan Xin An Kou Fu Ye is packaged as liquid extract in small vials, ten vials per box

Chinese medical action

Invigorates blood circulation in the chest, invigorates blood, benefits Heart qi

Biomedical action

Improves cardiac circulation, anti-platelet action

INDICATIONS

- Blood stasis affecting the Heart with chest pain, atherosclerosis and arteriosclerotic heart disease, angina pectoris.
- Cerebrovascular insufficiency, transient ischaemic attacks, cerebrovascular spasm.
- Poor peripheral circulation, early stage of peripheral vascular disease.

Composition (each vial contains extracts equivalent to dry)

Bupleurum falcatum (chai hu, bupleurum) 2.91g, *Ligusticum wallichi* (chuan xiong, ligusticum) 2.31g, *Chrysanthemum indicum* (ye ju hua, wild chrysanthemum) 2.01g, *Poria cocos* (fu ling, hoelen) 1.89g, *Dalbergia odorifera* (jiang xiang, dalbergia wood) 1.79g, *Polygonum multiflorum* (he shou wu, polygonum root) 1.51g, *Zizyphus jujuba* (da zao, chinese dates) 1.47g, *Achyranthes bidentata* (niu xi, achyranthes) 1.41g, *Glycyrrhiza uralensis* (gan cao, licorice) 803mg, *Panax notoginseng* (tian qi, tian qi ginseng) 616mg, *Cinnamomum cassia* (gui zhi, cinnamon twigs) 411mg

Combine with

- **5.2 Dan Shen Pill** or **5.7 Sunho Multi Ginseng Tablets** for frequent angina
- **13.14 Ching Wan Hung** for venous ulcers in a patient with blood stasis and cold accumulation

Dosage and method of administration

One vial, 2-3 times daily.

Pattern identifying features

- **blood stasis in the chest and Heart**

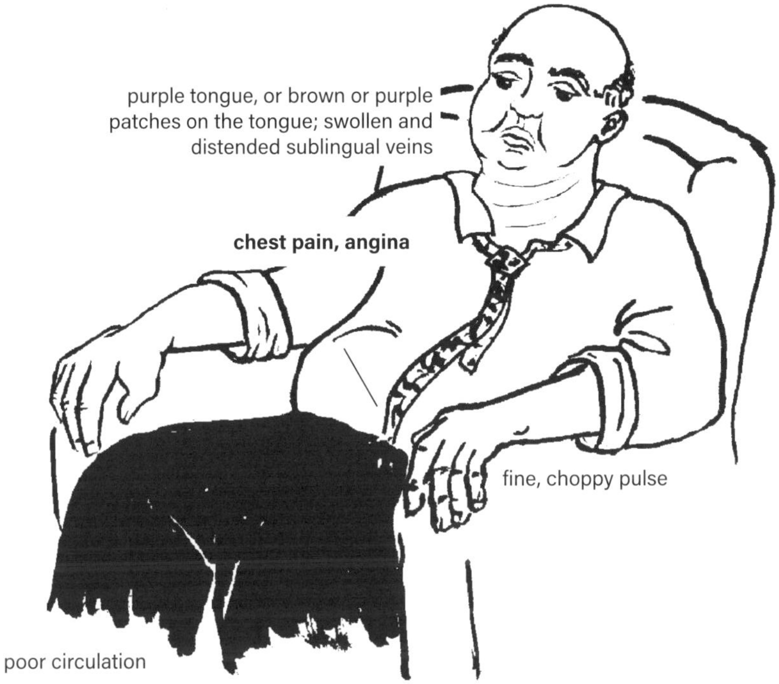

Cautions and contraindications

Contraindicated during pregnancy and for patients with low platelet count, internal bleeding (as in a bleeding gastric ulcer) or heavy menstrual periods. Caution in patients who are also taking anticoagulant therapy as clotting time may be reduced.

5.7 SUNHO MULTI GINSENG TABLETS

三参健康丸

(*San Shen Jian Kang Wan*)
Sunho Traditional Medicine Co. (Australia)
'Health [Promoting] Pills Composed of Three Roots'
Sunho Multi Ginseng Tablets are packaged in bottles of 80 tablets

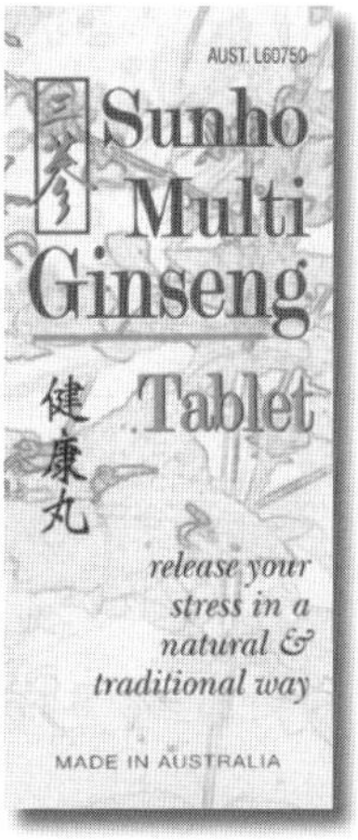

Chinese medical action

Invigorates blood, dispels static blood, tonifies qi and yin

Biomedical action

Anti-platelet action, vasodilator, lowers cholesterol and triglycerides, improves coronary circulation

INDICATIONS

- Blood stasis with qi deficiency. Improves and strengthens cardiac function, dilates coronary arteries. Useful for preventative maintenance of healthy cardiovascular and cerebrovascular circulation. Can be used to alleviate mild angina.
- For maintenance of peripheral circulation and treatment of blood stasis in the extremities. This includes disorders such as varicose veins, spider vessels or discoloration around the ankles and mild peripheral vascular disease. Useful for peripheral or diabetic neuropathy.
- Tonifies Lung and Spleen qi and calms the *shén*. Useful as an energy tonic to improve endurance and stamina, or for the treatment of fatigue and lack of vitality.
- Various types of pain associated with blood stasis, including epigastric, hypochondriac and cardiac.
- Chronic liver disease, such as hepatitis and mild cirrhosis.
- Elevated blood cholesterol and high blood pressure.

Composition (each tablet contains powdered)

Panax quinquefolium (xi yang shen, american ginseng) 120mg, *Panax notoginseng* (tian qi, tianqi ginseng) 120mg, *Salvia miltiorrhiza* (dan shen, salvia) 60mg

Combine with

- **5.1 Xue Fu Zhu Yu Wan** for cardiac disease and cerebrovascular insufficiency. This combination is also used for chronic liver disease with cirrhosis
- **6.1 Xiao Chai Hu Wan** for chronic hepatitis C with blood stasis
- **3.18 Tung Hsuan Li Fei Pien** for gastric ulcers with fixed, boring pain
- **2.18 Bao He Wan** for hypercholesterolemia
- **15.7 Yang Yin Jiang Ya Wan** for resistant hypertension
- **7.26 Reishi Mushroom** as adjunct treatment for symptoms of fatigue and immune weakness in patients being treated with chemotherapy or radiotherapy
- **5.8 Bu Yang Huan Wu Wan** for hemiplegia following a stabilized wind stroke

Pattern identifying features

- **blood stasis; qi deficiency**
- fixed recurrent pain

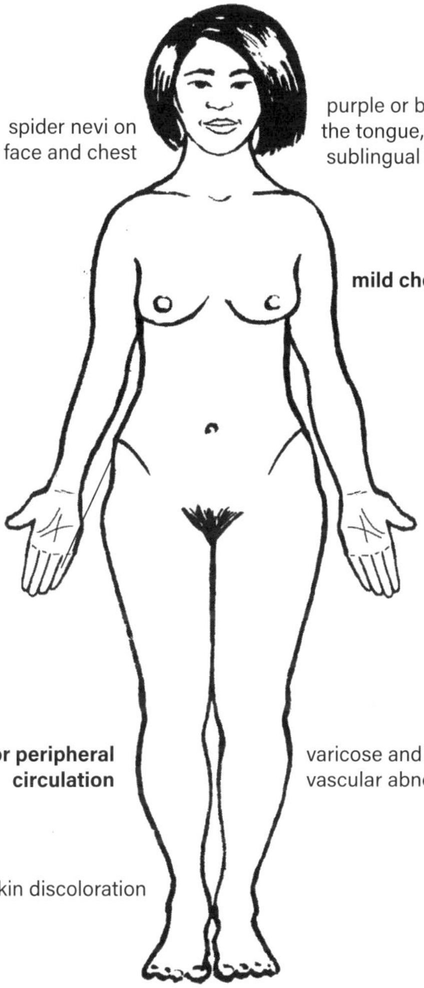

Dosage and method of administration

The dose for general cardiovascular maintenance is two tablets twice daily. In the early stages of treatment for disease, the dose can be doubled until results are noticed, then reduced to the maintenance dose.

Cautions and contraindications

Contraindicated during pregnancy and in patients taking warfarin (coumarin). Caution in patients taking mild anticoagulant therapy such as aspirin and fish oil as clotting time can be reduced.

5.8 BU YANG HUAN WU WAN

补阳还五丸

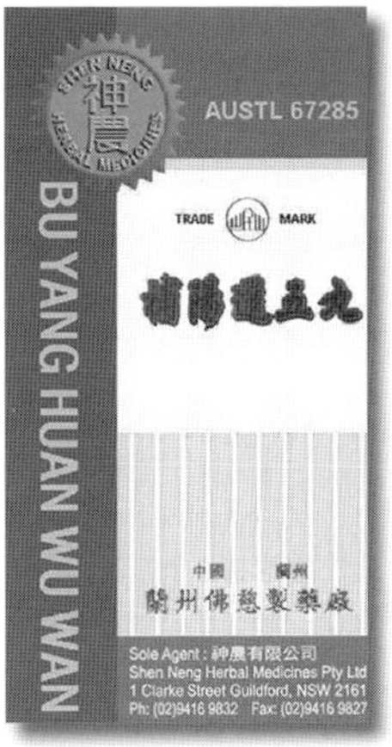

Lanzhou Foci Pharmaceutical Factory (Gansu)
'Pills to Tonify Yang and Restore the Other Half'
Bu Yang Huan Wu Wan is packaged in bottles of 200 pills
Also available as: Great Yang Restoration Teapills (PF), Astragalus and Peony Combination (conc. extract)

Chinese medical action

Tonifies qi, invigorates blood, unblocks channels and collaterals

Biomedical action

Improves circulation to the periphery, anti-platelet action

INDICATIONS

- Sequelae of wind-stroke in patients with qi and/or yang deficiency complicated by blood stasis. Features include hemiplegia, facial paralysis, slurred speech, drooling, incontinence, exhaustion and wasting. Widely used and effective (when used early enough) for convalescence following a stabilized wind-stroke, but needs to be used for some months. Also useful for loss of function, weakness and wasting following cranial surgery or head injury.
- Sequelae of poliomyelitis and other atrophy and muscular weakness syndromes with wasting and weakness of the peripheral muscles, such as myasthenia gravis and multiple sclerosis.
- Peripheral or diabetic neuropathy with altered sensation, paresthesia or loss of sensation in the extremities, usually the lower limbs.
- Peripheral vascular disease and insufficiency, deep venous thrombosis, diabetic and stasis ulcers, varicose veins.

Composition (each pill contains powdered)

Astragalus membranaceous (huang qi, astragalus) 54mg, *Spatholobus suberectus* (ji xue teng, spatholobus) 27mg, *Prunus persica* (tao ren, peach seed) 27mg, *Crocus sativus* (xi hong hua, crocus stamen) 23.4mg, *Paeonia rubra* (chi shao, red peony) 18mg, *Angelica sinensis* (dang gui, chinese angelica) 18mg, *Ligusticum wallichii* (chuan xiong, ligusticum) 12.6mg

Combine with

- **5.1 Xue Fu Zhu Yu Wan** or **5.7 Sunho Multi Ginseng Tablets** to enhance the blood invigorating action in chronic or resistant cases
- **10.11 Shu Jin Huo Xue Wan** for paralysis and pain that is worse in the lower limbs from wind damp and blood stasis
- **11.8 Kang Wei Ling Wan** for pronounced or difficult facial paralysis
- **2.22 Er Chen Wan** for complication by residual phlegm (thick greasy tongue coat, dizziness)

Pattern identifying features

- **blood stasis with qi deficiency**
- sequelae of stroke
- atrophy and muscular weakness syndrome
- easy sweating
- fatigue, breathlessness

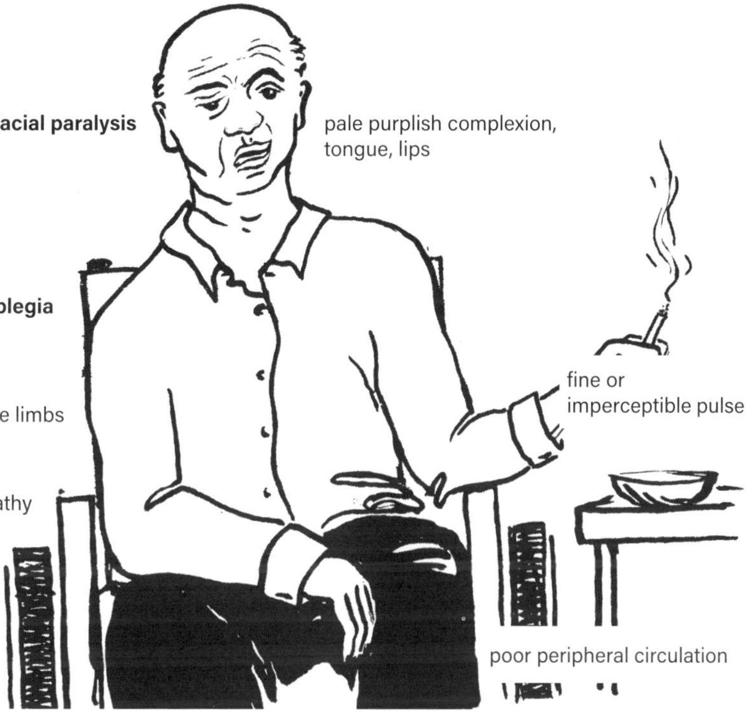

- **2.11 Bu Zhong Yi Qi Wan** or **7.17 Hua Tuo Shi Quan Da Bu Jiu** for atrophy and muscular weakness syndrome associated with qi deficiency
- **10.16.1 Zhuang Yao Jian Shen** or **10.18 Jian Bu Qiang Shen Wan** for atrophy and muscular weakness syndrome patterns associated with Kidney deficiency

Dosage and method of administration

12-15 pills three times daily on an empty stomach. The dose can be spread out, or two lots of 18-22 pills taken, morning and evening. In severe cases or during the early stages of treatment (the first few weeks), a 50% increase in dose can be used, then reduced as treatment takes effect. The pills may need to be softened and mashed to a slurry with hot water before ingestion.

Cautions and contraindications

Contraindicated during pregnancy, and in the first two weeks following stroke to avoid aggravation of bleeding from a cerebral hemorrhage. The patient must be stable before beginning treatment. Contraindicated in hemiplegic patients with ascendant Liver yang (*see* **15.4 Tian Ma Gou Teng Wan** or **15.6 Zhen Gan Xi Feng Wan**), or Liver and Kidney deficiency with residual wind (*see* **15.5 Tian Ma Wan**).

GMP

5.9 DANG GUI SI NI WAN

当归四逆丸

1-3/12

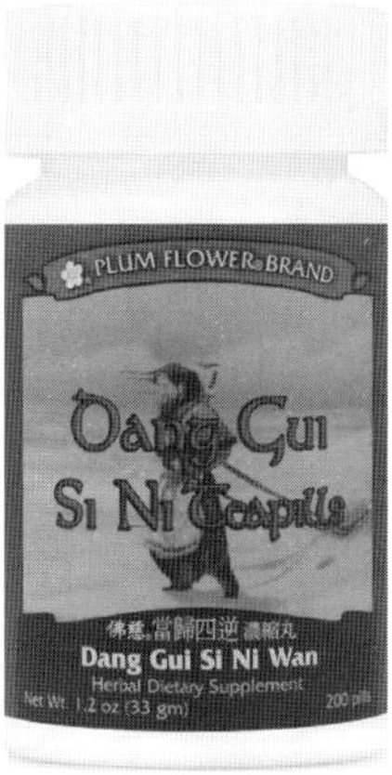

Lanzhou Foci Pharmaceutical Factory (Gansu)
'Dang Gui Pills for Frigid Extremities'
Dang Gui Si Ni Wan is packaged in bottles of 200 pills
Also available as: Tangkuei and Jujube Combination (conc. extract)

Chinese medical action

Warms and opens the channels and collaterals, dispels cold, nourishes blood and unblocks blood vessels

Biomedical action

Vasodilator, promotes circulation to the extremities

INDICATIONS

- Cold obstructing and congealing circulation of qi and blood in channels, collaterals and blood vessels of the periphery, manifesting primarily as chronic, icy cold hands and feet that may be pale or purple pale. May also be cramping and pain in the affected limbs. The focus of the pathology, the cold, is mostly confined to the hands and feet, thus this pattern differs from that in which yang is systemically weak and unable to reach the limbs (*see* **7.9 Jin Gui Shen Qi Wan** and **2.14 Li Chung Yuen Medical Pills**), in which case the whole limb is cold and there are systemic signs of yang deficiency.
- For joint pain, lower back pain, abdominal pain and dysmenorrhea from blood deficiency and cold accumulation.
- With the appropriate identifying features, this formula can assist in the treatment of conditions such as Raynaud's syndrome, frostbite, sciatica, scleroderma, thrombophlebitis and intestinal adhesions.

Composition

Angelica sinensis (dang gui, chinese angelica), *Paeonia lactiflora* (bai shao, white peony), *Cinnamomum cassia* (gui zhi, cinnamon twigs), *Asarum seiboldi* (xi xin, asarum), *Glycyrrhiza uralensis* (zhi gan cao, honey fried licorice), *Akebia trifoliata* (mu tong, akebia stem), *Zizyphus jujuba* (da zao, chinese dates)

Combine with

– **5.7 Sunho Multi Ginseng Tablets** or **10.2 Raw Tienchi Tablets** to enhance the blood moving action in chronic or resistant cases

Dosage and method of administration

8-12 pills three times daily on an empty stomach. The dose can be spread out, or taken in two lots of 12-18 pills, morning and evening. In severe cases or the early stages of treatment (the first few weeks), a 50% increase in dose can be used, then reduced as treatment takes effect.

Pattern identifying features

- **cold accumulation in the channels and vessels**
- pain and cramping in the limbs, aggravated by exposure to cold, better for heat

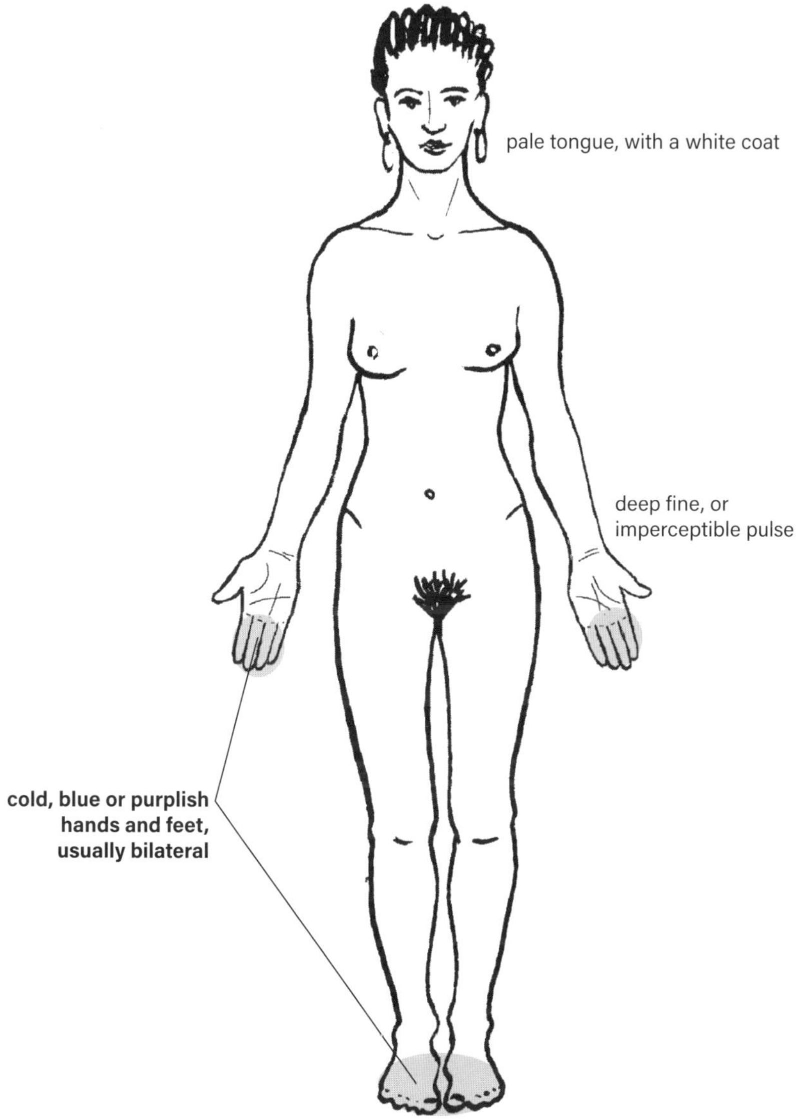

Cautions and contraindications

Contraindicated in patients with yin deficiency or internal heat causing cold extremities (*see* **6.2 Si Ni Wan**).

GMP

5.10 XIAO SHUAN ZAI ZAO WAN

1-3/12

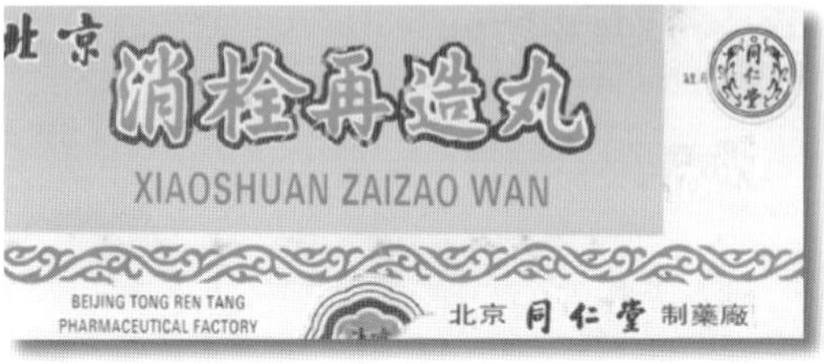

消栓再造丸

Tong Ren Tang (Beijing)
'Pills to Remove the Plug and Give a New Lease on Life'
Xiao Shuan Zai Zao Wan is packaged as 55 small pills in a wax ball, ten balls per box

Chinese medical action

Invigorates blood, dispels static blood, extinguishes wind, opens the channels and collaterals, tonifies qi and blood

Biomedical action

Improves circulation, anti-cholesterol, anti-thrombus, anti-platelet action.

INDICATIONS

- Sequelae of wind-stroke–hemiplegia, slurred speech, drooling, facial paralysis etc. This is a broad spectrum formula, designed to address a variety of pathological conditions that may occur in the aftermath of a stabilized stroke.
- Acute facial paralysis, Bell's palsy.
- Atrophy and muscular weakness syndrome.

Composition (each dose contains powdered)

Astragalus membranaceous (huang qi, astragalus) 231mg, *Angelica polymorpha* (dang gui, chinese angelica) 198mg, *Atractylodes macrocephala* (bai zhu, atractylodes) 137.5mg, *Achyranthes bidentata* (niu xi, achyranthes) 121mg, *Citrus aurantium* (zhi ke, aurantium) 121mg, *Clematis sinensis* (wei ling xian, chinese clematis) 110mg, *Ophiopogon japonicus* (mai dong, ophiopogon) 99mg, *Ligusticum wallici* (chuan xiong, ligusticum) 93.5mg, *Poria cocos* (fu ling, hoelen) 93.5mg, *Panax notoginseng* (tian qi, tian qi ginseng) 82.5mg, *Curcum longa* (yu jin, curcuma) 71.5mg, *Salvia miltiorrhiza* (dan shen, salvia) 71.5mg, *Schizandra chinensis* (wu wei zi, schizandra) 71.5mg, *Stephania tetrandra* (han fang ji, stephania) 71.5mg, *Drynaria fortunei* (gu sui bu, drynaria rhizome) 71.5mg, *Gastrodia elata* (tian ma, gastrodia) 71.5mg, *Cinnamomum cassia* (rou gui, cinnamon bark) 66mg, *Sophora japonica* (huai hua mi, sophora seed) 44mg, *Ammomum cardamomum* (bai dou kou, amomum) 44mg, *Daemonorops draco* (xue jie, dragons blood) 44mg, *Crategus pinnatifida* (shan zha, crategus) 44mg, *Commiphora myrhha* (mo yao, myrhh) 44mg, *Paeonia veitchii* (chi shao, red peony) 44mg, *Panax ginseng* (ren shen, ginseng) 38.5mg, *Aquilaria sinensis* (chen xiang, aquilaria wood) 38.5mg, *Chaenomeles speciosa* (mu gua, chinese quince) 22mg, *Styrax tonkinensis* (an xi xiang, styrax resin) 22mg, *Liquidamber orientalis* (su he xiang, liquidamber resin) 11mg, Borneol 5.5mg, honey

Pattern identifying features

- **sequelae of wind-stroke**

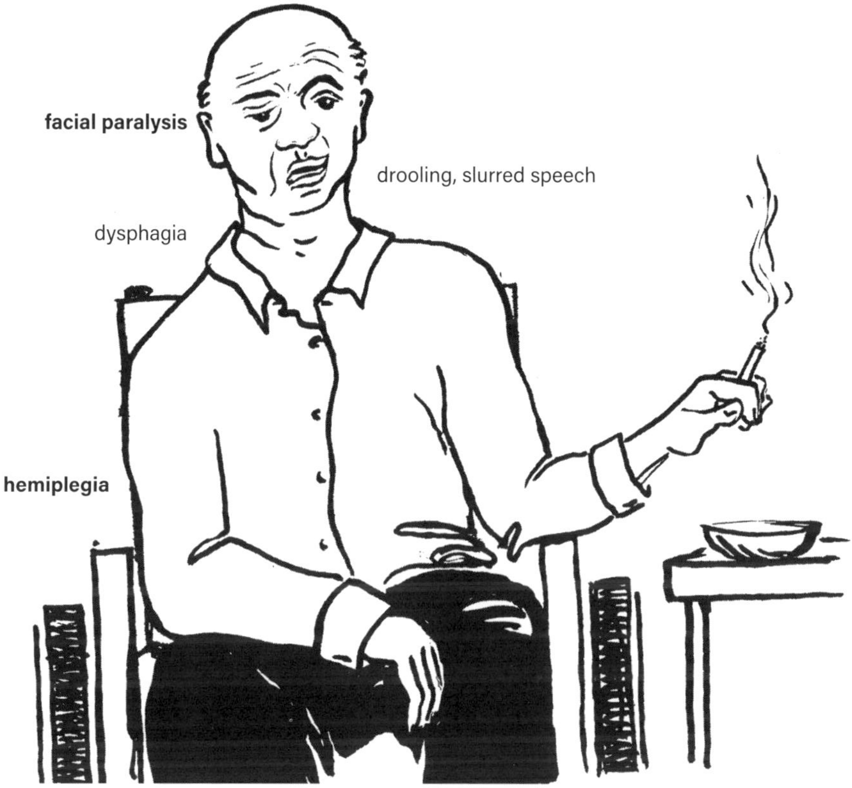

Dosage and method of administration

The recommended dose is one ball (55 pills) twice daily with warm water or a little alcohol (vodka or sherry is good). Take for one month, then stop for one week, then repeat. A course of treatment is 1-3 months, although patients should notice some improvement after a month or so. Physical therapy must be maintained during the treatment period.

Cautions and contraindications

Contraindicated during pregnancy. The patient must be stable before beginning this treatment. Contraindicated in patients with residual ascendant Liver yang (*see* **15.4 Tian Ma Gou Teng Wan** or **15.6 Zhen Gan Xi Feng Wan**).

T G A

5.11 HUA TUO ZAI ZAO WAN

华佗再造丸

1-3/12

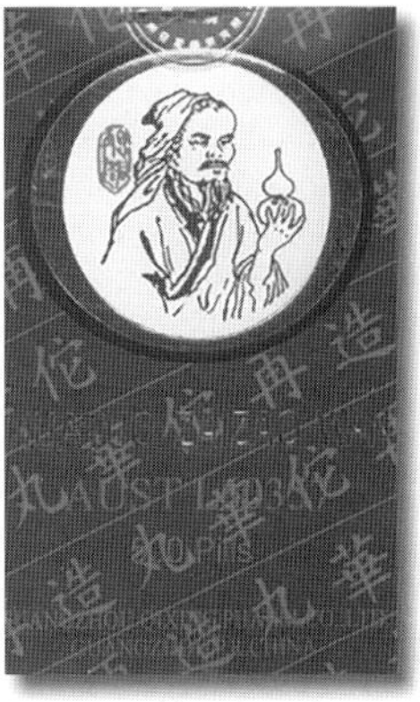

Guangzhou Qixing Pharmaceutical Co. (Guangzhou)
'Hua Tuo's Restorative Pills'
Hua Tuo Zai Zao Wan is packaged in bottles of 500 small pills with a slotted measuring spoon

Chinese medical action

Tonifies qi, yin and blood, dispels wind damp, promotes circulation of qi and blood in the channels

Biomedical action

Tonic, circulatory stimulant

INDICATIONS

- Atrophy and muscular weakness with spastic or flaccid paralysis and hemiplegia. Used for patterns associated with qi and yin deficiency following wind-stroke or associated with a variety of wasting disorders.
- Chronic or persistent tremors, tics, spasms and cramps resulting from yin and blood deficiency.
- Poor circulation in the extremities in a patient with deficient qi, yang and yin.
- With the appropriate identifying features, this formula can assist in treatment of conditions such as post stroke hemiplegia, dysphagia and aphasia, Bell's palsy, peripheral neuropathy, fibromyalgia, Raynaud's syndrome, chilblains and frostbite. Also for chronic headaches or migraines that are worse with exposure to cold, facial pain, chronic trigeminal neuralgia, coldness and discomfort in the external genitals and chronic neck pain. May assist in conditions such as Amyotrophic Lateral Sclerosis (ALS), multiple sclerosis and Parkinson's disease.

Composition (each pill contains extracts equivalent to dry)

Gentiana macrophylla (qin jiao, gentiana chin chiu) 89.6mg, *Panax ginseng* (ren shen, ginseng) 89.6mg, *Ophiopogon japonicus* (mai dong, ophiopogon) 89.6mg, *Schizandra chinensis* (wu wei zi, schizandra) 89.6mg, *Sophora japonica* (huai hua, sophora flower) 89.6mg, *Angelica dahurica* (bai zhi, angelica) 35.2mg, *Ligusticum wallichi* (chuan xiong, ligusticum) 35.2mg, *Angelica polymorpha* (dang gui, chinese angelica) 35.2mg, *Cinnamomum cassia* (rou gui, cinnamon bark) 19.2mg, *Evodia rutaecarpa* (wu zhu yu, evodia) 19.2mg

Combine with

- **15.9 Headache and Dizziness Reliever** for chronic neck and upper back pain from fibromyalgia
- **2.11 Bu Zhong Yi Qi Wan** or **2.12 Shen Ling Bai Zhu Wan** for atrophy and muscular weakness from Spleen qi and yin deficiency with damp
- **10.18 Jian Bu Qiang Shen Wan** or **10.16.2 Zhuang Yao Jian Shen Tablet** for atrophy and muscular weakness from Kidney qi and yin deficiency

Pattern identifying features

- **qi and yin deficiency, wind damp**
- cold intolerance
- poor peripheral circulation
- wasting and weakness of the extremities
- dysphagia, aphasia

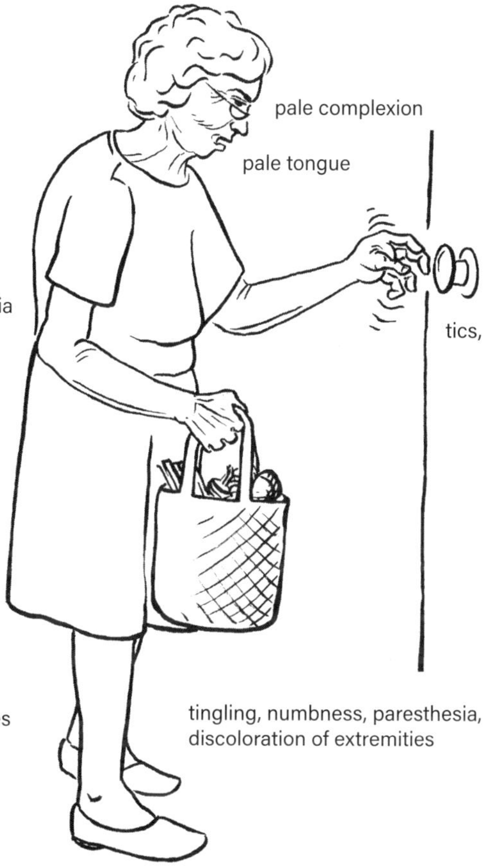

- **1.2 Si Wu Wan** or **7.16 Shi Quan Da Bu Wan** for atrophy and muscular weakness with significant muscle spasm, fasciculations and tics
- **5.7 Sunho Multi Ginseng Tablets** for concurrent blood stasis

Dosage and method of administration

The recommended dose is fifty (50) pills twice daily for ten days (the equivalent of two jars), then break for a day, then repeat twice for a total of six jars. Alternatively, fewer pills, to a total of 100, can be consumed over the course of a day. This formula comes with a neat slotted spoon device that takes 12 pills, so four spoons is close enough to a single dose. After the first six jars, or when an improvement is noticed, reduce the dose by half. The pills can be soaked in hot water and mashed to ease ingestion.

Cautions and contraindications

Contraindicated during the early phase of acute illness such as colds and flu.

肝胆病 6

Liver and Gallbladder

6.1 XIAO CHAI HU WAN

小柴胡丸

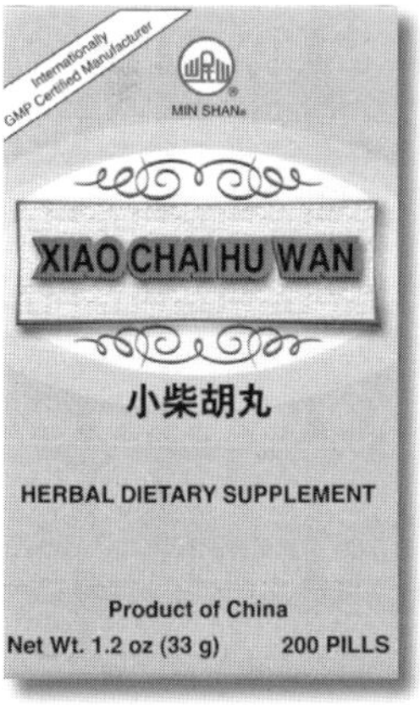

Lanzhou Foci Pharmaceutical Factory (Gansu)
'Minor Bupleurum Pills'
Xiao Chai Hu Wan is packaged in bottles of 200 pills
Also available as: Minor Bupleurum Combination (conc. extract)

Chinese medical action

Harmonizes *shào yáng*, tonifies qi, transforms phlegm, dredges the Liver and regulates qi, clears heat

Biomedical action

Hepatoprotective, enhances digestive function, strengthens immunity, aids clearance of residual pathogens

INDICATIONS

- *Shào yáng* syndrome (*see* glossary). The classical formula for *shào yáng* syndrome, used extensively to treat chronic or persistent viral, parasitic, or otherwise mysterious low grade infections of a *shào yáng* type.
- Gastrointestinal, chronic inflammatory and allergic disorders from Liver qi constraint, Spleen deficiency and heat (the primary pathological triad, *see* glossary).
- With the appropriate identifying features, this formula can assist in the treatment of conditions such as post viral syndrome, chronic fatigue syndrome, post acute Ross River fever and glandular fever, symptoms that occur in the post acute stage of a febrile illness or upper respiratory tract infection, acute and chronic hepatitis, acute mastitis, recurrent glue ear, otitis media, malaria, postpartum fever and common cold, bronchitis, pleurisy, hay fever and other allergies, acute pyelonephritis and cystitis, intercostal neuralgia, pleurisy, gallstones, cholecystitis and menstrual disorders.

Composition (each pill contains powdered)

Bupleurum falcatum (chai hu, bupleurum), *Pinellia ternata* (zhi ban xia, processed pinellia), *Scutellaria baicalensis* (huang qin, scute), *Codonopsis pilosula* (dang shen, codonopsis), *Zizyphus jujuba* (da zao, chinese dates), *Glycyrrhiza uralensis* (gan cao, licorice), *Zingiber officinalis* (sheng jiang, ginger)

Combine with

- **1.2 Si Wu Wan** for colds and flu in menstruating or run down women
- **14.5 Chuan Xin Lian Antiphlogistic Tablets**, **14.8 Wu Wei Xiao Du Wan** or **13.1 Lien Chiao Pai Tu Pien** for acute mastitis or ear infections
- **6.9 Jigucao Wan** for chronic hepatitis
- **7.22 Shen Qi Da Bu Wan** for pronounced qi deficiency
- **3.2 Gan Mao Zhi Ke Chong Ji** to assist in rooting out deeply buried or hidden pathogens

Pattern identifying features

- ***shào yáng* syndrome**
- **never well since a severe flu, gastroenteritis or other infection**
- **alternating fever and chills (or 'flu like' feelings, especially when fatigued)**
- **fatigue and irritability**
- **primary pathological triad and chronic inflammatory disorders**

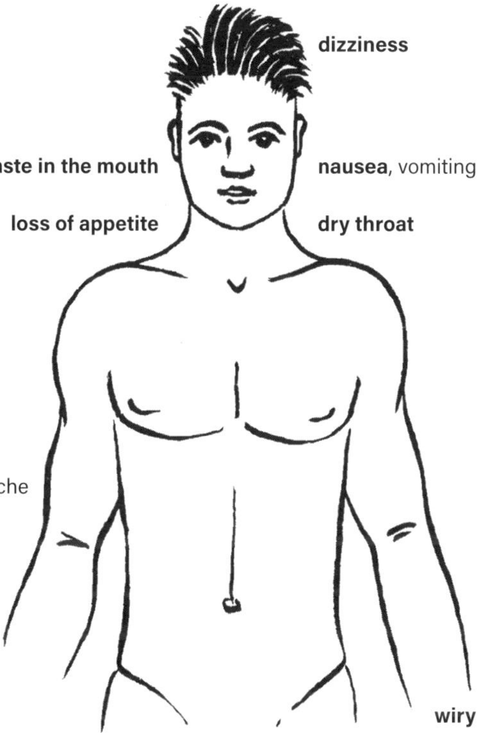

Dosage and method of administration

8-12 pills three times daily on an empty stomach. The dose can be spread out, or two lots of 12-18 pills may be taken, morning and evening. In severe cases or during the early stages of treatment (the first few weeks), a 50% increase in dose can be used, then reduced as the effects are felt.

Cautions and contraindications

Contraindicated for patients taking interferon. In general **6.1 Xiao Chai Hu Wan** is a very safe and well tolerated formula, but can cause energy to rise in some patients causing headaches or dizziness, especially when used long term. Any side effects cease when the formula is stopped. Patients with chronic fatigue or post viral patterns may experience a temporary recurrence of the initial disorder as the pathogen is eliminated from the body.

GMP

6.2 SI NI WAN

四逆丸

3+/12

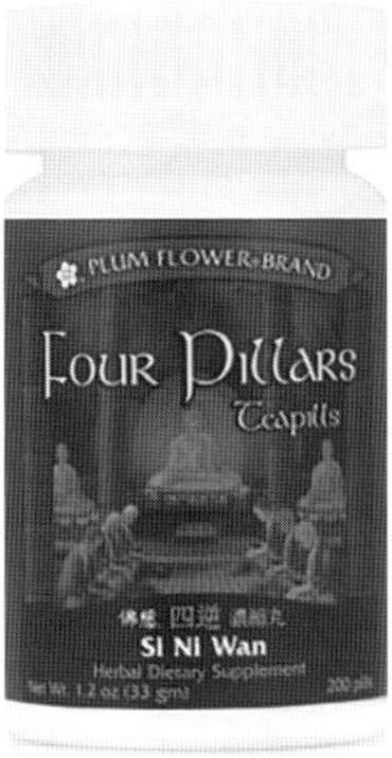

Lanzhou Foci Pharmaceutical Factory (Gansu)
'Frigid Extremities Pills'
Si Ni Wan is packaged in bottles of 200 pills
Also available as: Bupleurum and Aurantium Immaturus Formula (conc. extract)

Chinese medical action

Dredges and softens the Liver and regulates qi, harmonizes the Liver and Spleen and restores the qi dynamic

Biomedical action

Antispasmodic, benefits digestion, carminative, alleviates depression

INDICATIONS

- Liver qi constraint. This is the base formula on which all other Liver qi moving formulas are built. Its main focus is on moving qi in the Liver and gastrointestinal system, and ensuring proper distribution of qi and blood to the extremities. One of the main features pointing to the use of this formula reflects this unequal distribution–stagnant qi and pent up heat from the constraint trapped in the interior obstruct the movement of qi and blood to the tips of the extremities so the that fingers and toes are quite cold while the trunks feels quite warm–hence the name Frigid Extremities Pills.
- Liver invading Spleen and Stomach patterns characterized by hypochondriac, abdominal and epigastric pain and distension. The combination of honey fried licorice and white peony is especially good at alleviating smooth muscle spasm and pain, while the ascending action of bupleurum and the descending action of aurantium create a dynamic flow through the middle burner to drive and restore the qi dynamic (*see* glossary).

Composition

Paeonia alba (bai shao, white peony), *Bupleurum falcatum* (chai hu, bupleurum), *Citrus aurantium* (zhi shi, aurantium), *Glycyrrhiza uralensis* (zhi gan cao, honey fried licorice)

Combine with

– **2.26 Xiang Lian Wan** for heartburn from Liver invading the Spleen
– **6.11 Li Dan Tablets** for gallstones or chronic cholecystitis from qi constraint and damp heat
– **4.10 Shi Lin Tong** for gallstones from qi constraint
– **2.18 Bao He Wan** for irritable bowel syndrome characterized by abdominal bloating and indigestion
– **2.38 Hua Zhi Ling Tablet** for rectal bleeding or colitis from qi constraint
– **1.34 Hai Zao Jing Wan** or **1.33 Ru Jie Xiao Tablet** for breast and ovarian cysts
– **2.30 Chen Xiang Hua Qi Wan** for constipation

Pattern identifying features

- **Liver qi constraint**
- **symptoms worse with emotion or stress**
- **irritability, depression, mood swings**
- cyclical symptoms in an otherwise robust patient
- premenstrual syndrome
- tooth grinding

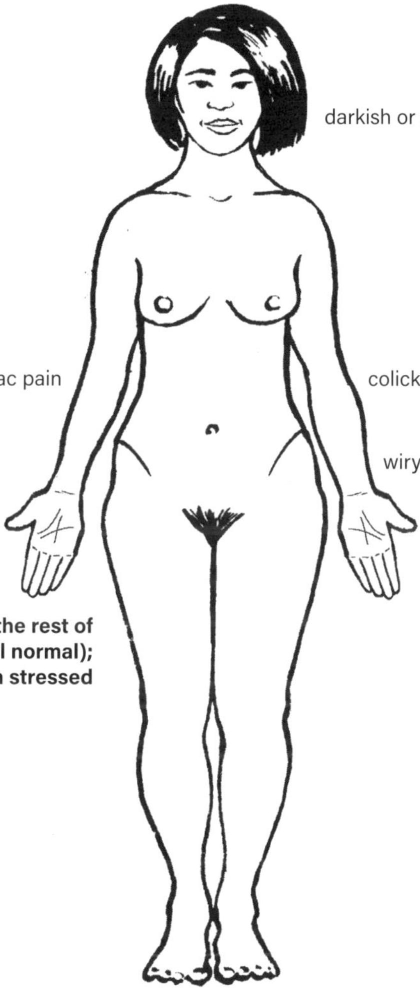

Dosage and method of administration

8-12 pills three times daily on an empty stomach. The dose can be spread out, or two lots of 12-18 pills may be taken, morning and evening. In severe cases, premenstrually, or during the early stages of treatment a 50% increase in dosage can be used, then reduced as treatment takes effect.

Cautions and contraindications

Contraindicated for cold extremities associated with yang or blood deficiency. Not suitable for weak or deficient patients.

6.3 CHAI HU SHU GAN WAN

柴胡疏肝丸

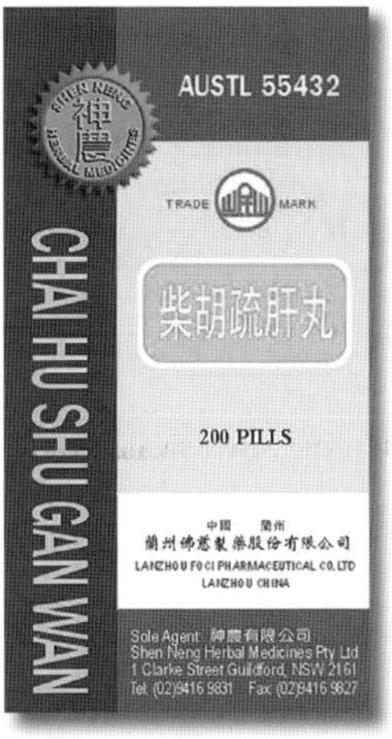

Lanzhou Foci Pharmaceutical Factory (Gansu)
'Bupleurum Liver Soothing Pills'
Chai Hu Shu Gan Wan is packaged in bottles of 200 pills
Also available as: Bupleurum Shu Gan Teapills (PF), Bupleurum and Cyperus Combination (conc. extract)

Chinese medical action

Dredges the Liver and regulates qi, harmonizes the Liver and Spleen and restores the qi dynamic

Biomedical action

Antispasmodic, benefits digestion, carminative, alleviates depression

INDICATIONS

- Liver qi constraint with little or no deficiency; especially indicated for patterns with pain or distension. A variation of **6.2 Si Ni Wan**, with the addition of three herbs to enhance qi and blood regulating activity.
- Gastrointestinal pain, distension and spasm, gas build up or ulceration from Liver qi constraint and Liver invading the Spleen or Stomach.
- Gynecological disorders of a Liver qi constraint type. Useful following lumpectomy or mastectomy to prevent complications and future stagnation.
- Painful conditions with an emotional component, in particular those along the Liver or Gallbladder channel pathways, including intercostal neuralgia, hypochondriac pain, genital pain, qi stagnation type painful urination, tension and migraine headaches.
- Poor peripheral circulation associated with constrained qi – usually only the fingers and toes are cold and the body is warm.
- Depression, mood swings, irritability, 'plum pit qi' (globus hystericus).
- With the appropriate identifying features, this formula may be used to treat irritable bowel syndrome, gastritis, nervous stomach, peptic ulcers, bruxism, temporomandibular joint dysfunction, chronic cholecystitis, gallstones, biliary spasm, hepatitis, fibrocystic breast disease and lumps associated with the menstrual cycle, ovarian cysts, irregular menstruation, premenstrual syndrome, premenstrual headaches and dysmenorrhea.

Composition (each pill contains powdered)

Bupleurum falcatum (chai hu, bupleurum) 33mg, *Paeonia alba* (bai shao, white peony) 33mg, *Cyperus rotundus* (xiang fu, cyperus) 33mg, *Citrus aurantium* (zhi shi, aurantium) 23mg, *Ligusticum wallichi* (chuan xiong, ligusticum) 23mg, *Citrus reticulata* (qing pi, immature citrus) 23mg, *Glycyrrhiza uralensis* (gan cao, licorice) 16mg

Pattern identifying features

- **Liver qi constraint; symptoms worse with emotion or stress**
- cyclical symptoms in an otherwise robust patient
- **irritability, depression, mood swings**
- premenstrual syndrome

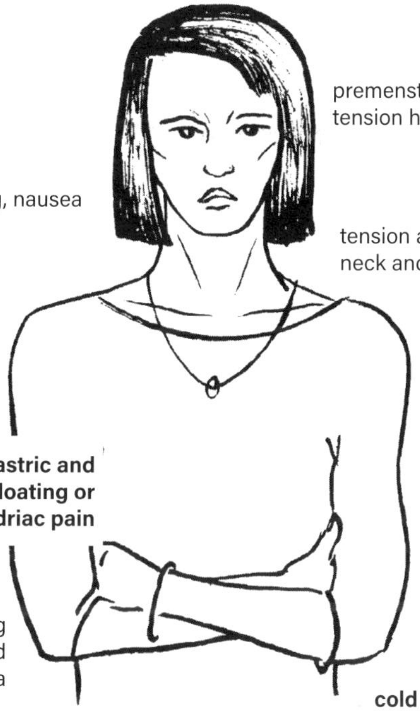

Combine with

- **2.26 Xiang Lian Wan** for heartburn from Liver qi invading the Spleen
- **6.11 Li Dan Tablets** for gallstones or chronic cholecystitis from qi constraint with damp heat
- **2.23 Ping Wei San** for mild ascites from qi and damp stagnation
- **10.22 Shao Yao Gan Cao Wan** for severe colicky abdominal or epigastric pain
- **1.34 Hai Zao Jing Wan** or **1.33 Ru Jie Xiao Tablet** for breast lumps
- **2.30 Chen Xiang Hua Qi Wan** for dry constipation
- **2.38 Hua Zhi Ling Tablet** for rectal bleeding and colitis from stress

Dosage and method of administration

8-12 pills three times daily on an empty stomach. The dose can be spread out, or two lots of 12-18 pills may be taken, morning and evening. With severe constraint, before a menstrual period, or during the early stages of treatment a 50% increase in dosage can be used, then reduced as treatment takes effect.

Cautions and contraindications

Not suitable for weak or deficient patients.

6.4 XIAO YAO WAN

逍遥丸

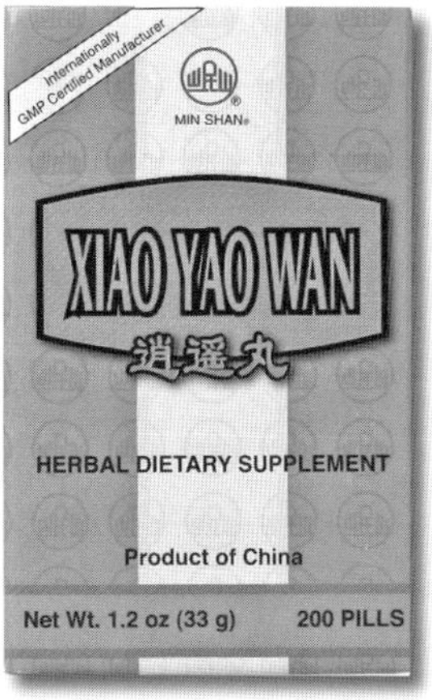

Lanzhou Foci Pharmaceutical Factory (Gansu)
'Free and Easy Wanderer Pills', 'Rambling Pills'
Xiao Yao Wan is packaged in bottles of 200 pills
Also available as: Free and Easy Wanderer Teapills (PF), Hsiao Yao Wan, Liv-Ease Pill (BE), Bupleurum and Tangkuei Formula (conc. extract)

Chinese medical action

Softens the Liver, regulates Liver qi, nourishes blood, strengthens the Spleen, harmonizes the Liver and Spleen

Biomedical action

Regulates the hormones that influence the menstrual cycle, emmenagogue, relieves depression and emotional stress

INDICATIONS

- Liver qi constraint with Liver blood and Spleen qi deficiency. An important formula for menstrual disorders with an emotional component. Specifically used for irregular menstruation, late periods, premenstrual syndrome, breast tenderness or lumps, fibrocystic breast disease, premenstrual irritability, headaches, depression, constipation and insomnia, dysmenorrhea and chronic pelvic inflammatory disease.
- For the effects of stress on the body in general, and the gastrointestinal system in particular. Liver and Spleen disharmony. The key feature for the use of this formula is the relationship of the emotional state of the patient to the onset or aggravation of symptoms.
- In addition to the gynecological conditions noted above, with the appropriate identifying features, this formula can assist in the treatment of irritable bowel syndrome, chronic gastritis, peptic ulcers, chronic tension in the gastrointestinal system, biliary spasm, chronic hepatitis, the early stages of liver cirrhosis, anemia, neurasthenia, menopausal syndrome, depression, tension headaches and migraines, bruxism, chronic neck and upper back pain and globus hystericus ('plum pit qi').

Composition (each pill contains powdered)

Bupleurum falcatum (chai hu, bupleurum), *Angelica sinensis* (dang gui, chinese angelica), *Paeonia alba* (bai shao, white peony), *Atractylodes macrocephala* (bai zhu, atractylodes), *Poria cocos* (fu ling, hoelen), *Zingiber officinalis* (sheng jiang, ginger), *Glycyrrhiza uralensis* (gan cao, licorice), *Mentha haplocalycis* (bo he, mint)

Combine with

- **1.1 Ba Zhen Wan** or **1.9 Gui Pi Wan** from the end of the period to mid-cycle to nourish blood and yin, then **6.4 Xiao Yao Wan** from mid-cycle to menstruation, as part of a cyclical treatment (*see* glossary)
- **1.33 Ru Jie Xiao Tablet** for breast cysts and thyroid nodules

Pattern identifying features

- **Liver qi constraint with Spleen qi and blood deficiency; Liver Spleen disharmony**
- **symptoms worse with stress or emotional upset**
- **premenstrual syndrome, irregular menses**
- **irritability, depression, mood swings**
- vague nonspecific aches and pains
- variable energy levels
- frequent sighing
- tooth grinding

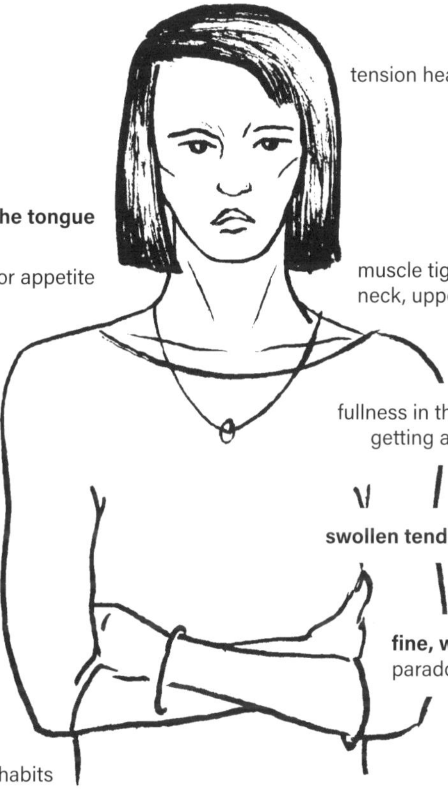

– **1.2 Si Wu Wan** for irregular menses from blood deficiency and qi constraint
– **4.2 Wu Ling Wan** for premenstrual fluid retention

Dosage and method of administration

8-12 pills three times daily on an empty stomach. The dose can be spread out, or taken in two lots of 12-18 pills, morning and evening. In severe cases or during the early stages of treatment (the first few weeks), a 50% increase in dose can be used, then reduced as treatment takes effect.

Cautions and contraindications

Contraindicated during the early phase of acute illness such as colds and flu. Very occasionally a sensitive patient may experience mild nausea or loose stools in the early stages of treatment. This can be alleviated by reducing the dose or by adding a few pills of **2.9 Xiang Sha Liu Jun Wan**.

6.5 JIA WEI XIAO YAO WAN
加味逍遥丸

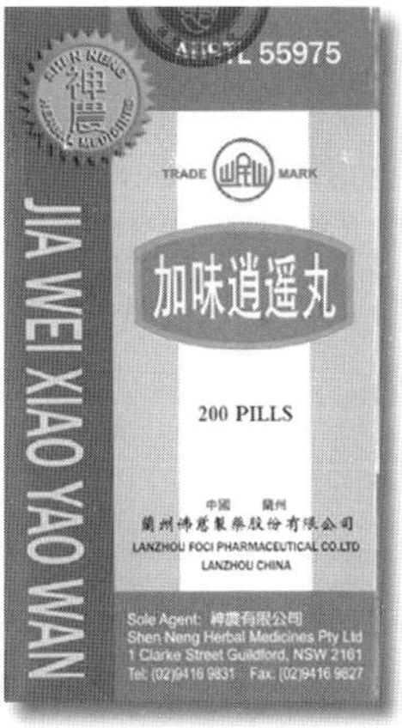

Lanzhou Foci Pharmaceutical Factory (Gansu)
'Augmented Free and Easy Wanderer Pills'
Jia Wei Xiao Yao Wan is packaged in bottles of 200 pills
Also available as: Free and Easy Wanderer Plus Teapills (PF), Dan Zhi Xiao Yao Wan, Liv-Ease Plus Pill (BE), Bupleurum and Peony Formula (conc. extract)

Chinese medical action
Softens the Liver, regulates Liver qi, nourishes the blood and strengthens the Spleen, clears heat from the Liver

Biomedical action
Regulates the hormones that influence the menstrual cycle, relieves depression and emotional stress, cools the body

INDICATIONS

- Liver qi constraint with heat. A variation of **6.4 Xiao Yao Wan**, the addition being two herbs to clear heat. The key feature for the use of this formula (and others used to treat Liver qi constraint), is the clear relationship between the initiation or aggravation of symptoms and the emotional state of the patient.
- Menstrual disorders from qi constraint with heat, including irregular menstruation, especially shortened cycles, menorrhagia or abnormal uterine bleeding, premenstrual syndrome with heat symptoms (fever, flushing, redness), bruxism, migraine headaches, rashes, acne, red, sore eyes, mouth ulcers, galactorrhea and nonspecific vaginitis.
- An important formula for inflammatory skin disorders with an emotional component, such as premenstrual acne or rashes, eczema, dermatitis, psoriasis.
- Chronic sinus congestion and headaches (including migraines) that are worse with stress.

Composition (each pill contains powdered)
Bupleurum falcatum (chai hu, bupleurum), *Paeonia suffruticosa* (mu dan pi, moutan), *Gardenia jasminoides* (shan zhi zi, gardenia), *Angelica sinensis* (dang gui, chinese angelica), *Paeonia lactiflora* (bai shao, white peony), *Atractylodes macrocephala* (bai zhu, atractylodes), *Poria cocos* (fu ling, hoelen), *Glycyrrhiza uralensis* (gan cao, licorice), *Zingiber officinalis* (sheng jiang, ginger), *Mentha haplocalycis* (bo he, mint)

Combine with
- **10.2 Raw Tienchi Tablets** for uterine bleeding or menorrhagia from qi stagnation with heat from constraint
- **13.2 Xiao Feng Wan** for psoriasis, eczema or dermatitis worse for stress and before a menstrual period

Pattern identifying features

- **Liver qi constraint with heat**
- **cyclical symptoms with heat signs, aggravated by stress**
- **irritability, anger outbursts**
- premenstrual syndrome
- tooth grinding

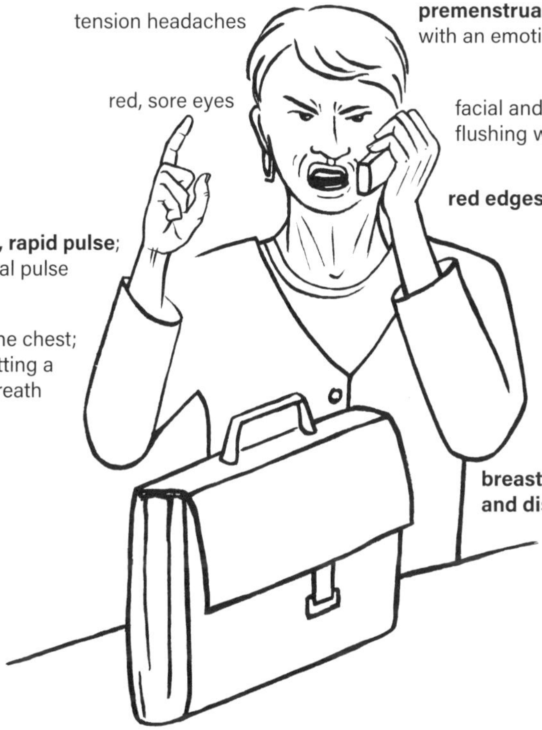

- **14.2 Huang Lian Su Tablets** for stubborn pustular acne in teenagers
- **9.17 Qian Bai Bi Yan Pian** for chronic sinusitis
- **1.12 Shi Xiao Wan** for mild blood stasis
- **13.11 Dan Shen Huo Xue Wan** for chronic qi and blood stasis and hot blood type skin diseases

Dosage and method of administration

8-12 pills three times daily on an empty stomach. The dose can be spread out, or taken in two lots of 12-18 pills, morning and evening. In severe cases or during the early stages of treatment (the first few weeks), a 50% increase in dose can be used, then reduced as treatment takes effect.

Cautions and contraindications

Caution during pregnancy. Very occasionally a sensitive patient may experience mild nausea, diarrhea or loose stools in the early days of treatment. This can be alleviated by reducing the dose or by adding a few pills of **2.9 Xiang Sha Liu Jun Wan**.

6.6 LONG DAN XIE GAN WAN

龙胆泻肝丸

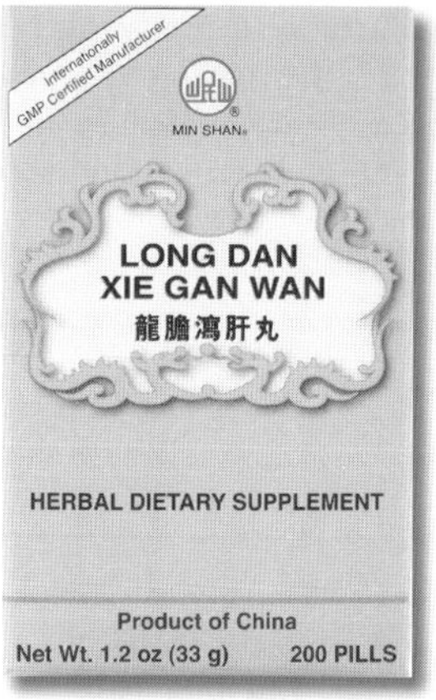

Lanzhou Foci Pharmaceutical Factory (Gansu)
'Gentiana Pills to Drain the Liver'
Long Dan Xie Gan Wan is packaged in bottles of 200 pills
Also available as: Snake and Dragon Teapills (PF), Lung Tan Hsieh Kan Wan, Wetness Heat Pill, Gentiana Liver-Drain Pill (BE), Gentiana Combination (conc. extract)

Chinese medical action

Clears damp heat from the Liver system (where heat is greater than damp), cools Liver fire

Biomedical action

Bitter tonic, depurative, anti-inflammatory, detoxicant, cholagogue

INDICATIONS

- Liver fire or Liver and Gallbladder damp heat affecting those areas that are controlled by the Liver and Gallbladder systems–the ears, eyes, flanks and urogenital system.
- With the appropriate identifying features, this formula can assist in the treatment of the following conditions:
  - **Liver fire rising through the Liver and GB channels**: acute otitis media and externa, conjunctivitis, glaucoma, uveitis, corneal ulcers, migraine headache, ocular or aural herpes, acute sinusitis, hypertension and hyperthyroidism.
  - **damp heat or fire in the flanks**: hepatobiliary infections (acute cholecystitis and hepatitis), jaundice, abscess and other swellings associated with infection, intercostal neuralgia, shingles.
  - **damp heat in the lower burner**: acute genital herpes, acute cystitis or urethritis, pyelonephritis, pelvic inflammatory disease, vulvitis, Bartholin's cyst, acute prostatitis, orchitis, epididymitis, genital eczema and pruritus. (*see also* **1.37 Bi Xie Sheng Shi Wan** for similar patterns with damp greater than heat)

Composition

Gentiana scabra (long dan cao, gentiana), *Bupleurum falcatum* (chai hu, bupleurum), *Alisma plantago-aquatica* (ze xie, alisma), *Rehmannia glutinosa* (sheng di, raw rehmannia), *Gardenia jasminoides* (shan zhi zi, gardenia), *Scutellaria baicalensis* (huang qin, scute), *Plantago asiatica* (che qian zi, plantago), *Akebia trifolata* (mu tong, akebia stem), *Angelica sinensis* (dang gui, chinese angelica), *Glycyrrhiza uralensis* (gan cao, licorice)

Combine with

- **9.9 Superior Sore Throat Powder** topically for otitis or shingles
- **6.11 Li Dan Tablets** for damp heat jaundice (acute hepatitis)
- **14.5 Chuan Xin Lian Antiphlogistic Tablets** or **14.6 Fu Fang Nan Ban Lan Gen** for herpes zoster or simplex

Pattern identifying features

- **Liver fire, damp heat in the Liver and Gallbladder**
- redness, swelling, pain or yellow mucopurulent discharges in a hot, robust patient
- pounding headache, migraine
- jaundice

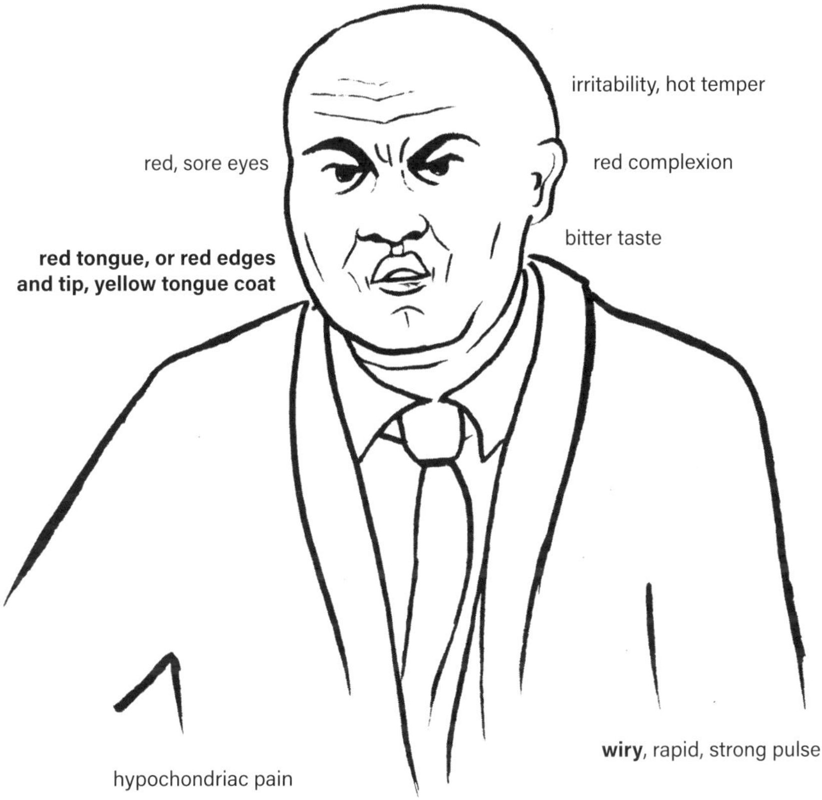

– **1.2 Si Wu Wan** for nonspecific vaginitis or genital eczema with a component of Liver fire and blood deficiency
– **1.38 Yu Dai Wan** for yellow vaginal discharge from Liver fire or damp heat

Dosage and method of administration

The recommended dose is 8-12 pills three or four times daily on an empty stomach, however in severe cases this can be doubled or trebled. The dose can be spread out evenly, or taken every two hours. Generally not recommended for use longer than a few weeks, other than at a low dose on the rare occasions that constitutional use is warranted.

Cautions and contraindications

Caution during pregnancy. Can weaken the Spleen and damage yin and yang when overused.

GMP

6.7 DA CHAI HU WAN

大柴胡丸

1-3/12

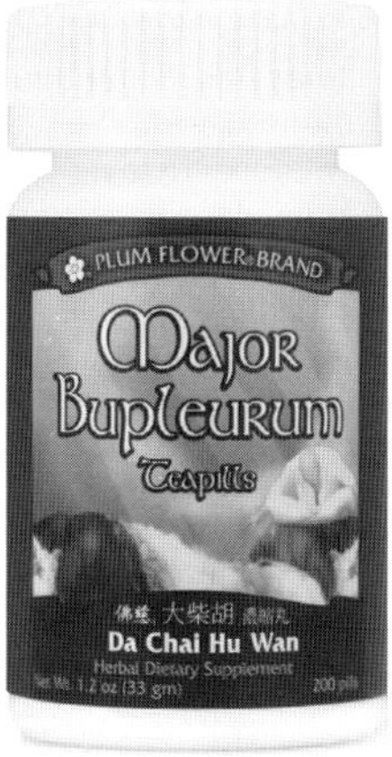

Lanzhou Foci Pharmaceutical Factory (Gansu)
'Major Bupleurum Pills'
Da Chai Hu Wan is packaged in bottles of 200 pills
Also available as: Major Bupleurum Combination (conc. extract)

Chinese medical action

Harmonizes *shào yáng*, dredges the Liver and regulates qi, purges heat and stagnation from *yáng míng*

Biomedical action

Hepatoprotective, aids clearance of residual pathogens, laxative, cholagogue

INDICATIONS

- *Shào yáng – yáng míng* overlap syndrome, an acute pattern characterized by relatively severe fever and gastrointestinal symptoms which follow a few days (or slightly longer) of malaise and flu like (*tài yáng*) symptoms. The main features are alternating fever and chills, nausea and vomiting, abdominal and epigastric pain and constipation or urgent diarrhea. There may be jaundice.
- Chronic damp heat with constrained qi in the Liver and Gallbladder causing accumulation and congealing of damp into gallstones. Used to gradually improve Gallbladder function and assist in breakdown and expulsion of small gallstones. Some of the main features may be absent in chronic cases, but the practitioner would still expect to see constipation, intermittent hypochondriac and abdominal pain, nausea, aversion to fats and oils, a strong wiry pulse and greasy, yellow tongue coat.
- With the appropriate identifying features, this formula can assist in the treatment of conditions such as acute and chronic cholecystitis, acute pancreatitis, hepatitis, dysentery, gallstones, malaria, migraine headaches and hypertension.

Composition

Bupleurum falcatum (chai hu, bupleurum), *Pinellia ternata* (zhi ban xia, processed pinellia), *Scutellaria baicalensis* (huang qin, scute), *Rheum palmatum* (da huang, rhubarb), *Citrus aurantium* (zhi shi, aurantium), *Paeonia alba* (bai shao, white peony), *Zingiber officinalis* (sheng jiang, ginger), *Zizyphus jujuba* (da zao, chinese dates)

Combine with

- **6.10 Qing Gan Li Dan Tablets** or **4.10 Shi Lin Tong** for gallstones
- **14.5 Chuan Xin Lian Antiphlogistic Tablets** or **14.8 Wu Wei Xiao Du Wan** for acute infectious hepatitis or cholecystitis
- **2.26 Xiang Lian Wan** for severe vomiting, both formulas crushed and decocted together, then sipped slowly through a straw to facilitate ingestion

Pattern identifying features

- ***Shào yáng - yáng míng* overlap syndrome; damp heat/excess heat in the Gallbladder and Stomach**
- **alternating fever and chills**
- irritability, manic behavior
- bitter taste in the mouth
- jaundice

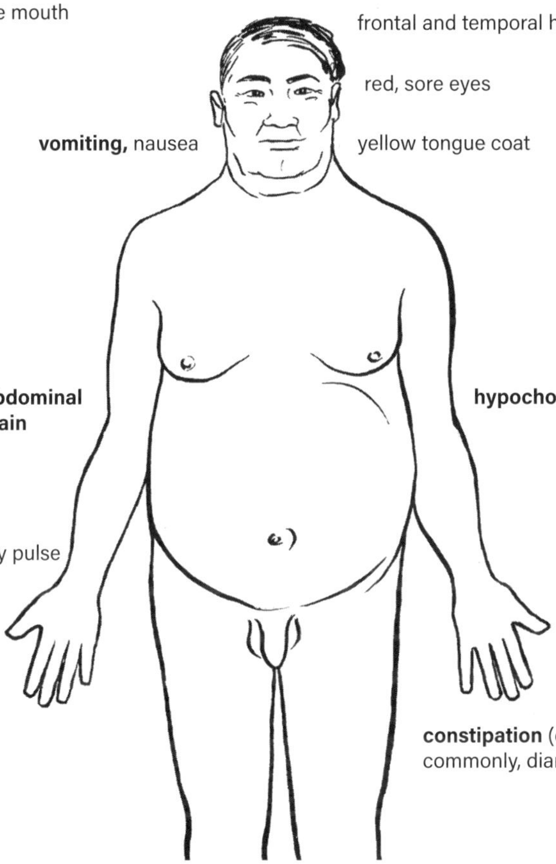

Dosage and method of administration

The recommended dose is 8-12 pills three or four times daily on an empty stomach, however in acute and severe cases this can be doubled or trebled. The dose should be spread out evenly, taken every two hours or so. When treating chronic problems such as gallstones, the dose is 4-6 pills three times daily, or sufficient to enable a smooth bowel movement with no abdominal cramping. After a month or two the patient should be rested off the formula for a few weeks as they may become habituated to the rhubarb.

Cautions and contraindications

Contraindicated during pregnancy and for patients taking interferon. Can weaken the Spleen and damage yin when overused.

GMP

6.8 YI GUAN JIAN WAN

一贯煎丸

3+ / 12

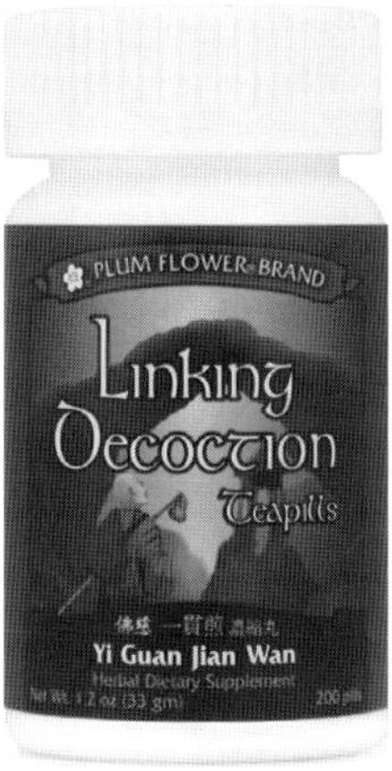

Lanzhou Foci Pharmaceutical Factory (Gansu)
'Linking Decoction Pills'
Yi Guan Jian Wan is packaged in bottles of 200 pills
Also available as: Linking Combination (conc. extract)

Chinese medical action

Tonifies Liver yin, nourishes Liver blood, dredges the Liver and regulates qi, benefits the Stomach

Biomedical action

Demulcent febrifuge, antispasmodic

INDICATIONS

- Liver and Stomach yin deficiency with qi constraint and rebellious Stomach qi, giving rise to upper gastrointestinal tract problems such as acid reflux and heartburn, epigastric pain, indigestion, belching, nausea and dry retching. Symptoms provoked by stress and emotional turmoil.
- Chronic dull hypochondriac discomfort, tightness or pain. Can be used for the same pathology causing pain anywhere along the course of the Liver channel pathway.
- With the appropriate identifying features, this formula can assist in the treatment of conditions such as chronic hepatitis, early hepatic cirrhosis, fatty liver, peptic ulcer disease, chronic atrophic gastritis, gastric neurosis, gastroesophageal reflux (GERD), intercostal neuralgia, costochondritis, essential hypertension, preeclampsia, hyperthyroidism and chronic testicular pain.

Composition

Rehmannia glutinosa (sheng di, raw rehmannia), *Lycium barbarum* (gou qi zi, lycium fruit), *Glehnia littoralis* (bei sha shen, glehnia), *Ophiopogon japonicus* (mai dong, ophiopogon), *Angelica sinensis* (dang gui, chinese angelica), *Melia toosendan* (chuan lian zi, melia fruit)

Combine with

- **10.22 Shao Yao Gan Cao Wan** for more intense cramping abdominal pain
- **3.38 Sheng Mai San Wan** for chronic hepatitis from yin and qi deficiency
- **2.26 Xiang Lian Wan** for severe heartburn
- **5.7 Sunho Multiginseng Tablets** for early cirrhosis with mild blood stasis
- A small dose of **2.31 Run Chang Wan** or **2.32 Wu Ren Wan** for constipation
- **2.18 Bao He Wan** for distension and food stagnation
- **15.7 Yang Yin Jiang Ya Wan** or **15.8 Fu Fang Jiang Ya Capsule** for hypertension
- **8.6 Suan Zao Ren Tang Pian** for insomnia and restlessness

Pattern identifying features

- **Liver yin deficiency with qi constraint**
- **Liver and Stomach yin deficiency**
- **symptoms aggravated or initiated by stress**
- indefinable epigastric discomfort
- muscle tightness, spasm, tics
- insomnia

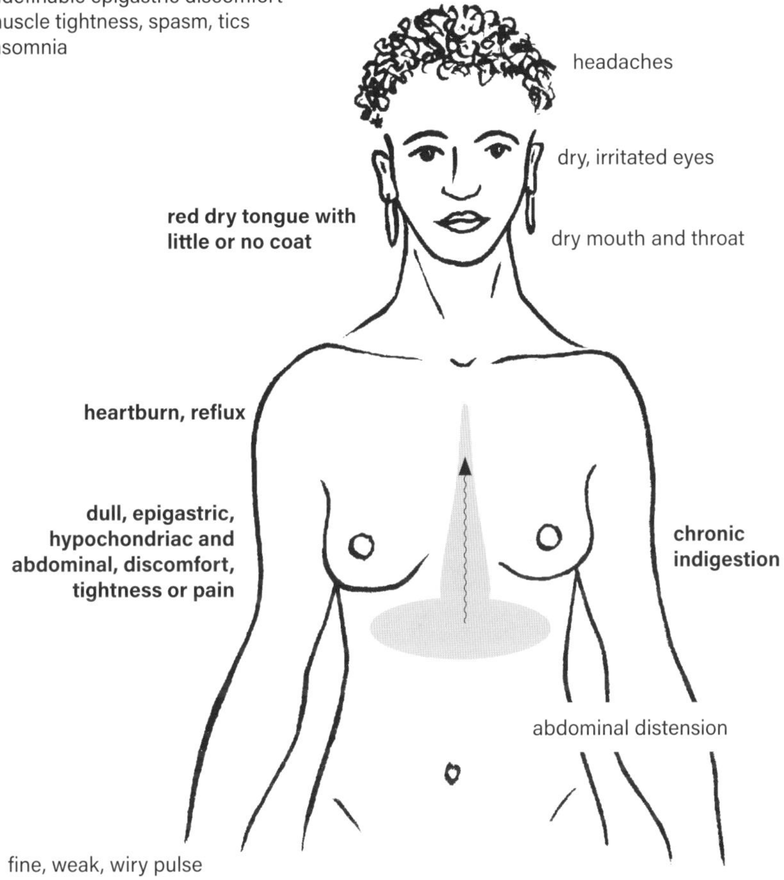

Dosage and method of administration

8-12 pills three times daily on an empty stomach. The dose can be spread out, or taken in two lots of 12-18 pills, morning and evening. In severe cases or during the early stages of treatment (the first few weeks), a 50% increase in dose can be used, then reduced as treatment takes effect.

Cautions and contraindications

Contraindicated during the early phase of acute illness such as colds and flu, and in phlegm damp patterns. Caution in patients with elevated liver enzyme (AST/ALT) levels, as the melia, even though the dose is small, can occasionally cause irritation of the liver and elevation of AST/ALT levels.

6.9 JIGUCAO WAN

鸡骨草丸

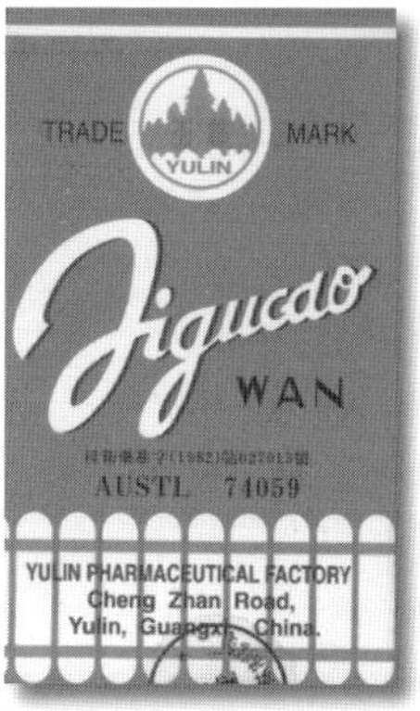

Yulin Pharmaceutical Factory (Guangxi)
'Abrus Pills'
Jigucao Wan is packaged in bottles of 50 capsules

Chinese medical action

Cools the Liver and benefits the Gallbladder, nourishes yin and blood, invigorates blood

Biomedical action

Hepatoprotective, cholagogue

INDICATIONS

- Acute and chronic Liver and Gallbladder disease from damp heat. A relatively mild formula suited to both acute and chronic problems, but best for chronic conditions. Used for chronic hepatitis, especially hepatitis C infection. Suitable for prolonged use.
- With the appropriate identifying features, this formula can assist in the treatment of conditions such as acute and chronic hepatitis, cholecystitis and jaundice.

Composition (each capsule contains)

Abrus cantoniensis (ji gu cao, abrus) 160mg, pearl powder (zhen zhu fen) 72mg, *Lycium chinensis* (gou qi zi, lycium fruit) 68mg, *Salvia miltorrhiza* (dan shen, salvia) 60mg, Bovine gallstone (niu huang) 40mg

Combine with

- **6.1 Xiao Chai Hu Wan** for chronic hepatitis (especially chronic asymptomatic hepatitis C)
- **14.5 Chuan Xin Lian Antiphogistic Tablets** for acute viral hepatitis
- **6.3 Chai Hu Shu Gan Wan**, **6.4 Xiao Yao Wan** or **6.5 Jia Wei Xiao Yao Wan** for chronic hepatitis of a Liver qi constraint type
- **2.12 Shen Ling Bai Zhu Wan**, **2.16 Zi Sheng Wan** or **2.13 Li Zhong Wan** for hepatitis patients with significant Spleen deficiency
- **2.24 Shu Gan Wan** for chronic hepatic disease and abdominal pain from qi constraint
- **6.6 Long Dan Xie Gan Wan** for acute or symptomatic hepatitis associated with Liver fire or marked damp heat

Dosage and method of administration

4 pills, three times daily on an empty stomach.

Pattern identifying features

- **Liver/Gallbladder damp heat, blood stasis**
- acute and **chronic liver disease**
- malaise, fatigue, lack of vitality
- jaundice

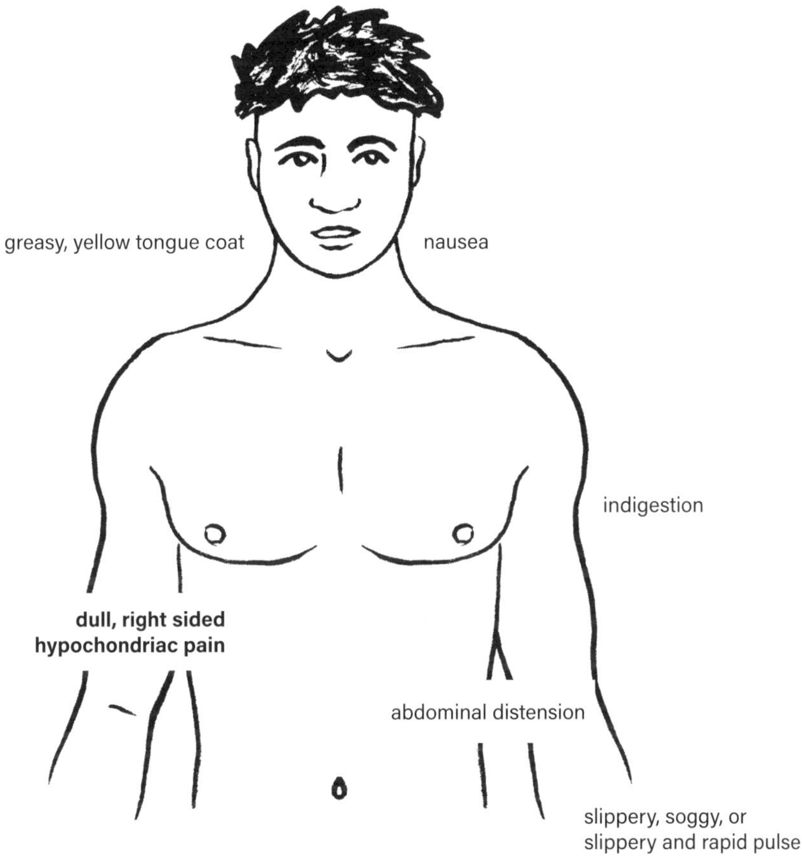

Cautions and Contraindications

Contraindicated during pregnancy and in patients taking warfarin (coumarin). Not suitable unmodified for cold damp patterns, with dull or sallow skin, 'dirty' yellow jaundice and significant digestive weakness. Caution in patients taking mild anticoagulants like aspirin and fish oil as clotting time can be reduced.

6.10 QING GAN LI DAN TABLETS

清肝利胆片

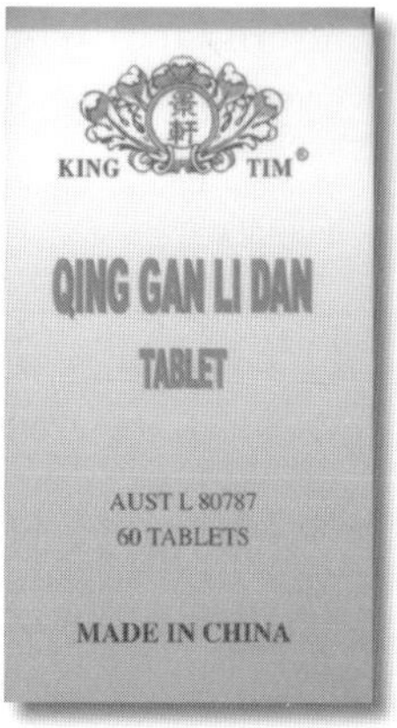

(*Qing Gan Li Dan Pian*)
'Cool the Liver and Benefit the Gallbladder Pills'
Qing Gan Li Dan Tablets are packaged in bottles of 60 tablet

Chinese medical action

Clears damp heat from the Liver and Gallbladder, regulates qi and invigorates blood, promotes urination, assists in expulsion of minor gall stones, opens the bowels

Biomedical action

Diuretic, cholagogue, laxative

INDICATIONS

- Damp heat (damp greater than heat) and qi constraint affecting the Gallbladder and Liver. Used for gallstones (less than 5mm diameter), sludge in the Gallbladder, colicky hypochondriac pain, indigestion with aversion to and intolerance of fats and oils, constipation or pasty stools. Similar to **6.11 Lidan Tablets** with less emphasis on cooling heat, and more on draining damp and descending and regulating qi. It is more focused on the gastrointestinal symptoms that accompany Gallbladder disease, such as abdominal distension and bloating, indigestion and nausea. Useful for chronic indigestion and gastrointestinal upsets from poor Gallbladder or Liver function, for biliousness in those who overindulge and for chronic Gallbladder disorders in obese patients.
- Chronic Gallbladder congestion and irritation, which in Chinese medical terms affects both the Gallbladder organ and structures along the course of the Gallbladder channel. Symptoms can be reflected along the course of the Gallbladder channel, manifesting as vague temporomandibular, jaw, hip or shoulder pain, ear problems or headaches.
- With the appropriate identifying features, this formula can assist in the treatment of conditions such as gallstones, chronic cholecystitis, biliary spasm, hepatitis and early hepatic cirrhosis.

Composition (each tablet contains extracts equivalent to dry)

Plantago asiatica (che qian zi, plantago) 576mg, *Salvia miltorrhiza* (dan shen, salvia) 576mg, *Citrus aurantium* (zhi shi, aurantium) 576mg, *Curcuma longa* (yu jin, curcuma) 480mg, *Lysimachia christina* (jin qian cao, lysimachia) 480mg, *Magnolia officinalis* (hou po, magnolia bark) 480mg, *Scutellaria baicalensis* (huang qin, scute) 432mg, *Areca catechu* (da fu pi, betel husk) 432mg, *Rheum officinale* (da huang, rhubarb) 40mg

Combine with

– **6.4 Xiao Yao Wan** for chronic hypochondriac ache and Gallbladder irritation (particularly in women) from qi and/or damp stagnation

Pattern identifying features

- **damp heat and qi constraint in the Gallbladder and Liver (damp > heat)**
- tenderness and pain along the course of the Gallbladder channel
- gallstones, cholecystitis, jaundice
- fat intolerance, loss of appetite
- heaviness, lethargy
- pain worse following fatty meals

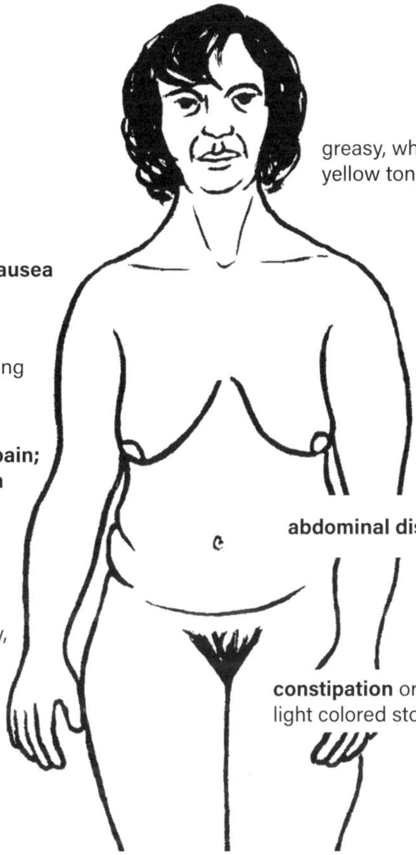

- **2.23 Ping Wei San** for marked distension and damp; for obese patients
- **6.7 Da Chai Hu Wan** for gallstones from lingering damp heat
- **4.10 Shi Lin Tong** to reinforce the stone dissolving action

Dosage and method of administration

3-5 tablets, three times daily on an empty stomach. For gall stones, prolonged administration (3-6 months), in association with appropriate dietary modification, is necessary. The patient should be advised to expect minor diarrhea initially. The dose can be adjusted until a smooth bowel movement is achieved.

Cautions and Contraindications

Contraindicated during pregnancy and in patients taking warfarin (coumarin). Not suitable unmodified for cold damp patterns, with dull or sallow skin, 'dirty' yellow jaundice and significant digestive weakness. Caution in patients taking mild anticoagulants like aspirin and fish oil as clotting time can be reduced.

3+/12

6.11 LIDAN TABLETS

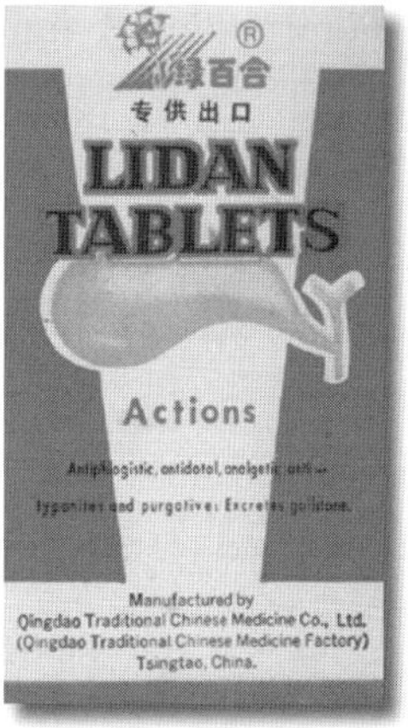

利胆片

(Li Dan Pian)
Qingdao Traditional Chinese Medicine Co. (Qingdao)
'Benefit the Gallbladder Pills'
Lidan Tablets are packaged in bottles of 120 tablets
Also available as: Li Dan Pian (PF)

Chinese medical action

Clears damp and toxic heat from Liver and Gallbladder, alleviates jaundice, assists in expulsion of minor gall stones, opens the bowels.

Biomedical action

Cholagogue, diuretic, anti-inflammatory, antipyretic, laxative

INDICATIONS

- Damp heat in the Liver and Gallbladder with inflammation and gallstones. This formula is quite cooling and is best suited to acute conditions with clear signs of heat such as fever, red eyes and a yellow tongue coat. It can, however, be used for chronic conditions with lingering heat. In general, similar in overall action to **6.10 Qing Gan Li Dan Tablets**, with a greater emphasis on cooling heat.
- With the appropriate identifying features, this formula can assist in the treatment of conditions such as gallstones, acute and chronic cholecystitis, cholangitis, inflammation of the bile duct, jaundice, acute hepatitis and early hepatic cirrhosis.

Composition

Scutellaria baicalensis (huang qin, scute) 30%, *Plantago asiatica* (che qian zi, plantago) 16%, *Bupleurum falcatum* (chai hu, bupleurum) 10%, *Artemesia capillaris* (yin chen, capillaris) 10%, *Lysimachia christina* (jin qian cao, lysimachia) 10%, *Isatis tinctora* (da qing ye, isatis) 10%, *Lonicera japonica* (jin yin hua, honeysuckle) 10%, *Rheum palmatum* (da huang, rhubarb) 4%

Combine with

- **2.24 Shu Gan Wan** or **10.21 Yan Hu Suo Zhi Tong Wan** for severe hypochondriac pain
- **6.6 Long Dan Xie Gan Wan** for acute hepatitis with jaundice
- **14.5 Chuan Xin Lian Antiphlogistic Tablets** to enhance the toxic heat clearing action for acute viral hepatitis or cholecystitis
- **6.1 Xiao Chai Hu Wan** for acute cholecystitis with alternating fever and chills

Pattern identifying features

- **damp heat in the Liver and Gallbladder (heat > damp)**
- **fever**
- irritability
- malaise
- pain worse following fatty or rich meals

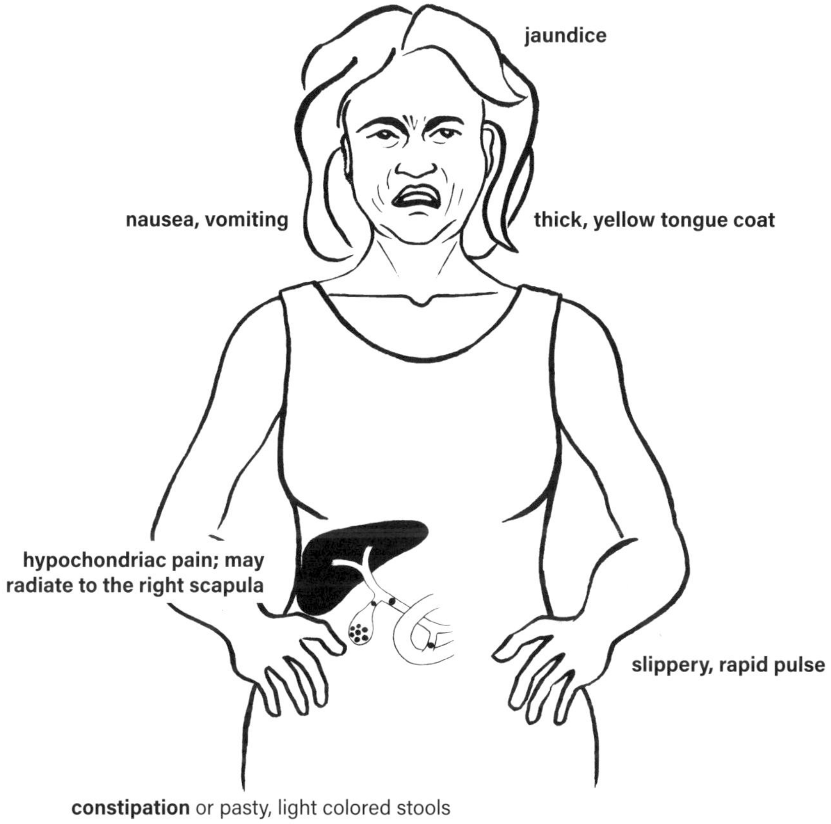

Dosage and method of administration

4-6 tablets three times daily on an empty stomach. The patient should be advised to expect diarrhea. The dose can be adjusted until a smooth bowel movement is achieved.

Cautions and contraindications

Contraindicated during pregnancy. Not suitable for cold damp patterns.

GMP

6.12 GE XIA ZHU YU WAN

膈下逐瘀丸

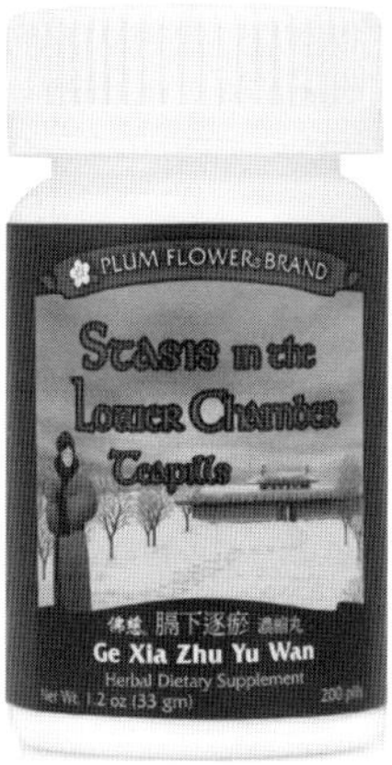

3+/12

Lanzhou Foci Pharmaceutical Factory (Gansu)
'Pills to Remove Static Blood from Beneath the Diaphragm'
Ge Xia Zhu Yu Wan is packaged in bottles of 200 pills
Also available as: Tangkuei and Corydalis Combination (conc. extract)

Chinese medical action

Invigorates the circulation of qi and blood, breaks up and dispels static blood, resolves masses, stops pain

Biomedical action

Vasodilator, analgesic, anti-platelet action, softens and resolves masses

INDICATIONS

- Masses and swelling in the upper abdomen from chronic Liver qi and blood stasis. A variation of the classic **5.1 Xue Fu Zhu Yu Wan** specifically targeted at painful masses or swellings of the Liver and Spleen.
- A powerful qi and blood 'breaking' formula, it can also be used for painful blood stasis masses in other locations within the abdomen, such as endometriosis and fibroids (but *see also* **1.18 Shao Fu Zhu Yu Wan**).
- With the appropriate identifying features, this formula can assist in the treatment of conditions such as hepatic cirrhosis, chronic malaria, liver abscess, hepatosplenomegaly, ascites secondary to liver disease, benign gynecological masses. Also uses for splenomegaly secondary to glandular fever, bacteremia, portal hypertension, systemic lupus erythematosus, leukemia, cysts or hemolytic anemia.

Composition

Angelica sinensis (dang gui, chinese angelica), *Prunus persica* (tao ren, peach seed), *Carthamus tinctorius* (hong hua, carthamus), *Lindera strychnifolia* (wu yao, lindera), *Ligusticum wallici* (chuan xiong, ligusticum), *Paeonia suffruticosa* (mu dan pi, moutan), *Paeonia veitchii* (chi shao, red peony), *Cyperus rotundus* (xiang fu, cyperus), *Citrus aurantium* (zhi ke, aurantium), *Corydalis turtschaninovii* (yan hu suo, corydalis), *Glycyrrhiza uralensis* (gan cao, licorice), *Boswellia carterii* (ru xiang*, frankincense), *Commiphora myrhha* (mo yao*, myrhh) [*substituted for the restricted *Trogopterus xanthipes* (wu ling zhi, flying squirrel feces) of the original formula]

Combine with

- **1.34 Hai Zao Jing Wan** for rubbery phlegm and blood stasis masses
- **1.2 Si Wu Wan** for patients with a greater degree of blood deficiency

Pattern identifying features

- **Liver/Spleen blood stasis**
- dull, sallow or darkish complexion; dark rings under the eyes; purplish lips and conjunctiva
- fatigue, listlessness, weakness
- mild feverishness at night
- possible jaundice
- weight loss

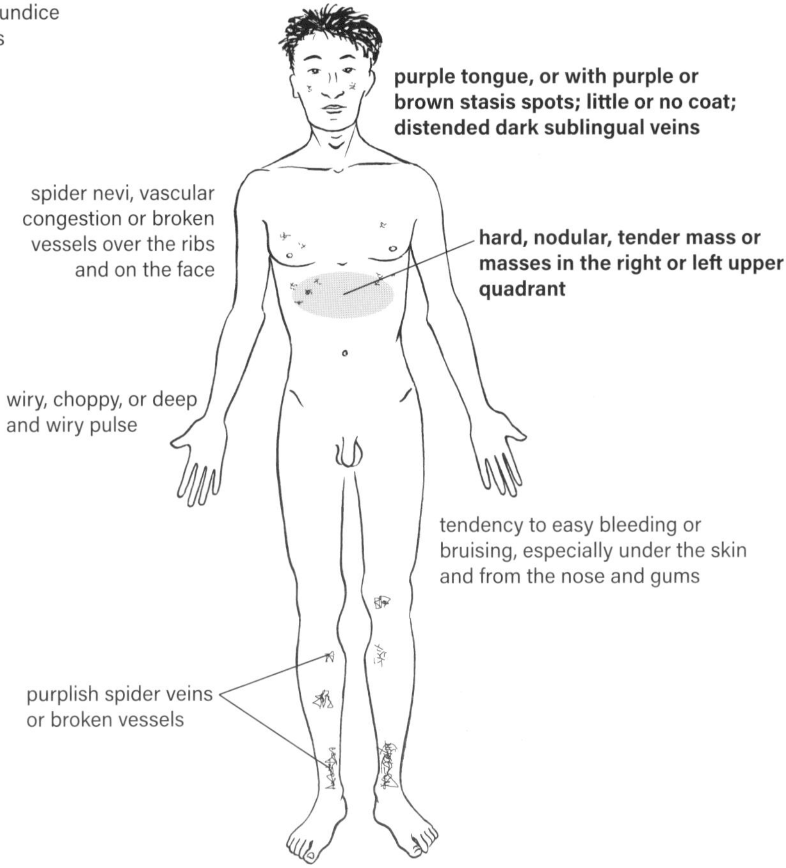

Dosage and method of administration

8-12 pills three times daily on an empty stomach. The dose can be spread out, or taken in two lots of 12-18 pills, morning and evening. In severe cases or during the early stages of treatment, a 50% increase in dose can be used, then reduced as the effects are felt.

Cautions and contraindications

Contraindicated during pregnancy, in menorrhagia, and patients with bleeding disorders. Caution in patients on anticoagulant therapy. Watch for bruising or increased tendency to bleeding. Prolonged use can deplete qi and blood, so breaking every 2-3 months with a change to a qi and blood tonifying strategy for a few weeks is recommended.

6.13 HERBA ABRI FRUTICULOSI BEVERAGE

鸡骨草精

(Ji Gu Cao Jing)
Guangdong Medicines and Health Products Co.
'Essence of *Abrus fruticulosus*'
Herba Abri Fruticulosi Beverage is packaged in 15 gram sachets of soluble granules, ten sachets per box

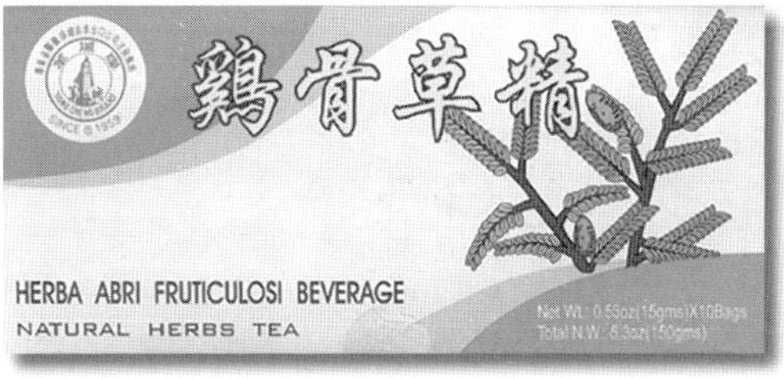

Chinese medical action

Clears damp heat from the Liver and Gallbladder, promotes urination, alleviates jaundice

Biomedical action

Hepatoprotective, diuretic, cholagogue

INDICATIONS

- Acute and chronic hepatitis. This formula has both preventive effects (for those in epidemic areas or in high risk) and therapeutic effects in cases of acute and chronic disease.

Composition

Abrus cantoniensis (ji gu cao, abrus), *Hypericum japonicum* (di er cao, hypericum), *Artemesia capillaris* (yin chen, capillaris), *Rhodomyrtus tomentosa* (tao jin tui gen, rose myrtle), *Artemesia anomala* (ya tui ai), *Zanthoxylum avicennae* (ying bu bo)

Dosage and method of administration

The recommended dose is one sachet, 2-3 times daily. In acute cases the dose may be increase 50-100%.

Cautions and contraindications

Contraindicated during pregnancy.

6.14 XI HUANG CAO

溪黄草

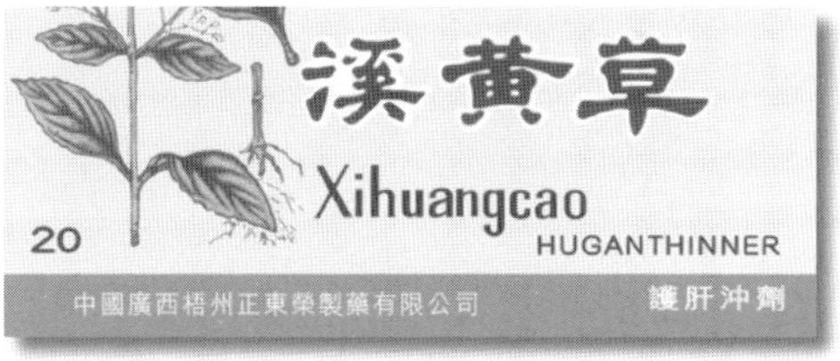

1-3/12

(*Xi Huang Cao Hu Gan Chong Ji*)
Wuzhou Traditional Medicine Factory (Guangxi)
'Rabdosia Liver Protecting Granules'
Xi Huang Cao is packaged in 10 gram sachets of soluble granules, twenty to a box

Chinese medical action

Clears damp heat from the Liver and Gallbladder, clears Toxic heat, strengthens the Liver and Spleen

Biomedical action

Hepatoprotective, antipyretic, immunomodulating

INDICATIONS

- Acute and chronic hepatitis. This formula has both preventive effects for those in epidemic areas or at high risk, and therapeutic effects in cases of acute and chronic disease. It is slightly more tonifying than **6.13 Herba Abri Fruticulosi Beverage** and good for chronic hepatitis with some qi deficiency.

Composition (each 10 gram sachet)

Rabdosia lophanthoides (xi huang cao, rabdosia) 40%, *Abrus cantoniensis* (ji gu cao, abrus) 15%, *Oldenlandia diffusa* (bai hua she she cao, oldenlandia) 15%, *Codonopsis pilosula* (dang shen, codonopsis) 15%, *Poria cocos* (fu ling, hoelen) 15%

Dosage and method of administration

The recommended dose is one or two sachets, 2-3 times daily. In acute cases the dose may be increased by 50%.

Cautions and contraindications

None noted.

补益成药 7

Tonics

7.1.1 LIU WEI DI HUANG WAN

六味地黄丸

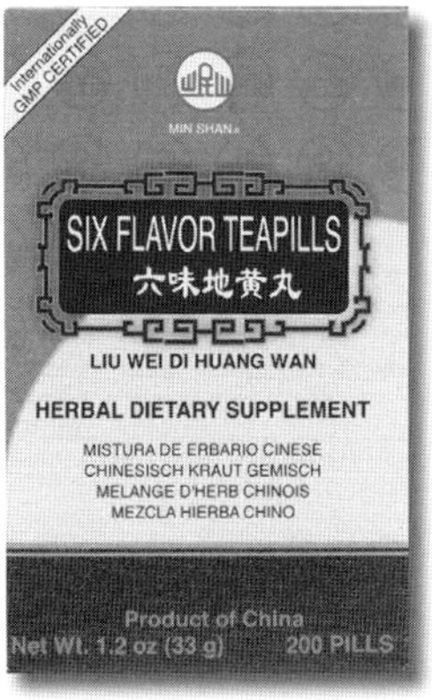

Lanzhou Foci Pharmaceutical Factory (Gansu)
'Six Ingredient Pills with Rehmannia'
Liu Wei Di Huang Wan is packaged in bottles of 200 pills
Also available as: Six Flavor Teapills (PF), Rehmannia Six Formula (conc. extract)

Chinese medical action

Tonifies Kidney yin

Biomedical action

Demulcent febrifuge, hypoglycemic, anti-hypertensive, improves kidney function

INDICATIONS

- Kidney yin deficiency. Base formula from which most Kidney yin and yang tonics are built and one of the most important formulas of Chinese medicine. Used for a wide variety of problems associated with Kidney yin deficiency in adults and children, first appearing in a pediatric text for slow closure of the fontanel and developmental delay.
- General Kidney support and tonic for older people and those at risk of Kidney yin depletion, such as the chronically overworked, night shift workers and patients taking steroids. Has a steroid sparing effect, and can help alleviate unwanted effects of prolonged steroid use, which tend to deplete yin.
- For those over 40 as a means of preserving yin from further depletion (by 40 half the yin is gone). Can assist in maintenance of good skin tone and elasticity, and retard development of wrinkles, loss of muscle mass and other signs of aging.
- Support for patients with diabetes. Clinical experience and studies have shown this formula and its derivatives to have a significant regulatory effect on blood glucose levels.
- With the appropriate identifying features, this formula can be used to treat conditions such as hypertension, anovulation, amenorrhea, menopausal syndrome, delayed development in children, hyperthyroidism, arteriosclerosis, impotence, type 2 diabetes mellitus, chronic asthma, optic neuritis and optic nerve atrophy, chronic nephritis, glomerulonephritis, chronic cystitis, polycystic kidneys and various yin deficiency type urinary disturbances.

Composition

Rehmannia glutinosa (shu di, processed rehmannia), *Cornus officinalis* (shan zhu yu, cornus), *Dioscorea opposita* (shan yao, dioscorea), *Poria cocos* (fu ling, hoelen), *Alisma orientalis* (ze xie, alisma), *Paeonia suffruticosa* (mu dan pi, moutan)

Combine with

- **7.11 Deer Velvet** or **7.12 Lu Rong Jiao** for failure to thrive, developmental delay or bone growth problems in children
- **2.35 Yu Quan Wan** or **2.36 Sugarid** for diabetes

Pattern identifying features

- **Kidney yin deficiency**
- **generalized dryness of the skin, hair, eyes, vagina, mouth and throat; premature wrinkles**
- tiredness and exhaustion with restlessness and agitation
- loss of hearing acuity
- heat intolerance
- mild night sweats
- afternoon fever
- poor libido

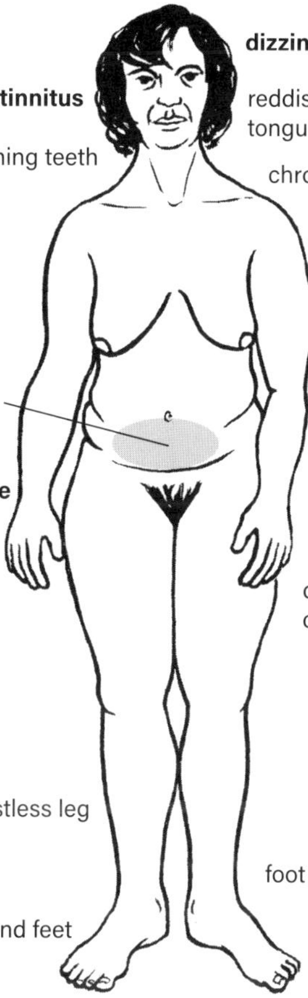

– **3.38 Sheng Mai San Wan** for chronic asthma from Lung and Kidney qi and yin deficiency
– **7.22 Shen Qi Da Bu Wan** for concurrent Spleen qi deficiency
– **4.10 Shi Lin Tong** for urinary calculi
– **3.33 Yang Yin Qing Fei Wan** or **2.32 Wu Ren Wan** for chronic dry constipation from yin deficiency

Dosage and method of administration

8-12 pills three times daily on an empty stomach. The dose can be spread out, or taken in two lots of 12-18 pills, morning and evening. In severe cases or during the early stages of treatment (the first few weeks), a 50% increase in dose can be used, then reduced as treatment takes effect.

Cautions and contraindications

Contraindicated during the early phase of acute illness such as colds and flu. This is a cooling formula and can weaken digestion in some people, so care in patients with a tendency to abdominal distension, loose stools or phlegm damp. This can usually be alleviated by taking it with a small dose (3-6 pills at the same time) of **2.18 Bao He Wan** or **2.9 Xiang Sha Liu Jun Wan**, or taking the pills after food.

7.1.2 LIU WEI DI HUANG WAN

六味地黄丸

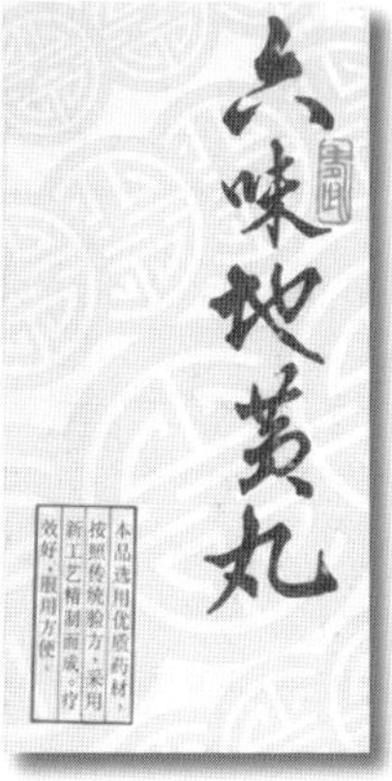

Tong Ren Tang (Beijing)
'Six Ingredient Pills with Rehmannia'
Liu Wei Di Huang Wan is packaged in bottles of 360 small honey pills

Chinese medical action

Tonifies Kidney yin

Biomedical action

Demulcent febrifuge, hypoglycemic, anti-hypertensive, improves kidney function

INDICATIONS

- As for **7.1.1 Liu Wei Di Huang Wan**

Composition (each dose [30 pills] contains powdered)

Rehmannia glutinosa (shu di, processed rehmannia) 1.6mg, *Cornus officinalis* (shan zhu yu, cornus) 810mg, *Dioscorea opposita* (shan yao, dioscorea) 810mg, *Poria cocos* (fu ling, hoelen) 600mg, *Alisma orientalis* (ze xie, alisma) 600mg, *Paeonia suffruticosa* (mu dan pi, moutan) 600mg

Dosage and method of administration

30 pills twice daily on an empty stomach.

Cautions and contraindications

As for **7.1.1 Liu Wei Di Huang Wan**.

7.1.3 TINNITUS HERBAL TREATMENT

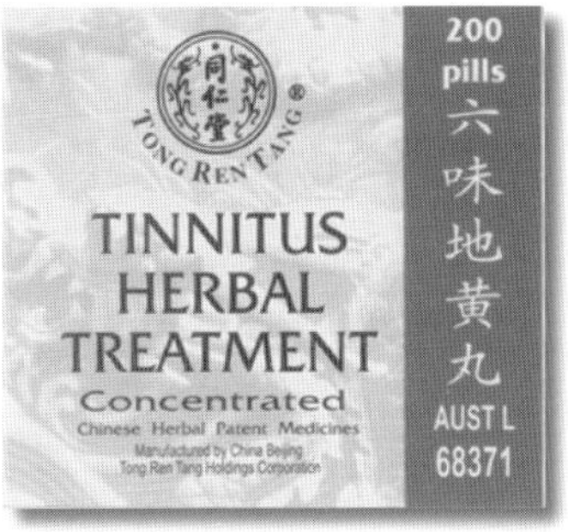

六味地黄丸

(*Liu Wei Di Huang Wan*)
Tong Ren Tang (Beijing)
'Six Flavour Pills with Rehmannia'
Tinnitus Herbal Treatment is packaged in bottles of 200 pills

Chinese medical action

Tonifies Kidney yin

Biomedical action

Demulcent febrifuge, hypoglycemic, anti-hypertensive, improves kidney function

INDICATIONS

- As for **7.1.1 Liu Wei Di Huang Wan**

Composition (each dose [8 pills] contains extracts equivalent to dry)

Rehmannia glutinosa (shu di, processed rehmannia) 960mg, *Cornus officinalis* (shan zhu yu, cornus) 480mg, *Dioscorea opposita* (shan yao, dioscorea) 480mg, *Poria cocos* (fu ling, hoelen) 360mg, *Alisma orientalis* (ze xie, alisma) 360mg, *Paeonia suffruticosa* (mu dan pi, moutan) 360mg

Dosage and method of administration

8 pills twice daily on an empty stomach.

Cautions and contraindications

As for **7.1.1 Liu Wei Di Huang Wan**.

7.1.4 LIU WEI DI HUANG PILLS

六味地黄丸

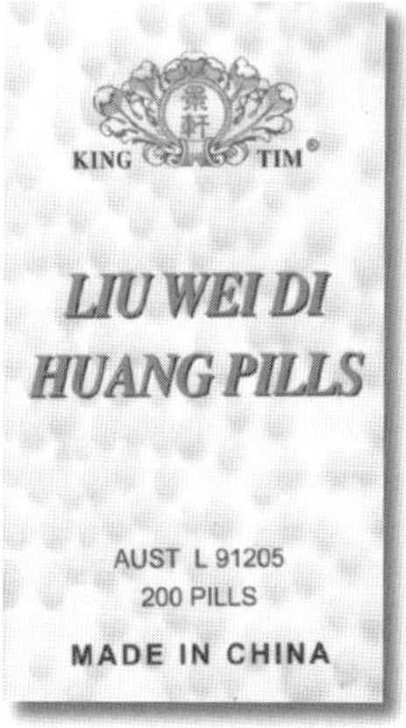

(*Liu Wei Di Huang Wan*)
Jing Xian Pharmaceutical Co. (Guangzhou)
'Six Ingredient Pills with Rehmannia'
Liu Wei Di Huang Pills are packaged in bottles of 200 pills

Chinese medical action

Tonifies Kidney yin

Biomedical action

Demulcent febrifuge, hypoglycemic, anti-hypertensive, improves kidney function

INDICATIONS

- As for **7.1.1 Liu Wei Di Huang Wan**

Composition (each pill contains extracts equivalent to dry)

Rehmannia glutinosa (shu di, processed rehmannia) 473mg, *Cornus officinalis* (shan zhu yu, cornus) 218mg, *Dioscorea opposita* (shan yao, dioscorea) 218mg, *Poria cocos* (fu ling, hoelen) 164mg, *Alisma orientalis* (ze xie, alisma) 164mg, *Paeonia suffruticosa* (mu dan pi, moutan) 164mg

Dosage and method of administration

8 pills, three times daily on an empty stomach.

Cautions and contraindications

As for **7.1.1 Liu Wei Di Huang Wan**.

7.2.1 QI JU DI HUANG WAN

杞菊地黄丸

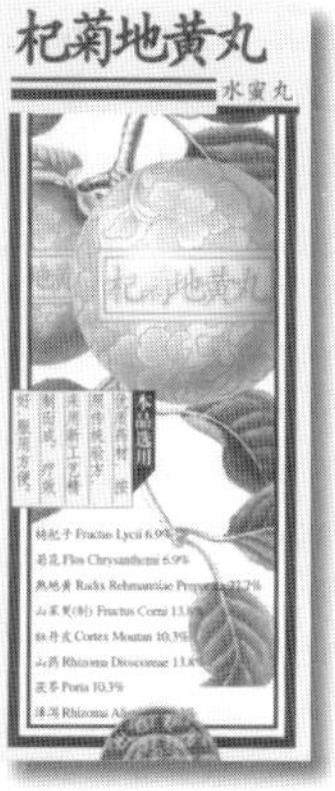

Tong Ren Tang (Beijing)
'Rehmannia Pills with Lycium Fruit and Chrysanthemum Flowers'
Qi Ju Di Huang Wan is packaged in bottles of 200 pills

Chinese medical action

Tonifies Liver and Kidney yin and brightens the eyes

Biomedical action

Demulcent febrifuge, hypoglycemic, anti-hypertensive, improves kidney and liver function

INDICATIONS

- As for **7.2.2 Qi Ju Di Huang Wan**

Composition

Rehmannia glutinosa (shu di, processed rehmannia) 27.7%, *Cornus officinalis* (shan zhu yu, cornus) 13.8%, *Dioscorea opposita* (shan yao, dioscorea) 13.8%, *Poria cocos* (fu ling, hoelen) 10.3%, *Alisma orientalis* (ze xie, alisma) 10.3%, *Paeonia suffruticosa* (mu dan pi, moutan) 10.3%, *Lycium barbarum* (gou qi zi, lycium fruit) 6.9%, *Chrysanthemun morifolium* (ju hua, chrysanthemum flower) 6.9%

Dosage and method of administration

30 pills, twice daily on an empty stomach.

Cautions and contraindications

Contraindicated during the early phase of acute illness such as colds and flu. This is a cooling formula and can weaken digestion in some people, so care in patients with a tendency to abdominal distension, loose stools or phlegm damp. This can usually be alleviated by taking it with a small dose (3-6 pills at the same time) of **2.18 Bao He Wan** or **2.9 Xiang Sha Liu Jun Wan**, or by taking the pills after food.

7.2.2 QI JU DI HUANG WAN

杞菊地黄丸

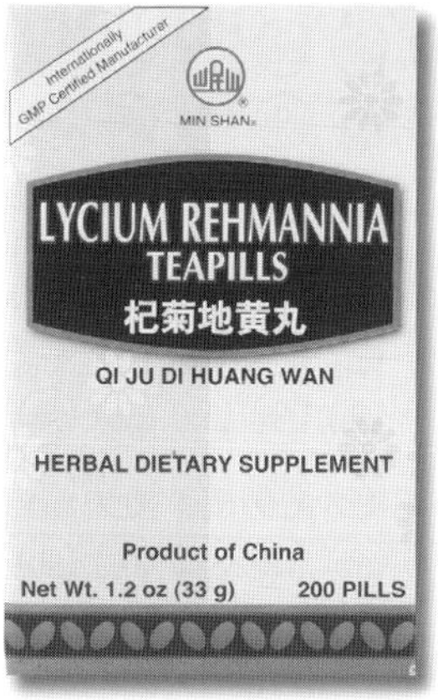

Lanzhou Foci Pharmaceutical Factory (Gansu)
'Rehmannia Pills with Lycium Fruit and Chrysanthemum Flowers'
Qi Ju Di Huang Wan is packaged in bottles of 200 pills
Also available as: Lycium, Chrysanthemum and Rehamannia Formula (conc. extract)

Chinese medical action

Tonifies Liver and Kidney yin and brightens the eyes

Biomedical action

Demulcent febrifuge, hypoglycemic, anti-hypertensive, improves kidney and liver function

INDICATIONS

- Liver and Kidney yin deficiency. A variation of **7.1 Liu Wei Di Huang Wan**, with the addition of chrysanthemum flower and lycium fruit to shift the focus of the formula towards the Liver. This formula is preferred for Liver yin specific problems such as visual weakness and eye disorders, headaches, chronic liver disease and tightness or stiffness of the sinews and muscles.
- With the appropriate identifying features, this formula can assist in the treatment of conditions such as keratitis sicca, chronic glaucoma, optic neuritis, optic nerve atrophy, essential hypertension, chronic migraine headaches, hyperthyroidism, diabetes mellitus and chronic hepatitis.

Composition

Rehmannia glutinosa (shu di, processed rehmannia), *Cornus officinalis* (shan zhu yu, cornus), *Dioscorea opposita* (shan yao, dioscorea), *Poria cocos* (fu ling, hoelen), *Alisma orientalis* (ze xie, alisma), *Paeonia suffruticosa* (mu dan pi, moutan), *Lycium barbarum* (gou qi zi, lycium fruit), *Chrysanthemun morifolium* (ju hua, chrysanthemum flower)

Combine with

- **15.4 Tian Ma Gou Teng Wan** or **15.7 Yang Yin Jiang Ya Wan** for Liver and Kidney yin deficiency with yang rising type hypertension, headaches, dizziness, transient ischaemic attacks (TIA's)
- **13.19 Pearl Powder** for yin deficient eye disorders

Dosage and method of administration

8-12 pills three times daily on an empty stomach. The dose can be spread out, or taken in two lots of 12-18 pills, morning and evening. In severe cases or during the early stages of treatment (the first few weeks), a 50% increase in dose can be used, then reduced as treatment takes effect.

Pattern identifying features

- **Liver and Kidney yin deficiency**
- irritability, anger, tinnitus, dizziness
- dull hypochondriac pain
- red dry tongue with little or no coat

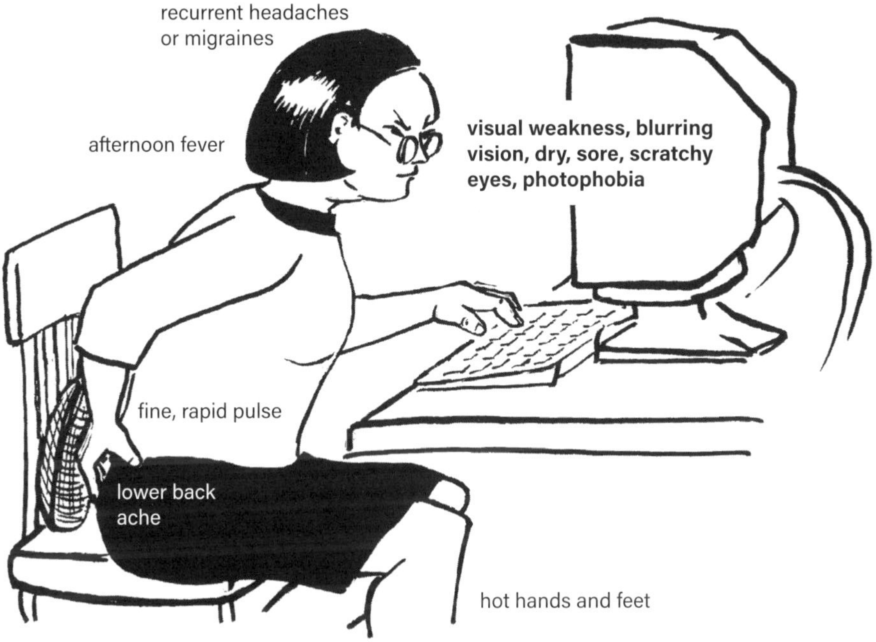

Cautions and contraindications

Contraindicated during the early phase of acute illness such as colds and flu. This is a cooling formula and can weaken digestion in some people, so care in patients with a tendency to abdominal distension, loose stools or phlegm damp. This can usually be alleviated by taking it with a small dose (3-6 pills at the same time) of **2.18 Bao He Wan** or **2.9 Xiang Sha Liu Jun Wan**, or by taking the pills after food.

7.3 ZUO GUI WAN

左归丸

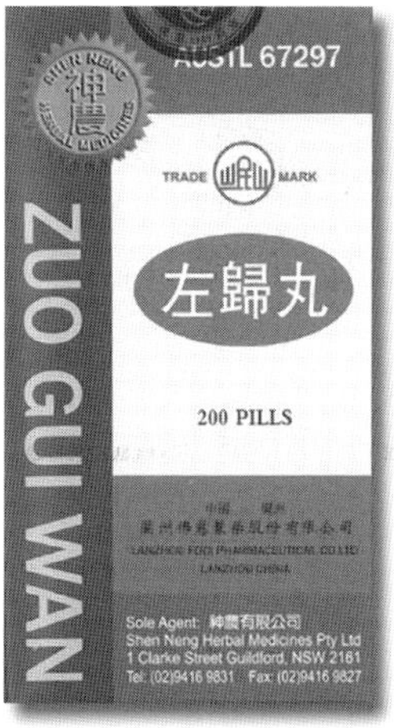

Lanzhou Foci Pharmaceutical Factory (Gansu)
'Left Returning Pills'
Zuo Gui Wan is packaged in bottles of 200 pills
Also available as: Left Side Replenishing Teapills (PF), Cyathula and Rehmannia Formula (conc. extract)

Chinese medical action

Tonifies Kidney yin, nourishes essence

Biomedical action

Demulcent febrifuge, hypoglycemic, anti-hypertensive, improves kidney function

INDICATIONS

- Kidney yin and essence deficiency. Similar to **7.1 Liu Wei Di Huang Wan**, without the 'draining' components that clear heat from deficiency, instead substituting additional tonic herbs. The variation creates a richer yin tonic suitable for marked yin and essence deficiency with mild to moderate heat from deficiency. Good as a general Kidney yin support in the elderly or in those at risk of Kidney yin depletion. The symptom picture reflect the deep level of Kidney deficiency, with weakness of the 'marrow' (memory, hearing, dizziness) and bones.
- With the appropriate identifying features, this formula can assist in treatment of conditions such as hypertension, delayed development in children, anovulation, amenorrhea, impotence, type 2 diabetes mellitus, chronic nephritis, glomerulonephritis, cystitis, polycystic kidneys and various yin deficiency type urinary disturbances and consumptive disorders.

Composition (each pill contains powdered)

Rehmannia glutinosa (shu di, processed rehmannia) 55.1mg, *Cornus officinalis* (shan zhu yu, cornus) 29.4mg, *Dioscorea opposita* (shan yao, dioscorea) 29.4mg, *Lycium barbarum* (gou qi zi, lycium fruit) 22mg, *Cuscuta hygrophilae* (tu si zi, cuscuta) 22mg, *Achyranthes bidentata* (huai niu xi, achyranthes) 22mg

Combine with

- **7.11 Deer Velvet** or **7.12 Lu Rong Jiao** for failure to thrive, learning difficulties or developmental delay in children with insufficient essence
- **1.2 Si Wu Wan** for the pre-ovulation phase of a cyclical infertility treatment
- **3.38 Sheng Mai San Wan** for qi and yin deficiency (dry, cracked tongue, easy sweating, breathlessness)
- **7.19 Shou Wu Pian**, **7.7 Qi Bao Mei Ran Dan** or **7.6 Yang Xue Sheng Fa Capsule** for prematurely graying or falling hair from Kidney essence deficiency

Pattern identifying features

- **Kidney yin and essence deficiency**
- fatigue, lack of vitality, exhaustion
- emaciation
- dry throat, skin and hair
- visual weakness
- insomnia

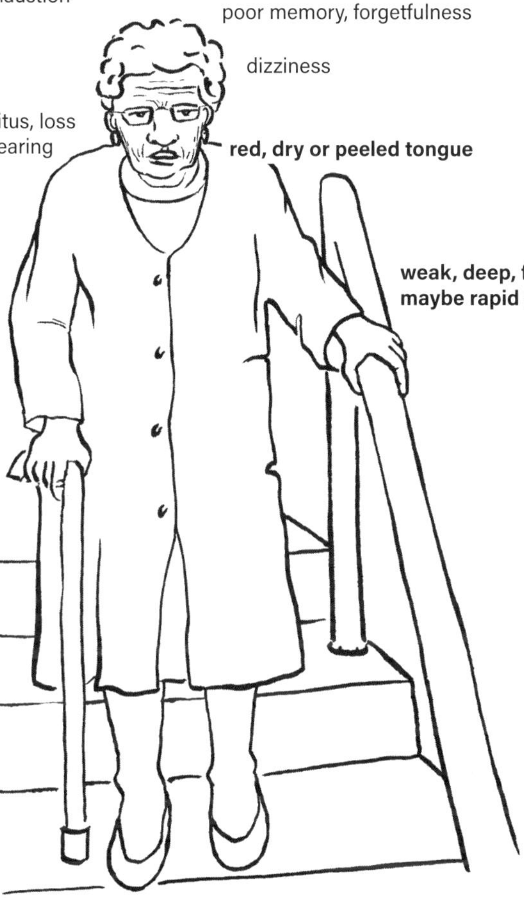

Dosage and method of administration

8-12 pills three times daily on an empty stomach. The dose can be spread out, or taken in two lots of 12-18 pills, morning and evening. In severe cases or during the early stages of treatment (the first few weeks), a 50% increase in dose can be used, then reduced to maintenance as treatment takes effect.

Cautions and contraindications

Contraindicated during the early phase of acute illness such as colds and flu. Care should be taken in patients with a tendency to abdominal distension, loose stools or mucus accumulation. Digestive upset can usually be alleviated by taking it with a small dose (3-6 pills at the same time) of **2.18 Bao He Wan** or **2.9 Xiang Sha Liu Jun Wan**, or taking after food.

GMP

7.4 DA BU YIN WAN

大补阴丸

3+/12

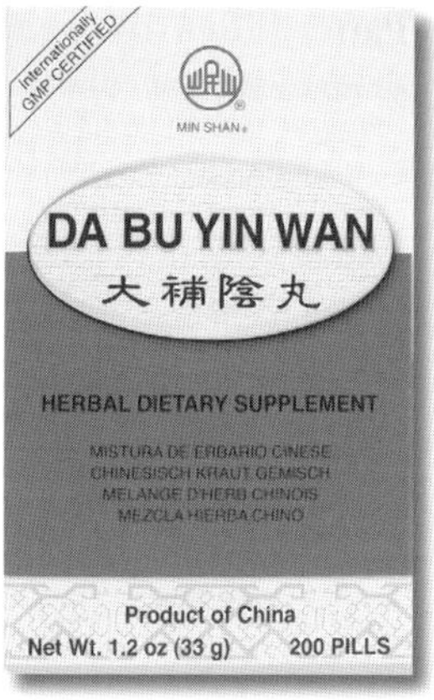

Lanzhou Foci Pharmaceutical Factory (Gansu)
'Major Yin Tonic Pills'
Da Bu Yin Wan is packaged in bottles of 200 pills
Also available as: Abundant Yin Teapills (PF), Rehmannia and Testudinis Combination (conc. extract)

Chinese medical action

Deeply enriches Kidney yin, clears heat from deficiency, cools the blood, alleviates bone steaming

Biomedical action

Demulcent febrifuge, hypoglycemic

INDICATIONS

- Liver and Kidney yin deficiency patterns with marked heat from deficiency causing bone streaming, afternoon or tidal fever, heat in the palms and soles, night sweats and facial flushing. The main focus of this formula is to cool the blood and alleviate heat, with yin nourishing secondary. Combines well with other constitutional formulas when a more profound yin tonifying and blood cooling effect is desired.
- Bleeding disorders associated with yin deficiency patterns. Especially indicated for hemoptysis.
- With the appropriate identifying features, this formula can assist in the treatment of conditions such as fever of unknown origin, menopausal syndrome, chronic consumptive or wasting diseases with fever (such as tuberculosis and AIDS), interstitial cystitis, bronchiectasis, hyperthyroidism, and diabetes mellitus.

Composition

Rehmannia glutinosa (shu di, processed rehmannia), *Chinemys reevesii* (gui ban, turtle shell), *Anemarrhena aspheloides* (zhi mu, anemarrhena), *Phellodendron amurense* (huang bai, phellodendron)

Combine with

- **3.34 Bai He Gu Jin Wan** for hemoptysis associated with Lung and Kidney yin deficiency; **10.2 Raw Tienchi Tablets** can be added when bleeding is persistent
- **7.1 Liu Wei Di Huang Wan** or **7.3 Zuo Gui Wan** for Kidney yin deficiency patterns with bone steaming fever and night sweats
- **3.41 Xu Han Ting** for copious sweating

Dosage and method of administration

8-12 pills three times daily on an empty stomach. The dose can be spread out, or taken in two lots of 12-18 pills, morning and evening. In severe cases or during the early stages of treatment (the first few weeks), a 50% increase in dose can be used, then reduced to maintenance as treatment takes effect.

Pattern identifying features

- **Liver and Kidney yin deficiency with marked heat from deficiency**
- **bone streaming, night sweats**
- **afternoon or tidal fever**
- insomnia
- irritability
- hemoptysis

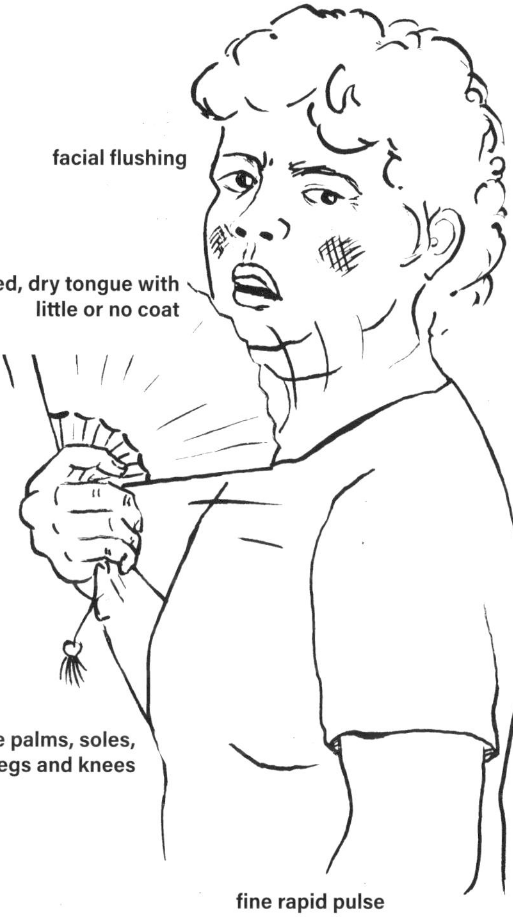

Cautions and contraindications

Contraindicated during the early phase of acute illness such as colds and flu. Care should be taken in patients with a tendency to abdominal distension, loose stools or mucus accumulation. Digestive upset can usually be alleviated by taking it with a small dose (3-6 pills at the same time) of **2.18 Bao He Wan** or **2.9 Xiang Sha Liu Jun Wan**, or taking after food.

7.5 GU BEN WAN

固本丸

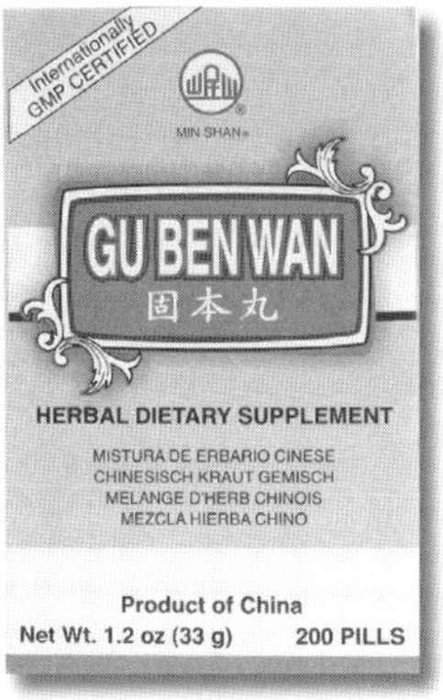

Lanzhou Foci Pharmaceutical Factory (Gansu)
'Secure the Root Pills'
Gu Ben Wan is packaged in bottles of 200 pills

Chinese medical action

Nourishes Lung, Stomach and Kidney yin and qi, generates body fluids

Biomedical action

Demulcent, anti-inflammatory, hypoglycemic

INDICATIONS

- Dryness of the skin and mucous membranes of the Lungs and Intestines, giving rise to cough, thirst, dry mouth and throat, constipation and indefinable epigastric discomfort. This is associated with yin deficiency and fluid damage predominantly affecting of the Lungs and Stomach. Can be combined with a constitutional or targeting formula to enhance the yin nourishing, fluid generating action of that formula.
- With the appropriate identifying features, this formula can assist in the treatment of conditions such as type 2 diabetes mellitus, persistent dry cough following an upper respiratory tract or febrile illness, smokers cough, chronic gastritis, dryness of the oral cavity following radiation treatment to the head and neck, dysphagia from dryness of the esophagus, glossitis, stomatitis, Sjogren's syndrome and xerostomia.

Composition

Rehmannia glutinosa (shu di, processed rehmannia), *Rehmannia glutinosa* (sheng di, raw rehmannia), *Asparagus lucidius* (tian dong, asparagus), *Ophiopogon japonicus* (mai dong, ophiopogon), *Codonopsis pilosula* (dang shen, codonopsis)

Combine with

- **7.1 Liu Wei Di Huang Wan** or **7.3 Zuo Gui Wan** for Kidney yin deficiency type 2 diabetes mellitus
- **3.35 Mai Wei Di Huang Wan** for chronic dry cough from Lung yin deficiency
- **2.11 Bu Zhong Yi Qi Wan** for chronic atrophic gastritis associated with Stomach qi and yin deficiency

Dosage and method of administration

When used alone, the recommended dose is 8-12 pills three times daily on an empty stomach. When used to augment another formula, 12-15 pills per day is generally sufficient.

Pattern identifying features

- **Lung and Stomach yin and fluid deficiency**
- dryness of the Lungs, Stomach and Intestines
- dryness of mucous membranes
- indefinable epigastric discomfort

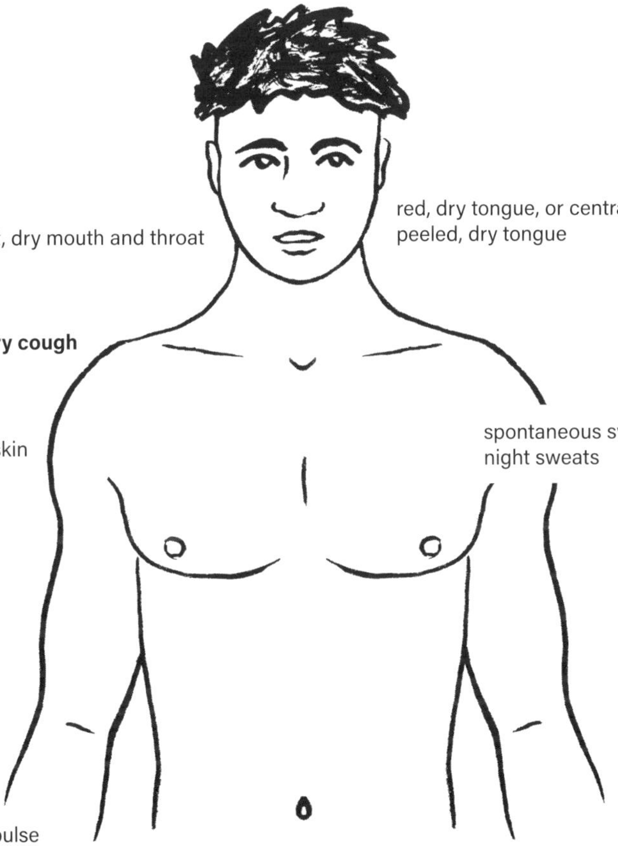

Cautions and contraindications

Contraindicated during the early phase of acute illness such as colds and flu. Care should be taken in patients with a tendency to abdominal distension, loose stools or mucus accumulation as rehmannia can aggravate these problems. Digestive distress can usually be alleviated by taking the pills with a small dose (3-6 pills at the same time) of **2.18 Bao He Wan** or **2.9 Xiang Sha Liu Jun Wan**, or taking after food.

7.6 YANG XUE SHENG FA CAPSULE

养血生发胶囊

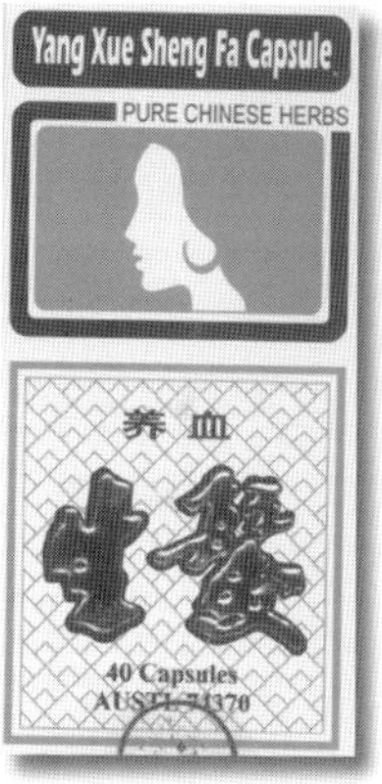

(*Yang Xue Sheng Fa Jiao Nang*)
Tianjin Drug Manufactory (Shandong)
'Blood Nourishing, Hair Generating Capsules'
Yang Xue Sheng Fa Capsules are packaged in bottles of 40 capsules

Chinese medical action

Tonifies Kidney yin and Liver blood, promotes hair growth

Biomedical action

Hematinic, antioxidant

INDICATIONS

- Liver and Kidney yin, essence and blood deficiency with falling hair, alopecia, dry lusterless hair, or premature graying of hair.
- Liver and Kidney deficiency with dizziness, weak or blurring vision, numbness in the extremities, chronic lower back weakness and ache, memory problems, poor hearing and fatigue. In women there may be menstrual disorders such as scanty periods or amenorrhea, long cycles and infertility.
- With the appropriate identifying features, this formula can assist in the treatment of conditions such as alopecia areata, postpartum alopecia, alopecia totalis, and hair loss following chemotherapy or radiation therapy.

Composition (each capsule contains)

Polygonum multiflorum (he shou wu, polygonum root) 160mg, *Rehmannia glutinosa* (shu di, processed rehmannia) 160mg, *Angelica polymorpha* (dang gui, chinese angelica) 80mg, *Chaenomeles lagenaria* (mu gua, chinese quince) 50mg, *Ligusticum wallichi* (chuan xiong, ligusticum) 35mg, *Cuscuta hygrophilae* (tu si zi, cuscuta) 15mg

Combine with

- **13.2 Xiao Feng Wan** or **13.3 Dang Gui Yin Zi Wan** for itchy skin diseases with underlying blood deficiency
- **7.3 Zuo Gui Wan** or **7.1 Liu Wei Di Huang Wan** for falling or prematurely graying hair from Kidney essence deficiency or following radiation therapy
- **1.2 Si Wu Wan** or **7.12 Lu Rong Jiao** for severe blood deficiency
- **7.10 You Gui Wan** for early graying or loss of hair in patients with a tendency to yang deficiency

Dosage and method of administration

4 capsules, twice daily on an empty stomach. The dose can be increased by 50% for the first week or two to get the treatment started. To nourish blood and assist the hair in cases with hair loss, **7.6 Yang Xue Sheng Fa Capsules** usually need to be taken for a minimum of 6 months.

Pattern identifying features

- **Liver and Kidney yin and blood deficiency**
- visual weakness
- lower back ache

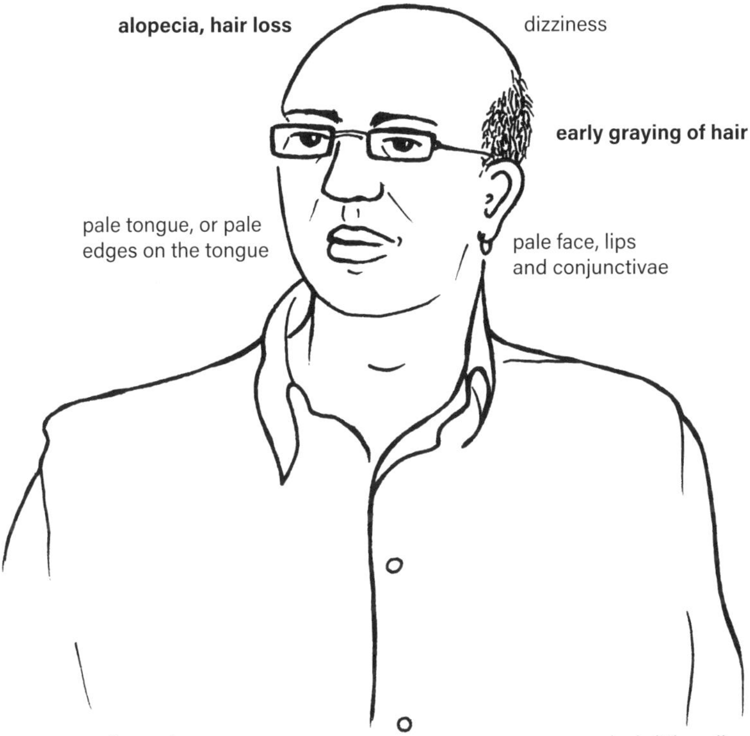

Cautions and contraindications

Contraindicated during the early phase of acute illness such as colds and flu. Care should be taken in patients with a tendency to abdominal distension, loose stools or mucus accumulation as rehmannia and chinese angelica can aggravate these problems. Digestive distress can usually be alleviated by taking it with a small dose (3-6 pills at the same time) of **2.18 Bao He Wan** or **2.9 Xiang Sha Liu Jun Wan**, or taking after food.

GMP

7.7 QI BAO MEI RAN DAN

七宝美髯丹

3+/12

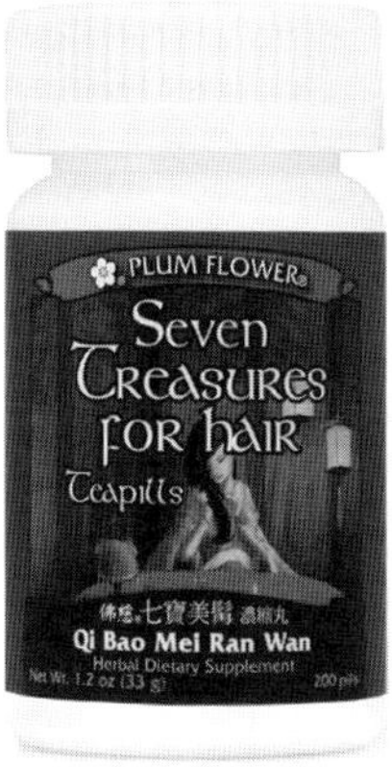

Lanzhou Foci Pharmaceutical Factory (Gansu)
'Seven Treasure Special Pill for Beautiful Whiskers'
Qi Bao Mei Ran Dan is packaged in bottles of 200 pills
Also available as: Seven Treasures Formula (conc. extract)

Chinese medical action

Tonifies and nourishes Kidney yin and Liver blood, promotes hair growth, strengthens sinews and bones

Biomedical action

Hematinic, antioxidant

INDICATIONS

- Hair loss or thinning hair, and premature graying of the hair from Liver and Kidney blood and yin deficiency. Can assist in encouraging hair regrowth following serious illness and cancer treatment.
- Can also be used for other Kidney related problems such as loose teeth or loss of teeth, visual weakness and memory problems associated with Kidney deficiency.
- With the appropriate identifying features, this formula can assist in the treatment of conditions such as alopecia areata, postpartum alopecia, alopecia totalis.

Composition

Polygonum multiflorum (he shou wu, polygonum root), *Angelica polymorpha* (dang gui, chinese angelica), *Lycium chinense* (gou qi zi, lycium fruit), *Achyranthes bidentata* (huai niu xi, achyranthes), *Poria cocos* (fu ling, hoelen), *Cuscuta hygrophilae* (tu si zi, cuscuta), *Psoralea corylifolia* (bu gu zhi, psoralea), *Sesamum indicum* (hei zhi ma, sesame seed)

Combine with

- **1.16 Tao Hong Si Wu Wan** for hair loss associated with a mild degree of blood stasis, or following a significant emotional trauma or shock
- **7.3 Zuo Gui Wan** or **7.1 Liu Wei Di Huang Wan** for falling or prematurely graying hair from Kidney essence deficiency or following radiation therapy
- **1.2 Si Wu Wan** or **7.12 Lu Rong Jiao** for profound blood deficiency
- **7.10 You Gui Wan** for early graying or loss of hair in patients with yang deficiency

Dosage and method of administration

8-12 pills three times daily on an empty stomach. The dose can be spread out, or taken in two lots of 12-18 pills, morning and evening. In severe cases or during the early stages of treatment (the first few weeks), a 50% increase in dose can be used, then reduced to maintenance as treatment takes effect. Patients often notice some improvement in hair quality, or the beginning of regrowth within a few weeks, however treatment should continue for several months at least.

Pattern identifying features

- **Liver blood and Kidney yin deficiency**
- poor memory and concentration
- loose and brittle teeth

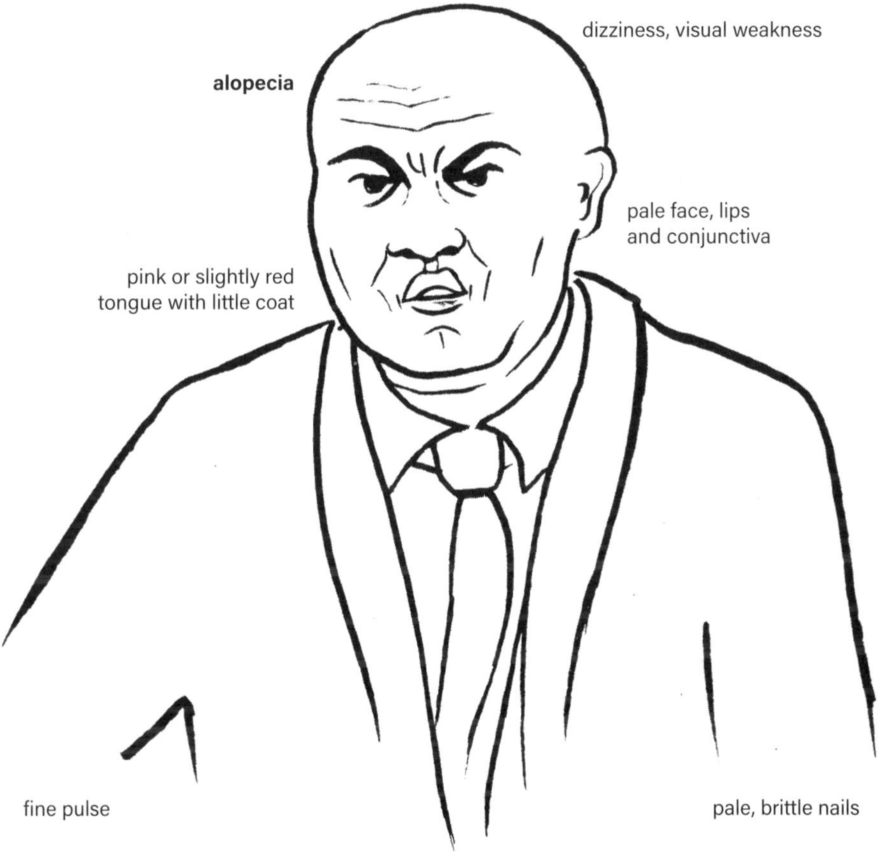

Cautions and contraindications

Contraindicated during the early phase of acute illness such as colds and flu. Care should be taken in patients with a tendency to abdominal distension, loose stools or phlegm damp.

1-3/12

7.8 SHOU WU CHIH

首乌汁

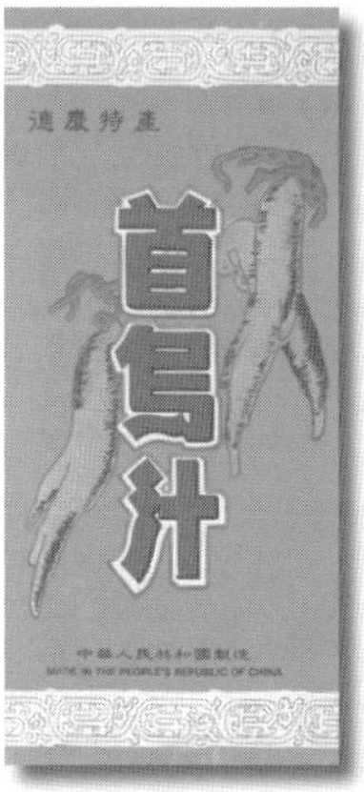

(*Shou Wu Zhi*)
United Pharmaceutical Manufactory (Guangzhou)
'Polygonum Root Juice'
Shou Wu Chih is packaged as a liquid in bottles of about 600ml

Chinese medical action

Tonifies and nourishes Kidney yin and Liver blood, regulates qi, promotes hair growth

Biomedical action

Hematinic, antioxidant

INDICATIONS

- Liver and Kidney yin and blood deficiency. Used for generalized and postpartum weakness and deficiency, anemia, menstrual disorders and convalescence from surgery or serious illness. Contains digestive qi regulating herbs (cardamom, cloves and finger citron) to improve absorption and digestibility of the richer tonic herbs, and thus is particularly good for patients requiring blood tonification but who have Spleen deficiency or a tendency to qi or damp stagnation in the Spleen.
- Good as a general tonic for the elderly, and for periods when demands on qi and blood are higher than normal.
- Menstrual disorders associated with qi and blood deficiency, including irregular menstruation, infertility, scanty periods or amenorrhea, premenstrual syndrome or post menstrual fatigue.
- Used to treat or prevent falling and thinning hair, and premature graying or loss of head hair.

Composition

Polygonum multiflorum (he shou wu, polygonum root) 25%, *Angelica sinensis* (dang gui, chinese angelica) 25%, *Polygonatum chinensis* (huang jing, polygonatum) 20%, *Rehmannia glutinosa* (sheng di, raw rehmannia) 10%, *Ligusticum wallichi* (chuan xiong, ligusticum) 10%, *Angelica dahurica* (bai zhi, angelica) 6.7%, *Ammomum villosum* (sha ren, cardamom) 1.6%, *Eugenia caryophyllata* (ding xiang, cloves) 0.85%, *Citrus medica* (fo shou, finger citron) 0.85%, rice or sorghum wine

Combine with

– **1.2 Si Wu Wan** for marked blood deficiency

Pattern identifying features

- **Liver and Kidney yin and blood deficiency**
- memory problems

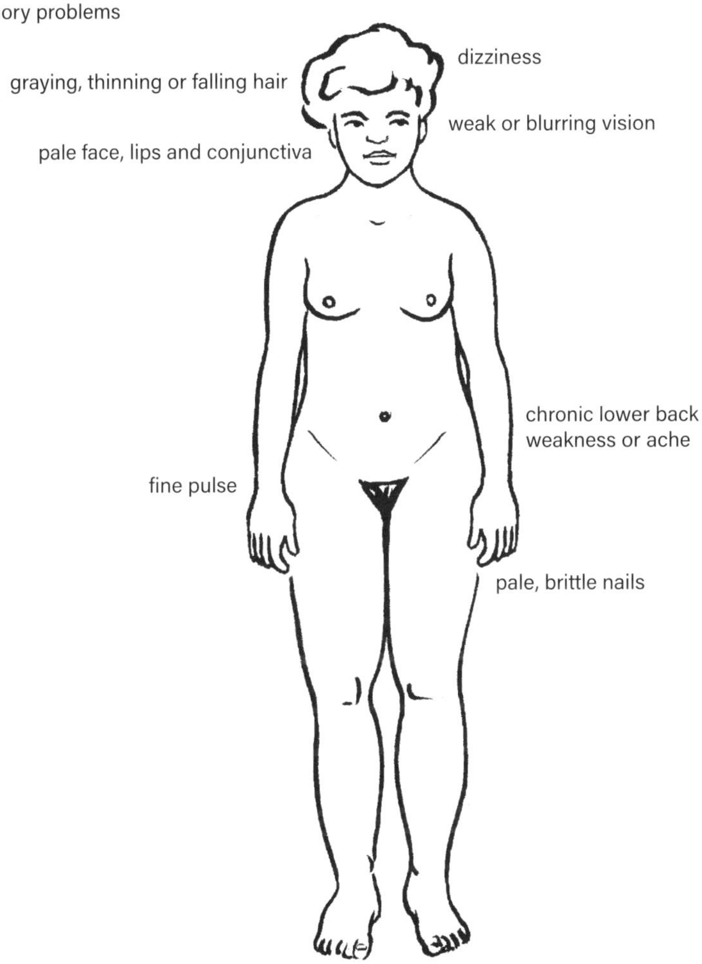

Dosage and method of administration

2-3 tablespoons, three times daily on an empty stomach.

Cautions and contraindications

Contraindicated during the early phase of acute illness such as colds and flu. Generally well tolerated but care should be taken in patients with a tendency to abdominal distension, loose stools or phlegm damp.

7.9 JIN GUI SHEN QI WAN

金匮肾气丸

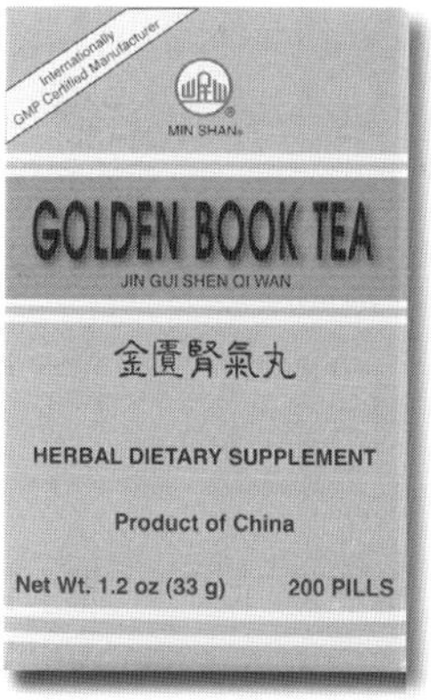

Lanzhou Foci Pharmaceutical Factory (Gansu)
'Kidney Qi Pill [from the *Jin Gui Yao Lue*])'
Jin Gui Shen Qi Wan is packaged in bottles of 200 pills
Also available as: Jin Kui Shen Qi Wan (HT, BE), Sexoton Pills, Golden Book Teapills (PF), Rehmannia Eight Formula (conc. extract)

Chinese medical action

Tonifies and warms Kidney yang

Biomedical action

Stimulates metabolism, promotes adrenal function, improves fluid metabolism, hypoglycemic, anti-hypertensive, improves kidney function

INDICATIONS

- Kidney yang deficiency. An important formula for hypofunction of Kidney yang with cold intolerance, poor circulation, fatigue and disturbances of fluid metabolism. Prized as a strengthening tonic for the elderly.
- Urinary disorders characterized by frequency or difficulty, including nocturia, daytime frequency, broken stream, or terminal dribbling. The converse of weak fluid metabolism may however be the opposite–scanty urine or oliguria with ankle or generalized edema.
- Sexual dysfunction, low libido, impotence, infertility, lower back ache.
- Chronic respiratory weakness and dyspnea from Kidney not grasping Lung qi
- With the appropriate identifying features, this formula can be used to alleviate a diverse range of conditions including benign prostatic hypertrophy, chronic nephritis, nephritic edema, poor adrenal function, chronic bronchitis and asthma, cardiac asthma, chronic fatigue syndrome, diabetes mellitus and insipidus, chronic arthritis, infertility, amenorrhea, menopausal syndrome, senile cataracts and hypothyroidism.

Composition

Rehmannia glutinosa (shu di, processed rehmannia), *Cornus officinalis* (shan zhu yu, cornus), *Dioscorea opposita* (shan yao, dioscorea), *Poria cocos* (fu ling, hoelen), *Alisma orientalis* (ze xie, alisma), *Paeonia suffruticosa* (mu dan pi, moutan), *Cinnamomum cassia* (rou gui, cinnamon bark), *Aconite carmicaheli* (zhi fu zi, processed aconite)

Combine with

- **4.14 Chin So Ku Ching Wan** or **4.11 Ba Ji Yin Yang Wan** for severe nocturia, frequency or incontinence of urine
- **2.11 Bu Zhong Yi Qi Wan** for uterine or bladder prolapse
- **11.5 Wu Zi Yan Zong Wan** for sperm disorders from yang deficiency
- **3.39 Yulin Bu Shen Wan** for chronic asthma
- **2.13 Li Zhong Wan** for Spleen and Kidney yang deficiency
- **1.34 Hai Zao Jing Wan** or **1.17 Gui Zhi Fu Ling Wan** for gynecological masses (such as fibroids and endometriosis) from Kidney yang deficiency

Pattern identifying features

- **Kidney yang deficiency**
- **cold intolerance, cold extremities**
- **fatigue, listlessness, exhaustion**

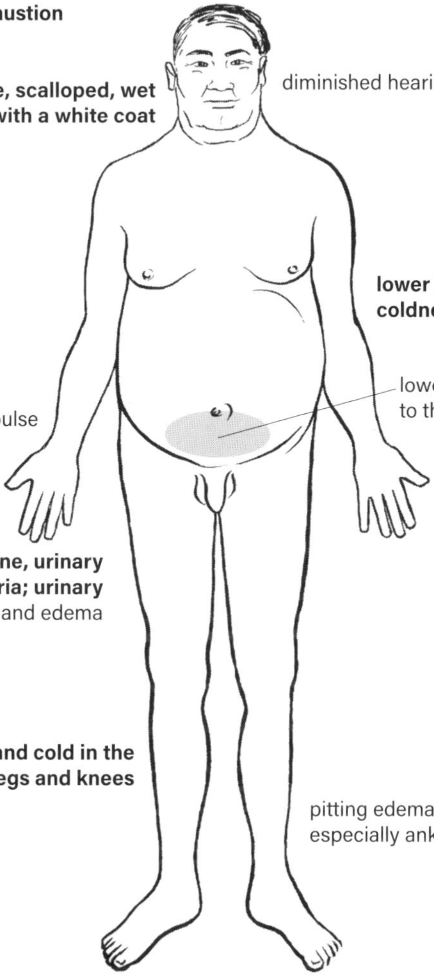

- **2.34 Cong Rong Bu Shen Wan** for cold atonic constipation
- **3.41 Xu Han Ting** for copious sweating from yang and defensive qi deficiency

Dosage and method of administration

8-12 pills three times daily on an empty stomach. The dose can be spread out, or taken in two lots of 12-18 pills, morning and evening. In severe cases or during the early stages of treatment (the first two weeks), a 50% increase in dose can be used, then reduced as treatment takes effect.

Cautions and contraindications

Contraindicated during pregnancy and during the early phase of acute illness such as colds and flu. Some patients may experience digestive upset or diarrhea which can be alleviated with a small dose of **2.13 Li Zhong Wan**.

7.10 YOU GUI WAN

右归丸

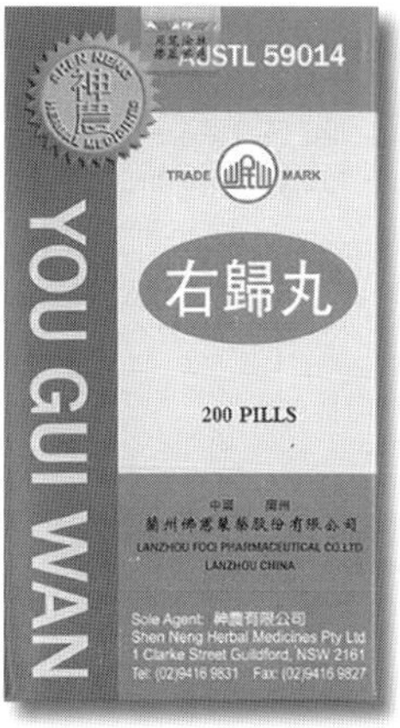

Lanzhou Foci Pharmaceutical Factory (Gansu)
'Right Returning Pills'
You Gui Wan is packaged in bottles of 200 pills.
Also available as: Right Side Replenishing Teapills (PF), Eucommia and Rehmannia Formula (conc. extract)

Chinese medical action

Warms and tonifies Kidney yang, nourishes essence, tonifies blood, strengthens sinews and bones

Biomedical action

Stimulant and tonic, strengthens adrenal function, adaptogenic, hematinic, warms the body

INDICATIONS

- Kidney yang and essence deficiency patterns with exhaustion and debility. Similar to **7.9 Jin Gui Shen Qi Wan**, without the 'draining' components, instead substituting additional yang tonic herbs, creating a stronger yang warming and essence tonic suitable for more severe deficiency patterns. Much prized by elderly Chinese as a general Kidney support and health promoting tonic.
- Congenital weakness of the Kidneys causing failure to thrive, learning difficulties and slow development. This may manifest as late descent of the testicles, delayed or absent menarche, or any of a series of disorders present from birth. Severe essence or yang deficiency may also follow severe or prolonged illness.
- Atrophy and muscular weakness syndromes associated with essence deficiency.
- With the appropriate identifying features, this formula can assist in the treatment of conditions such as leukopenia, anemia, diabetes mellitus, chronic nephritis, chronic asthma, benign prostatic hypertrophy, infertility, declining sexual function, progressive muscular dystrophy and multiple sclerosis.

Composition (each pill contains powdered)

Rehmannia glutinosa (shu di, processed rehmannia) 38.8mg, *Cornus officinalis* (shan zhu yu, cornus) 28.6mg, *Dioscorea opposita* (shan yao, dioscorea) 28.6mg, *Lycium barbarum* (gou qi zi, lycium fruit) 22.4mg, *Eucommia ulmoides* (du zhong, eucommia) 22.4mg, *Cuscuta hygrophilae* (tu si zi, cuscuta) 22.4mg, *Angelica polymorpha* (dang gui, chinese angelica) 22.4mg, *Cinnamomun cassia* (rou gui, cinnamon bark) 14.2mg

Combine with

- **7.12 Lu Rong Jiao** or **7.11 Deer Velvet** to enhance essence augmentation
- A small dose (around 2-4 pills per day) of **10.8 Xiao Huo Luo Wan** for those with severe cold signs and cold intolerance
- **11.5 Wu Zi Yan Zong Wan** for sperm disorders from essence deficiency
- **2.13 Li Zhong Wan** for Spleen and Kidney yang deficiency
- **10.16.1 Zhuang Yao Jian Shen** for chronic back, leg or joint ache and weakness

Pattern identifying features

- **Kidney yang deficiency**
- **cold intolerance, cold extremities**
- urinary frequency; or scanty urine and edema
- exhaustion, lassitude
- impotence, infertility

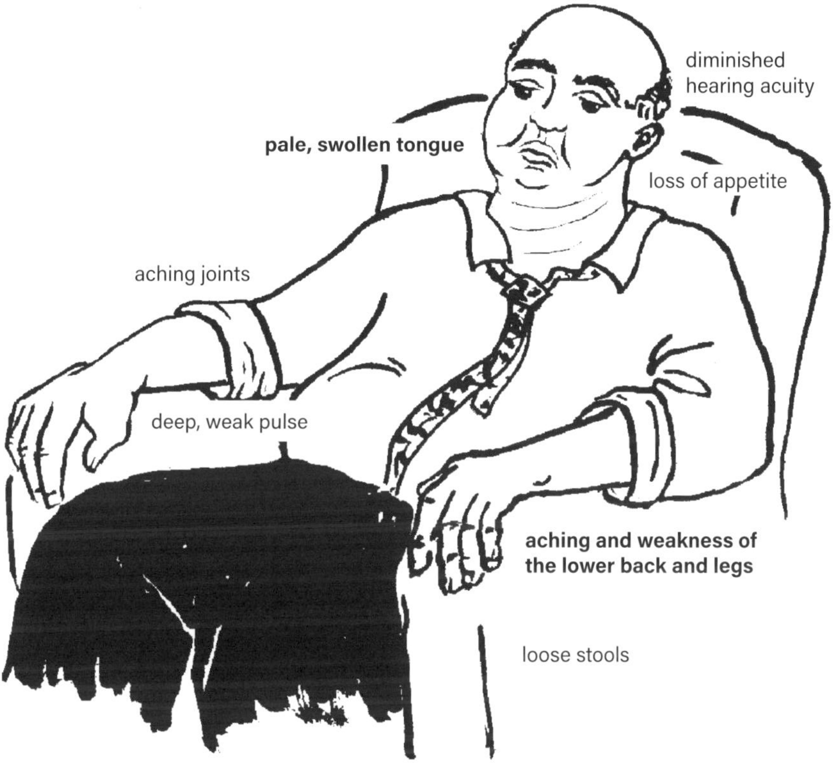

Dosage and method of administration

8-12 pills three times daily on an empty stomach. The dose can be spread out, or taken in two lots of 12-18 pills, morning and evening. In severe cases or during the early stages of treatment (the first two weeks), a 50% increase in dose can be used, then reduced to maintenance as treatment takes effect.

Cautions and contraindications

Contraindicated during the early phase of acute illness such as colds and flu. May occasionally cause digestive upset in sensitive individuals. This can usually be alleviated by taking it with a small dose (3-6 pills at the same time) of **2.13 Li Zhong Wan**.

7.11 DEER VELVET

鹿茸

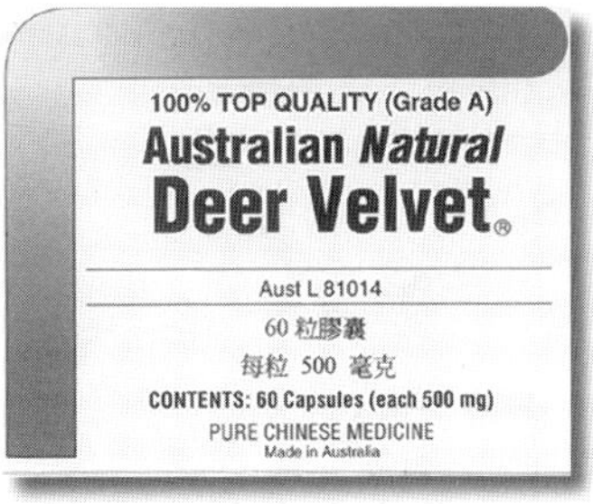

(*Lu Rong*)
Tong Ren Tang (Australia)
'Deer Velvet'
Deer Velvet is packaged in bottles of 60 capsules, 500mg per capsule

Chinese medical action

Warms and tonifies Kidney yang and essence, nourishes blood, strengthens sinews and bones

Biomedical action

Adaptogen, stimulant, increases metabolism, promotes hemopoiesis

INDICATIONS

- Important substance for augmenting essence in children and adults. Used to strengthen Kidney yang and augment essence and blood in the treatment of premature graying of the hair or hair loss, lower back ache, general debility, impotence, primary infertility, amenorrhea, anovulation, sperm abnormalities and low sperm count, hearing disorders and other signs and symptoms of yang deficiency.
- Essence deficiency problems such as failure to thrive, slow or retarded development, poor tooth development, failure of the fontanel to close, learning problems and other congenital problems.
- Joint pain associated with osteoarthritis. Recent research has shown that deer velvet and related deer horn products can stimulate the growth of cartilage in degenerate joints.
- Chronic non-healing ulcerations and sores, such as diabetic ulcers, bedsores or tropical ulcers.
- To enhance blood production in patients with severe or resistant blood deficiency.

Composition (each capsule contains)

Cervus nippon (lu rong, deer velvet) 500mg

Combine with

- **7.9 Jin Gui Shen Qi Wan** for yang deficiency with impotence and infertility
- **7.16.1 Shi Quan Da Bu Wan** for non healing ulcers and sores
- **7.1 Liu Wei Di Huang Wan** for children with essence deficiency developmental problems
- **1.1 Ba Zhen Wan** or **1.9 Gui Pi Wan** for resistant blood deficiency patterns
- **11.5 Wu Zi Yan Zong Wan** for sperm disorders

Pattern identifying features

- **yang, essence and blood deficiency**
- learning difficulties
- failure to thrive
- joint pain

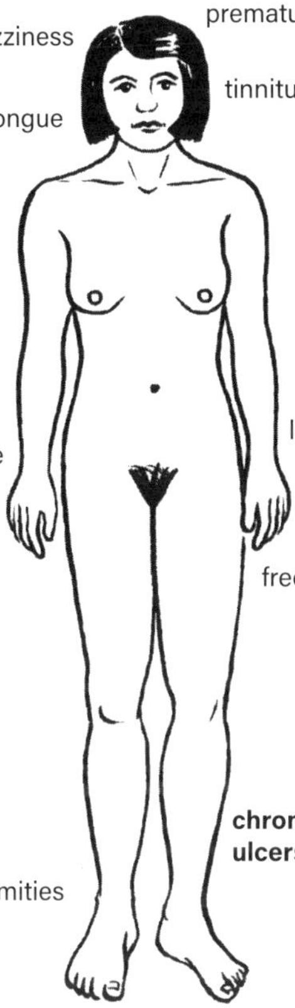

Dosage and method of administration

2 capsules per day. In severe cases the dose can be doubled to 4 capsules daily. Quarter to half dose for children. Generally best to begin with a small dose (1 capsule per day) and gradually increase it. **7.11 Deer Velvet** is very warm and can sometime cause overheating. Usually combined with a constitutional formula. Good for children as the capsules can be opened and the contents mixed with food to aid ingestion.

Cautions and contraindications

Contraindicated during the early phase of acute illness such as colds and flu. Not suitable for yin deficiency with heat, or excess heat patterns. Keep an eye on the patient at the start of therapy to make sure they don't overheat. Symptoms of overheating include facial flushing, insomnia, nosebleeds and dizziness.

7.12 LU RONG JIAO

鹿茸胶 [鹿角胶]

(also packaged as **Lu Jiao Jiao**)
Tong Fu Tang, Henan Lao Jun Tang Pharmaceutical Factory
'Deer Horn Resin'
Lu Rong Jiao is packaged in hard resinous blocks which can be pulverized to a fine powder in a coffee grinder and added to a liquid, or just taken as is

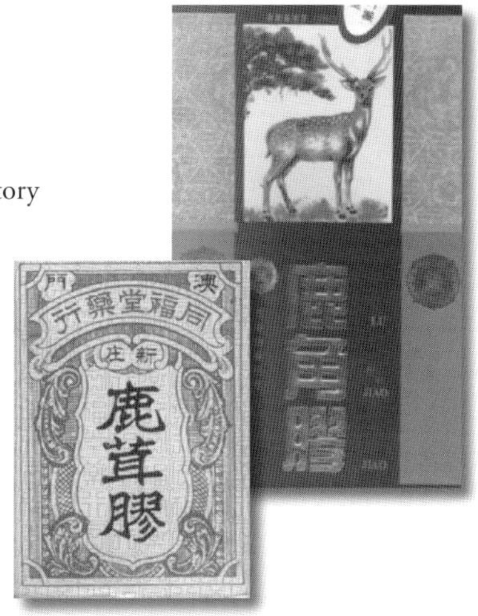

Chinese medical action

Warms and tonifies Kidney yang, augments essence and blood, strengthens sinews and bones

Biomedical action

Adaptogenic, stimulant, increases metabolism, promotes hemopoiesis

INDICATIONS

- As for **7.11 Deer Velvet**. The difference between this product and deer velvet is concentration and price. **7.11 Deer Velvet** is generally considered superior to **7.12 Lu Rong Jiao** for augmenting essence and blood, but is more expensive. **7.12 Lu Rong Jiao** is not as strong and more must be used, but is considered an affordable yet effective compromise.

Composition

Cervus nippon (lu jiao, deerhorn) boiled down to a hard resin.

Dosage and method of administration

The resinous block can be pulverized in a coffee grinder and packed into capsules. 5-10 grams per day. Generally best to begin with a small dose (2-3 grams per day) and gradually increase it. **7.12 Lu Rong Jiao** is quite warming and some people are easily overheated by it. Usually combined with a constitutional formula.

Cautions and contraindications

Contraindicated during the early phase of acute illness such as colds and flu. Not suitable for yin deficiency with deficient heat patterns, or excess heat patterns. Keep an eye on the patient when beginning therapy with **7.12 Lu Rong Jiao** to make sure the patient doesn't overheat. Symptoms of overheating include facial flushing, insomnia, nosebleeds and dizziness.

GMP

3+/12

7.13 HUAN SHAO WAN

还少丸

Lanzhou Foci Pharmaceutical Factory (Gansu)
'Miraculous Pills for the Recovery of Youth'
Also available as: Lycium Formula (conc. extract)

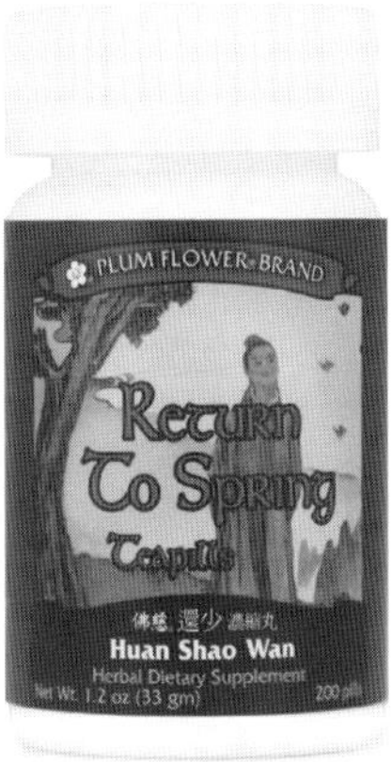

Chinese medical action

Tonifies the Liver and Kidneys, nourishes yin, warms yang, strengthens the Spleen, nourishes the Heart, benefits and calms the mind

Biomedical action

Strengthens digestion, memory and kidney function

INDICATIONS

- Heart and Kidney yang qi deficiency with chronic lower back ache, *shén* disturbance, memory problems, loss of hearing acuity, loss of appetite, weight loss, impotence, urinary frequency and loss of teeth.
- Prized in China for strengthening and invigorating the elderly, infirm or debilitated. Can assist in the treatment and prevention of the confusion and memory problems of old age.
- Infertility from Spleen and Kidney deficiency.

Composition

Zizyphus jujuba (da zao, chinese dates), *Rehmannia glutinosa* (shu di, processed rehmannia), *Lycium chinensis* (gou qi zi, lycium), *Poria cocos* (fu ling, hoelen), *Cistanche deserticola* (rou cong rong, cistanches), *Eucommia ulmoides* (du zhong, eucommia), *Morinda officinalis* (ba ji tian, morinda), *Foeniculum vulgarae* (xiao hui xiang, fennel seed), *Broussonetia papyrifera* (chu shi zi, broussonetia), *Achyranthes bidentata* (huai niu xi, achyranthes), *Polygala sibiricum* (yuan zhi, polygala), *Cornus officinalis* (shan zhu yu, cornus), *Schizandra chinensis* (wu wei zi, schizandra), *Dioscorea opposita* (shan yao, dioscorea)

Dosage and method of administration

8-12 pills three times daily on an empty stomach. In severe cases or during the early stages of treatment (the first few weeks), a 50% increase in dose can be used, then reduced as treatment takes effect.

Cautions and contraindications

Contraindicated during the early phase of acute illness such as colds and flu.

7.14 DEER ANTLER AND GINSENG

鹿角人参胶囊

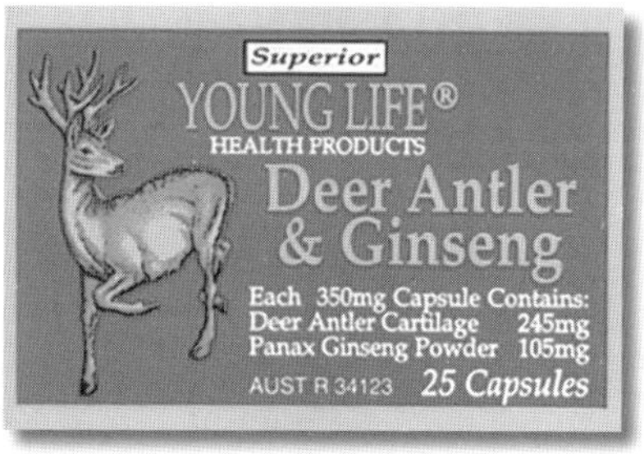

(*Lu Jiao Ren Shen Jiao Nang*)
ADP Pharmaceuticals Pty. Ltd (Australia)
Deer Antler and Ginseng is packaged in 350mg capsules, in jars of 25 or 50 capsules

Chinese medical action

Strengthens and tonifies the Spleen and Kidneys, tonifies qi and yang, augments essence

Biomedical action

Adaptogenic, stimulant, increases metabolism, immunomodulator

INDICATIONS

- Fatigue, lack of energy, vitality and stamina from yang qi and essence deficiency. Can assist in maintaining strength and well being and support the immune system in many situations where energy demands are high. These include chronic or serious illness and post surgical recovery.
- Essence disorders in children and adults, including failure to thrive, poor tooth development, slow development, failure of the fontanel to close, learning problems and other congenital problems.
- To strengthen Kidney yang and nourish blood for premature graying of the hair or hair loss, lower back ache, general debility, impotence, hearing disorders.
- Joint pain associated with osteoarthritis. Recent research has shown that deer antler and related deer horn products can stimulate the growth of cartilage in degenerate joints.
- Chronic non-healing sores, such as bedsores or tropical ulcers.
- Used to enhancing blood production in patients with severe or resistant blood deficiency.

Composition (each capsule contains)

Cervus nippon (lu jiao, deer antler cartilage) 245mg, *Panax ginseng* (ren shen, ginseng) 105mg

Combine with

- **7.9 Jin Gui Shen Qi Wan** or **7.10 You Gui Wan** for patients with yang deficiency infertility and reproductive problems
- **7.1 Liu Wei Di Huang Wan** for children with yin deficiency developmental problems, and for women with yang deficiency infertility (post-ovulation)
- **1.1 Ba Zhen Wan** or **1.9 Gui Pi Wan** for resistant blood deficiency patterns
- **11.5 Wu Zi Yan Zong Wan** for sperm disorders

Pattern identifying features

- **yang qi and essence deficiency**
- lack of stamina and vitality
- failure to thrive
- non healing sores
- fatigue

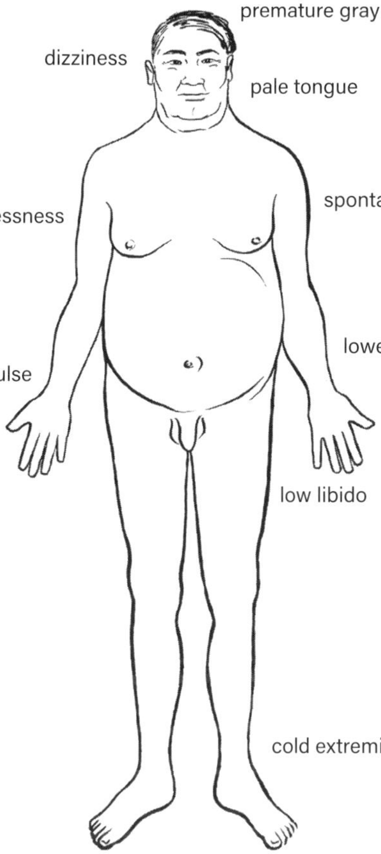

Dosage and method of administration

The adult dose is 1-4 capsules daily; for children ½-2 capsules daily. Usually best to begin with one capsule per day and build up gradually, as deer antler is very warming and can cause patients to overheat. For children the capsules can be opened and contents mixed with food to aid ingestion.

Cautions and contraindications

Contraindicated during the early phase of acute illness such as colds and flu, in patients with heat, yang rising or yin deficiency patterns, and in the absence of qi or yang deficiency. Contraindicated (without modification) in patients with hypertension, and gastric ulcers. Overdose can lead to headaches, insomnia, palpitations, hypertension, tremors, nervousness and anxiety. Concurrent consumption of other stimulants (e.g. coffee) can exacerbate the negative effects. Monitor patients closely at the start of therapy with **7.14 Deer Antler and Ginseng** to make sure they don't overheat. Symptoms of overheating include facial flushing, insomnia, nosebleeds and dizziness.

7.15 YULIN DA BU WAN

玉林大补丸

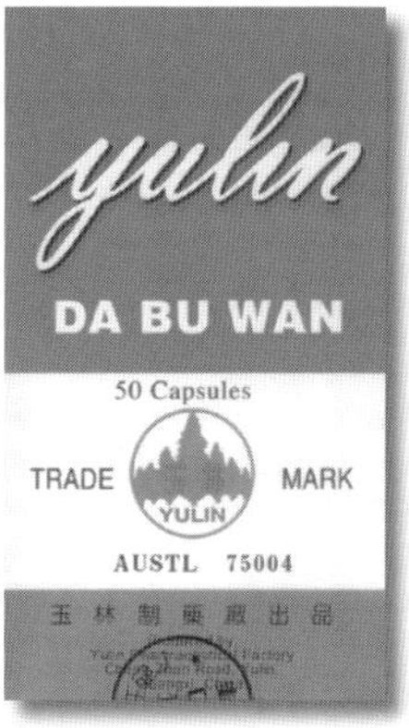

Yulin Pharmaceutical Factory (Guangxi)
'Great Tonic Pills from Yulin'
Yulin Da Bu Wan is packaged in bottles of 50 capsules.
Also available as: Gecko Tonic Teapills (PF), Ge Jie Da Bu Wan

Chinese medical action

Warms and tonifies Kidney yang, source qi and blood, strengthens the Spleen and Lungs

Biomedical action

Energy tonic and stimulant, promotes metabolism, improves respiratory, digestive and renal functions

INDICATIONS

- Loss of libido, infertility, impotence, urinary dysfunction, urinary frequency or nocturia, generalized weakness, fatigue and exhaustion from Kidney yang deficiency.
- Digestive problems such as early morning diarrhea (cock crow), diarrhea with undigested food, abdominal distension, loss of appetite, fluid metabolism problems and edema from Spleen and Kidney yang deficiency.
- Respiratory weakness, chronic wheezing, asthma, shortness of breath, frequent colds and chronic cough from Lung and Kidney deficiency and Kidney failure to grasp Lung qi. Used for emphysema and other chronic respiratory illnesses.
- A good general tonic for the elderly, and for those convalescing from a prolonged illness or surgical procedure that has damaged yang qi.

Composition (each capsule contains)

Gecko gecko (ge jie, gecko) 107.5mg, *Poria cocos* (fu ling, hoelen) 50mg, *Rehmannia glutinosa* (shu di, processed rehmannia) 34mg, *Polygonatum sibiricum* (huang jing, solomon seal rhizome) 28.5mg, *Dioscorea batatas* (shan yao, dioscorea) 26.5mg, *Ligustrum lucidum* (nu zhen zi, privet fruit) 26mg, *Dipsacus asper* (xu duan, dipsacus) 24mg, *Chaenomeles lagenaria* (mu gua, chinese quince) 23.5mg, *Astragalus membranaceous* (huang qi, astragalus) 21.5mg, *Atractylodes macrocephala* (bai zhu, atractylodes) 21.5mg, *Morinda officinalis* (ba ji tian, morinda) 21.5mg, *Eucommia ulmoides* (du zhong, eucommia) 21.5mg, *Codonopsis pilosula* (dang shen, codonopsis) 21.5mg, *Lycium barbarum* (gou qi zi, lycium fruit) 20.5mg, *Drynaria fortunei* (gu sui bu, drynaria) 20mg, *Angelica polymorpha* (dang gui, chinesc angelica) 19mg, *Glycyrrhiza uralensis* (gan cao, licorice) 14mg

Combine with

- **3.40 Bu Fei Wan** for chronic wheezing and cough from Lung and Kidney qi deficiency
- **7.11 Deer Velvet** to enhance the yang warming action of the formula

Pattern identifying features

- **Kidney, Spleen and Lung yang qi deficiency**
- wheezing, chronic cough, respiratory weakness
- fatigue, exhaustion

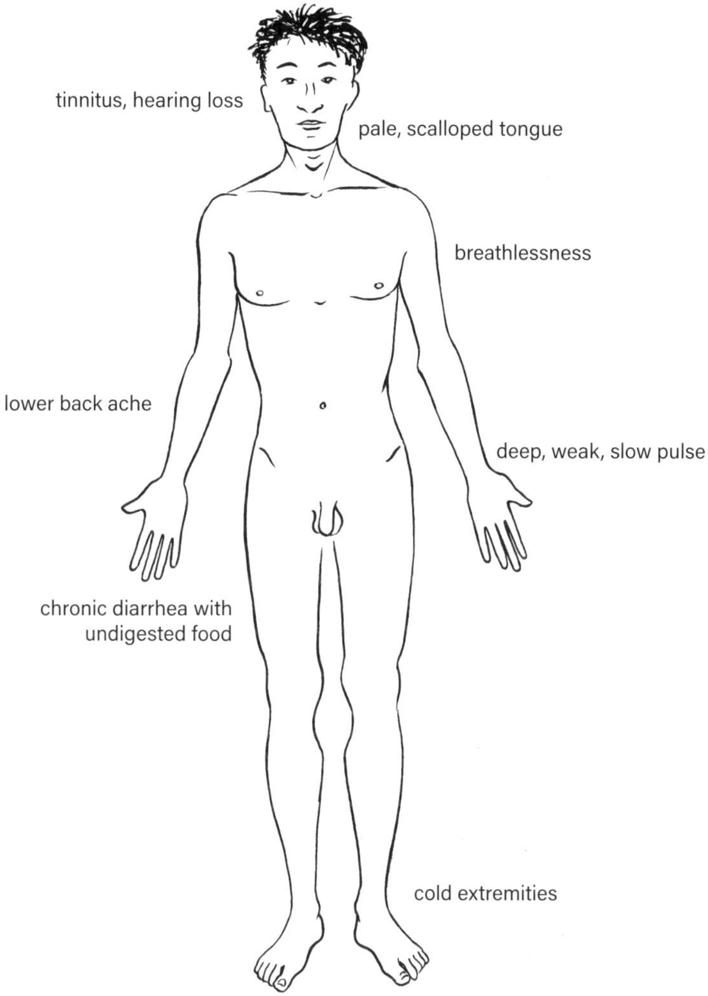

Dosage and method of administration

3-5 capsules twice daily on an empty stomach.

Cautions and contraindications

Contraindicated during the early phase of acute illness such as colds and flu. Contraindicated in patients with wheezing or other respiratory patterns associated with external pathogens or heat. This formula can be quite warming and may overheat some patients. Lowering the dosage usually alleviates the problem.

7.16.1 SHI QUAN DA BU WAN

十全大补丸

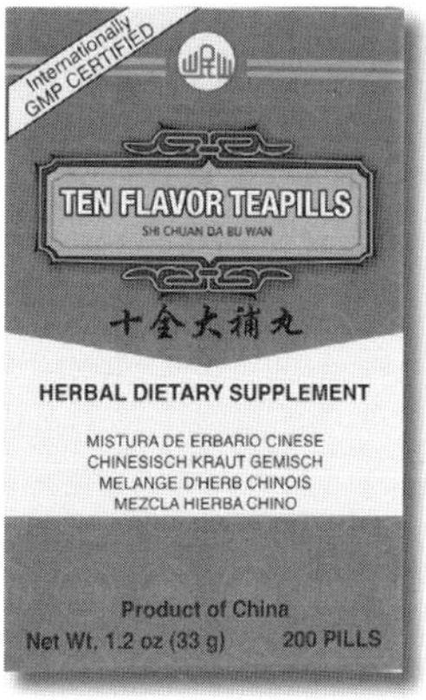

Lanzhou Foci Pharmaceutical Factory (Gansu)
'Ten Ingredient Pills for Complete Tonification'
Shi Quan Da Bu Wan is packaged in bottles of 200 pills.
Also available as: Ginseng and Dang Gui Ten Combination (conc. extract)

Chinese medical action

Warms and tonifies qi and blood, supports yang, fortifies defensive qi

Biomedical action

Energy tonic and stimulant, promotes metabolism, nourishes blood and regulates menstruation, promotes circulation to the extremities

INDICATIONS

- Qi and blood deficiency with cold. A variation of **1.1 Ba Zhen Wan**, with astragalus to increase defensive qi fortification, and cinnamon bark to warm the Kidneys and channels and stimulate transformation of qi into blood.
- Chronic yin sores or ulcers that are slow to heal, bedsores and tropical ulcers.
- Benign gynecological tumors, such as fibroids and ovarian cysts associated with weak movement of yang qi and blood deficiency in the lower burner.
- With the appropriate identifying features, this formula can be used to assist in convalescence following prolonged illness, hemorrhage, surgery or pregnancy, general weakness and exhaustion, consumptive disorders, chronic debility, malnutrition associated with deprivation or anorexia, anemia, chronic leukemia, scanty menstrual periods or amenorrhea, infertility, habitual miscarriage, abnormal uterine bleeding, long menstrual cycle or irregular menstruation, insufficient lactation, weakness during pregnancy and thrombocytopenic purpura.

Composition

Rehmannia glutinosa (shu di, processed rehmannia), *Angelica sinensis* (dang gui, chinese angelica), *Codonopsis pilosula* (dang shen, codonopsis), *Paeonia alba* (bai shao, white peony), *Atractylodes macrocephala* (bai zhu, atractylodes), *Poria cocos* (fu ling, hoelen), *Astragalus membranaceous* (huang qi, astragalus), *Ligusticum wallichi* (chuan xiong, ligusticum), *Glycyrrhiza uralensis* (gan cao, licorice), *Cinnamomum cassia* (rou gui, cinnamon bark)

Combine with

– **13.14 Ching Wan Hung** topically for chronic ulcers and bed sores

Pattern identifying features

- **qi and blood deficiency with cold**
- fatigue, weakness
- loss of appetite
- palpitations
- poor appetite
- cold intolerance
- poor concentration

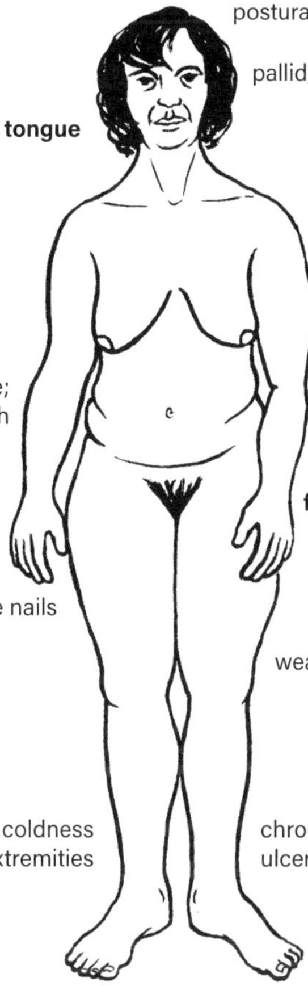

Dosage and method of administration

8-12 pills three times daily on an empty stomach. The dose can be spread out, or taken in two lots of 12-18 pills, morning and evening. In severe cases or during the early stages of treatment (the first few weeks), a 50% increase in dose can be used, then reduced as effects are felt.

Cautions and contraindications

Contraindicated during the early phase of acute illness such as colds and flu. Care in patients with a tendency to abdominal distension, loose stools or general digestive weakness. Some patients may find **7.16.1 Shi Quan Da Bu Wan** aggravates these symptoms. This can usually be alleviated by taking it with a small dose (3-6 pills at the same time) of **2.18 Bao He Wan** or **2.9 Xiang Sha Liu Jun Wan**.

7.16.2 SHI QUAN DA BU WAN

十全大补丸

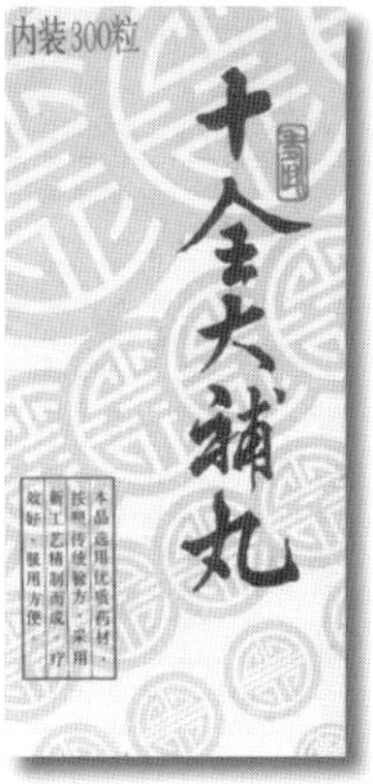

Tong Ren Tang (Beijing)
'Ten Ingredient Pills for Complete Tonification'
Shi Quan Da Bu Wan is packaged in bottles of 300 pills

Chinese medical action

Warms and tonifies qi and blood, supports yang, fortifies defensive qi

Biomedical action

Energy tonic and stimulant, promotes metabolism, nourishes blood and regulates menstruation, promotes circulation to the extremities

INDICATIONS

- As for **7.16.1 Shi Quan Da Bu Wan**

Composition (each dose of 30 pills contains powdered)

Rehmannia glutinosa (shu di, processed rehmannia) 696mg, *Angelica polymorpha* (dang gui, chinese angelica) 696mg, *Codonopsis pilosula* (dang shen, codonopsis) 462mg, *Paeonia alba* (bai shao, white peony) 462mg, *Atractylodes macrocephala* (bai zhu, atractylodes) 462mg, *Poria cocos* (fu ling, hoelen) 462mg, *Astragalus membranaceous* (huang qi, astragalus) 462mg, *Ligusticum wallichi* (chuan xiong, ligusticum) 234mg, *Glycyrrhiza uralensis* (gan cao, licorice) 234mg, *Cinnamomum cassia* (rou gui, cinnamon bark) 114mg, sucrose

Dosage and method of administration

30 pills, twice daily on an empty stomach. In severe cases or during the early stages of treatment (the first few weeks), a 50% increase in dose can be used, then reduced as treatment takes effect.

Cautions and contraindications

Contraindicated during the early phase of acute illness such as colds and flu. Care s in patients with a tendency to abdominal distension, loose stools or general digestive weakness. Although mostly well tolerated, some patients may find **7.16.2 Shi Quan Da Bu Wan** aggravates these symptoms. This can usually be alleviated by taking it with a small dose (3-6 pills at the same time) of **2.18 Bao He Wan** or **2.9 Xiang Sha Liu Jun Wan**.

7.17 HUA TUO SHI QUAN DA BU JIU

华佗十全大补酒

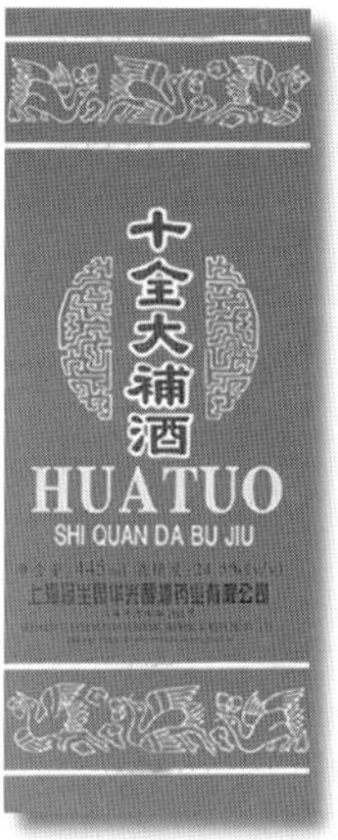

3+/12

Shanghai Guanshengyuan Huaguang Brewing and Medicine Company (Shanghai)
'Hua Tuo's Ten Ingredient Wine for Complete Tonification'
Hua Tuo Shi Quan Da Bu Jiu is packaged in 445ml bottles.

Chinese medical action

Warms and tonifies qi and blood, supports yang, fortifies defensive qi

Biomedical action

Energy tonic and stimulant, opens the channels, nourishes blood and regulates menstruation, promotes circulation to the extremities.

INDICATIONS

- Famous medicinal wine, identical in composition and action to **7.16.1 Shi Quan Da Bu Wan**. The wine makes this version a little warmer and more invigorating to the blood. It is thus ideal for painful obstruction and general aches and pains associated with qi and blood deficiency, as well as chronic ulcers, post-operative sores, bedsores and other non-healing wounds.
- An excellent restorative and preventative tonic for elderly patients and those recovering from a serious illness or surgery.

Composition

Rehmannia glutinosa (shu di, processed rehmannia), *Angelica sinensis* (dang gui, chinese angelica), *Codonopsis pilosula* (dang shen, codonopsis), *Paeonia alba* (bai shao, white peony), *Atractylodes macrocephala* (bai zhu, atractylodes), *Poria cocos* (fu ling, hoelen), *Astragalus membranaceous* (huang qi, astragalus), *Ligusticum wallichi* (chuan xiong, ligusticum), *Glycyrrhiza uralensis* (gan cao, licorice), *Cinnamomum cassia* (rou gui, cinnamon bark), *Shao Xing Jiu* (sorghum or rice wine) 24.5% (v/v)

Dosage and method of administration

50-80mls (2 small cups, supplied), daily.

Cautions and contraindications

As for **7.16.1 Shi Quan Da Bu Wan**, but rarely causes digestive upset.

GMP

7.18 YANG YING WAN

3+ / 12

养营丸

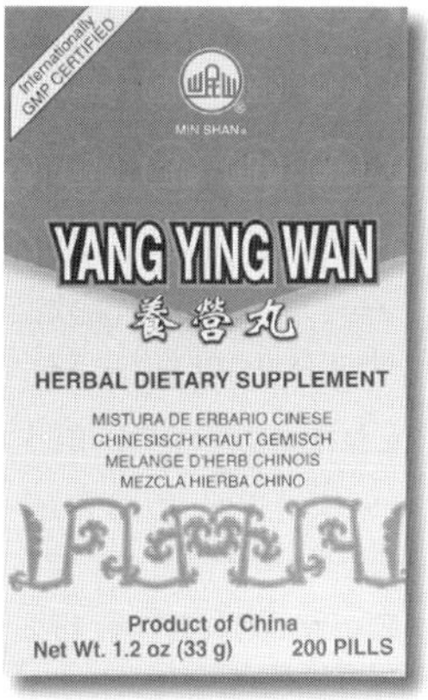

Lanzhou Foci Pharmaceutical Factory (Gansu)
'Nutritive Pills'
Yang Ying Wan is packaged in bottles of 200 pills

Chinese medical action

Warms and tonifies qi and blood, supports yang, fortifies defensive qi, calms the *shén*

Biomedical action

Energy tonic and stimulant, promotes metabolism, nourishes blood and regulates menstruation, promotes circulation to the extremities, sedative, tranquilizer

INDICATIONS

- Similar in actions and indications to **7.16.1 Shi Quan Da Bu Wan**, with the addition of herbs to calms the Heart and *shén*. Used for qi and blood deficiency patterns with *shén* disturbances, insomnia, palpitations, shortness of breath, chronic debility, exhaustion and loss of appetite.
- Convalescence from serious illness, surgery or pregnancy, as well as all chronic disorders of a qi and blood deficiency type.
- Chronic Hepatitis C infection of a qi and blood deficiency type.

Composition

Codonopsis pilosula (dang shen, codonopsis), *Atractylodes macrocephala* (bai zhu, atractylodes), *Poria cocos* (fu ling, hoelen), *Astragalus membranaceous* (huang qi, astragalus), *Glycyrrhiza uralensis* (gan cao, licorice), *Zizyphus jujuba* (da zao, chinese dates), *Angelica sinensis* (dang gui, chinese angelica), *Rehmannia glutinosa* (shu di, processed rehmannia), *Paeonia lactiflora* (bai shao, white peony), *Cinnamomum cassia* (rou gui, cinnamon bark), *Polygala sibiricum* (yuan zhi, polygala), *Citrus reticulata* (chen pi, citrus), *Schizandra chinensis* (wu wei zi, schizandra), *Zingiber officinale* (sheng jiang, ginger)

Dosage and method of administration

8-12 pills three times daily, on an empty stomach. Two lots of 12-18 pills can be taken, morning and evening. In the early stages of treatment (the first few weeks), a 50% increase in dose can be used, then reduced as treatment takes effect.

Cautions and contraindications

Contraindicated during the early phase of acute illness such as colds and flu.

7.19 SHOU WU PIAN

首乌片

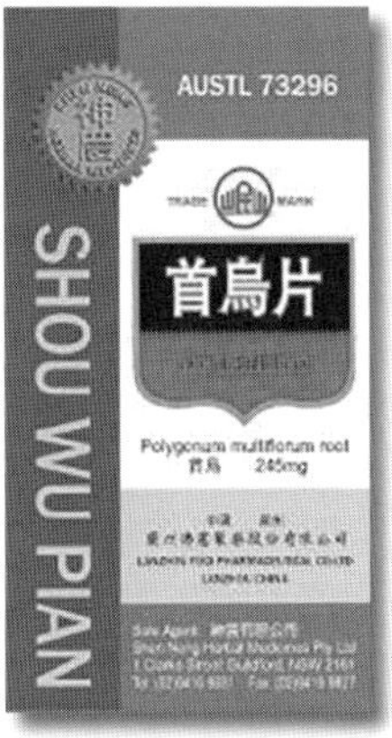

Lanzhou Foci Pharmaceutical Factory (Gansu)
'Polygonum Root Pills'
Shou Wu Pian is packaged in bottles of 100 coated tablets
Also available as: Shou Wu Pian (PF)

Chinese medical action

Tonifies the Liver and Kidneys, benefits essence and nourishes blood and hair

Biomedical action

Hematinic, antioxidant

INDICATIONS

- Liver and Kidney yin and blood deficiency with dizziness, weak or blurring vision, chronic lower back weakness or ache, memory problems and poor hearing, premature graying or loss of head hair, brittle nails and numbness in the extremities.
- Chronic itchy skin diseases and wind rash. Especially good when there is a component of blood deficiency.

Composition (each pill contains powdered)

Polygonum multiflorum (he shou wu, polygonum root) 245mg

Combine with

– **13.2 Xiao Feng Wan** for itchy skin diseases with underlying blood deficiency
– **7.3 Zuo Gui Wan** for falling or prematurely graying hair from Kidney essence deficiency

Dosage and method of administration

4-5 pills, three times daily on an empty stomach. The dose can be increased by 50% for the first week or two to get treatment started.

Cautions and contraindications

Contraindicated during the early phase of acute illness such as colds and flu. Care should be taken in patients with a tendency to abdominal distension, loose stools or phlegm damp.

7.20 CORDYCEPS ESSENCE OF CHICKEN

虫草鸡精

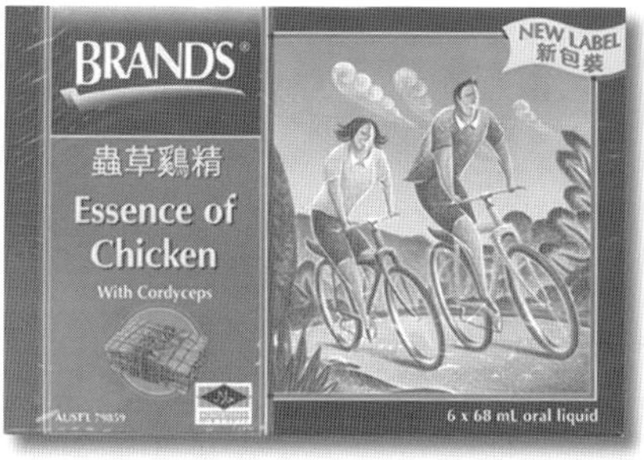

(*Chong Cao Ji Jing*)
Cerebos Thailand Ltd (Thailand)
Cordyceps Essence of Chicken is packaged in 68ml jars of liquid extract, six jars to a box

Chinese medical action

Tonifies the Kidneys and Lungs, warms yang, tonifies Lung qi and yin

Biomedical action

Nutritive to build energy and improve athletic performance, strengthens lung and kidney function, stimulates and protects the immune system

INDICATIONS

- Lung and Kidney yang, yin and qi deficiency. A well balanced nutritive tonic suitable for patients with generalized deficiency. The primary focus of the formula is towards warming and tonifying yang qi. An excellent tonic for the debilitated, elderly and those recovering from prolonged or severe illness, including major surgery and the after effects of radiotherapy of chemotherapy. Assists in strengthening immunity in weak and immunocompromised patients, thus a useful adjunct in conditions such as leukopenia and thrombocytopenia.
- Strengthens the Lungs and improves Lung function to assist in the treatment of chronic consumptive pulmonary diseases of a qi and yin deficiency type, such as pulmonary tuberculosis, sarcoidosis and silicosis, as well as emphysema and chronic asthma.
- Warms Kidney yang to assist in urinary and sexual disorders of a yang deficient type.
- Assists in the improvement of physical endurance, maintenance of peak performance and recovery time in athletes and others with high physical and stress demands.

Composition **(Each jar contains extracts equivalent to dry)**

Black foot chicken extract, *Cordyceps sinensis* (dong chong xia cao, cordyceps stroma) 6.8g, *Rehmannia glutinosa* (shu di, processed rehmannia) 950mg, *Polygonatum officinale* (yu zhu, polygonatum) 950mg, *Cistanches deserticola* (rou cong rong, cistanches) 815mg, *Astragalus membranaceous* (huang qi, astragalus) 540mg

Combine with

- **3.35 Mai Wei Di Huang Wan** or **3.34 Bai He Gu Jin Wan** for chronic respiratory disorders from Lung yin deficiency
- **7.23 Yu Ping Feng Wan**, **2.11 Bu Zhong Yi Qi Wan** or **3.41 Xu Han Ting** for severe spontaneous sweating and immune deficiency
- **3.18 Tung Hsuan Li Fei Pien** for a persistent cough

Pattern identifying features

- **Lung and Kidney yang qi and yin deficiency**
- **general debility, weakness and frailty**
- spontaneous sweating, night sweats
- breathlessness, dyspnea
- poor appetite
- loss of libido, impotence

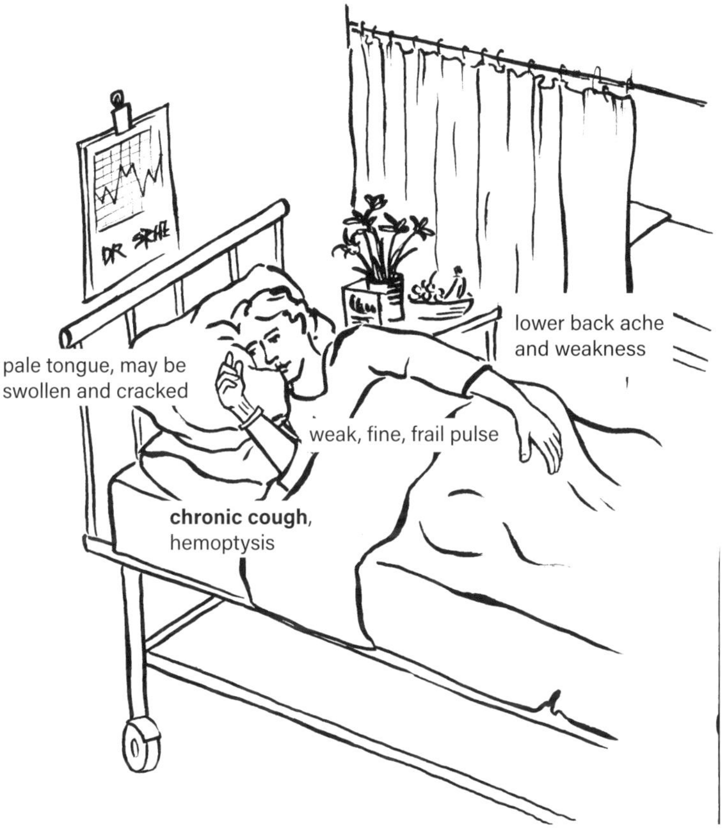

Dosage and method of administration

In the early days of treatment, 1-2 jars may be taken daily, diluted with warm water or straight, or used in cooking. As energy and symptoms improve, one jar every second or third day is usually sufficient.

Cautions and contraindications

Contraindicated during the early phase of acute illness such as colds and flu. Care should be taken in those patients with a tendency to abdominal distension, loose stools or nausea. Some patients may find **7.20 Cordyceps Essence of Chicken** aggravates these symptoms. This can usually be alleviated by dilution with a strong ginger root tea.

7.21 AMERICAN GINSENG ESSENCE OF CHICKEN

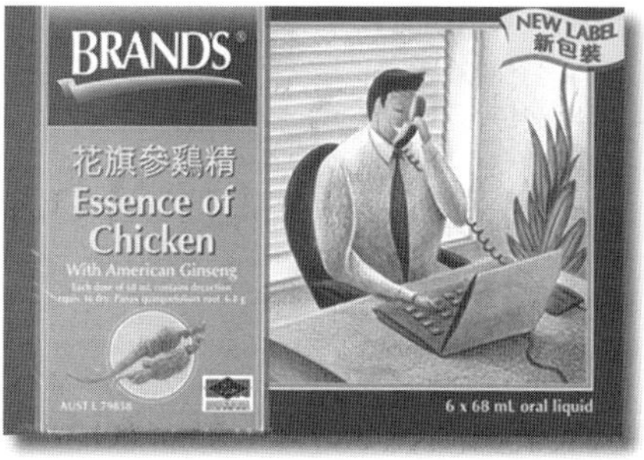

花旗参鸡精

(*Hua Qi Shen Ji Jing*)
Cerebos Thailand Ltd (Thailand)
American Ginseng Essence of Chicken is packaged in 68ml jars of liquid extract, six jars to a box

Chinese medical action

Tonifies qi and yin, generates fluids, strengthens the Lungs

Biomedical action

Tonic to build energy, strengthens the lungs, stimulates and protects the immune system

INDICATIONS

- Lung qi and yin deficiency. Used for chronic respiratory weakness or disease of a qi and yin deficient type. Useful for chronic respiratory irritation in smokers or others exposed to respiratory irritants that dry and damage Lung fluids.
- Used to support patients recuperating from a severe febrile or other illness including surgery, that has damaged qi and yin.
- For those with significant loss of appetite or enhanced nutritional needs, such as patients with cancer or other severe illness.
- For persistent low grade fever associated with qi and yin deficiency.
- Can assist in alleviating the side effects of chemotherapy or radiotherapy, especially dryness and damage to mucous membranes, oral ulceration, decreased salivation and fatigue.

Composition (Each jar contains extracts equivalent to dry)

Black foot chicken, *Panax quinquefolium* (xi yang shen, american ginseng) 6.8g

Combine with

- **7.1.1 Liu Wei Di Huang Wan** or **7.5 Gu Ben Wan** for type 2 diabetes
- **3.33 Yang Yin Qing Fei Wan** or **3.36 Luo Han Kuo Beverage** for severe or chronic dryness of the oral cavity
- **6.1 Xiao Chai Hu Wan** for post febrile fatigue and loss of appetite with mild alternating fever and chills

Pattern identifying features

- **Lung qi and yin deficiency**
- **fatigue, exhaustion**
- high stress
- convalescence following febrile illness

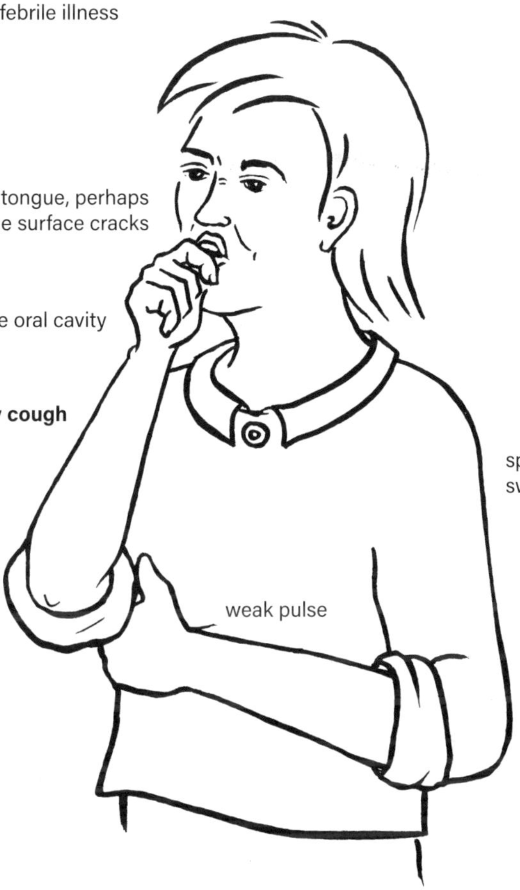

Dosage and method of administration

For recovery following illness, surgery, chemotherapy or radiotherapy, one jar may be taken daily, diluted with warm water. As energy improves, one jar every second or third day is sufficient. For general maintenance of health, one jar every 2-3 days is sufficient.

Cautions and contraindications

Contraindicated during the early phase of acute illness such as colds and flu.

7.22 SHEN QI DA BU WAN

参芪大补丸

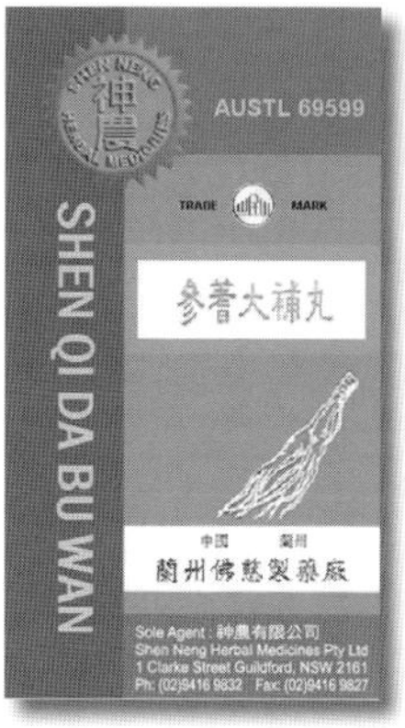

Lanzhou Foci Pharmaceutical Factory (Gansu)
'Codonopsis and Astragalus Major Tonic Pills'
Shen Qi Da Bu Wan is packaged in bottles of 200 pills
Also available as: Shen Qi Wan

Chinese medical action

Tonifies Spleen and Lung qi, fortifies defensive qi

Biomedical action

Energy tonic, immune stimulant, anhidrotic

INDICATIONS

- A general formula to strengthen Spleen and Lung qi and defensive qi. Can be used alone for this purpose, but more frequently is combined with another constitutional formula when an enhanced qi tonification effect is desired.

Composition (each pill contains powdered)

Astragalus membranaceous (huang qi, astragalus) 80mg, *Codonopsis pilosula* (dang shen, codonopsis) 80mg

Combine with

- **2.9 Xiang Sha Liu Jun Wan** for patients with significant deficiency, to enhance the qi tonifying and defensive qi fortifying effect
- **7.1.1 Liu Wei Di Huang Wan** for Kidney yin deficiency with elements of Spleen qi deficiency
- **1.2 Si Wu Wan** for patients with elements of qi deficiency within predominant blood deficiency
- **11.1 Qian Lie Xian Capsule** or **11.2 Prostate Gland Pills** for prostate swelling that is worse when fatigued, and following sex, in patients with Kidney qi deficiency
- **5.8 Bu Yang Huan Wu Wan** to enhance that formula's ability to penetrate through obstructions in the channels and relieve hemiplegia
- **7.23 Yu Ping Feng Wan** or **3.41 Xu Han Ting** for children with immune weakness, tendency to allergies and loss of appetite.

Dosage and method of administration

When used alone, the recommended dose is 8-12 pills three times daily on an empty stomach. When used to augment another formula, 12-15 pills per day is usually sufficient.

Pattern identifying features

- **Lung and Spleen qi deficiency**
- frequent colds, low immunity

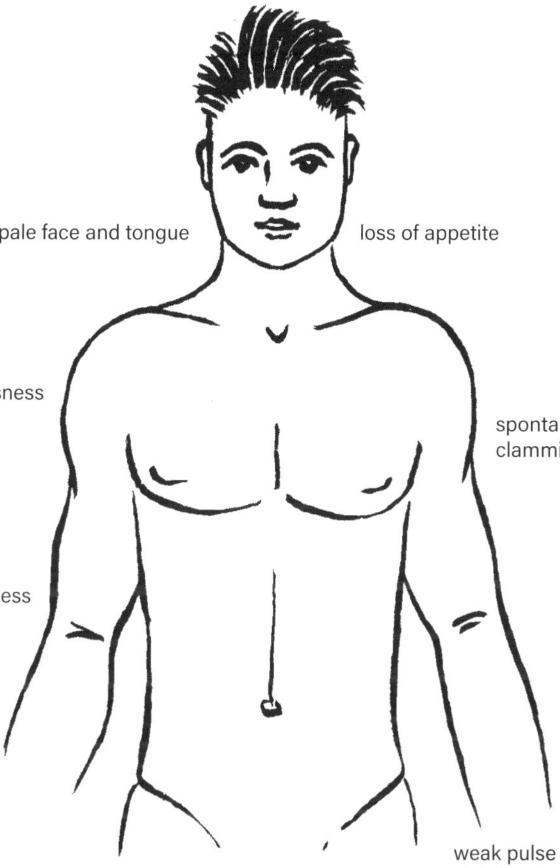

Cautions and contraindications

Contraindicated during the early phase of acute illness such as colds and flu.

7.23 YU PING FENG WAN

玉屏风丸

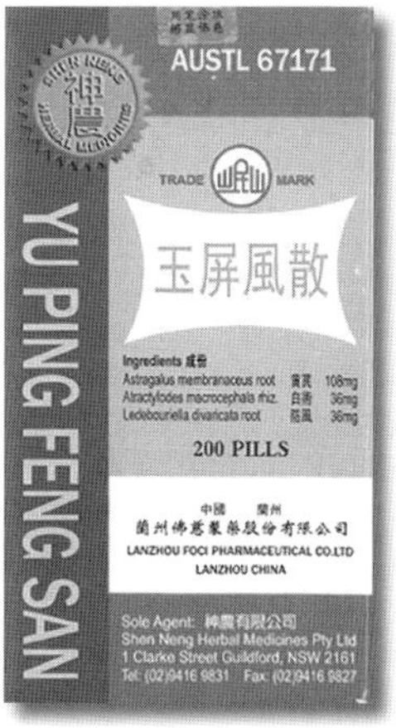

Lanzhou Foci Pharmaceutical Factory (Gansu)
'Jade Screen Wind Pills'
Yu Ping Feng Wan is packaged in bottles of 200 pills
Also available as: Jade Screen Teapills (PF), Astragalus and Siler Formula (conc. extract)

Chinese medical action

Fortifies defensive qi, tonifies the Spleen, secures the surface and stops sweating

Biomedical action

Immune stimulant, strengthens digestion, tones the mucous membranes, anhidrotic

INDICATIONS

- Lung qi and defensive qi deficiency with chronic retention of wind on the surface. **7.23 Yu Ping Feng Wan** strengthens qi and disperses pathogens at the same time. An important formula to strengthen defensive qi and improve the body's resistance to pathogenic invasion, widely used for patients prone to frequent colds and upper respiratory tract infection, or patients unable to shake off the last of a lingering cold. Mostly used in between infections. A popular formula to strengthen weak children.
- Chronic retention of wind in the respiratory system, mucous membranes and skin. This manifests as respiratory allergies–allergic and perennial rhinitis, atopic asthma and a tendency to allergic skin rashes, urticaria and itch.
- Excessive sweating from qi deficiency that occurs at rest and during the day.

Composition (each pill contains powdered)

Astragalus membranaceous (huang qi, astragalus) 108mg, *Atractylodes macrocephala* (bai zhu, atractylodes) 36mg, *Ledebouriella divaricata* (fang feng, siler) 36mg

Combine with

- **9.18 Xin Yi San** for chronic or allergic rhinitis in a patient with qi deficiency
- **4.11 Ba Ji Yan Yang Wan** to strengthen the Lung Kidney axis for patients with an atopic constitution
- **6.1 Xiao Chai Hu Wan** to strengthen immunity in children prone to middle ear infection
- **3.38 Sheng Mai San Wan** for hypo-tension
- **3.41 Xu Han Ting** for persistent sweating
- **7.22 Shen Qi Da Bu Wan** or **2.7 Si Jun Zi Wan** for pronounced Spleen qi deficiency

Pattern identifying features

- **Lung qi and defensive qi deficiency**
- **frequent colds and flu**
- chronic respiratory allergies
- weak immunity
- fatigue, run down
- sensitivity to wind
- breathlessness

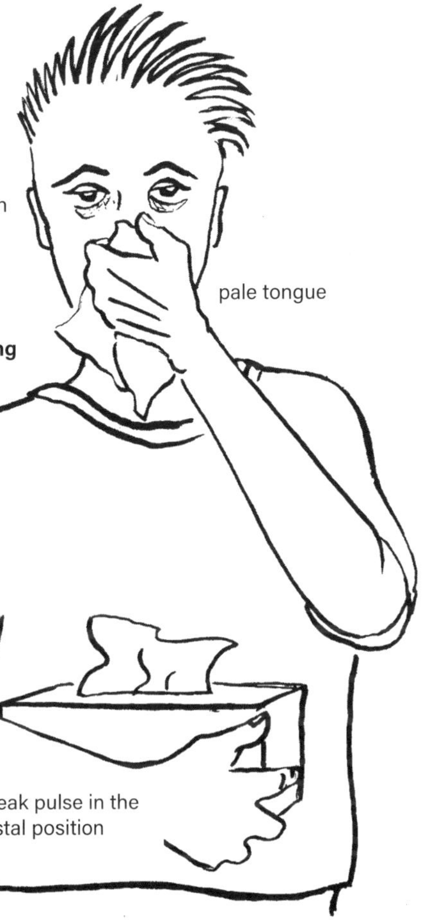

Dosage and method of administration

8-12 pills three times daily, before meals. The dose can be spread out, or taken in two lots of 12-18 pills, morning and evening. In severe cases or during the early stages of treatment (the first few weeks), a 50% increase in dose can be used, then reduced as treatment takes effect. One third to one half dose for children.

Cautions and contraindications

Contraindicated during the early phase of acute illness such as colds and flu, such as a full on wind cold or wind heat invasion.

7.24 PANAX GINSENG EXTRACTUM

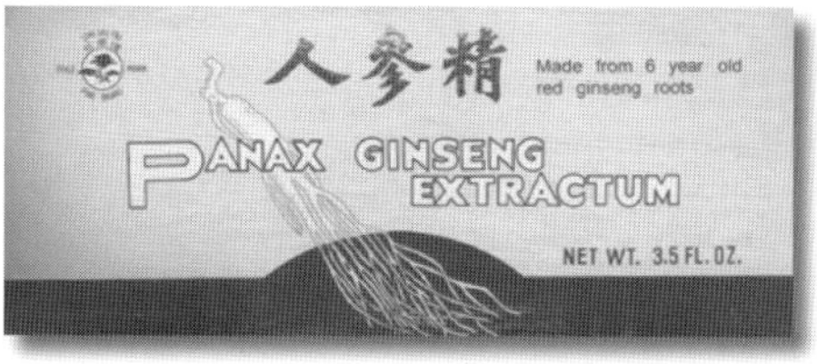

人参精

(Ren Shen Jing)
China National Native Produce and Animal By Products Import Export Corporation (Tianjin)
'Essence of Ginseng'
Panax Ginseng Extractum is packaged in 10ml vials of liquid extract, ten vials per box

Chinese medical action

Tonifies source qi, strengthens the Spleen and Lungs, generates fluids and stops thirst, calms the *shén*

Biomedical action

Immune stimulant, immunomodulating, adaptogenic, regulates adrenal function, lowers blood glucose

INDICATIONS

- Lung and Spleen qi deficiency. A good tonic for all qi deficiency patterns with fatigue, lack of energy, vitality and stamina. Can assist in maintaining strength and well being and augment the immune system in situations where energy demands are high. These include chronic or serious illness (cancer, auto-immune disorders) and post surgical recovery.
- Used to help moderate the negative effects of prolonged or severe stress; helps people adapt to changing conditions and stresses.
- Can help to better regulate and lower blood glucose in patients with hyperglycemia. Useful as an adjunct in the treatment of type 2 diabetes mellitus.
- Can assist recovery following a severe shock or emotional trauma that has dispersed qi, leading to shortness of breath, anxiety, insomnia, mood swings and lethargy.

Composition (each vial contains)

Panax ginseng (ren shen, ginseng) 1200mg

Dosage and method of administration

In the early stages of treatment, three or four vials per day can be used. As the symptoms improve, the dose can be reduced to a maintenance dose of one or two vials per day. The major benefits of ginseng are observed after prolonged and regular use, usually a minimum of two months.

Pattern identifying features

- **Lung and Spleen qi deficiency**
- **fatigue, lack of stamina**
- poor appetite
- hypotension
- immune weakness

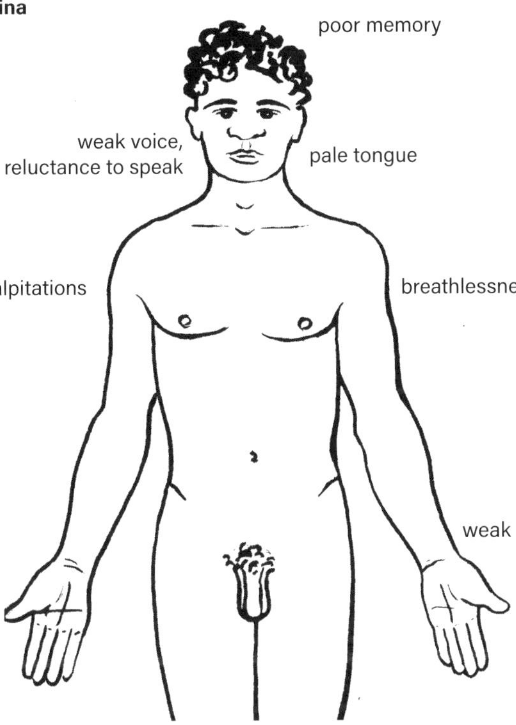

Cautions and contraindications

Contraindicated during the early phase of acute illness such as colds and flu, in patients with heat, yang rising or yin deficiency patterns and in the absence of qi deficiency. Also contraindicated when used alone for patients with a tendency to hypertension, and those with gastric ulcers. Overdose can lead to headaches, insomnia, palpitations, hypertension, tremors, nervousness and anxiety. Concurrent consumption of other stimulants (e.g. coffee) can exacerbate the negative effects. Caution in patients on anticoagulant therapy as ginseng can decrease the effectiveness of warfarin. Caution prior to surgical procedures, as in some patients ginseng can inhibit clotting.

Ginseng products are frequently abused in China and the West, especially by already healthy individuals looking for some sort of super health. Inappropriate use of ginseng by young and otherwise healthy individuals can generate excessive heat and contribute to yin damage.

7.25 PEKING GINSENG ROYAL JELLY

北京人参蜂王精

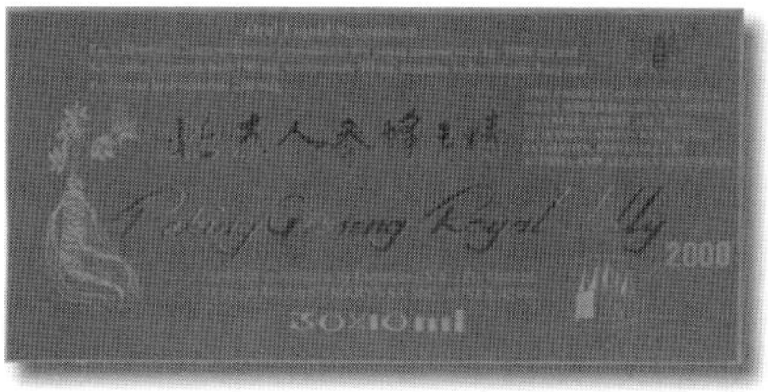

(Bei Jing Ren Shen Feng Wang Jing)
Laboratory de Tonique de Pekin (Beijing)
Peking Ginseng Royal Jelly is packaged in 10ml vials of liquid extract, ten vials per box

Chinese medical action

Tonifies source qi, warms and strengthens the Spleen, Lungs and Liver, generates fluids and stops thirst, calms the *shén*

Biomedical action

Immune stimulant, immunomodulator, adaptogen, lowers blood glucose

INDICATIONS

- A general tonic formula, with warming B vitamins combined with ginseng and royal jelly. Similar in action and indications to **7.24 Panax Ginseng Extractum**, but more warming. There are numerous varieties of royal jelly with and without additional herbs. Their functions are all quite similar. Royal jelly tonifies qi and blood, and strengthens the Liver and Spleen.

Composition (each vial contains)

Fresh Royal Jelly 2000mg, *Panax ginseng* (ren shen, ginseng) 1000mg, *Schizandra chinensis* (wu wei zi, schizandra) 100mg, Nicotinamide 10mg, Thiamine hydrochloride (Vit B1) 3mg, Pyridoxine hydrochloride (Vit B6) 200µg, Benzyl alcohol 100mg, Citric acid monohydrate 8mg, Agar 10mg, Caramel 200mg

Dosage and method of administration

One vial daily.

Cautions and contraindications

Contraindicated in patients with allergy to bee stings, atopic constitutions, and asthma. Although rare, there have been reported deaths from anaphylactic shock following use of royal jelly. Contraindicated during the early phase of acute illness such as colds and flu, in patients with heat yang rising or yin deficiency patterns and in the absence of qi deficiency. Caution in those on anticoagulant therapy as ginseng can decrease the effectiveness of warfarin. Caution prior to surgical procedures, as in some cases when large doses are used, ginseng can inhibit clotting.

Overdose can lead to headaches, insomnia, palpitations, hypertension, tremors, nervousness and anxiety. Concurrent consumption of other warming stimulants (e.g. coffee) can exacerbate the negative effects.

Pattern identifying features

- **fatigue, lack of stamina**
- cold intolerance
- poor appetite
- convalescence
- immune weakness

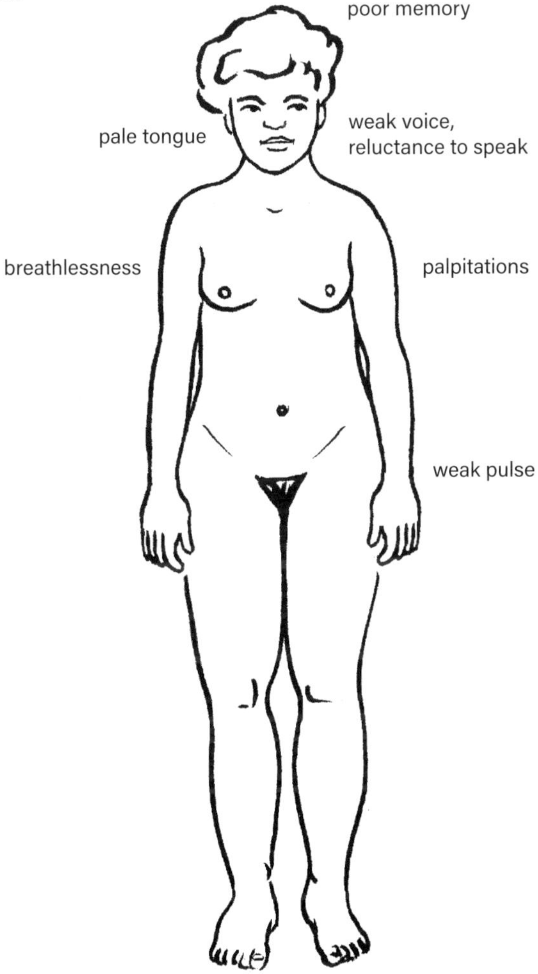

7.26 REISHI MUSHROOM

灵芝

(*Ling Zhi*)

Various manufacturers in Australia, Japan, Korea and China

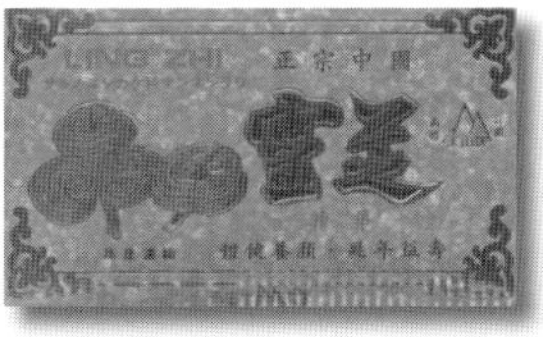

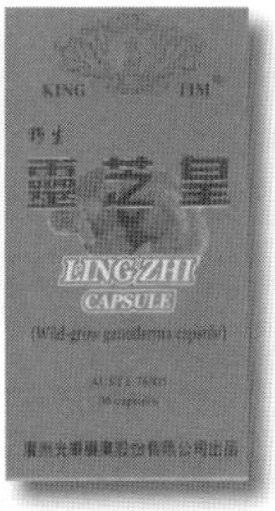

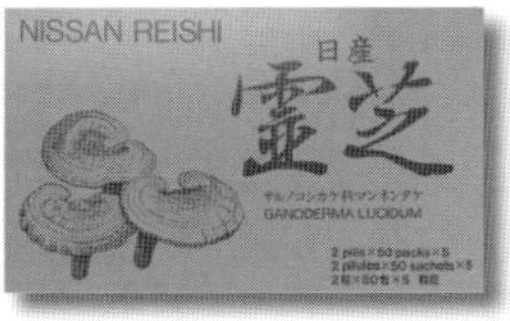

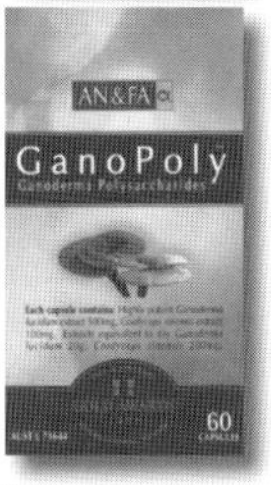

Chinese medical action

Nourishes the Heart and calms the *shén*, stops cough and alleviates wheezing, tonifies qi and blood

Biomedical action

Immune stimulant, adaptogen, immunomodulator, anti-platelet action, antitussive, sedative

INDICATIONS

- Reishi mushroom extract has been shown to exert many beneficial effects consistent with its reputation as an adaptogen. An adaptogen is defined as a substance which increases the resistance to stress and improves the general tone of the body and mind.
- Used to improve immune surveillance as an adjunct treatment for patients with cancer and chronic viral or auto-immune disease. Well designed studies have shown that reishi mushroom appears to improve not only quality of life for those undergoing chemotherapy or radiotherapy, but also can enhance survival and reduce the likelihood of metastasis, as well as help to prevent recurrence.
- May assist in connective tissue diseases such as rheumatoid arthritis, lupus (SLE), Beçhet's syndrome and scleroderma.
- For insomnia, high altitude sickness, sleep apnea, high cholesterol, chronic hepatitis, chronic cough and asthma, allergies and hypersensitive or weakened immune system problems like chronic fatigue syndrome.

Composition

Ganoderma lucidum or *G. japonicum* (ling zhi, reishi). **Note**: Not all available brands are listed with the TGA.

Combine with

- **6.1 Xiao Chai Hu Wan** to assist in maintaining the immune system in patients with chronic hepatitis and allergies
- **7.1.1 Liu Wei Di Huang Wan** for patients on high dose steroid treatment
- **2.11 Bu Zhong Yi Qi Wan** for patients undergoing chemotherapy or radiotherapy
- **3.38 Sheng Mai San Wan** for chronic respiratory diseases of a qi and yin deficient type
- **7.23 Yu Ping Feng Wan** or **3.41 Xu Han Ting** for atopic individuals with allergies, eczema and weak immunity
- **11.5 Wu Zi Yan Zong Wan** for antisperm antibodies or to enhance low sperm count

Pattern identifying features

- **immune weakness or hypersensitivity**
- adjunct to cancer therapy
- lack of vitality, malaise
- sleep apnea

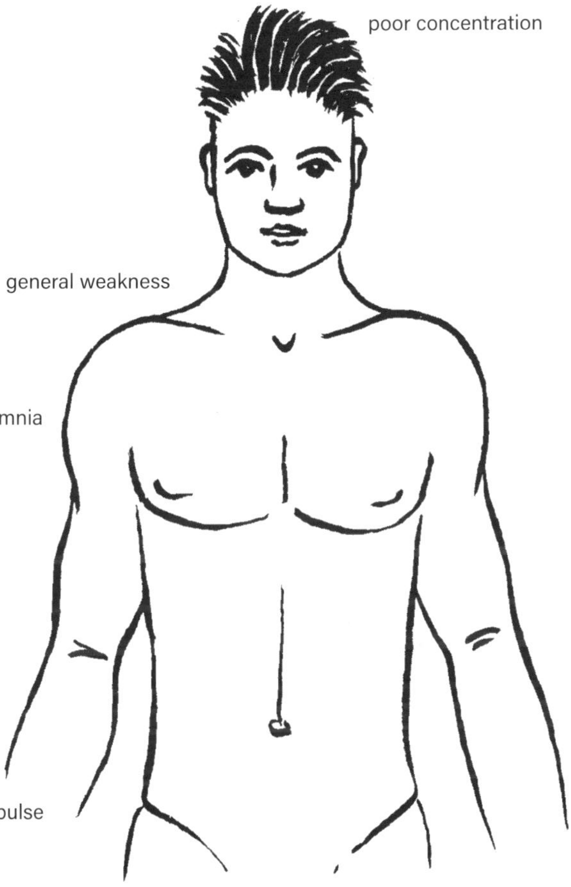

Dosage and method of administration

The manufacturers recommended dose is usually sufficient. Absorption and utilization of reishi mushroom is improved if taken with a dose of vitamin C (500mg is sufficient).

Cautions and contraindications

Reishi mushroom can occasionally cause dizziness, dry mouth and throat, nose bleeds and abdominal upset; these rare effects develop with continuous use over three to six months. As it can increase bleeding time, reishi mushroom is not recommended immediately prior to surgical procedures, or for those taking anticoagulant medications.

神病 8

Shén

8.1 TIAN WANG BU XIN DAN

天王补心丹

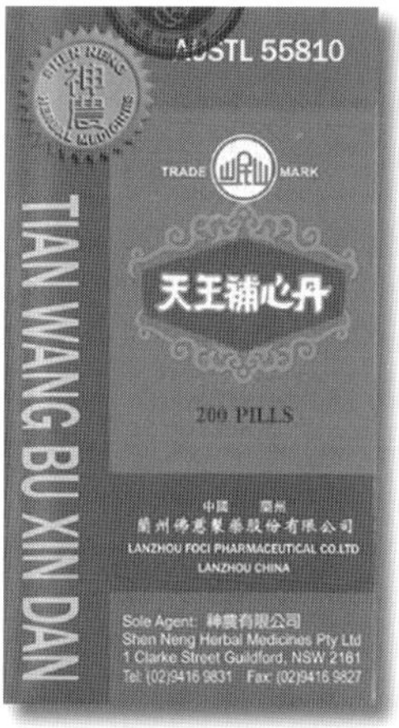

Lanzhou Foci Pharmaceutical Factory (Gansu)
'Heavenly King Heart Tonifying Special Pills'
Tian Wang Bu Xin Dan is packaged in bottles of 200 pills
Also available as: Emperor's Teapills (PF), Tian Wang Pu Hsin Tan, Ginseng and Zizyphus Formula (conc. extract)

Chinese medical action

Tonifies Heart and Kidney yin, nourishes blood, calms the *shén*, clears heat from deficiency

Biomedical action

Sedative and tranquilizer, nervine, calmative

INDICATIONS

- Heart and Kidney yin deficiency patterns with *shén* disturbances, in particular chronic insomnia and anxiety. This pattern is also described as Heart and Kidney not communicating and *shào yīn* syndrome of a heat transformation type. Not an especially cooling formula, it can be used for patterns of qi and yin deficiency, a common dual pathology often seen in *shén* disturbances.
- Used for those who have taken sedatives or tranquilizing drugs for so long the drugs have become ineffective. Also good for the physical and psychological damage inflicted by long term stimulant use (ice, amphetamines, cocaine etc.) including paranoia, agitation, anxiety and insomnia.
- Yin deficiency patterns complicated by a degree of phlegm or phlegm heat, seen in conditions such as chronic or recurrent oral ulceration, swellings in the neck and thyroid gland.
- With the appropriate identifying features, this formula can be used to assist the treatment of conditions such as acute and chronic anxiety states, panic attacks, chronic insomnia, memory problems, palpitations, tachycardia, cardiac arrhythmias, menopausal syndrome, chronic urticaria, chronic or recurrent apthous ulcers, stomatitis, Beçhet's syndrome, hyperthyroidism, benign thyroid nodules and neurasthenia.

Composition (each pill contains powdered)

Rehmannia glutinosa (sheng di, rehmannia) 60mg, *Angelica sinensis* (dang gui, chinese angelica) 15mg, *Schizandra chinensis* (wu wei zi, schizandra) 15mg, *Zizyphus spinoza* (suan zao ren, zizyphus) 15mg, *Biota orientalis* (bai zi ren, biota) 15mg, *Asparagus lucidius* (tian dong, asparagus) 15mg, *Ophiopogon japonicus* (mai dong, ophiopogon) 15mg, *Scrophularia ningpoensis* (xuan shen, scrophularia) 15mg, *Salvia miltorrhiza* (dan shen, salvia) 7mg, *Codonopsis pilosula* (dang shen, codonopsis) 7mg, *Poria cocos* (fu ling, hoelen) 7mg, *Platycodon grandiflorum* (jie geng, platycodon) 7mg, *Polygala sibirica* (yuan zhi, polygala) 7mg

Pattern identifying features

- **Heart and Kidney yin deficiency *shén* disturbances; Heart qi and yin deficiency**
- tiredness compounded by a sense of jitteriness that makes resting difficult
- waking feeling hot, night sweats, hot hands and feet, dry skin and hair
- patients tend to be thin, dry and nervy or agitated
- chronic or recurrent mouth ulcers

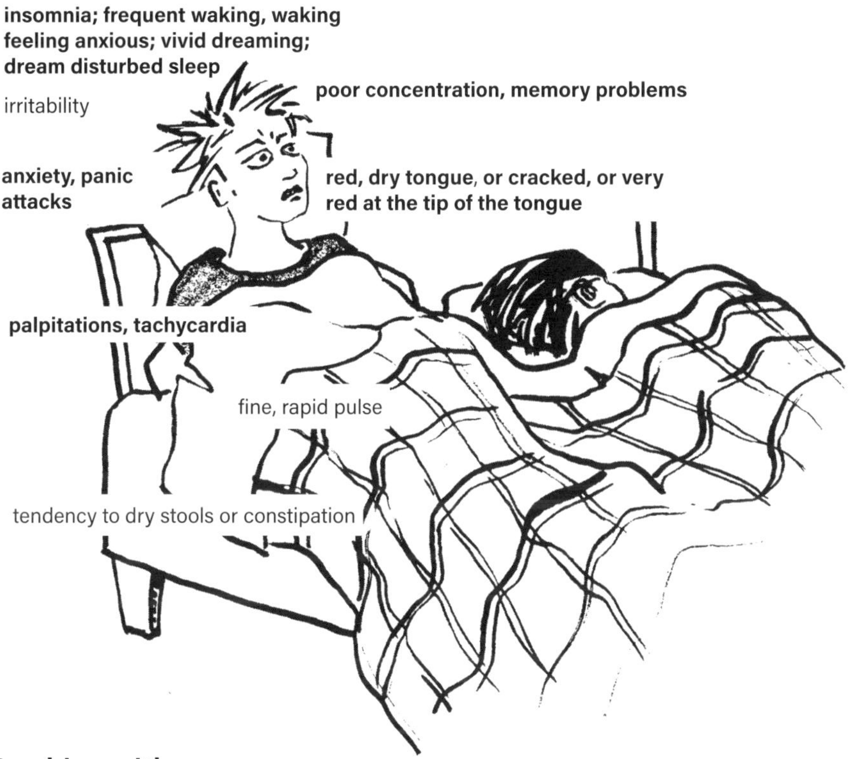

Combine with

– **9.10 Sanjin Watermelon Frost** for recurrent mouth ulcers

Dosage and method of administration

8-12 pills three times daily on an empty stomach. The dose can be spread out, or taken in two lots of 12-18 pills, morning and evening before bed. In severe cases or during the early stages of treatment (the first few weeks), a 50% increase in dose can be used, then reduced as treatment takes effect.

Cautions and contraindications

Contraindicated during the early phase of acute illness such as colds and flu. Generally well tolerated, but care should be taken in patients with a tendency to abdominal distension, loose stools or general digestive weakness. Digestive upsets can usually be alleviated by taking this formula with a small dose (3-6 pills at the same time) of **2.18 Bao He Wan** or **2.9 Xiang Sha Liu Jun Wan**.

8.2 BAI ZI YANG XIN WAN

柏子养心丸

3+/12

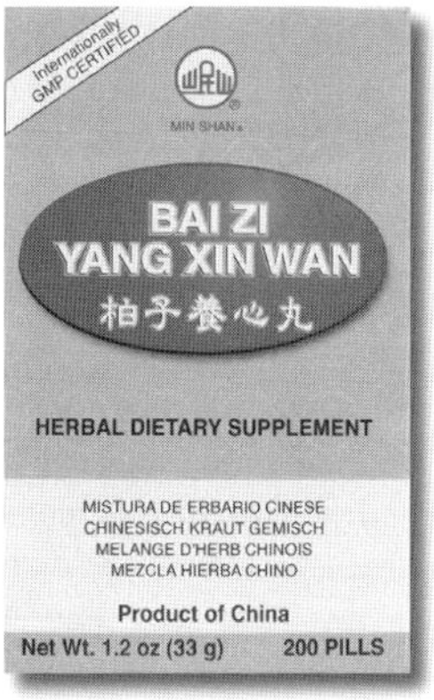

Lanzhou Foci Pharmaceutical Factory (Gansu)
'Biota Seed Pills to Nourish the Heart'
Bai Zi Yang Xin Wan is packaged in bottles of 200 pills
Also available as: Heavenly Heart Teapills (PF)

Chinese medical action
Tonifies Heart blood and yin, clears heat, calms the *shén*

Biomedical action
Sedative, tranquilizer

INDICATIONS
- *Shén* disturbances, in particular anxiety and insomnia, from Heart blood and/or yin deficiency.
- Night sweats from yin deficiency. Although on the cooling side, this formula is mild enough to be used for heat or thermally neutral presentations, and combines well with other constitutional formulas when additional *shén* calming action is desired.
- With the appropriate identifying features, this formula can assist in treating conditions such as neurasthenia, chronic anxiety states and insomnia, loss of memory, recurrent nightmares, palpitations, tachycardia and arrhythmias. Also useful for anxiety or insomnia that can occur in the aftermath of a febrile illness that has damaged yin and fluids.

Composition
Biota orientalis (bai zi ren, biota seed), *Rehmannia glutinosa* (shu di, prepared rehmannia), *Scrophularia ningpoensis* (xuan shen, scrophularia), *Acorus gramineus* (shi chang pu, acorus), *Poria cocos* (fu ling, hoelen), *Lycium chinensis* (gou qi zi, lycium fruit), *Ophiopogon japonica* (mai dong, ophiopogon), *Angelica sinensis* (dang gui, chinese angelica), *Glycyrrhiza uralensis* (gan cao, licorice)

Combine with
- **1.2 Si Wu Wan** for patients with a greater degree of blood deficiency
- **1.9 Gui Pi Wan** for Heart blood and Spleen qi deficiency
- **8.1 Tian Wang Bu Xin Dan** for marked insomnia from Heart yin deficiency
- **3.41 Xu Han Ting** for night sweats with insomnia and anxiety

Dosage and method of administration
8-12 pills three times daily on an empty stomach. In severe cases or during the early stages of treatment (the first few weeks), a 50% increase in dose can be used, then reduced as treatment takes effect.

Pattern identifying features

- **Heart blood and/or yin deficiency**
- **insomnia, nightmares, vivid or disturbing dreams**
- night sweats

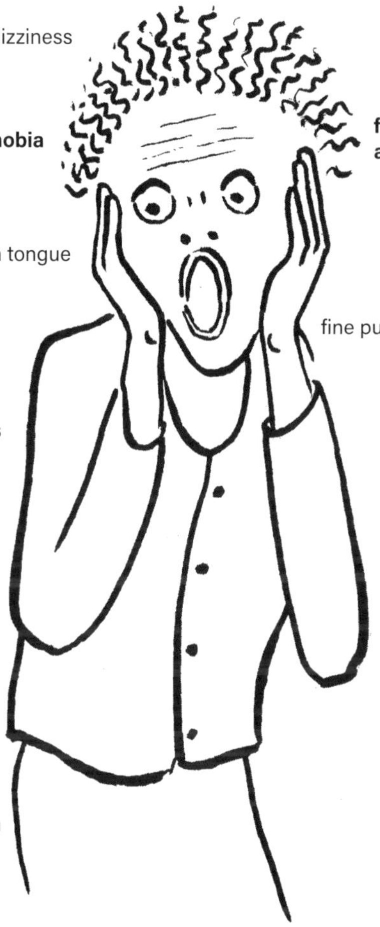

Cautions and contraindications

Contraindicated during the early phase of acute illness such as colds and flu. Generally well tolerated, but care should be taken in patients with a tendency to abdominal distension, loose stools or general digestive weakness. Digestive upsets can usually be alleviated by taking this formula with a small dose (3-6 pills at the same time) of **2.18 Bao He Wan** or **2.9 Xiang Sha Liu Jun Wan**.

8.3 AN SHEN DING ZHI WAN

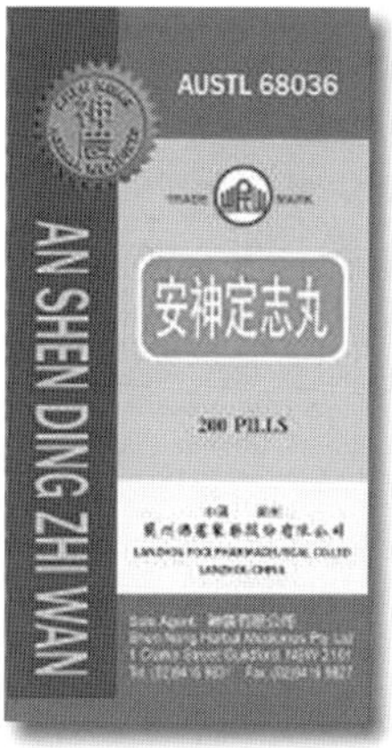

安神定志丸

Lanzhou Foci Pharmaceutical Factory (Gansu)
'Calm the *Shén* and Settle the *Zhì* Pills'
An Shen Ding Zhi Wan is packaged in bottles of 200 pills

Chinese medical action

Tonifies yin, qi and blood, calms the *shén* and *zhì*, transforms phlegm

Biomedical action

Sedative for anxiety and mild neurosis, nervine

INDICATIONS

- *Shén* disturbances, insomnia and anxiety states from qi, blood and/or yin deficiency, with or without insubstantial phlegm misting the Heart. A thermally neutral and broad acting *shén* calming formula, it can be combined with an appropriate constitutional formula where an increased *shén* calming effect is desired.

Composition (each pill contains powdered)

Zizyphus jujuba (da zao, chinese dates) 20.2mg, *Poria cocos* (fu ling, hoelen) 17.2mg, *Paeonia alba* (bai shao, white peony) 17.2mg, *Polygonum multiflorum* (ye jiao teng, polygonum vine) 17.2mg, *Glycyrrhiza uralensis* (gan cao, licorice) 16.1mg, *Ophiopogon japonica* (mai dong, ophiopogon) 13.7mg, *Zizyphus spinoza* (suan zao ren, zizyphus) 13.7mg, *Biota orientalis* (bai zi ren, biota seed) 13mg, *Curcuma longa* (yu jin, curcuma) 13mg, *Pinellia ternata* (zhi ban xia, processed pinellia) 13mg, *Polygala sibirica* (yuan zhi, polygala) 9.6mg, *Chrysanthemum sinensis* (ju hua, chrysanthemum) 9.6mg, *Schizandra chinensis* (wu wei zi, schizandra) 6.4mg

Combine with

- **1.9 Gui Pi Wan** for persistent anxiety states and insomnia from Spleen qi and Heart blood deficiency
- **8.1 Tian Wang Bu Xin Dan** for persistent anxiety states and insomnia from Heart and Kidney yin deficiency
- **6.4 Xiao Yao Wan** for anxiety and insomnia from constrained Liver qi

Dosage and method of administration

8-12 pills three times daily on an empty stomach, but when combining **8.3 An Shen Ding Zhi Wan** with a constitutional formula, a half dose is usually sufficient. In severe cases or during the early stages of treatment (the first few weeks), a 50% increase in dose can be used, then reduced to a maintenance dose as treatment takes effect.

Pattern identifying features

- **blood, qi and yin deficiency; phlegm misting the Heart**
- **insomnia**
- dream disturbed sleep, nightmares
- racing mind at night; difficulty settling to sleep

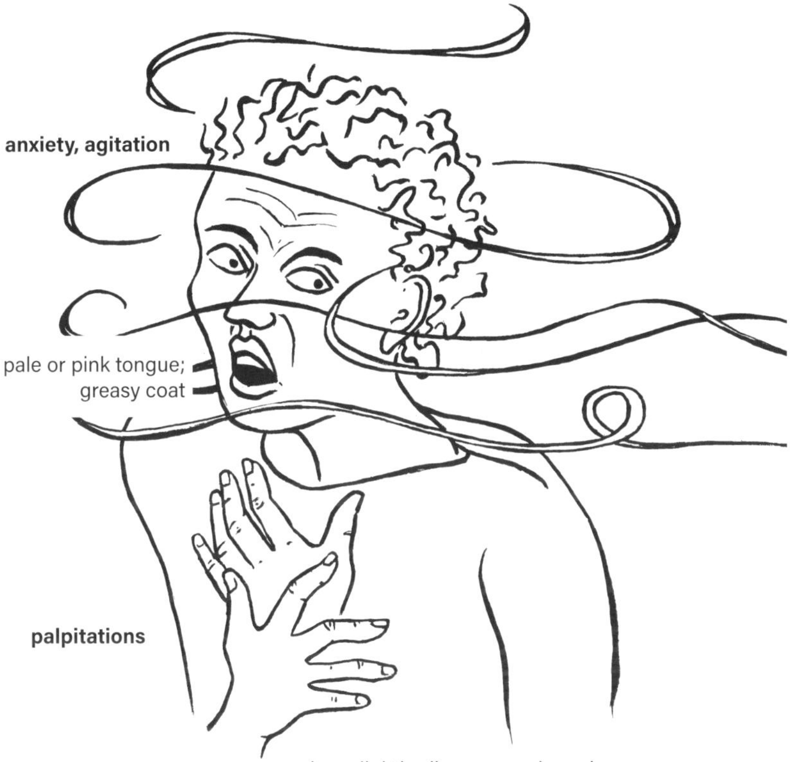

Cautions and contraindications

Contraindicated during the early phase of acute illness such as colds and flu.

GMP

8.4 AN SHEN BU XIN WAN

安神补心丸

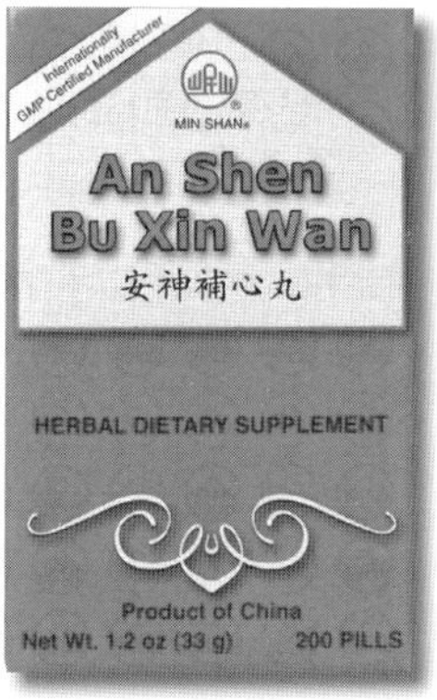

Lanzhou Foci Pharmaceutical Factory (Gansu)
'Calm the *Shén* and Tonify the Heart Pills'
An Shen Bu Xin Wan is packaged in bottles of 200 pills
Also available as: An Shen Bu Xin Teapills (PF)

Chinese medical action

Calms the *hún* and *shén*, tonifies yin and blood, regulates qi and invigorates blood

Biomedical action

Sedative, tranquilizer

INDICATIONS

- Heart and Liver yin and blood deficiency patterns with relatively severe *shén* and/or *hún* disturbance. This formula utilizes a high proportion of the mineral sedative, mother of pearl, to weigh down and anchor the *hún* and *shén*. The main focus of the formula is to quickly sedate and calm, while secondarily tonifying the underlying deficiency. Being able to sedate yang and regulate qi and blood, it is also good for *shén* and *hún* disturbances as a result of stress or emotional trauma.
- Used for irritability, restlessness, resistant insomnia or nightmare disturbed sleep, stress induced insomnia or palpitations, insomnia or panic attacks following trauma, post traumatic stress disorder, hypertension, sleepwalking, palpitations and anxiety.

Composition

Pteria martensii (zhen zhu mu, mother of pearl), *Polygonum multiflorum* (ye jiao teng, polygonum vine), *Ligustrum lucidum* (nu zhen zi, privet fruit), *Eclipta prostrata* (han lian cao, eclipta), *Salvia miltiorrhiza* (dan shen, salvia), *Cuscuta chinensis* (tu su zi, cuscuta), *Albizzia julibrissin* (he huan pi, albizzia), *Rehmannia glutinosa* (shu di, processed rehmannia), *Schizandra chinensis* (wu wei zi, schizandra), *Acorus gramineus* (shi chang pu, acorus)

Combine with

– **6.4 Xiao Yao Wan** or **8.7 An Shen Jie Yu Capsule** for anxiety and insomnia from constrained Liver qi

Dosage and method of administration

8-12 pills three times daily on an empty stomach, best towards the end of the day or before bedtime. In severe cases or during the early stages of treatment (the first few weeks), a 50% increase in dose can be used, then reduced to a maintenance dose as treatment takes effect. Generally only used for a few weeks, or until the *shén* and *hún* have settled, after which a more constitutional approach should be phased in.

Pattern identifying features

- **Yin and blood deficiency with unsettled *hún* and *shén***
- **insomnia, dream disturbed sleep, nightmares**
- **irritability, restlessness**
- heat intolerance
- facial flushing
- emotional instability

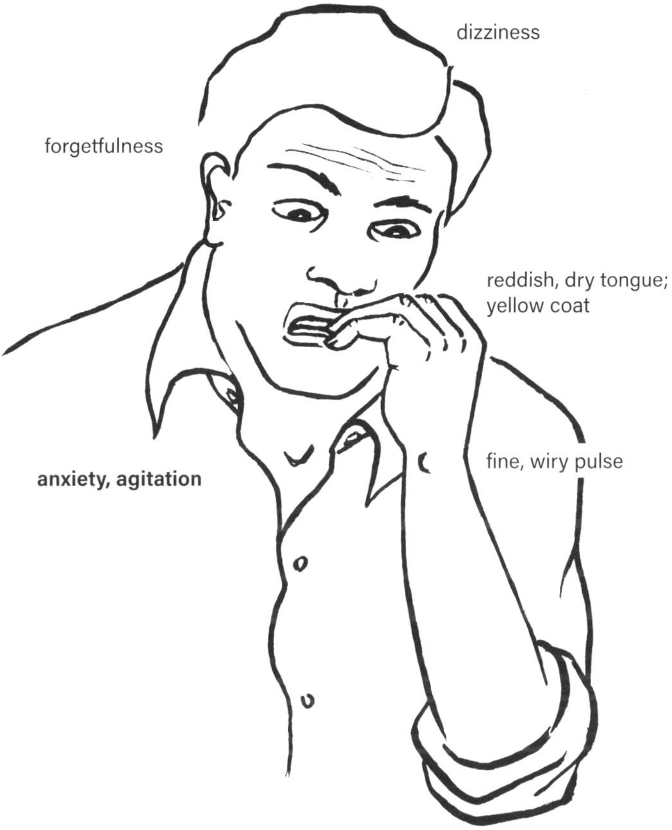

Cautions and contraindications

Contraindicated during pregnancy. Caution in patients on anticoagulant therapy. Watch for bruising or increased tendency to bleeding.

8.5 SHUIAN CAPSULE

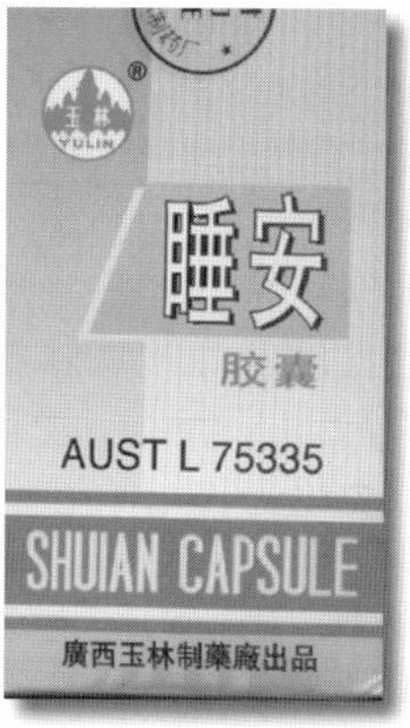

睡安胶囊

(*Shui An Jiao Nang*)
Yulin Drug Manufactory (Guangxi)
'Peaceful Sleep Capsules'
Shuian Capsules are packaged in bottles of 30 capsules
A formula with similar intent is available as: An Shui Teapills (PF)

Chinese medical action

Nourishes blood, settles the Heart, calms the *shén*

Biomedical action

Mild sedative, tranquilizer

INDICATIONS

- Insomnia, nervous tension and mild anxiety from blood and yin deficiency. May be used alone for mild patterns or added to a constitutional formula when enhanced *shén* calming action is desired.

Composition (each capsule contains extracts equivalent to)

Zizyphus spinoza (suan zao ren, zizyphus) 125mg, *Poria cocos* (fu ling, hoelen) 100mg, *Polygonum multiflorum* (ye jiao teng, polygonum vine) 100mg, *Schizandra chinensis* (wu wei zi, schizandra) 95mg, *Polygala sibirica* (yuan zhi, polygala) 80mg

Combine with

- **1.9 Gui Pi Wan** for persistent anxiety states and insomnia from Spleen qi and Heart blood deficiency
- **8.1 Tian Wang Bu Xin Dan** for relatively severe anxiety states and insomnia from Heart and Kidney yin deficiency
- **6.4 Xiao Yao Wan** or **6.5 Jia Wei Xiao Yao Wan** for anxiety and insomnia from constrained Liver qi

Dosage and method of administration

3 capsules, three times daily, preferably later in the day or close to bedtime.

Cautions and contraindications

Contraindicated during the early phase of acute illness such as colds and flu.

GMP

3+/12

8.6 SUAN ZAO REN TANG PIAN

酸枣仁汤片

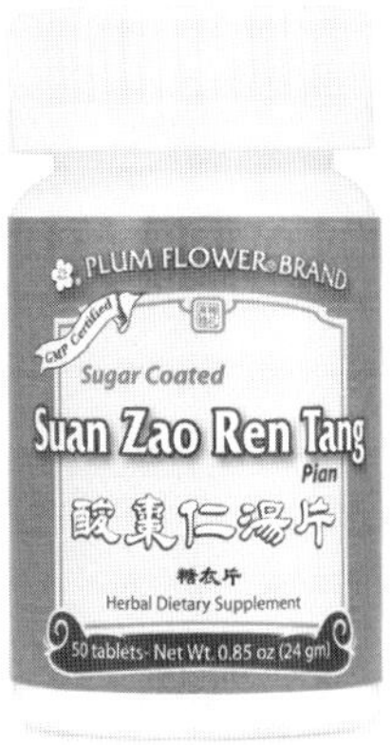

Guangzhou Qixing Pharmaceutical Co. (Guangzhou)
'Zizyphus Pills'
Suan Zao Ren Wan is packaged in bottles of 50 sugar coated tablets
Also available as: Zizyphus Combination (conc. extract)

Chinese medical action

Nourishes Liver blood, calms the *shén* and *hún*, clears heat, alleviates irritability

Biomedical action

Sedative, tranquilizer

INDICATIONS

- Sleep disturbance from Liver blood and yin deficiency. The bulk of this formula is composed of zizyphus, a gentle and effective sedative herb that nourishes the Liver and Heart, and is suitable for mild *shén* and *hún* disturbances. On balance, this formula is cooling, and is considered best for patterns with a degree of heat, although it can also be for patterns without heat. When the deficiency does generate some heat, there may also be night sweats, irritability, dryness of the mouth and throat and a red tongue. Commonly used for menopausal syndrome with sleep disturbances and irritability. Can be added to a constitutional formula when enhanced *shén* and *hún* calming and sedative action is required.

Composition

Zizyphus spinoza (suan zao ren, zizyphus), *Poria cocos* (fu ling, hoelen), *Ligusticum wallichi* (chuan xiong, ligusticum), *Anemarrhena aspheloides* (zhi mu, anemarrhena), *Glycyrrhiza uralensis* (gan cao, licorice)

Combine with

– **1.25 Er Xian Wan** or **1.23 Zhi Bai Di Huang Wan** for anxiety during menopause
– **6.4 Xiao Yao Wan** for anxiety and insomnia from constrained Liver qi

Dosage and method of administration

2-3 pills three times daily on an empty stomach, preferably towards the end of the day or close to bedtime. In severe cases a 50% increase in dose can be used, then reduced as treatment takes effect.

Cautions and contraindications

None noted.

8.7 AN SHEN JIE YU CAPSULE

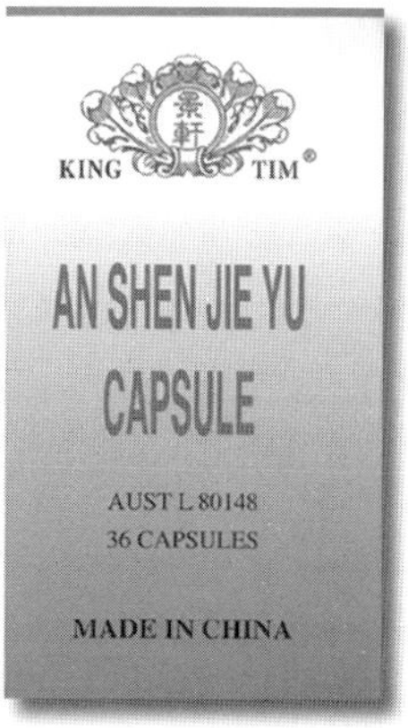

安神解郁丸

(*An Shen Jie Yu Wan*)
Jing Xian Pharmaceutical Co. (Guangzhou)
'Calm the *Shén* and Alleviate [Qi] Constraint Pills'
An Shen Jie Yu Capsules are packaged in bottles of 36 capsules

Chinese medical action

Soothes the Liver and regulates qi, calms the *shén* and settles the *hún*

Biomedical action

Sedative, tranquilizer

INDICATIONS

- *Shén* disturbances associated with constrained Liver qi. Liver qi constraint influences the Heart and *shén* via the generating cycle, and this type of *shén* disturbance typically occurs during periods of increased stress and emotional tension, or during the premenstrual period. Typical features include insomnia accompanied by headaches, stiff neck and muscular tension. Patient typically wake between 1-3am. Because the Liver and thus the *hún* is involved, some patients experience sleepwalking.
- With the appropriate identifying features, this formula can assist in treating conditions such as bruxism, stress induced sleep disturbances and premenstrual insomnia.

Composition (each capsule contains extracts equivalent to)

Schizandra chinensis (wu wei zi, schizandra) 765mg, *Polygala sibirica* (yuan zhi, polygala) 382mg, *Lycium barbarum* (gou qi zi, lycium fruit) 382mg, *Atractylodes macrocephala* (bai zhu, atractylodes) 340mg, *Bupleurum falcatum* (chai hu, bupleurum) 306mg, *Zizyphus spinoza* (suan zao ren, zizyphus) 306mg, *Poria cocos* (fu shen, hoelen spirit) 306mg

Combine with

- **6.4 Xiao Yao Wan** for more severe Liver qi constraint
- **6.5 Jia Wei Xiao Yao Wan** for more severe insomnia and restlessness due to qi constraint with heat

Dosage and method of administration

3 capsules, three times daily. The days dose can also be taken later in the day, close to bedtime.

Pattern identifying features

- ***Shén* and *hún* disturbance associated with Liver qi constraint**
- insomnia, easy waking (especially around 1-3am), vivid dreaming
- irritability, anger outbursts, depression
- frequent sighing

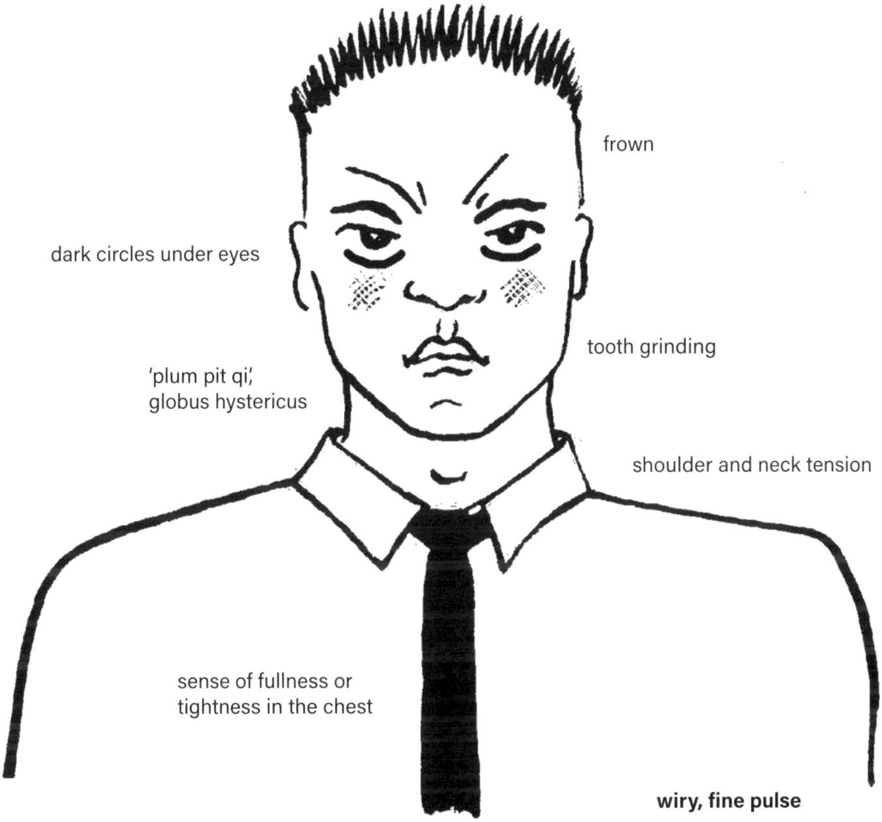

Cautions and contraindications

None noted.

8.8 WEN DAN WAN

温胆丸

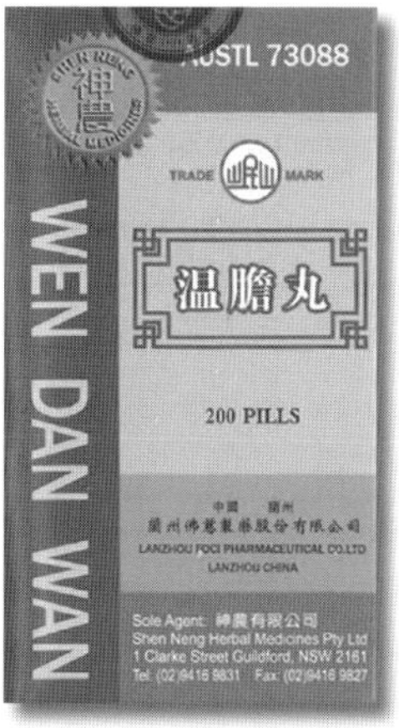

Lanzhou Foci Pharmaceutical Factory (Gansu)
'Warm Gallbladder Pills'
Wen Dan Wan is packaged in bottles of 200 pills
Also available as: Rising Courage Teapills (PF), Poria and Bamboo Combination (conc. extract)

Chinese medical action

Clears and transforms phlegm heat, regulates qi, harmonizes the Stomach and Gallbladder, calms the *shén*

Biomedical action

Sedative, tranquilizer, expectorant

INDICATIONS

- Phlegm heat. An important formula for phlegm heat affecting the Heart and *shén*, Gallbladder and Stomach. Used for a wide variety of mental emotional complaints of a phlegm heat type, especially those characterized by anxiety and insomnia.
- Nausea, vomiting and morning sickness, indigestion and indefinable epigastric discomfort from Stomach and Gallbladder disharmony with phlegm heat clogging the digestion.
- Dizziness, vertigo, fuzzy head and poor concentration from phlegm heat in the head. In severe cases, phlegm heat in the head can contribute to tremor and convulsion patterns, as well as epilepsy or absences.
- Fatigue, insomnia, restlessness, depression and anxiety states in the aftermath of a serious febrile illness that consumes yin and congeals fluids into phlegm. Also for residual cough or wheezing from phlegm heat following an upper respiratory tract infection.
- With the appropriate identifying features, this formula can assist in the treatment of Meniere's disease, the early stages of schizophrenia and other mental disorders, anxiety states, arrhythmias, acute and chronic gastritis, hypertension, post febrile insomnia and anxiety and chronic bronchitis.

Composition (each pill contains powdered)

Bambusa textilis (zhu ru, bamboo shavings) 24.8mg, Citrus aurantium (zhi shi, aurantium) 24.8mg, Pinellia ternata (zhi ban xia, processed pinellia) 24.8mg, Citrus reticulata (chen pi, citrus) 24.8mg, Poria cocos (fu ling, hoelen) 24.8mg, Zingiber officinale (sheng jiang, ginger) 12mg, Zizyphus jujuba (da zao, chinese dates) 12mg

Combine with

- A small dose of **14.2 Huang Lian Su Tablets** for severe phlegm heat
- **7.22 Shen Qi Da Bu Wan** for qi deficiency
- **15.4 Tian Ma Gou Teng Wan** for vertigo
- **3.21 She Dan Chuan Bei Ye** for residual cough from phlegm heat congestion in the Lungs

Pattern identifying features

Phlegm heat affecting the Heart and *shén*; Stomach and Gallbladder disharmony

- **insomnia, waking early in the morning**
- restlessness, irritability
- bitter taste in the mouth
- indefinable epigastric discomfort
- tinnitus

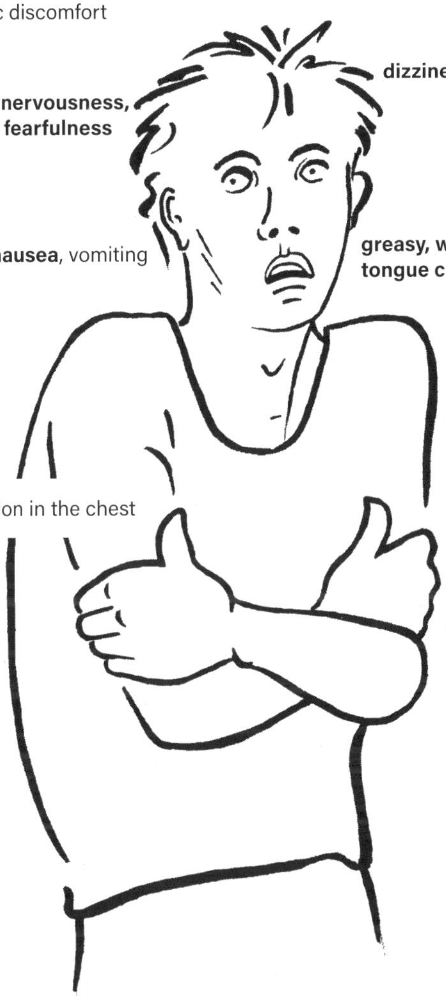

– **8.3 An Shen Ding Zhi Wan** for severe insomnia or anxiety

Dosage and method of administration

8-12 pills three times daily on an empty stomach. The dose can be spread out, or taken in two lots of 12-18 pills, morning and evening. In severe cases or during the early stages of treatment (the first few weeks), a 50% increase in dose can be used, then reduced as treatment takes effect.

Cautions and contraindications

Contraindicated in *shén* disturbances from yin or blood deficiency.

GMP

8.9 CHAI HU LONG GU MU LI WAN

柴胡龙骨牡蛎丸

1-3/12

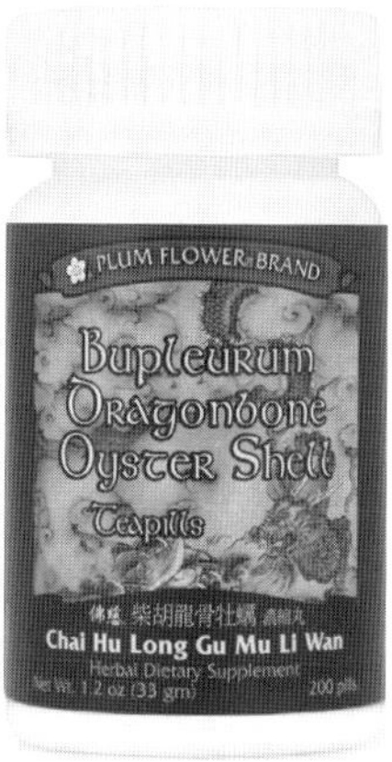

Lanzhou Foci Pharmaceutical Factory (Gansu)
'Bupleurum, Dragon Bone and Oyster Shell Pills'
Chai Hu Long Gu Mu Li Wan is packaged in bottles of 200 pills
Also available as: Bupleurum and Dragon Bone Combination (conc. extract)

Chinese medical action

Harmonizes *shào yáng*, clears heat from the Liver and Intestines, restrains ascendant yang, clears phlegm heat, sedates the *shén* and *hún*

Biomedical action

Sedative, nervine, sedates the sympathetic nervous system

INDICATIONS

- Liver qi constraint, phlegm heat, ascendant Liver yang and/or Liver and Heart fire giving rise to relatively severe emotional or psychological pathology, manifesting as severe irritability, agitation or manic behavior. Patients are usually robust, and display clear signs of excess. Traditionally used for simultaneous pathology of the three yang levels of the Six Level disease differentiation system (*see* glossary) following iatrogenic purgation of a superficial pathogen.
- Used to alleviate the symptoms of drug withdrawal (including tobacco, narcotics and stimulants), in particular the agitation and irritability, insomnia, anxiety, palpitations and tachycardia.
- Palpitations or cardiac arrhythmia that occur at rest (cf. **8.1 Tian Wang Bu Xin Dan** and **1.9 Gui Pi Wan** for palpitations that occur with exertion).
- Seizures or tremors associated with Liver fire and phlegm accumulation.
- With the appropriate identifying features, this formula can assist in treating conditions such as hypertension, hyperthyroidism, epilepsy, cardiac arrhythmia, withdrawal from narcotics and other drugs of addiction, post traumatic stress disorder, schizophrenia and manic depressive psychosis.

Composition

Bupleurum falcatum (chai hu, bupleurum), *Pinellia ternata* (zhi ban xia, processed pinellia), *Poria cocos* (fu ling, hoelen), *Cinnamomum cassia* (gui zhi, cinnamon twigs), *Scutellaria baicalensis* (huang qin, scute), *Zizyphus jujuba* (da zao, chinese dates), *Codonopsis pilosula* (dang shen, codonopsis), *Os Draconis* (duan long gu, calcined dragon bone), *Ostrea gigas* (duan mu li, calcined oyster shell), *Zingiber officinale* (sheng jiang, ginger), *Rheum palmatum* (da huang, rhubarb)

Combine with

– **6.2 Si Ni Wan** for relatively severe Liver qi constraint
– **6.6 Long Dan Xie Gan Wan** for relatively severe Liver fire
– **8.8 Wen Dan Wan** for relatively severe phlegm heat

Pattern identifying features

- **Liver qi constraint with phlegm heat and ascendant Liver yang; Liver and Heart fire**
- insomnia, restlessness
- anxiety, agitation
- heaviness in the body
- patients may exude a scorched smell

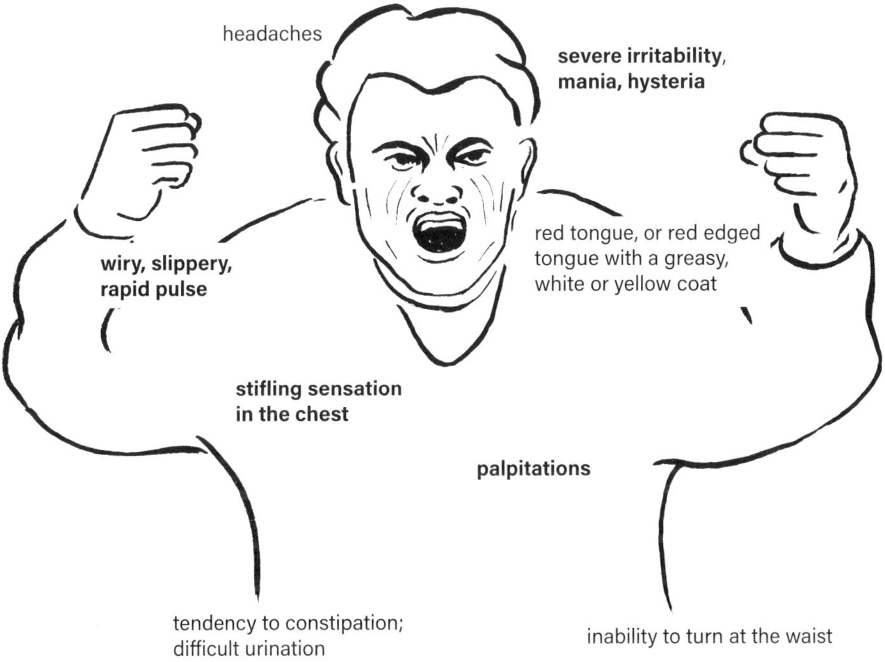

Dosage and method of administration

8-12 pills three times daily on an empty stomach. The dose can be spread out, or taken in two lots of 12-18 pills, morning and evening before bed. In severe cases or during the early stages of treatment (the first few weeks), a 50% increase in dose can be used, then reduced as treatment takes effect. Not suitable for prolonged use.

Cautions and contraindications

Contraindicated during pregnancy. Although generally well tolerated by the patients this formula is appropriate for, some caution should be exercised in patients with Spleen weakness as this formula can be hard on digestion.

8.10 BU NAO PIAN

补脑片

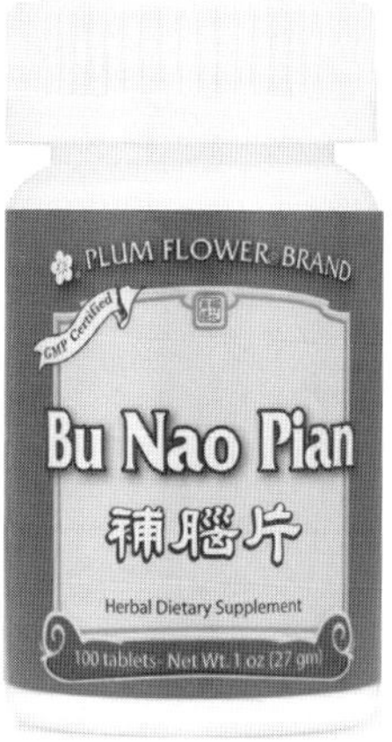

Guangzhou Qixing Pharmaceutical Co. (Guangzhou)
'Brain Tonic Pills'
Bu Nao Pian are packaged in bottles of 100 tablets

Chinese medical action

Calms the *shén*, transforms phlegm, extinguishes wind, strengthens the Kidneys, nourishes blood, benefits and clears the brain

Biomedical action

Sedative and tranquilizer, nervine, sedates the sympathetic nervous system

INDICATIONS

- Concentration and memory problems, confusion and disorientation from phlegm misting the mind and obscuring clear perception. A complex formula that supports the Kidneys and blood, while transforming phlegm, it is especially suited to the elderly, the Kidney deficient and weakened patients with elements of phlegm accumulation, cognitive impairment and *shén* disturbance.
- Anxiety and nervousness or depression and gloominess with palpitations, insomnia and mental agitation from phlegm misting the Heart.

Composition

Schizandra chinensis (wu wei zi, schizandra), *Zizyphus spinoza* (suan zao ren, zizyphus), *Angelica sinensis* (dang gui, chinese angelica), *Cynomorium songaricum* (suo yang, cynomorium), *Juglans regia* (hu tao ren, walnut), *Lycium barbarum* (gou qi zi, lycium fruit), *Biota orientalis* (bai zi ren, biota seed), *Uncaria rhyncophylla* (gou teng, gambir), *Arisaema cosanguinium* (zhi tian nan xing, processed arisaema), *Polygala sibirica* (yuan zhi, polygala), *Acorus gramineus* (shi chang pu, acorus), *Albizzia julibrissin* (he huan pi, albizzia), *Cristaria plicata* (zhen zhu, pearl)

Combine with

- **8.8 Wen Dan Wan** for marked phlegm heat
- **2.23 Ping Wei San** for cognitive problems and brain fog in patients with gastrointestinal disturbances, bloating and heaviness
- **6.1 Xiao Chai Hu Wan** for memory and cognitive problems as a result of an unresolved or lingering pathogen
- **2.18 Bao He Wan** for brain fog from persistent overeating

Dosage and method of administration

2-3 pills two or three times daily on an empty stomach. In the early stages of treatment (the first two weeks or so) the dose can be increased by 50% until results are noticed, then reduced to the maintenance dose.

Pattern identifying features

- **phlegm misting the mind, senses and *shén***
- **cognitive impairment, memory problems, poor concentration**
- confusion, disorientation
- insomnia, dream disturbed sleep
- anxiety, nervousness

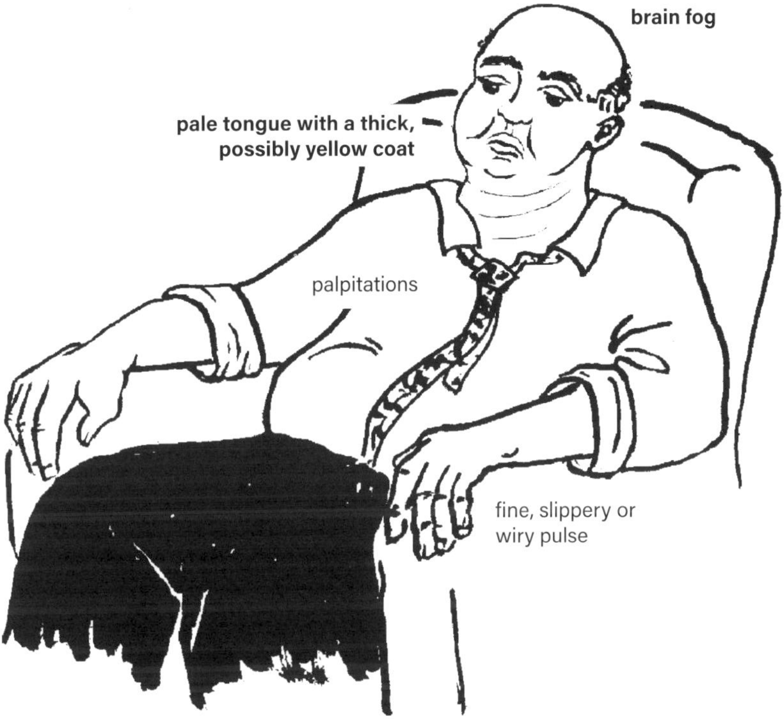

Cautions and contraindications

Contraindicated during pregnancy. Not suitable for cognitive problems from yin deficiency

8.11 JIAN NAO YI ZHI CAPSULE

健脑益智丸

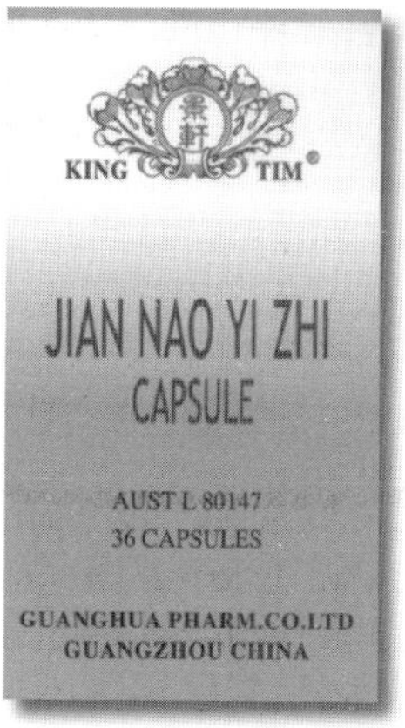

(*Jian Nao Yi Zhi Wan*)
Guanghua Pharmaceutical Co. (Guangzhou)
'Strengthen the Brain and Benefit the Mind Pills'
Jian Nao Yi Zhi Capsules are packaged in bottles of 36 capsules

Chinese medical action

Tonifies qi, nourishes the Heart, strengthens the brain and benefits the mind, invigorates blood, calms the *shén*

Biomedical action

Improves circulation, mild sedative, energy stimulant

INDICATIONS

- Forgetfulness and memory problems. Improves concentration and sharpens the mind for periods of intensive brain and memory work such as periods of intensive study at exam time. Also used for mental exhaustion and burn out following periods of intensive mental activity.
- Used as a preventive against the memory problems of the elderly.

Composition (each capsule contains extracts equivalent to dry)

Panax ginseng (ren shen, ginseng) 556mg, *Poria cocos* (fu shen, hoelen spirit) 556mg, *Polygala sibirica* (yuan zhi, polygala) 371mg, *Salvia miltorrhiza* (dan shen, salvia) 371mg

Combine with

- **7.10 You Gui Wan** or **7.13 Huan Shao Dan** for memory problems in elderly patients with Kidney yang deficiency
- **7.3 Zuo Gui Wan** for memory problems in elderly patients with Kidney yin or essence deficiency

Dosage and method of administration

2-3 capsules, two or three times daily on an empty stomach.

Cautions and contraindications

Contraindicated during the early phase of acute illness such as colds and flu, in patients with heat, yang rising or yin deficiency patterns. Caution in patients with hypertension, those with gastric ulcers, and patients on anticoagulant therapy.

8.12 ZAO REN AN SHEN YE

枣仁安神液

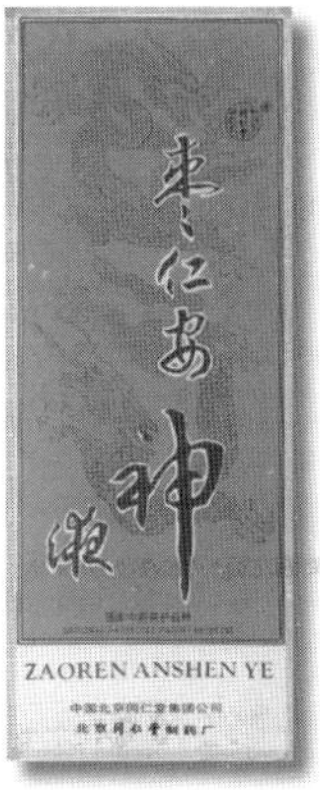

Tong Ren Tang (Beijing)
'Zizyphus Drink to Calm the *Shén*'
Zao Ren An Shen Ye is packaged as a liquid extract in 10 ml vials, ten vials per box

Chinese medical action
Calms the *shén* and *hún*, nourishes the Heart and Liver

Biomedical action
Sedative, tranquilizer, mild astringent

INDICATIONS

- A mild *shén* calming sedative for insomnia, dream disturbed sleep and neurasthenia associated with Heart and Liver blood deficiency. The main advantage of this formula is its ease of use and mild taste. Gentle enough for restless infants and children.
- May be of assistance in sweating disorders.

Composition (each 10 ml contains)
Zizyphus spinoza (suan zao ren, zizyphus) 500mg, *Schizandra chinensis* (wu wei zi, schizandra) 250mg, *Salvia miltorrhiza* (dan shen, salvia) 250mg

Combine with
– Any other *shén* calming formula to enhance the sedative effect
– **1.23 Zhi Bai Di Huang Wan** for insomnia and night sweats from yin deficiency

Dosage and method of administration
One or two vials before bed or upon waking during the night.

Cautions and contraindications
Caution in patients on anticoagulant therapy.

GMP

8.13 GAN MAI DA ZAO WAN

甘麦大枣丸

3+/12

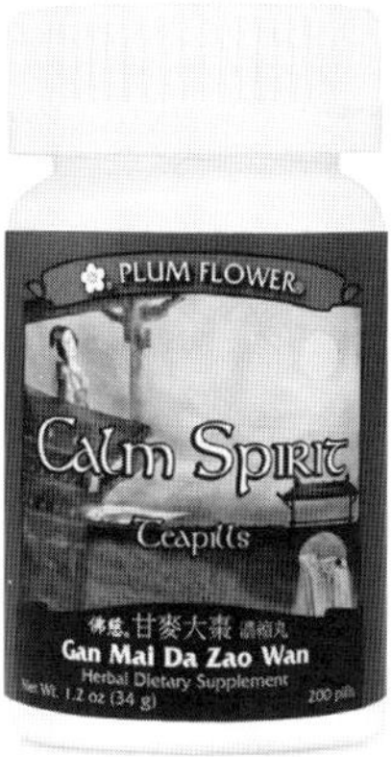

Lanzhou Foci Pharmaceutical Factory (Gansu)
'Licorice, Wheat and Chinese Date Pills'
Gan Mai Da Zao Wan is packaged in bottles of 200 pills
Also available as: Licorice and Jujube Combination (conc. extract)

Chinese medical action

Nourishes the Heart, calms the *shén* and *hun*, harmonizes the middle burner, strengthens the Spleen

Biomedical action

Sedative, tranquilizer

INDICATIONS

- Restless organ disorder (*zàng zào*). This is a type of emotional disorder associated with Heart and Spleen deficiency, characterized by intermittent depression, hysteria, mood swings, behavioral changes, anxiety, hypersensitivity and sleep disturbances. Considered to be most common in women and frequently associated with hormonal changes, it can be applied to any situation where emotional or physical trauma has led to emotional instability. Commonly combined with other constitutional formulas for disorders such as menopausal syndrome, postpartum depression, premenstrual syndrome, post traumatic stress disorder and neurosis.

Composition

Polygonum multiflorum (ye jiao teng, polygonum vine), *Triticum aestivum* (fu xiao mai, wheat), *Zizyphus jujuba* (da zao, chinese dates), *Poria cocos* (fu shen, hoelen spirit), *Lilium brownii* (bai he, lily), *Glycyrrhiza uralensis* (zhi gan cao, honey fried licorice), *Albizzia julibrissin* (he huan pi, albizzia)

Combine with

- **1.9 Gui Pi Wan** for severe anxiety from Heart and Spleen deficiency
- **1.23 Zhi Bai Di Huang Wan** or **1.25 Er Xian Wan** for agitation, insomnia and night sweats from yin deficiency

Dosage and method of administration

8-12 pills three times daily on an empty stomach. In severe cases or the early stages of treatment a 50% increase in dose can be used, reduced as treatment takes effect.

Cautions and contraindications

None noted.

耳鼻喉眼科 9

Ear, Nose, Throat and Eyes

9.1 ER LONG ZUO CI WAN

耳聋左慈丸

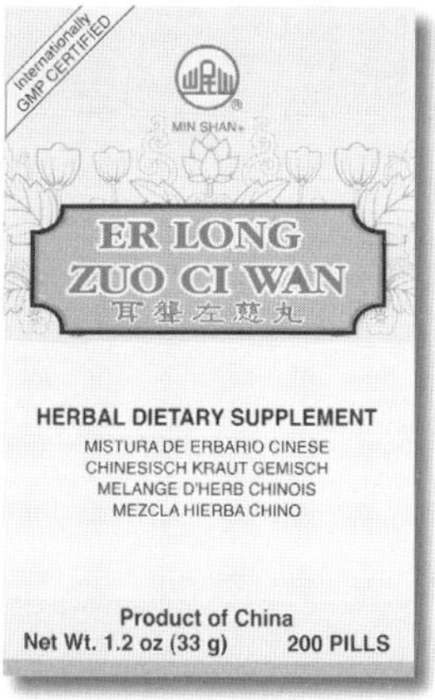

3+/12

Lanzhou Foci Pharmaceutical Factory (Gansu)
'Left Supporting Pills for Deafness'
Er Long Zuo Ci Wan is packaged in bottles of 200 pills
Also available as: Er Ming Zuo Ci Wan, Tso-Tzu Otic Pills

Chinese medical action

Tonifies Kidney yin, regulates qi and restrains ascendant yang

Biomedical action

Demulcent febrifuge, hematinic, hypoglycemic, anti-hypertensive, improves kidney function

INDICATIONS

- Kidney yin deficiency giving rise to hearing problems, specifically tinnitus and gradual loss of hearing. A variation of **7.1.1 Liu Wei Di Huang Wan**, most frequently used for chronic tinnitus with a high pitch that is worse with fatigue, exertion and at night.
- Liver and Kidney yin deficiency patterns with a degree of Liver qi constraint. This may include some visual problems like optic neuritis, optic nerve atrophy and central retinitis.
- With the appropriate identifying features, this formula can assist in treatment of conditions such as tinnitus in the elderly, chronic labyrinthitis, Ménière's disease and hypertension.

Composition

Rehmannia glutinosa (shu di, processed rehmannia), *Dioscorea opposita* (shan yao, dioscorea), *Poria cocos* (fu ling, hoelen), *Paeonia suffruticosa* (mu dan pi, moutan), *Cornus officinalis* (shan zhu yu, cornus), *Alisma orientalis* (ze xie, alisma), *Bupleurum chinensis* (chai hu, bupleurum), *Magnetitum* (ci shi, magnetite)

Combine with

– **15.4 Tian Ma Gou Teng Wan** with a component of ascendant Liver yang
– **8.1 Tian Wang Bu Xin Dan** if the tinnitus keeps the patient awake at night

Dosage and method of administration

8-12 pills three times daily on an empty stomach. The dose can be spread out, or two lots of 12-18 pills taken, morning and evening. In severe cases or during the early stages of treatment (the first few weeks), a 50% increase in dose can be used, then reduced as treatment takes effect.

Pattern identifying features

- **Liver and Kidney yin deficiency hearing disorders**

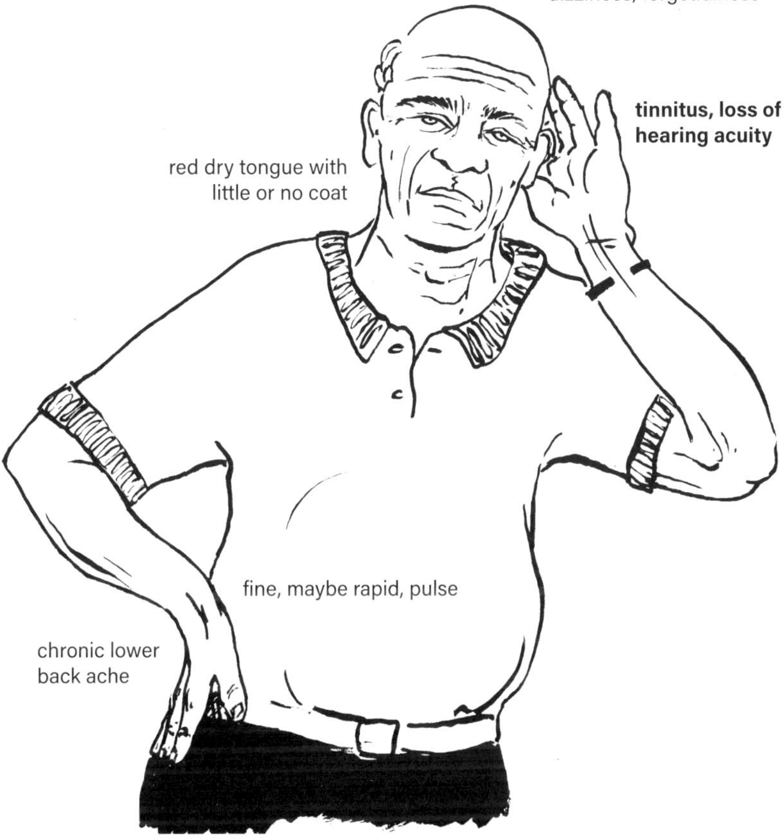

Cautions and contraindications

Contraindicated during the early phase of acute illness such as colds and flu. Care in patients with a tendency to abdominal bloating, loose stools or phlegm damp. This can usually be alleviated by taking a small dose (3-6 pills at the same time) of **2.18 Bao He Wan** or **2.9 Xiang Sha Liu Jun Wan**.

GMP

9.2 TONG QIAO HUO XUE WAN

通窍活血丸

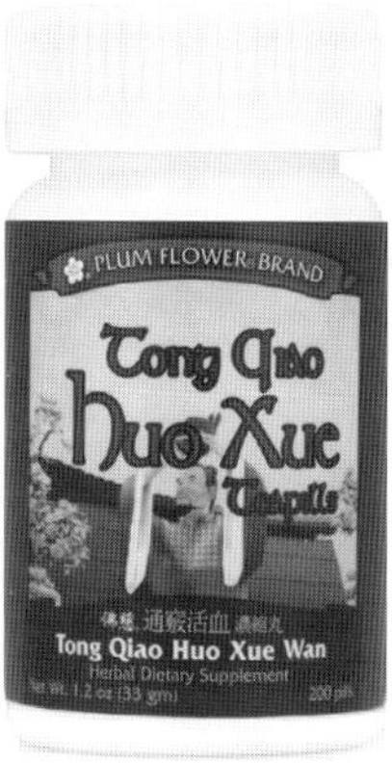

Lanzhou Foci Pharmaceutical Factory (Gansu)
'Blood Regulating, Orifice Opening Pills'
Tong Qiao Huo Xue Wan is packaged in bottles of 200 pills
Available as: Persica and Ligusticum Combination (conc. extract)

Chinese medical action

Invigorates blood and disperses stagnant blood, opens the sensory orifices

Biomedical action

Vasodilator, antispasmodic, anti-platelet action

INDICATIONS

- Blood stasis affecting the head. Used for blood stasis problems of the ears and other sensory structures, associated with chronic pathology or traumatic injury to the head. Direct injury to the ear includes etiology such as exposure to loud noise or sudden pressure changes when flying or scuba diving. The resulting tinnitus and/or hearing loss is persistent, and may be associated with pain and a dark or black discharge from the ear, or dark matter mixed in with the ear wax.
- Acute or chronic focal headaches including migraine and cluster headaches, post surgical, post traumatic and headache associated with drug reaction.
- Purple discoloration of the face and nose, 'brandy nose', hair and eyebrow loss and dark rings around the eyes.
- With the appropriate identifying features, this formula can assist in the treatment of disorders such as post concussion headache and dizziness, migraine and cluster headaches, vitiligo, epilepsy or seizures following head trauma, somnolence, memory loss, dizziness and vertigo.

Composition

Prunus persica (tao ren, peach seed), *Carthamus tinctorius* (hong hua, carthamus), *Paeonia veitchii* (chi shao, red peony), *Ligusticum wallici* (chuan xiong, cnidium), *Acorus gramineus* (shi chang pu, acorus), *Angelica dahurica* (bai zhi, angelica) , *Zingiber officinale* (sheng jiang, ginger), *Zizyphus jujuba* (da zao, chinese dates)

Dosage and method of administration

8-12 pills three times daily on an empty stomach. The dose can be spread out, or two lots of 12-18 pills taken, morning and evening. In severe cases or during the early stages of treatment, a 50% increase in dose can be used, then reduced as treatment takes effect.

Pattern identifying features

- **blood stasis in the head and sense organs**
- dry, scaly skin
- swollen, purple nose
- purple or dark complexion
- vitiligo

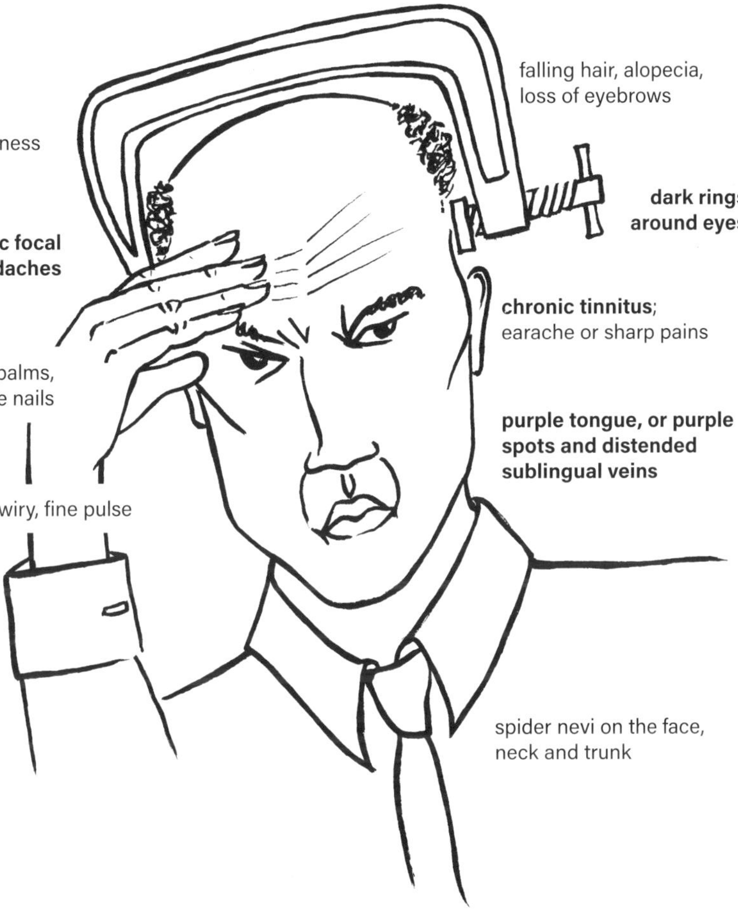

Cautions and contraindications

Contraindicated during pregnancy, in women with menorrhagia, and in patients with bleeding disorders. Caution in patients on anticoagulant therapy. Watch for bruising or increased tendency to bleeding. Prolonged use can deplete qi and blood, so a break every 2-3 months, with a change to a qi and blood tonifying strategy for a few weeks is recommended.

9.3 PEKING NIU HUANG JIE DU PIAN

北京牛黄解毒片

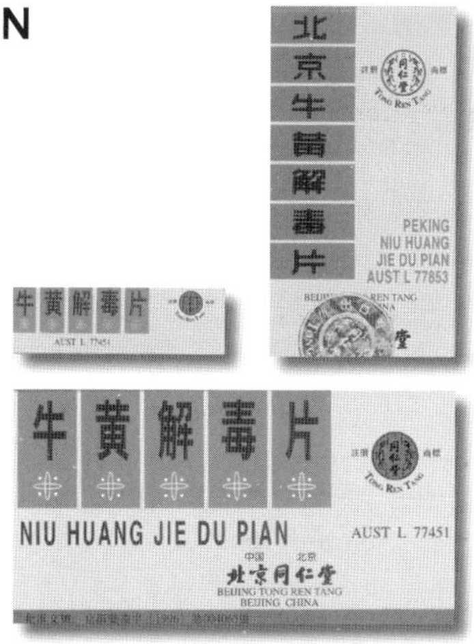

(Beijing Niu Huang Jie Di Pian)
Tong Ren Tang (Beijing)
'Cow Gallstone Anti-Toxic Pills'
Peking Niu Huang Jie Du Pian is packaged in bottles of 20 coated tablets and in vials of 8 uncoated pills, 12 vials to a box

Chinese medical action

Clears heat and toxic heat from the head and upper body and the *yáng míng* organs, dispels wind, stops pain and opens the bowels

Biomedical action

Anti-inflammatory, detoxicant, antibiotic, antiviral, laxative

INDICATIONS

- Toxic heat pathology of the head and upper body. An important formula for acute suppurative and febrile disorders, **9.3 Peking Niu Huang Jie Du Pian** is especially good for infection of the oral cavity, throat, ear and facial skin, including conditions such as tonsillitis, strep throat, acne and boils on the face and neck, folliculitis, acne rosacea, herpes simplex, acute otitis media and externa, acute sinusitis, conjunctivitis, stye, gingivitis, dental abscess, toothache and mouth ulcers.
- Acute wind heat, warm disease or toxic heat type fever, especially when accompanied by constipation. Can be used for disorders such as mumps, scarlet fever, measles and chicken pox.

Composition (each tablet contains extracts equivalent to)

Bovine gallstone (niu huang) 13.8mg, *Lonicera japonica* (jin yin hua, honeysuckle) 726mg, *Forsythia suspensa* (lian qiao, forsythia) 726mg, *Mentha haplocalycis* (bo he, mint) 240mg, *Schizonepeta tenuifolia* (jing jie, schizonepeta) 240mg, *Platycodon grandiflorum* (jie geng, platycodon) 360mg, *Glycyrrhiza uralensis* (gan cao , licorice) 240mg, *Gardenia florida* (shan zhi zi, gardenia) 360mg, *Siler divaricum* (fang feng, siler) 180mg, *Ligusticum wallichi* (chuan xiong, cnidium) 240mg, *Inula britannica* (xuan fu hua, inula flower) 360mg, *Rheum officinale* (da huang, rhubarb) 492mg, *Chrysanthemum sinense* (ju hua, chrysanthemum flower) 492mg, *Angelica dahurica* (bai zhi, angelica) 306mg, *Vitex trifolia* (man jing zi, vitex fruit) 180mg, *Gypsum fibrosum* (shi gao, gypsum) 36mg

Combine with

- **9.10 Sanjin Watermelon Frost** topically for mouth ulcers
- **9.9 Superior Sore Throat Powder** topically for tonsillitis or otitis media or externa
- **3.1.1 Yin Chiao Chieh Tu Pien** for acute seasonal febrile illness
- A saline eyewash or decocted chrysanthemum flowers for acute conjunctivitis

Pattern identifying features

- **toxic heat in the head and upper body**
- **localised suppuration, redness, swelling and pain**
- acute heat and inflammation in the head and upper body
- constipation

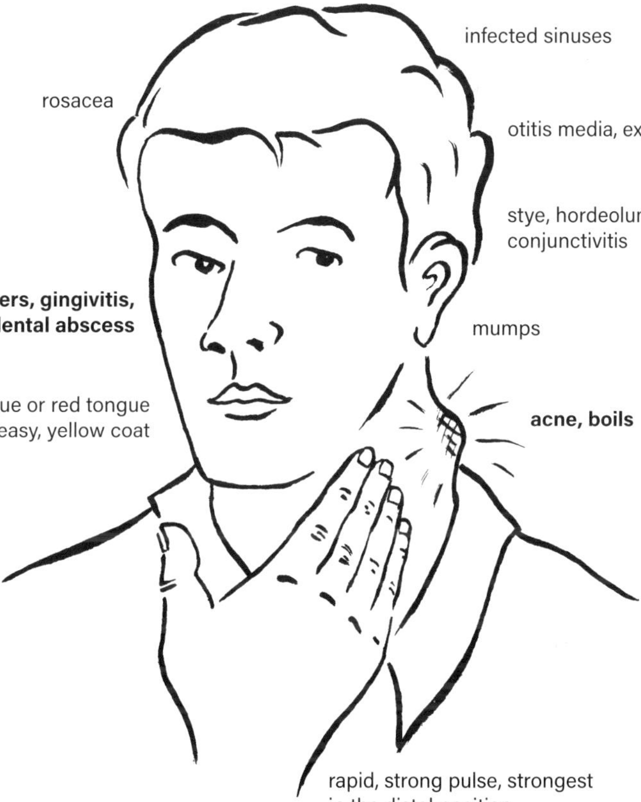

Dosage and method of administration

2 pills twice daily on an empty stomach (1 pill twice daily crushed for children). This may be safely doubled in adults and in severe cases. May cause diarrhea. For rosacea, **9.3 Peking Niu Huang Jie Du Pian** can be used for 1-3 months at a half or quarter dose. Do not take within one hour of eating rich or oily foods.

Cautions and contraindications

Contraindicated during pregnancy. Not suitable for prolonged use (except as noted above) or for deficient patients without toxic heat.

9.4.1 HUANG LIEN SHANG CHING PIEN

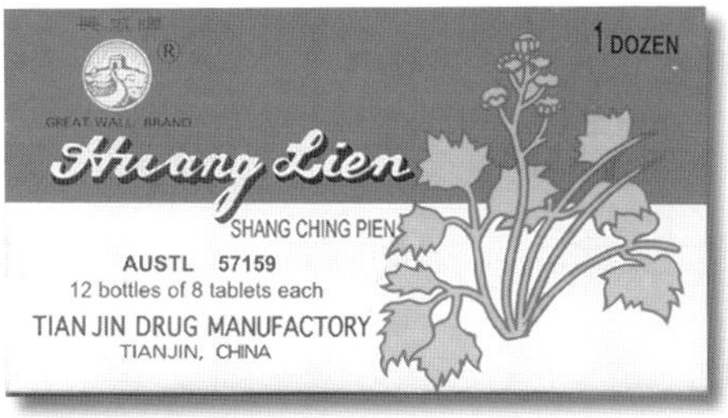

黄连上清片

(*Huang Lian Shang Qing Pian*)
Tianjin Drug Manufactory (Shandong)
'Coptis Pill to Clear [Heat from] the Upper Body'
Huang Lien Shang Ching Pien is packaged in vials of eight pills, twelve vials per box

Chinese medical action

Dispels wind heat and clears toxic heat, fire and damp heat from the upper body, cools the blood, clears heat from *yáng míng*, opens the bowels

Biomedical action

Antipyretic, anti-inflammatory, antibiotic, laxative

INDICATIONS

- Wind heat, toxic heat and damp heat type focal infections of the head and upper body. Especially good for infection and inflammation of the eyes associated with wind heat, fire or heat in the Liver channel. With the appropriate identifying features, this may include such biomedical disorders as acute conjunctivitis, hordeolum, stye, blepharitis, excessive lacrimation and orbital cellulitis.
- Wind heat or toxic heat affecting the throat causing acute sore throat, tonsillitis and laryngitis.
- Inflammatory or suppurative skin disorders of the head and upper body, including eczema, urticaria, pityriasis rosea, dermatitis, acne, abscesses, boils and cellulitis.
- Heat in the Stomach and *yáng míng* channel and organ system causing constipation, halitosis, gingivitis, ulcerations of the oral cavity, tooth infection or dental abscess.
- Headache, dizziness and tinnitus from wind heat or Liver fire rising up through the Liver/Gallbladder channel.

Composition (each tablet contains extracts equivalent to dry)

Chrysanthemum sinense (ju hua, chrysanthemum flower) 1.1g, *Vitex trifolia* (man jing zi, vitex fruit) 773mg, *Platycodon grandiflorum* (jie geng, platycodon) 591mg, *Schizonepeta tenuifolia* (jing jie, schizonepeta) 507mg, *Coptis chinensis* (huang lian, coptis) 364mg, *Scutellaria baicalensis* (huang qin, scute) 273mg, *Ledebouriella divaricata* (fang feng, siler) 253mg, *Rheum palmatum* (da huang, rhubarb) 148mg, *Angelica dahurica* (bai zhi, angelica) 53mg, *Glycyrrhiza uralensis* (gan cao, licorice) 18mg, Calcium sulphate 18mg

Combine with

– **9.10 Sanjin Watermelon Frost** topically for mouth ulcers
– **9.9 Superior Sore Throat Powder** topically for tonsillitis or otitis media or otitis externa

Pattern identifying features

- **wind heat and toxic heat in the head and upper body**
- inflammatory and suppurative disorders of the oral cavity, eyes, head and face
- mouth ulcers, gingivitis, toothache, dental abscess
- fever

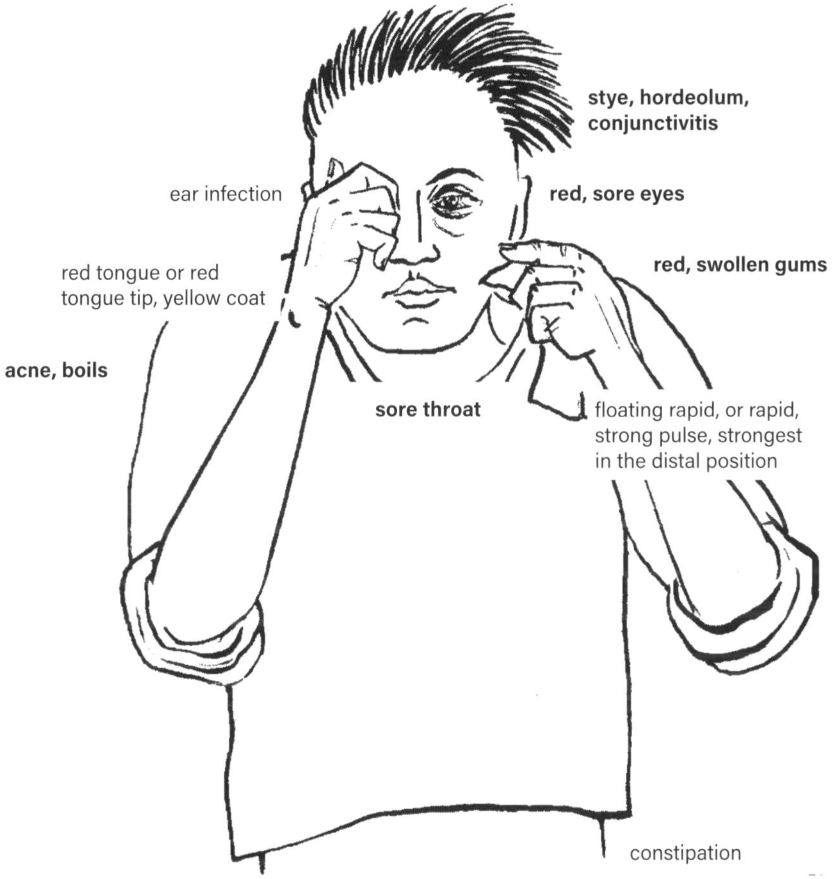

Dosage and method of administration

The recommended dose is 4 pills twice daily, on an empty stomach. In severe cases the dose can be increased by 50%. Usually not necessary for more than 4-7 days. Generally not recommended for children under 5 years old. May cause diarrhea.

Cautions and contraindications

Contraindicated during pregnancy. This formula is bitter and cold and can easily damage the Spleen and Stomach, and consume yin. It should only be used for the duration of the acute excess heat pattern. Overdose can cause dizziness and vomiting.

9.4.2 HUANG LIAN SHANG QING TABLET

黄连上清片

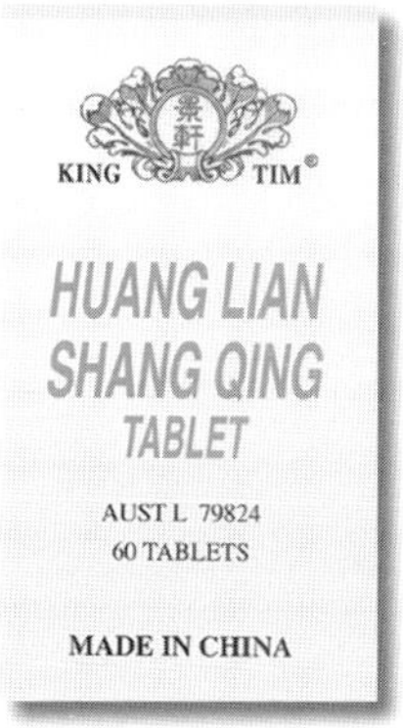

(*Huang Lian Shang Qing Pian*)
Jing Xian Pharmaceutical Co. (Guangzhou)
'Coptis Pill to Clear [Heat from] the Upper Body'
Huang Lian Shang Qing Tablets are packaged in bottles of 60 tablets

Chinese medical action

Dispels wind heat and clears toxic heat, fire and damp heat from the upper body, cools the blood, clears heat from *yáng míng*, opens the bowels

Biomedical action

Antipyretic, anti-inflammatory, antibiotic, laxative

INDICATIONS

- As for **9.4.1 Huang Lien Shang Ching Pien**

Composition (each tablet contains extracts equivalent to dry)

Chrysanthemum sinense (ju hua, chrysanthemum flower) 949mg, *Phellodendron amurense* (huang bai, phellodendron) 474mg, *Forsythia suspensa* (lian qiao, forsythia) 474mg, *Angelica dahurica* (bai zhi, angelica) 474mg, *Platycodon grandiflorum* (jie geng, platycodon) 474mg, *Scutellaria baicalensis* (huang qin, scute) 474mg, *Gardenia florida* (shan zhi zi, gardenia) 474mg, *Siler divaricum* (fang feng, siler) 238mg, *Rheum palmatum* (da huang, rhubarb) 20mg, *Coptis chinensis* (huang lian, coptis) 6.6mg, *Mentha haplocalycis* (bo he, mint) 26.4mg

Dosage and method of administration

3-5 tablets, three times daily, on an empty stomach.

Cautions and contraindications

As for **9.4.1 Huang Lien Shang Ching Pien**.

9.5 PU JI XIAO DU WAN

GMP

1/52

普济消毒丸

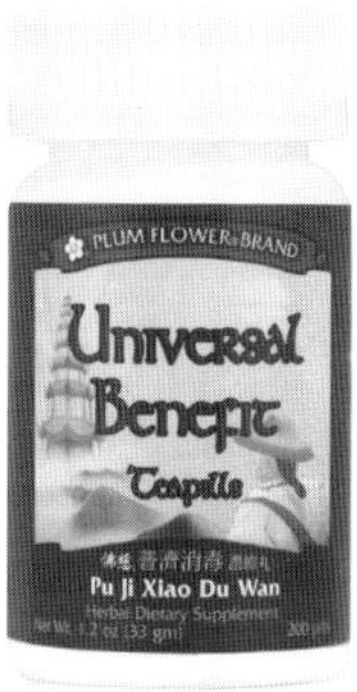

Lanzhou Foci Pharmaceutical Factory (Gansu)
'Universal Benefit Pills to Eliminate Toxin'
Available as: Scute and Cimicifuga Combination (conc. extract)

Chinese medical action
Clears toxic heat and fire, benefits the throat

Biomedical action
Antipyretic, anti-inflammatory, antibiotic

INDICATIONS

- Acute warm disease. Used for infection of the throat and/or other structures of the head – the parotid and salivary glands, subcutaneous connective tissues etc. Main features include acute high fever and chills or rigors, redness, swelling and burning pain of the throat, head or face, thirst, a red or red tipped tongue with dry coat and a rapid floating pulse.
- With the appropriate identifying features, this formula can assist in treatment of disorders such as infectious parotitis (mumps), erysipelas or cellulitis of the face and head, streptococcal tonsillitis, measles, infectious meningitis, scarlet fever, lymphadenitis and otitis media.

Composition
Coptis chinensis (huang lian, coptis), *Scutellaria baicalensis* (huang qin, scute), *Scrophularia ningpoensis* (xuan shen, scrophularia), *Platycodon grandiflorum* (jie geng, platycodon), *Citrus reticulata* (chen pi, citrus), *Bupleurum falcatum* (chai hu, bupleurum), *Glycyrrhiza uralensis* (gan cao, licorice), *Arctium lappa* (niu bang zi, burdock seeds), *Forsythia suspensa* (lian qiao, forsythia), *Mentha haplocalycis* (bo he, mint), *Lasiosphaera femslii* (ma bo, puffball), *Isatis tinctora* (ban lan gen, isatis root), *Cimicifuga foetida* (sheng ma, cimicifuga), *Bombyx mori* (bai jiang can, silkworm)

Dosage and method of administration
The recommended dose is 8-12 pills three times daily, however to get a good result a larger dose usually needs to be taken: 8-15 pills every 2 hours depending on severity and size of patient.

Cautions and contraindications
Reserved for relatively severe heat patterns. Can easily damage Spleen yang if overused.

9.6 BAN LAN GEN CHONG JI
板蓝根冲剂

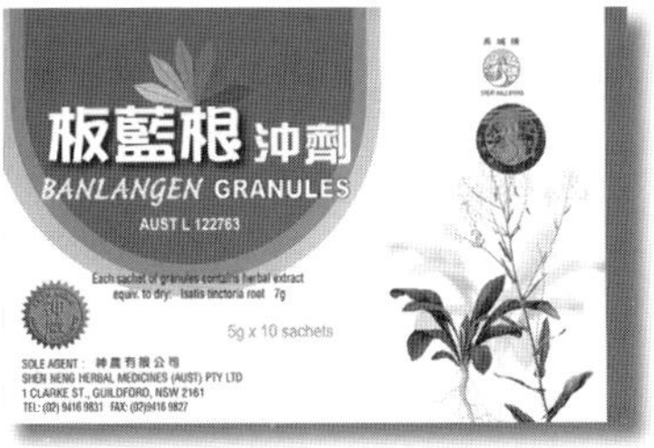

Tong Ren Tang (Beijing)
'Isatis granules'
Ban Lan Gen Chong Ji is packaged in 12 gram sachets of soluble granules, ten sachets per box
Also available as: Ban Lan Gen Ke Li

Chinese medical action
Clears toxic heat, dispels wind heat

Biomedical action
Anti-inflammatory, detoxicant, antibiotic, antiviral

INDICATIONS

- Acute throat and upper respiratory tract infections, especially viral, such as sore throat, tonsillitis and pharyngitis.
- Disorders that classified as warm diseases, such as mumps, measles, infectious meningitis, scarlet fever and hepatitis.
- Skin diseases such as herpes zoster (shingles), herpes simplex (cold sores), warts, pityriasis rosea and acne rosacea.
- Used preventively against hepatitis and meningitis during outbreaks.

Composition (each sachet contains extract equivalent to)
Isatis tinctoria (ban lan gen, isatis root) 12.5g, sucrose

Combine with
- **9.9 Superior Sore Throat Powder** for tonsillitis or otitis; this combination is also effective for shingles
- **3.1.1 Yin Chiao Chieh Tu Pien** or **3.4 Gan Mao Ling** for the early stage of an acute seasonal febrile illness or warm disease
- **6.6 Long Dan Xie Gan Wan** for shingles from Liver fire or damp heat

Dosage and method of administration
4-6 sachets per day, dissolved in hot water. Halve the dose for children.

Cautions and contraindications
Not suitable for use in the absence of heat or toxic heat symptoms.

9.7 JIE GENG WAN

桔梗丸

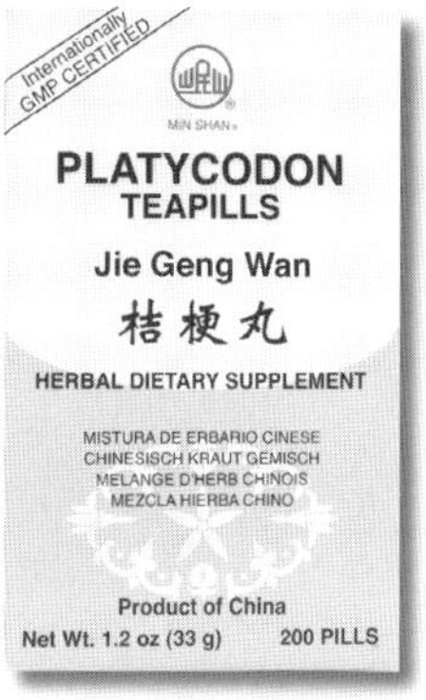

Lanzhou Foci Pharmaceutical Factory (Gansu)
'Platycodon Pills'
Jie Geng Wan is packaged in bottles of 200 pills

Chinese medical action

Expels phlegm and stops cough, eases the throat, aids in the discharge of pus, directs other herbs to the upper body

Biomedical action

Expectorant, antitussive

INDICATIONS

- Sore throat from any cause, including heat, phlegm heat and yin deficiency.
- Productive cough from both excess and deficiency.
- Helps to discharge pus. Used for suppurative disorders such as Lung abscess and throat abscess.
- Usually added to a targeting formula to enhance the throat easing and cough stopping effect.

Composition (each pill contains powdered)

Platycodon grandiflorum (jie geng, platycodon)

Combine with

- **3.31.1 Zhi Sou Wan** for persistent cough following unresolved wind invasion
- **3.15 Qing Qi Hua Tan Wan** for acute cough from severe phlegm heat

Dosage and method of administration

8 pills three times daily, on an empty stomach.

Cautions and contraindications

Contraindicated for patients with hemoptysis. Caution in nauseous patients as the elevating nature of platycodon can cause Stomach qi to rise.

GMP

9.8 QING WEI WAN

清胃丸

(1-3/52)

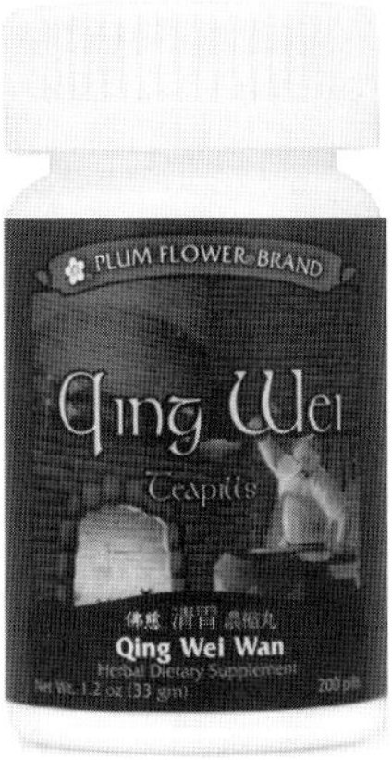

Lanzhou Foci Pharmaceutical Factory (Gansu)
'Stomach Cooling Pills'
Qing Wei Wan is packaged in bottles of 200 pills
Also available as: Coptis and Rehmannia Formula (conc. extract)

Chinese medical action

Clears heat and cools the Stomach, cools, nourishes and regulates the blood

Biomedical action

Anti-inflammatory

INDICATIONS

- Stomach heat type oral disorders. Used to treat acute, chronic or recurrent inflammation, ulceration and pain of the oral cavity. Ulcers may be single, or more usually, multiple and tend to be concentrated on the gums or buccal cavity which, in severe cases, may coalesce into a large ulcerated area. Ulcers are burning and painful, with a yellow or white floor and a red, swollen margin. They can be initiated or aggravated by overindulgence in heating foods and substances, and alleviated somewhat by the application of ice.
- Toothache and facial pain or swelling from heat in the Stomach channel.
- Epigastric pain from Stomach heat.
- With the appropriate identifying features, this formula can assist in the treatment of conditions such as apthous stomatitis, post radiation stomatitis, ulcerative stomatitis, dental caries, periodontal disease, acute episode of Beçhet's syndrome or Reiter's syndrome, trigeminal neuralgia, glossitis and gingivitis.

Composition

Cimicifuga foetida (sheng ma, cimicifuga), *Coptis chinensis* (huang lian, coptis), *Paeonia suffruticosa* (mu dan pi, moutan), *Rehmannia glutinosa* (sheng di, raw rehmannia), *Angelica sinensis* (dang gui, chinese angelica)

Combine with

- **9.10 Sanjin Watermelon Frost** or **9.9 Superior Sore Throat Powder** topically on ulcerated areas
- **7.1.1 Liu Wei Di Huang Wan** for post radiation stomatitis
- **14.2 Huang Lian Su Tablets** for intense Stomach fire with bleeding
- **10.21 Yan Hu Suo Zhi Tong Wan** for facial pain from heat

Pattern identifying features

- **Stomach heat/fire**
- frequent hunger
- tendency to constipation or dry stools
- thirst, desire for cold drinks
- dry mouth and lips
- belching, heartburn, reflux

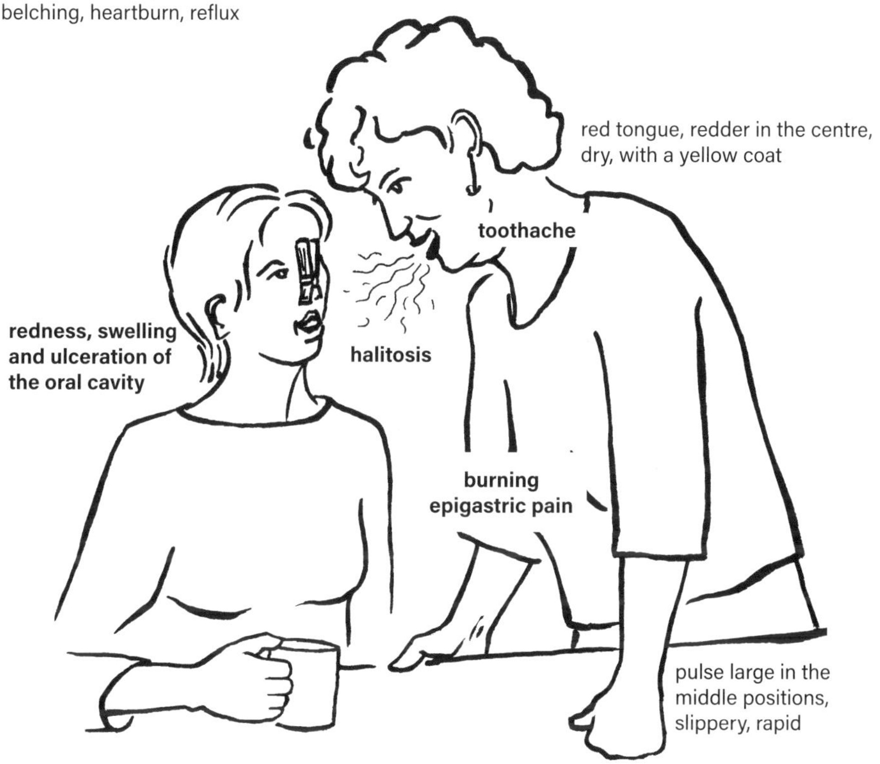

Dosage and method of administration

The recommended dose for chronic or recurrent cases is 8-12 pills three times daily, however, in acute or severe disorders a higher dose is required to be effective, in general, 16-24 pills three times daily (or about 12 pills every two hours), on an empty stomach.

Cautions and contraindications

Contraindicated in oral disorders associated with deficient heat or without excess heat. In patients with constipation, *see* **14.10 Liang Ge Wan**.

9.9 SUPERIOR SORE THROAT POWDER

双料喉风散

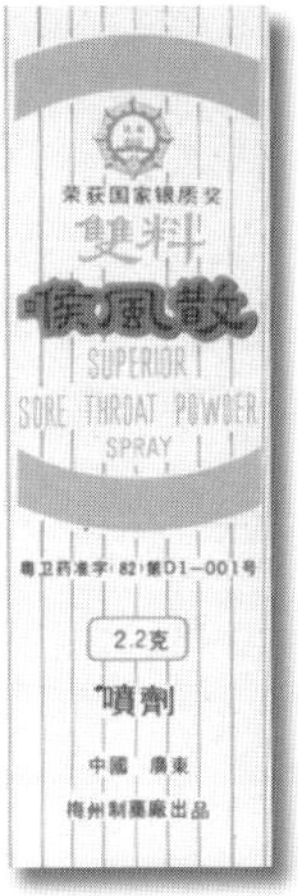

(*Shuang Liao Hou Feng San*)
Meichou Medicine Factory (Guandong)
'Superior Throat Wind Powder'
Superior Sore Throat Powder is packaged in 2.2 gram bottles of powder to be puffed onto the affected area

Chinese medical action

Clears toxic heat and damp heat from the throat and skin, relieves inflammation and stops pain

Biomedical action

Anti-inflammatory, vulnerary, promotes healing

INDICATIONS

- Topical application for inflammation and toxic heat patterns of the mouth and throat, especially tonsillitis, pharyngitis, mouth ulcers and gingivitis. Can be applied with a clean finger to the mouths of babies and infants with mouth ulcers.
- Can be applied to other sites of infection and inflammation. Can be blown up the nose for acute sinusitis or into the ear for suppurative otitis media and externa. Applied topically to ulcerative dermatitis or other open suppurative lesions, as well as the lesions of shingles and other viral infections of the skin.

Composition

Coptis chinensis (huang lian, coptis) 30%, Borneol (bing pian) 25%, *Glycyrrhiza uralensis* (gan cao, licorice) 15%, *Sophora subprostrata* (shan dou gen, sophora) 15%, Bovine gallstone (niu huang) 5%, Pearl (zhen zhu) 5%, *Indigo Pulverata Levis* (qing dai, indigo) 5%

Combine with

- **9.3 Peking Niu Huang Jie Du Pian**, **9.4.1 Huang Lien Shang Ching Pien** or **14.6 Fu Fang Nan Ban Lan Gen** for tonsillitis with suppuration
- **3.1.1 Yin Chiao Chieh Tu Pien** for tonsillitis without suppuration
- **6.6 Long Dan Xie Gan Wan** or **9.3 Peking Niu Huang Jie Du Pian** for acute otitis
- **6.6 Long Dan Xie Gan Wan** for shingles from damp heat in the Liver

Pattern identifying features

- **toxic heat in the throat and mouth**
- inflammation, suppuration and pain in the **mouth, throat**, ear, sinus or skin

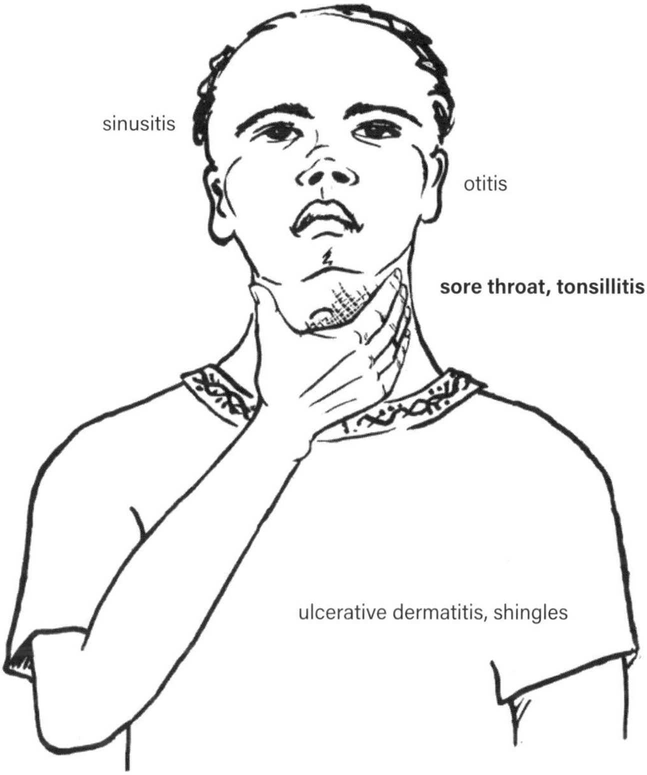

Dosage and method of administration

Spray on to the affected area 3-5 times daily. For mouth ulcers in infants, the powder can be rubbed over the affected area with a clean finger. For suppurative skin lesions, wash the affected area with strong black tea first, then spray. For otitis, rinse the ear with 3% hydrogen peroxide solution first, then spray. Only used for a short time during the acute phase (usually 5-7 days).

Cautions and contraindications

None noted.

9.10 SANJIN WATERMELON FROST

三金西瓜霜

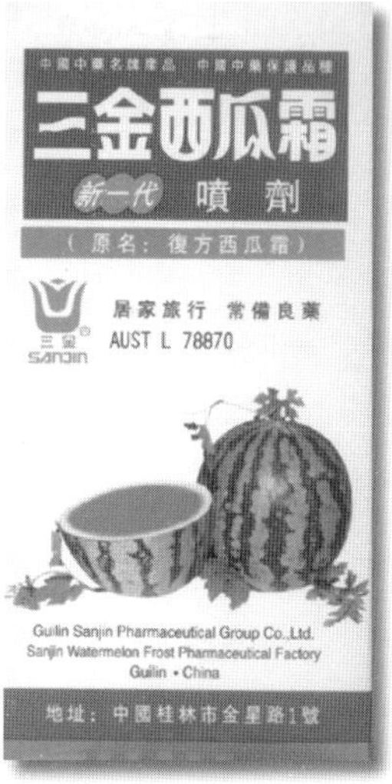

1-3/52

(*San Jin Xi Gua Shuang* – powder, *Xi Gua Pian* – lozenges)
Guilin Drug Manufactory (Guangxi province)
Sanjin Watermelon Frost is packaged either in powder form to be sprayed on directly or in blister packs of lozenges that can be dissolved slowly in the mouth

Chinese medical action

Clears heat and toxic heat from the mouth, stops pain and bleeding, promotes healing

Biomedical action

Anti-inflammatory, antibiotic, analgesic, soothing to mucous membranes, demulcent, vulnerary, promotes healing

INDICATIONS

- Inflammation and/or ulceration of the mouth and throat, especially mouth ulcers, apthous stomatitis, gingivitis and toothache. Even though the powder is cooling, it can be used topically for ulcers associated with deficient and cold patterns. Also useful to soothe a sore throat, laryngitis and tonsillitis.
- Can be sprayed onto open wounds to stop bleeding.
- Topically for burns and scalds (*see also* **13.14 Ching Wan Hung** and **13.17 Xiao Yan Tang Shang Cream**), and insect stings and bites.

Composition (each gram of powder contains)

Citrullus vulgaris (xi gua shuang, watermelon frost) 510mg, *Fritillaria cirrhosa* (chuan bei, fritillaria) 150mg, *Belamcanda chinensis* (she gan, belamcanda) 60mg, *Sophora subprostrata* (shan dou gen, sophora) 60mg, *Siraitia grosvenorii* (luo han guo, momordica fruit) 60mg, *Scutellaria baicalensis* (huang qin, scute) 60mg, *Indigo Pulverata Levis* (qing dai, indigo) 40mg, *Dryobalanops camphora* (bing pian, borneol) 30mg, Menthol (bo he, mint oil) 30mg

Combine with

- **9.3 Peking Niu Huang Jie Du Pian** for acute Hot type mouth ulcers or tonsillitis
- **8.1 Tian Wang Bu Xin Dan** for chronic or recurrent mouth ulcers from Heart and Kidney yin deficiency
- **2.13 Li Zhong Wan** or **2.14 Li Chung Yuen Medical Pills** for chronic mouth ulcers from Spleen yang deficiency
- **7.1.1 Liu Wei Di Huang Wan** or **3.33 Yang Yin Qing Fei Wan** for mouth ulcers following chemotherapy or radiotherapy
- **12.7 Xiao Er Gan Mao Chong Ji** for acute febrile illness with mouth ulcers in babies
- **10.2 Raw Tienchi Tablet** (internally) for bleeding from trauma

Pattern identifying features

- **toxic heat in the mouth and throat**
- inflammation, pain and ulceration of the **mouth, gums**, tongue and throat

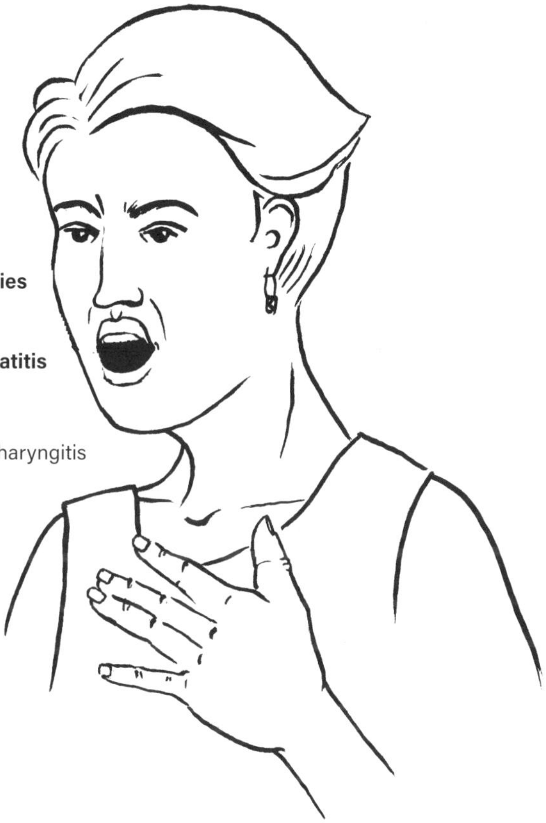

Dosage and method of administration

Powder: For problems in the throat and nose, spray a puff of powder directly onto the affected area. For gum disease the powder can be massaged into the area with a clean finger. Repeat every 2-4 hours. For burns and scalds mix some powder with an oil (olive or apricot) and apply to the affected area. For bleeding, wash away excess blood and spray on the affected area, and bind lightly with sterile gauze.

Lozenges: For throat disorders and mouth ulcers, dissolve one tablet in the mouth at a time.

Cautions and contraindications

None noted.

9.11 QING YIN WAN

清音丸

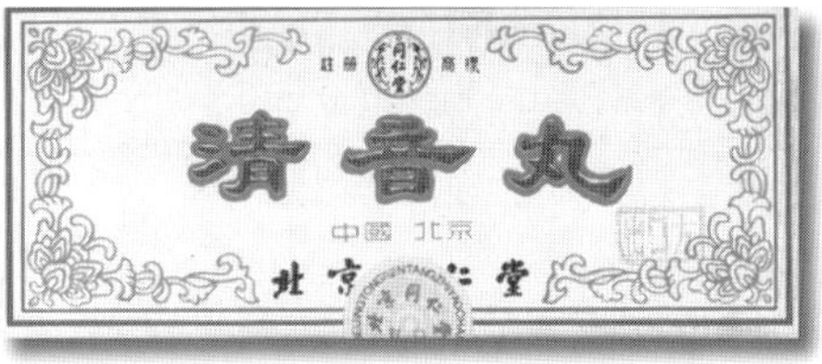

Tong Ren Tang (Beijing)
'Pure Sound Pills'
Qing Yin Wan is packaged in 3 gram honey pills sealed in wax balls, ten pills per box

Chinese medical action

Clears heat from the throat and Lungs, benefits the throat, generates fluids and saliva, moistens dryness and stops thirst

Biomedical action

Demulcent, soothes and lubricates the throat

INDICATIONS

- Hoarse or raspy voice, or loss of voice following an upper respiratory tract infection, overuse or smoking. Popular with singers, teachers and public speakers for voice strain and discomfort from prolonged vocal activity. May be useful in the prevention or alleviation of discomfort from polyps on the vocal cords.
- Recurrent or chronic soreness and irritation of the throat.
- Dryness of the oral cavity, either from local pathology, the after effects of radiation treatment, or systemic pathology such as diabetes and Sjogren's syndrome.

Composition (each pill contains powdered)

Pueraria lobata (ge gen, pueraria) 228mg, *Fritillaria cirrhosa* (chuan bei mu, fritillaria) 228mg, *Trichosanthes kirilowii* (tian hua fen, trichosanthes root) 114mg, *Terminalia chebula* (he zi rou, terminalia) 114mg, *Poria cocos* (fu ling, hoelen) 114mg, *Prunus mume* (wu mei, umeboshi plum) 114mg, *Glycyrrhiza uralensis* (gan cao, licorice), honey

Combine with

- **3.33 Yang Yin Qing Fei Wan**, **7.5 Gu Ben Wan** or **3.35 Mai Wei Di Huang Wan** for chronic hoarse or raspy voice from Lung yin deficiency
- **3.38 Sheng Mai San Wan** for lingering throat problems following an upper respiratory tract infection
- A large dose of **7.2.2 Qi Ju Di Huang Wan**, or **9.22 Ming Mu Di Huang Wan** for systemic, ocular and oral dryness from Liver and Kidney yin deficiency, as seen in conditions such as Sjogren's syndrome

Dosage and method of administration

1-2 pills dissolved slowly in the mouth and run over the throat and vocal cords, two or three times daily.

Pattern identifying features

- **heat and dryness of the throat and Lungs**
- chronic heat and dryness in the throat
- discomfort associated with nodules or polyps

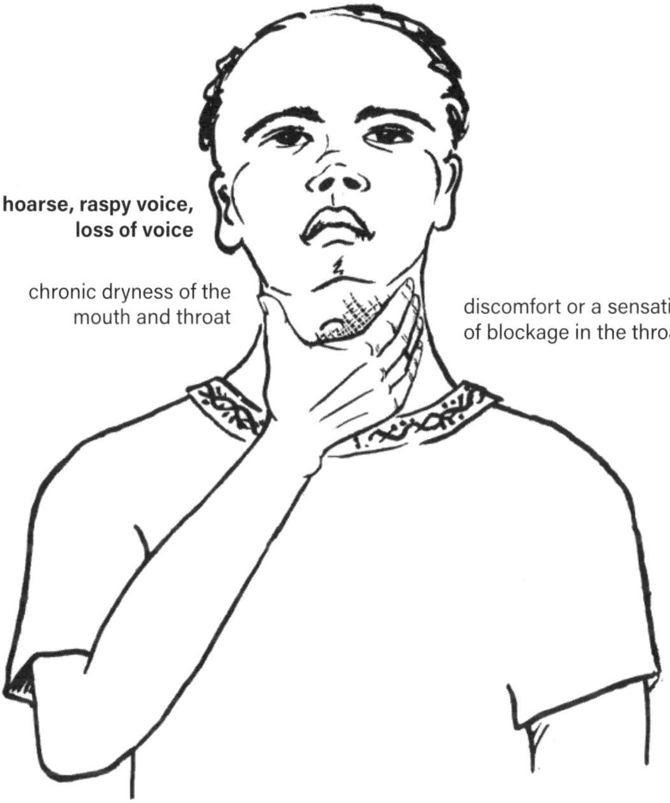

Cautions and contraindications

Avoid spicy or excessively greasy foods and other obvious irritants, such as cigarettes and other inhaled substances, while using this formula.

GMP

9.12 BAN XIA HOU PO WAN

1-3 / 12

半夏厚朴丸

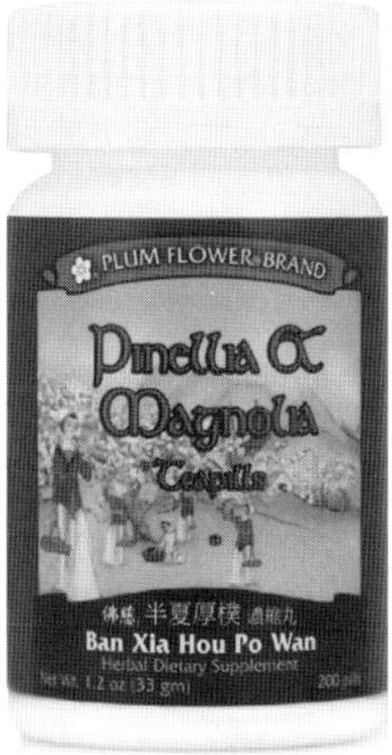

Lanzhou Foci Pharmaceutical Factory (Gansu)
'Pinellia and Magnolia Pills'
Ban Xia Hou Po Wan is packaged in bottles of 200 pills.
Also available as: Pinellia and Magnolia Combination (conc. extract)

Chinese medical action

Invigorates qi, transforms phlegm, directs qi downwards and dissipates nodules

Biomedical action

Sedative, mucolytic, anti-emetic

INDICATIONS

- Qi and phlegm stagnation affecting the throat and esophagus, known as 'plum pit qi'. The characteristic feature of plum pit qi is the sensation of something lodged in the throat that cannot be swallowed or cleared. The sensation has an emotional component, appearing and disappearing with changes in the emotional state of the patient. The pattern is associated with dysfunction of the Liver and Spleen. Typically, constrained Liver qi invades and weakens the Spleen creating the conditions for accumulation of damp and phlegm, which are then carried along the Liver channel to catch in the throat. The qi constraint may have its roots in an inability to express or vocalize feelings of anger or frustration–this especially affects the area of the larynx and throat. Similarly, difficulty in accepting (or swallowing) change or a new situation can create constraint in the throat. Patients may be stressed and under pressure; they may be fed up with various elements of their lives – 'I can't swallow any more!'.
- With the appropriate identifying features, this formula can be used to treat conditions such as globus hystericus, neurosis, assertiveness issues, anxiety, esophageal spasm, chronic laryngitis or pharyngitis.

Composition

Pinellia ternata (jiang ban xia, ginger processed pinellia), *Magnolia officinalis* (hou po, magnolia bark), *Poria cocos* (fu ling, hoelen), *Perilla frutescens* (zi su ye, perilla leaf), *Zingiber officinale* (sheng jiang, ginger)

Combine with

- **6.3 Chai Hu Shu Gan Wan** or **6.2 Si Ni Wan** for marked qi constraint
- **2.22 Er Chen Wan** for predominant phlegm

Pattern identifying features

- **qi and phlegm stagnation**
- cough or vomiting
- frequent sighing
- throat clearing

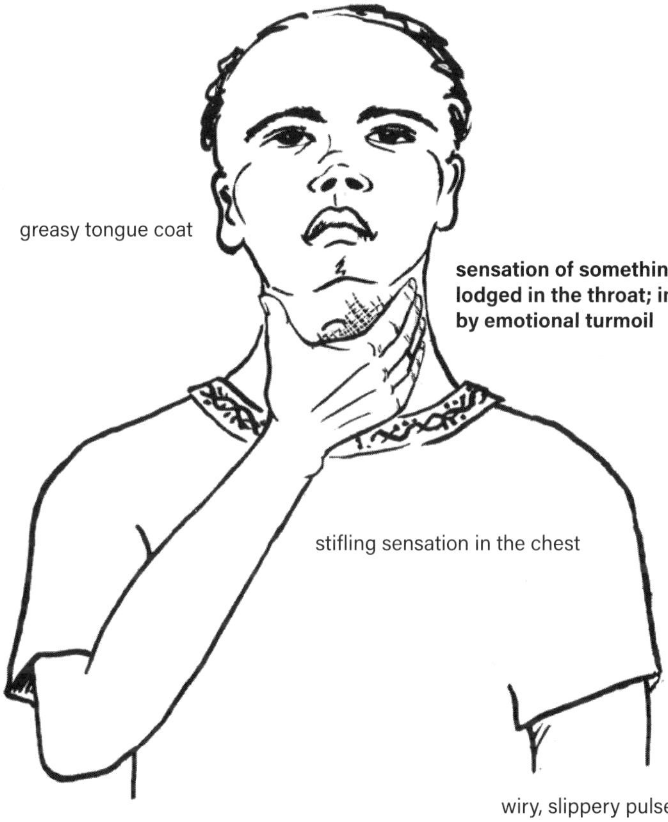

Dosage and method of administration

8-12 pills three times daily on an empty stomach. The dose can be spread out, or two lots of 12-18 pills taken, morning and evening. In severe cases or the early stages of treatment (the first few weeks), a 50% increase in dose can be used, then reduced as treatment takes effect.

Cautions and contraindications

Contraindicated in yin deficiency and dryness patterns.

1-3/12

9.13 PE MIN KAN WAN

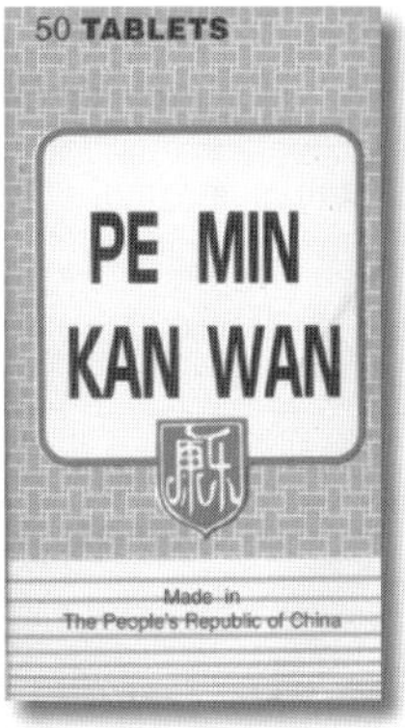

鼻敏感丸

(*Bi Min Gan Wan*)
Guandong Shaoqing Pharmaceutical Factory
'Nasal Allergy Pills'
Pi Min Kan Wan is packaged in bottles of 50 pills

Chinese medical action

Dispels wind, dries damp, unblocks the nasal passages

Biomedical action

Anti-inflammatory, mucolytic

INDICATIONS

- Allergic rhinitis, hay fever, perennial rhinitis. This formula is basically symptomatic, and used for acute attacks of sneezing, nasal congestion and discharge with non specific heat or cold signs, that is, acute wind in the nasal passages.

Composition

Magnolia liliflora (xin yi hua, magnolia flower), *Xanthium sibiricum* (cang er zi, xanthium), *Paeonia suffruticosa* (mu dan pi, moutan), *Agastache rugosa* (huo xiang, agastache), *Schizonepeta tenuifolia* (jing jie, schizonepeta), *Angelica dahurica* (bai zhi, angelica)

Combine with

- **7.9 Jin Gui Shen Qi Wan**, **4.11 Ba Ji Yin Yang Wan** or **7.10 You Gui Wan** for patients with a lifetime history of allergic rhinitis (indicating a congenital Lung and Kidney yang qi deficiency). Add **7.11 Deer Velvet** or **7.12 Lu Rong Jiao** for essence deficiency patterns
- **7.23 Yu Ping Feng Wan** for defensive qi deficiency
- **2.11 Bu Zhong Yi Qi Wan** for failure of Spleen qi to rise to the nasal mucous membranes, with chronic recurrent allergy and weak immunity

Dosage and method of administration

3 pills three times daily, on an empty stomach. In severe cases the dose may be increased by 50%. For chronic cases, the dose should be reduced as the patient improves, to a level that maintains a clear airway. For chronic cases some weeks of treatment may be necessary. Better and faster results are obtained when combined with a sinus wash. Generally not used for children.

Pattern identifying features

- **wind in the nasal passages**
- **sneezing**
- hypersensitive mucous membranes

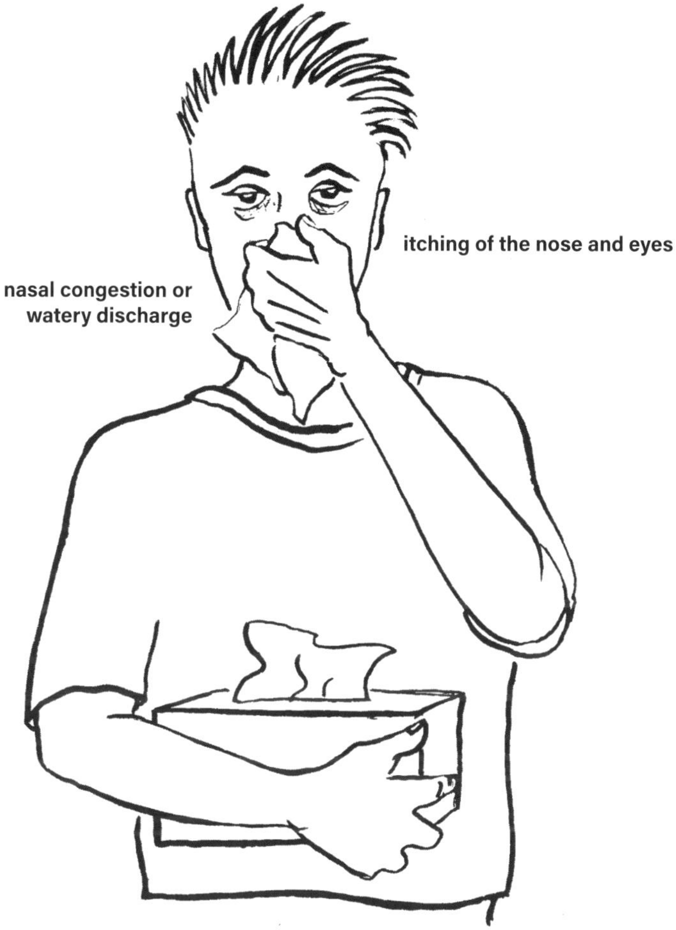

Cautions and contraindications

9.13 Pe Min Kan Wan is quite parching and may dry the nasal mucous membranes excessively in some patients.

1-3/12

9.14 PE MIN KAN WAN

鼻宁丸

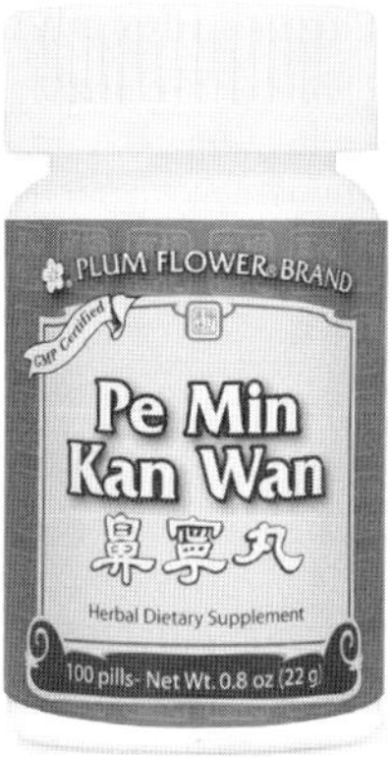

(*Bi Ning Wan*)
Guangzhou Qixing Pharmaceutical Factory (Guangzhou)
'Calm Nose Pill'
Pe Min Kan Wan is packaged in bottles of 100 and 500 pills

Chinese medical action

Clears heat, unblocks the nasal passages, reduces swelling and stops pain

Biomedical action

Anti-inflammatory, mucolytic, antibacterial

INDICATIONS

- Acute and chronic sinusitis and rhinitis from heat or phlegm heat accumulation in the nose and sinuses. Particularly good for chronic and stubborn sinus congestion with heat signs.
- Allergic sinusitis and rhinitis, seasonal and perennial nasal allergies with thick, sticky nasal discharge or nasal congestion, itching, irritation and sneezing.

Composition

Magnolia liliflora (xin yi hua, magnolia flower), *Xanthium sibiricum* (cang er zi, xanthium), *Isatis indigotica* (ban lan gen, woad root), *Agastache rugosa* (huo xiang, agastache), *Chrysanthemum sinense* (ju hua, chrysanthemum flower), *Ledebouriella divaricata* (fang feng, siler), *Centipeda minima* (e bu shi cao, centipeda), *Mentha haplocalycis* (bo he, mint), *Perilla frutescens* (zi su ye, perilla)

Combine with

- **6.5 Jia Wei Xiao Yao Wan** for sinus congestion or sinusitis worse with stress. Continue the **6.5 Jia Wei Xiao Yao Wan** after the sinus has resolved to prevent recurrence

  6.6 Long Dan Xie Gan Wan for acute sinus infection of a Liver fire type
- **3.16 Ching Fei Yi Huo Pien** or **9.3 Peking Niu Huang Jie Du Pian** for acute sinusitis
- **2.18 Bao He Wan** for chronic phlegm heat in the sinuses associated with food allergies or intolerances. The sinus congestion is worse with certain foods, especially alcohol and rich or greasy foods
- A few drops of **10.30 Po Sum On Medicated Oil** on a tissue to help open the sinuses and relieve congestion

Pattern identifying features

- heat, phlegm heat in the sinuses
- allergies; allergic sinusitis and rhinitis
- sneezing, nasal itch and irritation; watery irritated eyes

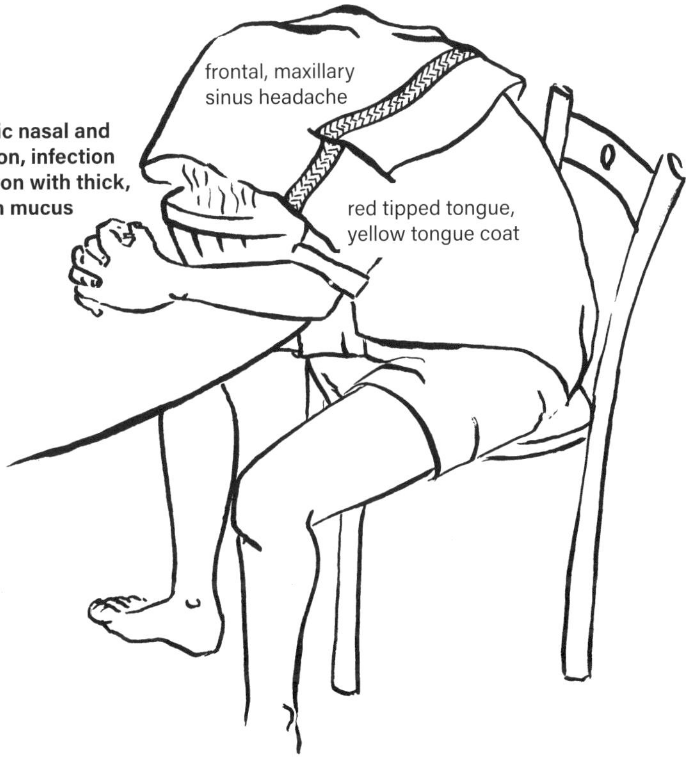

Dosage and method of administration

Two or three pills, three times daily on an empty stomach. In severe cases the dose can be increased by 50%. For chronic cases, the dose should be reduced as the patient improves, to a level that maintains a clear airway. For chronic cases some weeks of treatment may be necessary. Better and faster results are obtained when combined with a sinus wash.

Cautions and contraindications

Only used when there is colored mucus or chronic congestion. Not suitable for nasal problems with thin watery mucus. **9.14 Pe Min Kan Wan** is quite drying and excess use, or use unmodified in between episodes of sinus, can dry mucous membranes.

1-3/12

9.15 PE MIN KAN WAN (Nasal Clear)

鼻敏感丸

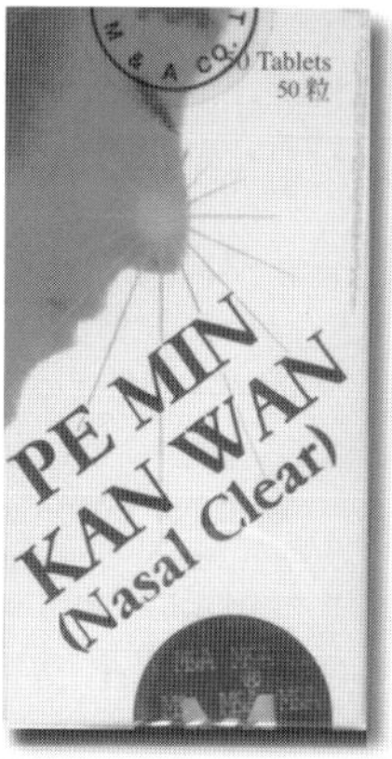

(*Bi Min Gan Wan*)
Wild Plants Research Centre, PRC
'Nasal Allergy Pills'
Pi Min Kan Wan is packaged in bottles of 50 pills

Chinese medical action

Clears heat, unblocks the nasal passages, reduces swelling and stops pain

Biomedical action

Anti-inflammatory, antibacterial, mucolytic

INDICATIONS

- Acute and chronic sinusitis and rhinitis. Particularly good for chronic and stubborn sinus congestion with heat signs. The nasal mucus will be sticky, yellow or green and hard to eliminate, or the patient may simply be more or less permanently congested.

Composition

Scutellaria baicalensis (huang qin, scute) 26%, *Xanthium sibiricun* (cang er zi, xanthium) 25%, *Agastache rugosa* (huo xiang, agastache) 25%, *Centipeda minima* (e bu shi cao, centipeda) 14%, *Angelica sinensis* (dang gui, chinese angelica) 10%

Dosage and method of administration

2-3 pills three times daily on an empty stomach. In acute or severe cases the dose can be increased by 50%. For chronic cases, the dose should be reduced after the first few weeks or as the patient improves, to a level that maintains a clear airway. For chronic cases some months of treatment are usually necessary. Better and faster results are obtained when combined with a sinus wash and constitutional formula. Generally not used for children.

Cautions and contraindications

Only used when there is coloured mucus or chronic congestion. **9.15 Pe Min Kan Wan** is quite drying and excessive use or use alone between episodes of sinus, can dry the mucous membranes.

9.16 HAY FEVER TABLET

鼻敏感片

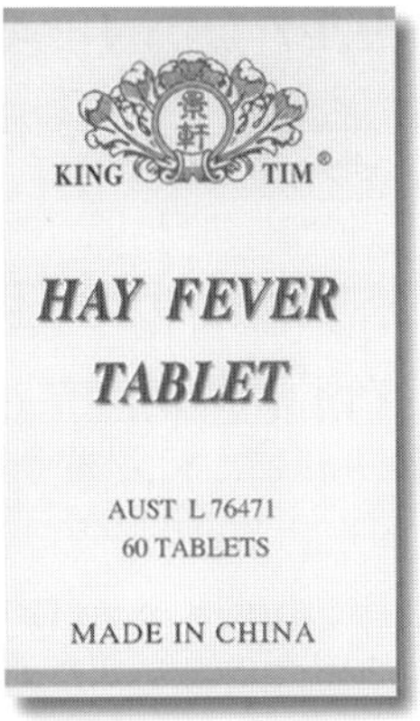

(*Bi Min Gan Pian*)
Jing Xian Pharmaceutical Co. (Guangzhou)
'Nasal Allergy Pills'
Hay Fever Tablets are packaged in bottles of 60 pills

Chinese medical action

Clears heat, unblocks the nasal passages, reduces swelling and stops pain

Biomedical action

Anti-inflammatory, antibacterial, mucolytic

INDICATIONS

- Acute and chronic sinusitis and rhinitis with heat signs. The nasal mucus will be sticky, yellow or green and hard to eliminate, or the patient may simply be more or less permanently congested.

Composition (each tablet contains extracts equivalent to dry)

Lonicera japonica (jin yin hua, honeysuckle) 830mg, *Xanthium sibiricum* (cang er zi, xanthium) 830mg, *Chrysanthemum indicum* (ye ju hua, wild chrysanthemum) 415mg, *Angelica dahurica* (bai zhi, angelica) 415mg, *Centipeda minima* (e bu shi cao, centipeda) 332mg, *Mentha haplocalycis* (bo he, mint) 83mg

Dosage and method of administration

3-5 tablets, three times daily on an empty stomach. For chronic cases, the dose should be reduced after the first few weeks or as the patient improves, to a level that maintains a clear airway. For chronic cases some months of treatment are usually necessary. Better and faster results are obtained when combined with a sinus wash and constitutional formula. Generally not used for children.

Cautions and contraindications

Only used when there is colored mucus or chronic congestion. **9.16 Hay Fever Tablets** are quite drying and excessive use or use alone between episodes of sinus, can dry the mucous membranes.

9.17 QIAN BAI BI YAN PIAN

千柏鼻炎片

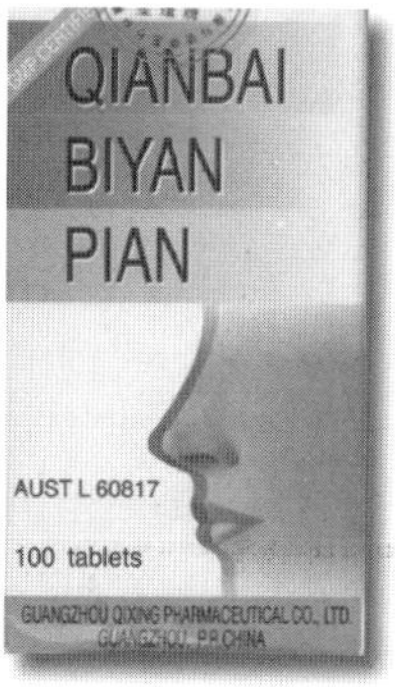

Guangzhou Qixing Pharmaceutical Co. (Guangzhou)
'Senecio and Selaginella Sinusitis Pills'
Qian Bai Bi Yan Pian is packaged in bottles of 30 capsules

Chinese medical action

Dispels wind, clears toxic heat, cools the Liver, dries phlegm damp, unblocks the nasal passages, stops pain

Biomedical action

Anti-inflammatory, analgesic, antibacterial, mild laxative

INDICATIONS

- Heat in the sinuses and nasal cavity. Used for acute and chronic sinusitis and rhinitis, with nasal and sinus congestion, sinus pain and headaches. This formula focuses primarily on the pain and inflammation associated with sinus congestion. Even though primarily targeted at heat patterns, it can be combined with an appropriate targeting formula to treat sinus pain and frontal headaches from cold or thermally neutral patterns.

Composition (each tablet contains extracts equivalent to dry)

Senecio scandens (qian li guang, senecio) 140mg, *Selaginella tamariscana* (juan bai, selaginella) 100mg, *Notopterygium incisum* (qiang huo, notopterygium) 76mg, *Ligusticum sinense* (gao ben, ligusticum) 53.6mg, *Angelica dahurica* (bai zhi, angelica) 50.8mg, *Cassia tora* (jue ming zi, cassia seed) 23mg

Combine with

- **6.5 Jia Wei Xiao Yao Wan** for sinus congestion and pain worse with stress
- **6.6 Long Dan Xie Gan Wan** for acute sinus infection of a Liver fire type
- **3.15 Qing Qi Hua Tan Wan** for chronic phlegm heat congestion in the sinuses
- **3.9 Chuan Xiong Cha Tiao Wan** for acute frontal headaches from wind cold congesting the sinuses
- **2.9 Xiang Sha Liu Jun Wan** for chronic sinus congestion and frontal headaches associated with Spleen qi deficiency and phlegm accumulation

Pattern identifying features

- **heat, phlegm heat in the sinuses**

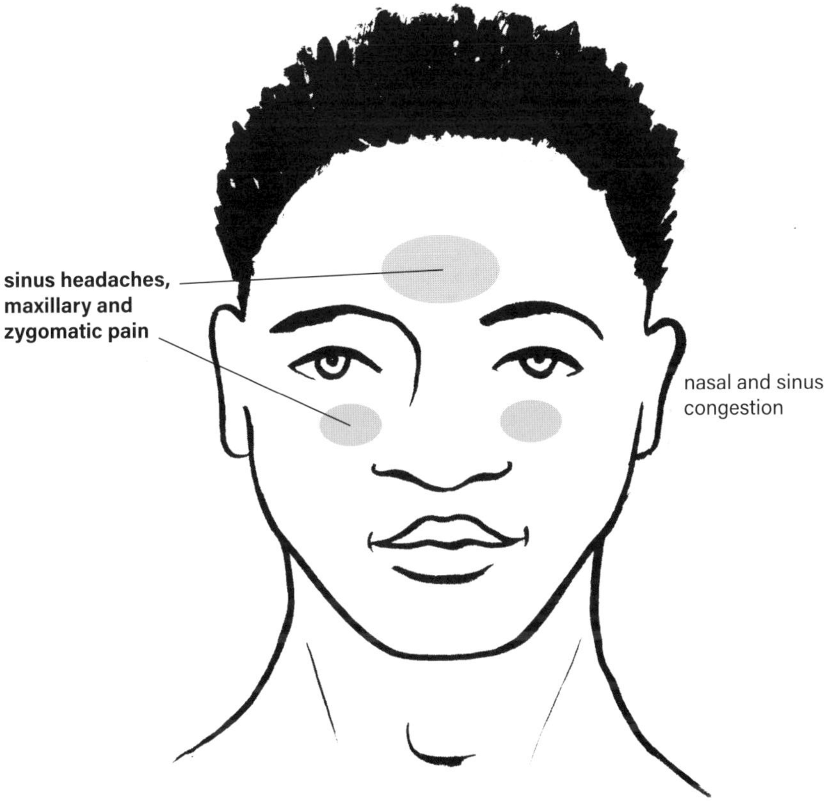

Dosage and method of administration

4 tablets three times daily on an empty stomach. After the condition begins to improve, the dose can be decreased to maintenance.

Cautions and contraindications

None noted.

9.18 XIN YI SAN

辛夷散

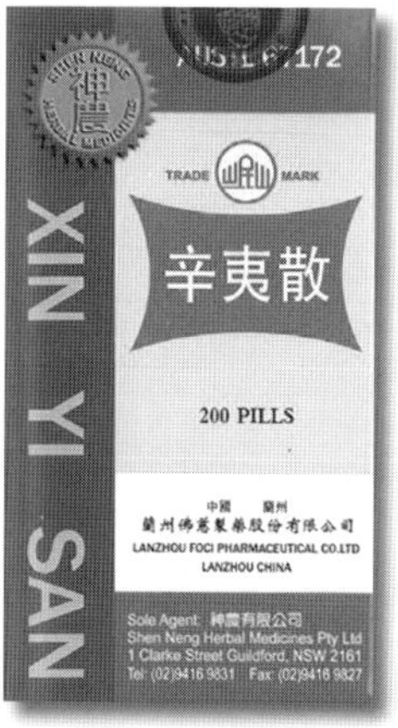

Lanzhou Foci Pharmaceutical Factory (Gansu)
'Magnolia Flower Powder'
Xin Yi San is packaged in bottles of 200 pills
Also available as: Magnolia Flower Teapills (PF), Magnolia Flower Formula (conc. extract)

Chinese medical action

Dispels wind cold, dries damp, unblocks the nasal passages and stops pain

Biomedical action

Diaphoretic, anti-inflammatory, analgesic

INDICATIONS

- Wind cold invasion or persistent cold lingering in the sinus cavity causing acute or chronic sinus congestion, sinusitis or rhinitis. Particularly good for chronic and stubborn sinus congestion with no heat signs, or with white or watery nasal discharge and postnasal drip.
- Sinus or frontal headaches.

Composition (each pill contains powdered)

Magnolia liliflora (xin yi hua, magnolia flower) 25.2mg, *Atractylodes macrocephala* (bai zhu, atractylodes) 21.6mg, *Ledebouriella divaricata* (fang feng, siler) 18mg, *Cimicifuga heraclefolia* (sheng ma, cimicifuga) 18mg, *Clematis armandii* (mu tong, akebia) 18mg, *Ligusticum wallici* (chuan xiong, cnidium) 18mg, *Asarum heterotropoides* (xi xin, asarum) 16.2mg, *Ligusticum sinense* (gao ben, ligusticum) 16.2mg, *Glycyrrhiza uralensis* (gan cao, licorice) 14.4mg, *Notopterygium incisum* (qiang huo, notopterygium) 14.4mg

Combine with

- **3.9 Chuan Xiong Cha Tiao Wan** for frontal headache and sinus congestion from wind cold invasion
- **2.9 Xiang Sha Liu Jun Wan** for chronic sinus congestion from phlegm damp accumulation in the sinuses
- **7.23 Yu Ping Feng Wan** for perennial rhinitis and sinusitis from defensive qi deficiency
- **4.11 Ba Ji Yin Yang Wan** for lifetime atopic rhinitis from congenital deficiency of Lung and Kidney qi

Pattern identifying features

- **wind cold invasion of the nasal passages and sinus cavity**
- postnasal drip
- decreased, or loss of, sense of smell

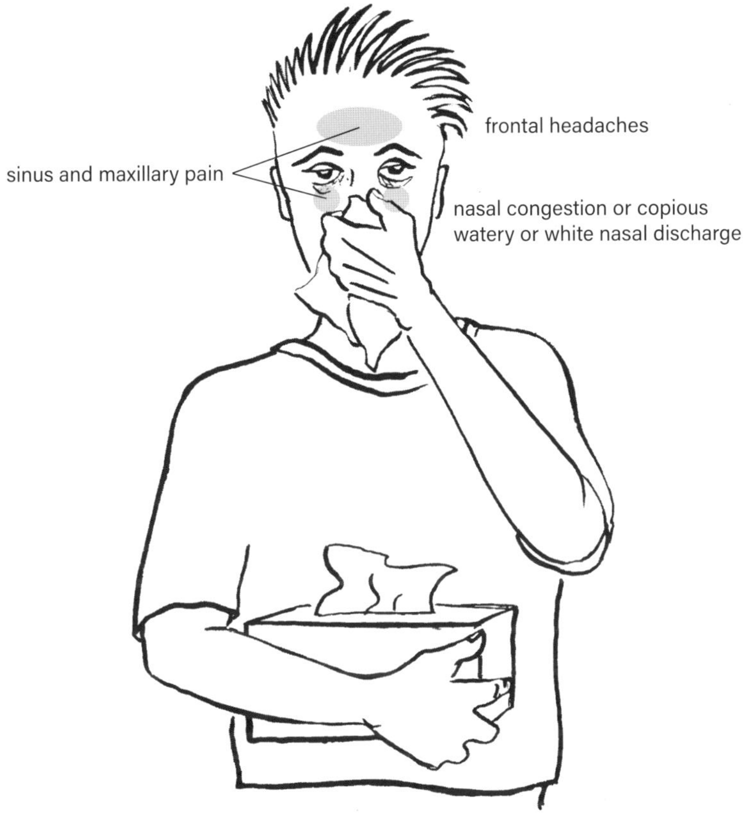

Dosage and method of administration

The recommended dose is 8-15 pills three times daily, on an empty stomach. Once the symptoms are controlled, the dose can be reduced until a comfortable maintenance level is reached.

Cautions and contraindications

Contraindicated in sinus congestion from heat.

GMP

9.19 CANG ER ZI WAN

苍耳子丸

1-3/52

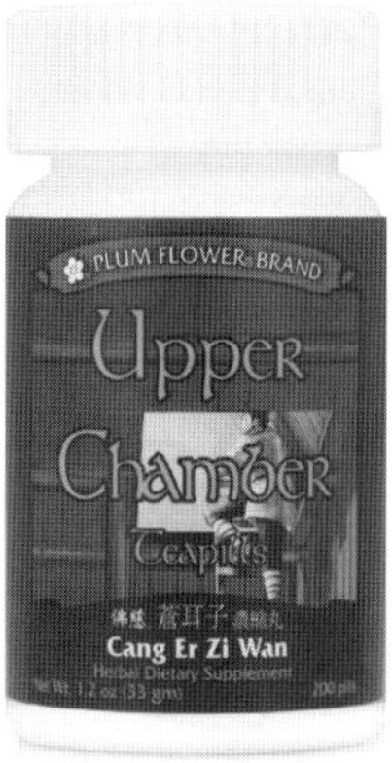

Lanzhou Foci Pharmaceutical Factory (Gansu)
'Xanthium Pills'
Cang Er Zi Wan is packaged in bottles of 200 pills
Available as: Xanthium Formula (conc. extract)

Chinese medical action
Dispels wind, clears heat, unblocks the nasal passages

Biomedical action
Diaphoretic, anti-inflammatory, analgesic

INDICATIONS
- Wind heat lingering in the nose and sinuses, causing sinus and nasal congestion, pain and discharge. This pattern typically follows an acute invasion of wind heat (or cold that transforms into heat) that congeals fluids to phlegm heat or stirs up existing phlegm. Although **9.19 Cang Er Zi Wan** is best for heat patterns, it can be combined with other formulas not specifically for heat when enhanced nasal and sinus decongestion is desired.
- With the appropriate identifying features, this formula can be used to treat conditions such as acute and chronic sinusitis and rhinitis, perennial and allergic rhinitis.

Composition
Xanthium sibiricum (cang er zi, xanthium), *Angelica dahurica* (bai zhi, angelica), *Magnolia liliflora* (xin yi hua, magnolia flower), *Mentha arvensis* (bo he, mint)

Combine with
- **2.11 Bu Zhong Yi Qi Wan** for chronic sinus congestion from retention of wind in a patient with qi deficiency
- **7.1.1 Liu Wei Di Huang Wan** for sinus congestion in patients with a tendency to yin deficiency
- **6.5 Jia Wei Xiao Yao Wan** for sinus congestion or sinusitis which is initiated or aggravated by stress. Continue the **6.5 Jia Wei Xiao Yao Wan** after the sinus has resolved to prevent recurrence
- **3.16 Ching Fei Yi Huo Pien** or **9.3 Peking Niu Huang Jie Du Pian** for acute sinusitis
- **2.18 Bao He Wan** for chronic phlegm heat in the sinuses associated with food allergies or intolerances. The sinus congestion is worse with certain foods, especially alcohol and rich or greasy foods

Pattern identifying features

- **wind heat and phlegm heat in the sinuses**
- reduction or loss of sense of smell, nasal voice
- inflamed and swollen nasal mucous membranes
- cough with yellow sputum
- in the early stages there may be fever, or fever and chills
- thirst

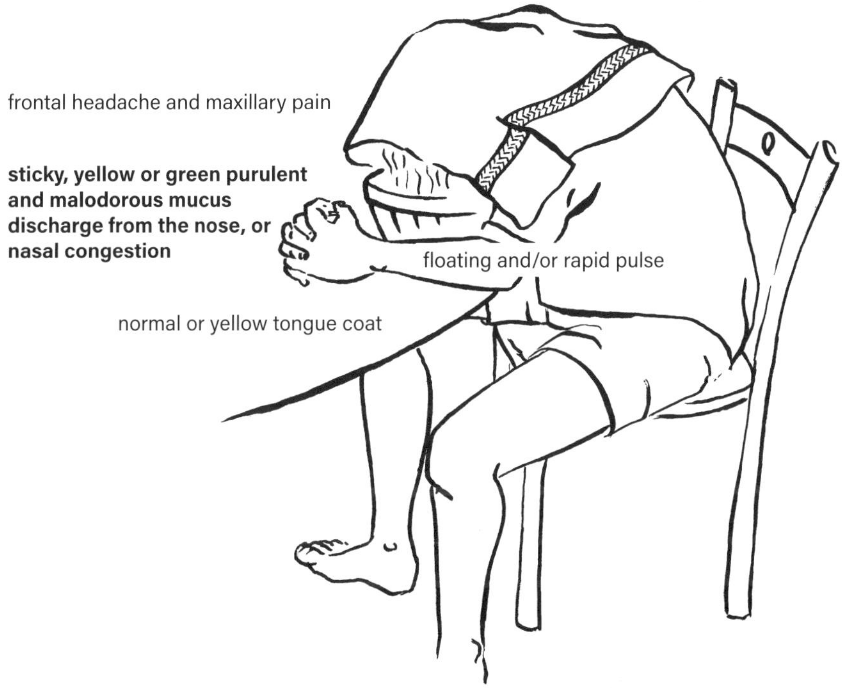

Dosage and method of administration

8-12 pills three times daily on an empty stomach. The dose can be spread out, or two lots of 12-18 pills taken, morning and evening. In severe cases or during the early stages of treatment (the first few weeks), a 50% increase in dose can be used, then reduced as treatment takes effect.

Cautions and contraindications

9.19 Cang Er Zi Wan is quite drying and excess use or use alone in between episodes of sinus, can dry and damage mucous membranes.

9.20 HAY FEVER RELIEVING TEA

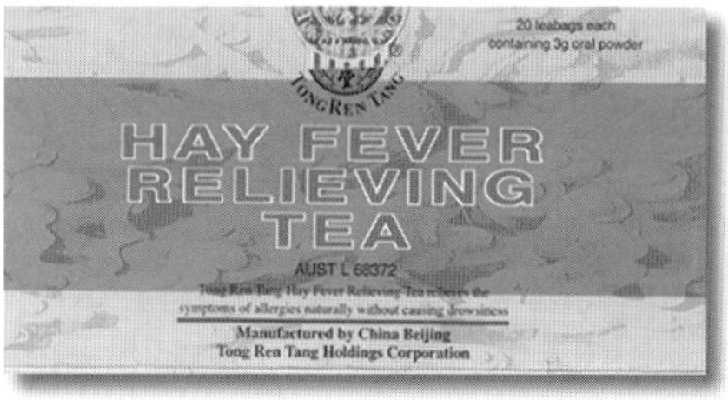

过敏鼻炎茶

(*Guo Min Bi Yan Cha*)
Tong Ren Tang (Beijing)
Hay Fever Relieving Tea is packaged in boxes of 20 teabags

Chinese medical action

Clears phlegm heat, dries damp and transforms phlegm, stops cough

Biomedical action

Decongestant, expectorant, antitussive

INDICATIONS

- Sinus and nasal congestion or sticky, yellow nasal discharge associated with phlegm heat congestion in the sinus cavity.
- Cough and wheezing from acute and chronic phlegm heat in the Lungs.
- With the appropriate identifying features, this formula can assist in the treatment of conditions such as acute and chronic sinusitis, hay fever, bronchitis, bronchiectasis, mild pneumonia and bronchial asthma.

Composition (each teabag [3g] contains extracts equivalent to dry)

Fritillaria thunbergii (zhe bei mu, fritillaria) 1.23g, *Scutellaria baicalensis* (huang qin, scute) 1.05g, *Eriobotrya japonica* (pi pa ye, loquat leaf) 877mg, *Cynanchum stauntonii* (bai qian, cynanchum) 877mg, *Morus alba* (sang bai pi, mulberry root bark) 877mg, *Perilla frutescens* (zi su ye, perilla) 877mg, *Glycyrrhiza uralensis* (gan cao, licorice) 877mg, *Poria cocos* (fu ling, hoelen) 877mg, *Citrus reticulata* (chen pi, citrus) 702mg, *Peucedanum praeruptorum* (qian hu, peucedanum) 526mg, *Angelica dahurica* (bai zhi, angelica) 351mg, *Xanthium sibiricun* (cang er zi, xanthium) 351mg, *Pinellia ternata* (zhi ban xia, processed pinellia) 526mg, *Ephedra sinica* (ma huang*, ephedra) 3mg [**Restricted use in some jurisdictions; may be subject to substitution*]

Combine with

– **9.17 Qian Bai Bi Yan Pian** for severe cases with frontal headache

Dosage and method of administration

The adult dose is 1-2 teabags steeped for 5 minutes in a cup of boiling water. More water can be added to the teabag until all taste is gone. In severe cases, up to six teabags can be used daily.

Pattern identifying features

- **phlegm heat accumulation in the Lung system**
- sinus congestion
- sneezing

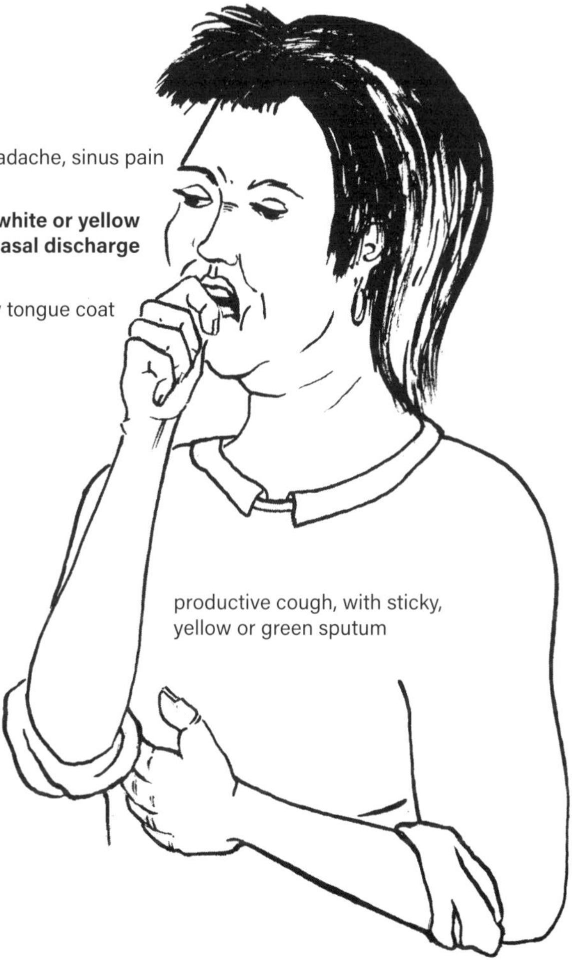

Cautions and contraindications

Not suitable for wind cold type cough or sinus congestion, with thin watery phlegm, or cough from yin deficiency. Caution in patients with hypertension. May cause or aggravate insomnia in some patients due to presence of ephedra.

9.21 MING MU SHANG CHING PIEN

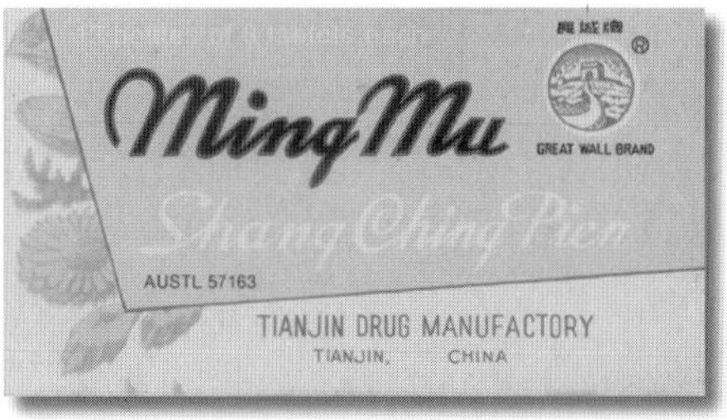

明目上清片

(*Ming Mu Shang Qing Pian*)
Tianjin Drug Manufactory (Shandong)
'Brighten the Eyes, Clear (Heat from) the Upper (Body) Pills'
Ming Mu Shang Ching Pien is packaged in vials of eight uncoated pills, twelve vials per box

Chinese medical action

Clears heat and damp heat from the Liver and Liver channel, dispels wind heat, brightens the eyes, benefits vision

Biomedical action

Anti-inflammatory, antibiotic, diuretic

INDICATIONS

- Inflammatory eye disorders from wind heat, damp heat, toxic heat, heat in the Liver channel or ascendant Liver yang. These are generally acute and associated with infection, eyestrain, stress and diet (especially alcohol). They may be diagnosed as conditions such as acute conjunctivitis, blepharitis, uveitis, glaucoma, dacryocystitis, urticaria, hordeolum, stye, pterygia and orbital cellulitis.
- Infections of the head, including skin, ear and oral infection and inflammation from Liver and Gallbladder heat, damp heat or Heart fire.
- Urinary tract infection, cystitis, urethritis or prostatitis from heat, damp heat or Heart fire invading the Small Intestine.
- Boils, acne, eczema, urticaria and dermatitis and other itchy, inflamed or suppurative skin disorders from damp heat or toxic heat in the skin.

Composition (each tablet contains extract equivalent to dry)

Gardenia florida (shan zhi zi, gardenia) 2.22g, *Angelica polymorpha* (dang gui, chinese angelica) 909mg, *Chrysanthemum sinense* (ju hua, chrysanthemum flower) 443mg, *Forsythia suspensa* (lian qiao, forsythia) 369mg, *Tribulus terrestris* (bai ji li, tribulus) 296mg, *Lophatherum elatum* (dan zhu ye, bamboo leaves) 296mg, *Ophiopogon japonicus* (mai dong, ophiopogon) 296mg, *Coptis chinensis* (huang lian, coptis) 273mg, *Scutellaria baicalensis* (huang qin, scute) 273mg, *Plantago asiatica* (che qian zi, plantago) 182mg, *Rheum palmatum* (da huang, rhubarb root) 36mg, Calcium sulphate 30mg

Combine with

- **13.19 Pearl Powder** for cataracts or inflamed pterygium from Liver fire
- **7.2.2 Qi Ju Di Huang Wan** for red, sore, irritated eyes from Liver yin deficiency and ascendant yang
- **6.6 Long Dan Xie Gan Wan** for acute exacerbation of glaucoma from Liver fire

Pattern identifying features

- **wind heat, Liver heat, damp heat or toxic heat eye disorders**
- fever

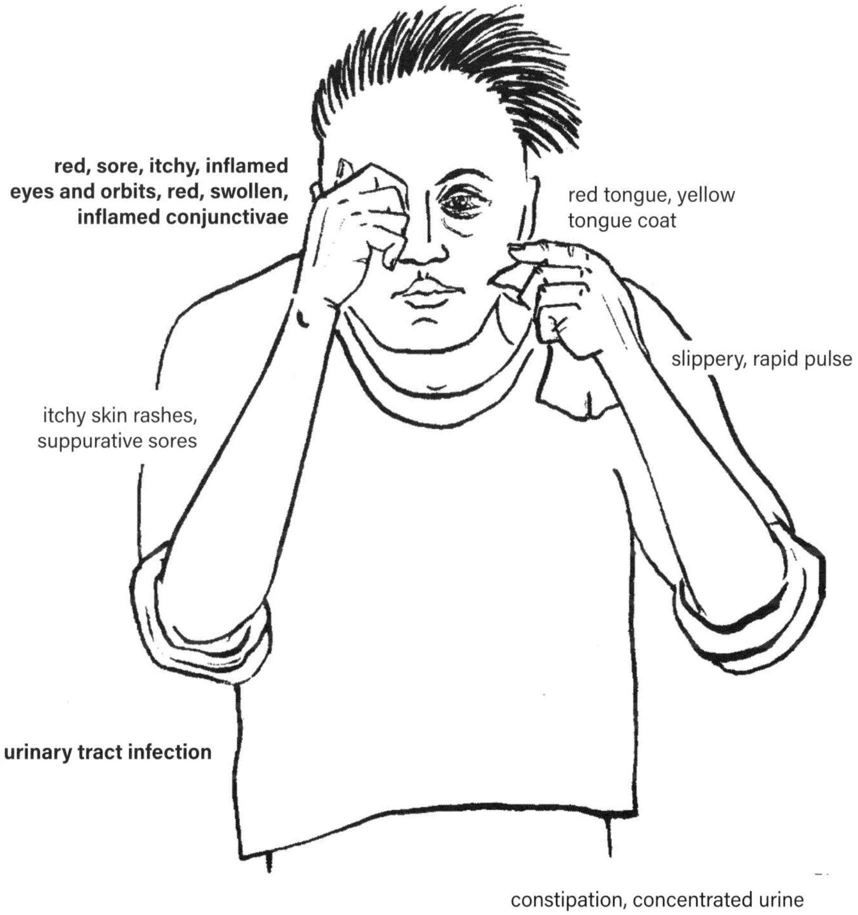

Dosage and method of administration

4-8 pills twice daily. In acute or severe cases, take one vial every 2-3 hours. May cause diarrhea.

Cautions and contraindications

Contraindicated during pregnancy.

9.22 MING MU DI HUANG WAN

明目地黄丸

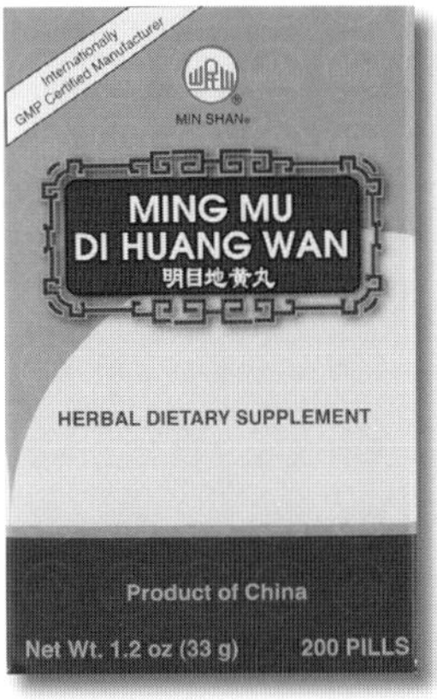

Lanzhou Foci Pharmaceutical Factory (Gansu)
'Rehmannia Pills to Brighten the Eyes'
Ming Mu Di Huang Wan is packaged in bottles of 200 pills
Also available as: Ming Mu Di Huang Teapills (PF)

Chinese medical action

Tonifies Liver and Kidney yin and blood, restrains Liver yang, brightens the eyes and improves vision

Biomedical action

Demulcent febrifuge, hypoglycemic, anti-hypertensive, improves kidney function

INDICATIONS

- Liver and Kidney yin and blood deficiency type chronic visual and eye disorders. These include weakness of vision, floaters, chronically sore dry irritated eyes, bloodshot eyes, photo-phobia, excessive lacrimation, night blindness, opacity of the vitreous humour, Sjogren's syndrome, keratitis sicca, non-acute glaucoma, optic neuritis, retinitis, retinal degeneration, myopia and atrophy of the optic nerve. May also be useful for strengthening the eyes in patients prone to conjunctivitis when used in between episodes of infection, or degenerative visual disorders.
- Dizziness, vertigo or hypertension from yin deficiency with ascendant yang.

Composition (each pill contains powdered)

Rehmannia glutinosa (shu di, processed rehmannia), *Cornus officinalis* (shan zhu yu, cornus), *Dioscorea opposita* (shan yao, dioscorea), *Poria cocos* (fu ling, hoelen), *Alisma orientalis* (ze xie, alisma), *Paeonia suffruticosa* (mu dan pi, moutan), *Lycium barbarum* (gou qi zi, lycium fruit), *Chrysanthemum morifolium* (ju hua, chrysanthemum flower), *Paeonia lactiflora* (bai shao, white peony), *Tribulus terrestris* (bai ji li, tribulus), *Uncaria rhyncophylla* (gou teng, gambir), *Angelica polymorpha* (dang gui, chinese angelica), *Glycyrrhiza uralensis* (gan cao, licorice)

Combine with

- **13.19 Pearl Powder** for cataracts
- **1.2 Si Wu Wan** for yin and blood deficient eye disorders
- **15.4 Tian Ma Gou Teng Wan** for severe dizziness, vertigo or headaches from Liver yin deficiency with ascendant yang
- **15.7 Yang Yin Jiang Ya Wan** for resistant hypertension from Liver yin deficiency with ascendant yang
- **9.11 Qing Yin Wan** or **7.21 American Ginseng Essence of Chicken** for the oral and ocular dryness associated with Sjogren's syndrome or other systemic patterns that dry the mucous membranes

Pattern identifying features

- **Liver and Kidney yin and blood deficiency visual disorders**
- heat, flushing, night sweats
- vision worse with overuse of the eyes
- red, thread-like capillaries in otherwise normal looking conjunctivae

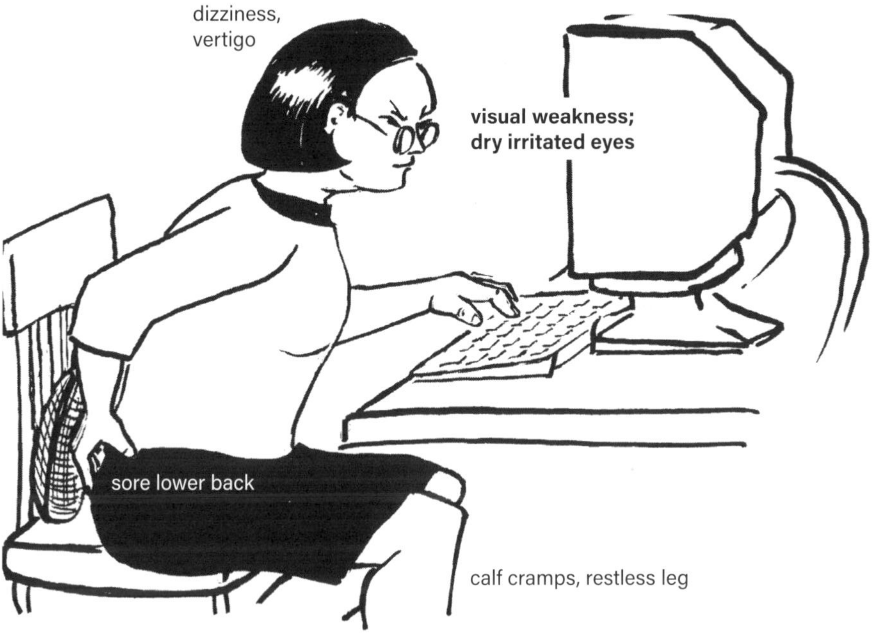

Dosage and method of administration

8-12 pills three times daily before meals. The dose can be spread out, or two lots of 12-18 pills taken, morning and evening. In severe cases or during the early stages of treatment (the first few weeks), a 50% increase in dose can be used, then reduced as treatment takes effect.

Cautions and contraindications

Not suitable for acute inflammatory eye disorders. Contraindicated during the early phase of acute illness such as colds and flu. Care should be taken in patients with a tendency to abdominal bloating, loose stools or mucus accumulation. Digestive distress can usually be alleviated by taking it with a small dose (3-6 pills at the same time) of **2.18 Bao He Wan** or **2.9 Xiang Sha Liu Jun Wan**.

9.23 MING MU CAPSULE

明目丸

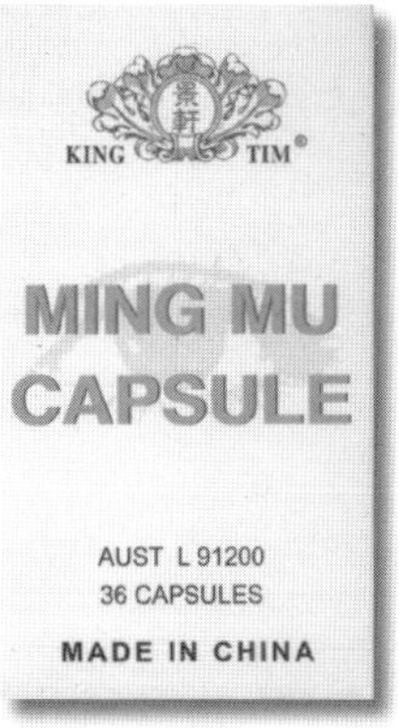

(*Ming Mu Wan*)
'Eye Brightening Capsules'
Jing Xian Pharmaceutical Co. (Guangzhou)
Ming Mu Capsule is packaged in bottles of 36 capsules

Chinese medical action

Tonifies the Liver and Kidneys, nourishes yin and blood, clears heat, brightens the eyes and improves vision

Biomedical action

Anti-inflammatory, improves kidney function, anti-hypertensive

INDICATIONS

- Visual disorders associated with Liver and Kidney yin and blood deficiency. This includes conditions such as loss of visual acuity, blurring vision following reading, eyestrain, photophobia, floaters, dry irritated eyes, excessive lacrimation and cataracts. Similar in scope and action to **9.22 Ming Mu Di Huang Wan**.
- Hypertension associated with Liver yin deficiency with ascendant yang.

Composition (each capsule contains extracts equivalent to dry)

Rehmannia glutinosa (shu di, processed rehmannia) 440mg, *Dendrobium nobile* (shi hu, dendrobium) 440mg, *Paeonia lactiflora* (bai shao, white peony) 365mg, *Schizandra chinensis* (wu wei zi, schizandra) 365mg, *Cornus officinalis* (shan zhu yu, cornus) 260mg, *Chrysanthemum sinense* (ju hua, chrysanthemum flower) 125mg, *Lycium barbarum* (gou qi zi, lycium fruit) 80mg, *Cuscuta hygrophila* (tu su zi, cuscuta) 80mg, *Achyranthes bidentata* (huai niu xi, achyranthes) 80mg, *Astragalus complanatus* (sha yuan ji li, astragalus seed) 80mg, *Angelica polymorpha* (dang gui, chinese angelica) 80mg, *Lycium chinense* (di gu pi, lycium root bark) 80mg

Dosage and method of administration

3–4 capsules, three times daily on an empty stomach

Cautions and contraindications

Not suitable for acute inflammatory eye disorders. Caution in patients with digestive weakness and Spleen deficiency.

跌打风湿 10

Pain and Trauma

10.1 YUNNAN PAIYAO

云南白药

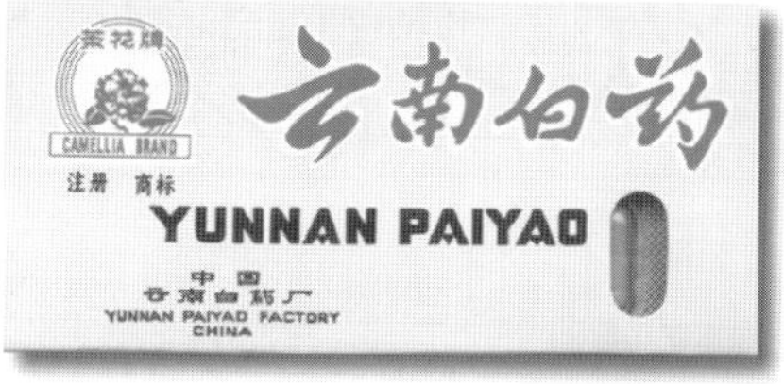

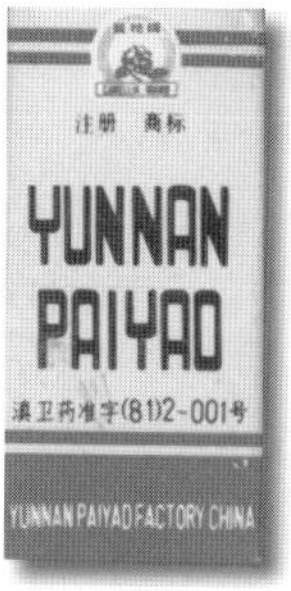

(*Yun Nan Bai Yao*)
Yunnan Paiyao Factory (Yunnan)
'White Powder from Yun Nan Province'
Yunnan Paiyao is packaged in two different forms, blister sheets of 16 x 250mg capsules, and small bottles of 4 grams loose powder. Both have a single peppercorn sized red pill reserved for serious hemorrhage and shock

Chinese medical action

Stops bleeding, invigorates blood and disperses static blood

Biomedical action

Hemostatic, invigorates local circulation, analgesic

INDICATIONS

- Bleeding. An important first aid remedy for all types of bleeding, regardless of etiology. Used to arrest internal and external bleeding from trauma, as well as conditions such as bleeding gastric ulcers and gums, hematemesis, hematuria, hemoptysis, epistaxis, rectal bleeding, bronchiectasis and purpura. Can be applied topically as well as taken internally for traumatic hemorrhage
- Gynecological conditions with blood stagnation or bleeding, including menorrhagia and dysmenorrhea from fibroids, amenorrhea, postpartum or post termination blood stagnation and hemorrhage, placental retention and painful gynecological masses
- Suppurative skin infections such as abscesses, boils, carbuncles and ulcers, both acute and chronic non-healing
- May be useful in alleviating bleeding and pain associated with certain types of neoplasm, such as those of the bladder and prostate.
- Used post-operatively to reduce keloid scarring, arrest bleeding, accelerate hemolysis and promote healing

Composition (each capsule [250mg] contains)

Panax notoginseng (tian qi, tian qi ginseng) 99mg, *Arjuga reptans* (jin gu cao, common bugle) 42.08mg, *Dioscorea batatas* (shan yao, dioscorea) 32.92mg, *Dioscorea japonica* (chuan shan long, japanese dioscorea) 24.75mg, *Erodium stephanianum* (lao guan cao, cranebill) 17.82mg, *Diospyros kaki* (shi shu gen, persimmon root) 14.85mg, *Inula cappa* (bai niu dan, inula) 12.38mg, *Cinnamomum camphora* (zhang nao, camphor) 3.71mg
Note: The ingredient listed, supplied by the manufacturer on application for listing with the TGA, are those in the powder. The contents of the red pill remain undisclosed at the time of printing.

Pattern identifying features

- **all types of bleeding** – uterine, hematemesis, hemoptysis, rectal, etc.

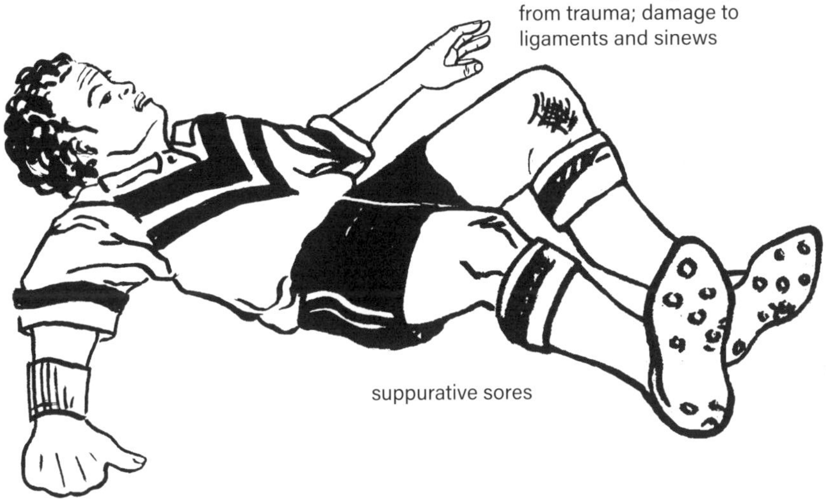

Combine with

- **10.23 Zheng Gu Shui** topically for bruising from trauma
- **1.9 Gui Pi Wan** for uterine bleeding or menorrhagia of a deficient type
- **14.1 Huang Lian Jie Du Wan** for sudden bleeding due to heat in the blood
- **2.37 Huai Jiao Di Yu Wan** or **2.38 Hua Zhi Ling Tablet** and **13.14 Ching Wan Hung** topically for painful bleeding hemorrhoids

Dosage and method of administration

The recommended dose is 2 capsules four times daily; for children 2-5 years old half a capsule four times daily; for children 5-12 years old one capsule four times daily. In serious cases the dose can be safely doubled for a few days to a week. A capsule can be broken and the wound sprinkled with powder, then held closed until bleeding ceases. For bleeding take with water; for blood stasis take with a little alcohol such as vodka or sherry.

The red pill is reserved for serious wounds and is used for patients about to go into shock.

Cautions and contraindications

Contraindicated during pregnancy. Avoid broad beans, fish, crustaceans and sour and cold foods while using this product.

GMP

10.2 RAW TIENCHI TABLETS

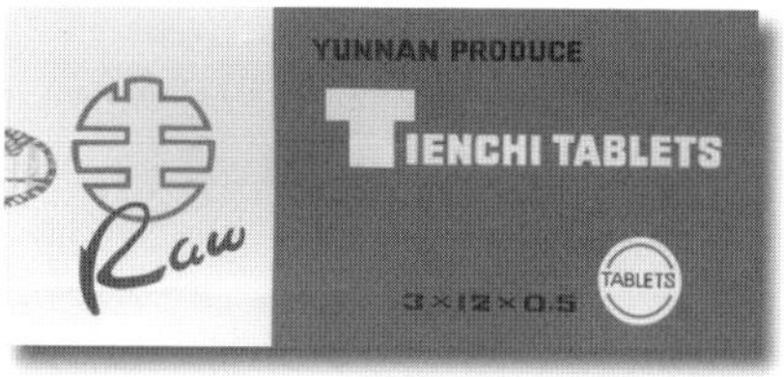

生田七片

(*Sheng Tian Qi Pian*)
Yunnan Medicines and Health Products Corp.
(Yunnan)
Tienchi Tablets are packaged in blister sheets, 36 tablets per box
A similar product available as: Tian Qi Teapills (PF), Pseudoginseng Capsules (Raw)

Chinese medical action

Invigorates blood, disperses static blood, stops bleeding

Biomedical action

Hemostatic, dilates coronary arteries, lower cholesterol and triglycerides, improves micro-circulation

INDICATIONS

- Bleeding with blood stasis. Has the unique property of being able to arrest bleeding without causing blood stasis, and disperse static blood without causing potential bleeding problems. An important herb for a variety of traumatic and cardiovascular problems. The subject of considerable research in China, tian qi ginseng has been shown to dilate coronary arteries and stimulate new micro-circulation thus improving cardiac function. It is also able to decrease blood lipids. Can be used post surgically to improve healing.
- Used in large doses for a few days to a few weeks for hemorrhagic disorders and acute trauma with bruising and hemorrhage, both internally and topically.
- Preventative for patients at risk of ischaemic cardiovascular and cerebrovascular disease. Used for conditions such as transient ischaemic attacks, angina, hyperlipidemia, retinal hemorrhage, sequelae of cerebrovascular hemorrhage, hemiplegia, thrombophlebitis and deep venous thrombosis.

Composition (each tablet contains)

Panax notoginseng (tian qi, tian qi ginseng) 500mg

Dosage and method of administration

Preventively for cardiovascular and cerebrovascular disease, hyperlipidemia: 2-4 tablets, 3 times daily. Bleeding and trauma: 4-8 tablets three times daily. The crushed tablet can be applied topically to a bleeding wound.

Cautions and contraindications

Contraindicated during pregnancy.

10.3 DIE DA ZHI TONG CAPSULE

跌打止痛丸

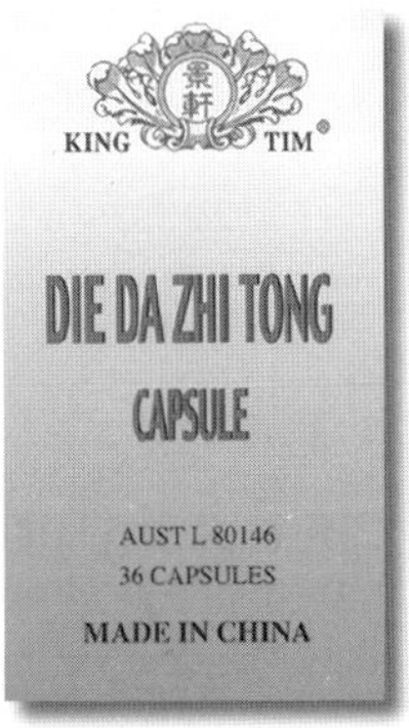

(*Die Da Zhi Tong Wan*)
Jing Xian Pharmaceutical Co. (Guangzhou)
'Trauma and Analgesic Pills'
Die Da Zhi Tong Capsules are packaged in bottles of 36 capsules

Chinese medical action

Invigorates circulation of qi and blood, disperses static blood, alleviates swelling and stops pain

Biomedical action

Analgesic, dissipates bruising, enhances circulation, promotes healing

INDICATIONS

- Pain, swelling, bruising and soft tissue damage from traumatic injury. This is quite a strong blood invigorating formula, and in conjunction with a topical liniment can significantly alleviate pain and swelling, and accelerate healing and recovery.
- For uncomplicated fractures, a few weeks of treatment to disperse as much blood stasis as possible, can be followed, once bruising has subsided, by **1.30 Bu Gai Zhuang Gu Capsule** or similar to encourage bone repair.

Composition (each capsule contains)

Salvia miltiorrhiza (dan shen, salvia) 90mg, *Paeonia lactiflora* (bai shao, white peony) 78mg, *Panax notoginseng* (tian qi, tian qi ginseng) 50mg, *Angelica polymorpha* (dang gui, chinese angelica) 35mg, *Corydalis turtschaninovii* (yan hu suo, corydalis) 35mg, *Dalbergia odorifera* (jiang xiang, dalbergia wood) 35mg, *Sparganium stoloniferum* (san leng, sparganium) 32mg, *Curcuma zedoaria* (e zhu, curcuma) 32mg, *Boswellia carterii* (ru xiang, frankincense) 25mg, *Rheum officinale* (da huang, rhubarb root) 15mg

Combine with

– **10.23 Zheng Gu Shui** or **10.32 Die Da Jiu** topically for bruising and pain

Dosage and method of administration

2-3 capsules, three times daily on an empty stomach. May cause diarrhea.

Cautions and contraindications

Contraindicated during pregnancy, where there is continuing bleeding or open wounds and in patients taking warfarin (coumarin). Caution in patients using mild anticoagulants such as aspirin and fish oil, as clotting time can be reduced.

10.4 CHIN GU TIE SHANG WAN

筋骨跌伤丸

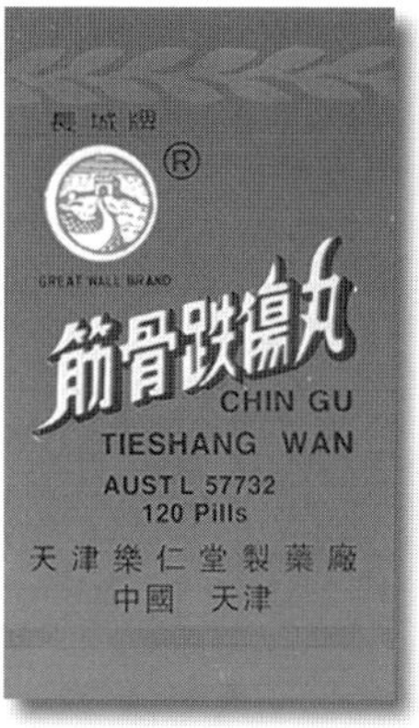

(*Jin Gu Die Shang Wan*)
Tianjin Lerentang Pharmaceutical Factory
'Sinew and Bone Trauma Pills'
Chin Gu Tie Shang Wan is packaged in bottles of 120 pills.
A similar formula available as: The Great Mender Teapills (PF)

Chinese medical action

Invigorates circulation of qi and blood, disperses static blood, alleviates swelling and stops pain

Biomedical action

Analgesic, dissipates bruising, enhances circulation, promotes healing

INDICATIONS

- Pain, swelling, spasm and bruising from traumatic injury. Used for soft tissue injury, sprains, strains, ligamentous damage, bruising and fracture.
- Assists in encouraging the healing of slow to heal fractures. Similar in most respects to **10.3 Die Da Zhi Tong Capsule** but more suited to prolonged use and better for bony lesions.
- For internal blood stasis patterns with pain, including chest and epigastric pain, dysmenorrhea and pelvic pain.
- Can assist in chronic skin diseases with purple or dark discoloration from blood stasis, including chronic abscesses and ulcers, psoriasis and rosacea.

Composition (each pill contains powdered)

Panax notoginseng (tian qi, tian qi ginseng) 30mg, *Angelica polymorpha* (dang gui, chinese angelica) 22.5mg, *Boswellia carterii* (ru xiang, frankincense) 22.5mg, *Daemonorops draco* (xue jie, dragons blood) 22.5mg, *Dipsacus asper* (xu duan, dipsacus) 22.5mg, *Commiphora myrhha* (mo yao, myrhh) 15mg, *Carthamus tinctorius* (hong hua, carthamus) 15mg

Combine with

- **10.23 Zheng Gu Shui** topically for the bruising and pain of traumatic injury
- **10.11 Shu Jin Huo Xue Wan** or **5.1 Xue Fu Zhu Yu Wan** for non-healing or slow healing fractures in patients with marked blood stasis, and severe pain in the joints and muscles from blood stasis following trauma
- **1.30 Bu Gai Zhuang Gu Capsule** for slow healing fractures with minor residual blood stasis
- **7.16.1 Shi Quan Da Bu Wan** for non-healing of fractures in patients with qi and blood deficiency
- **1.15 Tong Jing Wan**, **1.13 Woo Garm Yuen Medical Pills** or **1.18 Shao Fu Zhu Yu Wan** for severe dysmenorrhea
- **13.2 Xiao Feng Wan** for bleeding or chronic non-healing eczema and dermatitis

Pattern identifying features

- **blood stasis; bruising, sprains and fractures from traumatic injury**

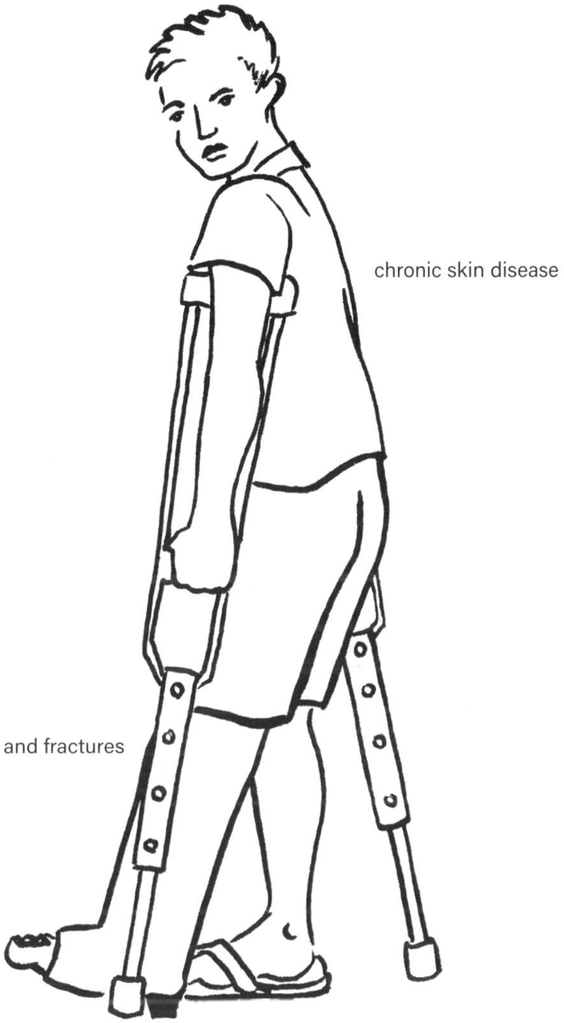

Dosage and method of administration

8 pills three times daily on an empty stomach. The dose can be spread out, or two lots of 12 pills may be taken morning and evening.

Cautions and contraindications

Contraindicated during pregnancy.

GMP

10.5 HUO LUO XIAO LING WAN

活络效灵丸

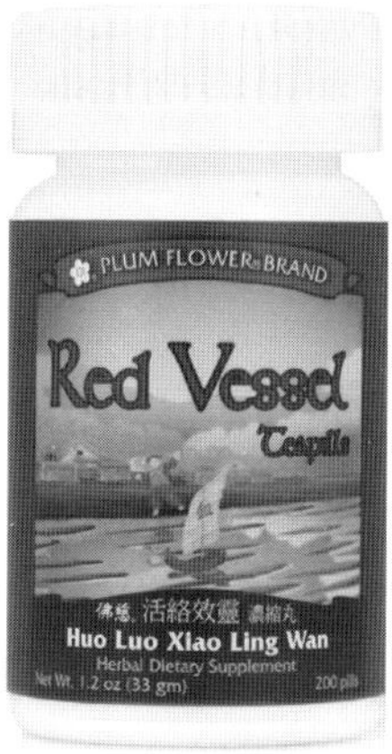

1-3/12

Lanzhou Foci Pharmaceutical Factory (Gansu)
'Miraculously Effective Collateral Regulating Pill'
Huo Luo Xiao Ling Wan is packaged in bottles of 200 pills

Chinese medical action

Invigorates circulation of qi and blood, disperses static blood, alleviates swelling and stops pain

Biomedical action

Analgesic, dissipates bruising, enhances circulation, promotes healing

INDICATIONS

- Pain from qi and blood stasis. For acute and chronic blood stasis type pain, regardless of location. A versatile formula that can be added to other targeting formulas when an extra analgesic or blood stasis dispersing action is desired.
- Fixed, painful abdominal masses.
- Purple or dark skin lesions associated with blood stasis, including internal and external suppurative lesions that may be acute and inflamed, or chronic and non-healing, chronic psoriasis and dermatitis, and rosacea.
- With the appropriate identifying features, this formula can assist in the treatment of conditions such as acute traumatic injury and bruising, angina pectoris, endometriosis, fibroids and cysts, hepatic abscess, hepatic cirrhosis, hepatosplenomegaly, chronic appendicitis, chronic abscess, chronic osteomyelitis, diverticulosis, diabetic ulcers, chronic fixed pain, postherpetic, intercostal or trigeminal neuralgia, 'fifty year shoulder' and sciatica.

Composition

Angelica polymorpha (dang gui, chinese angelica), *Salvia miltiorrhiza* (dan shen, salvia), *Commiphora myrhha* (mo yao, myrhh), *Boswellia carteri* (ru xiang, frankincense)

Combine with

- **1.16 Tao Hong Si Wu Wan** for dysmenorrhea and endometriosis
- **5.4 Xin Mai Ling** for diabetic ulcers and peripheral vascular disease
- **5.1 Xue Fu Zhu Yu Wan** for focal blood stasis pain in the chest or head; this combination also used for postherpetic neuralgia, migraine, angina and abdominal masses, such as hepatic cirrhosis
- **10.23 Zheng Gu Shui** topically for pain and bruising from trauma
- **13.2 Xiao Feng Wan** for chronic eczema, dermatitis or psoriasis with stubborn, purplish lesions
- **7.12 Lu Rong Jiao** or **7.16.1 Shi Quan Da Bu Wan** for deeply rooted yin type chronic abscesses or ulcerations

Pattern identifying features

- **blood stasis type pain**
- **abdominal, chest, peripheral pain**
- fixed masses

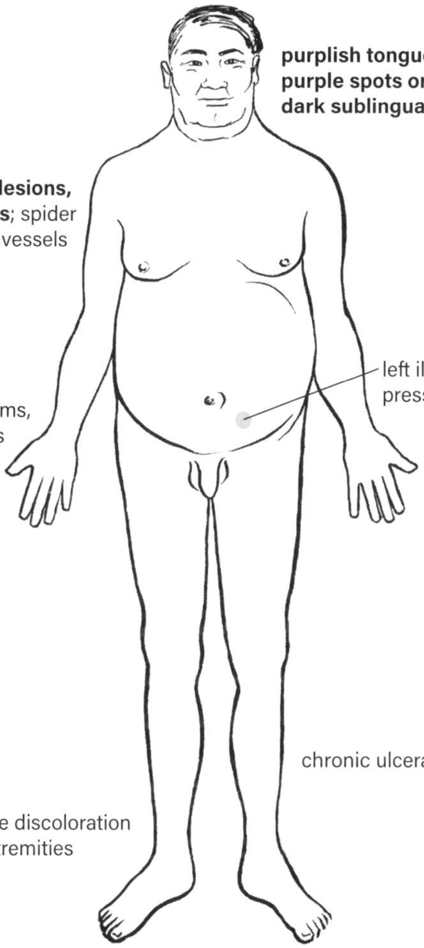

– **10.12 Shen Tong Zhu Yu Wan** for chronic blood stasis painful obstruction
– **14.8 Wu Wei Xiao Du Wan** for acute superficial painful abscesses and sores

Dosage and method of administration

8 pills three times daily on an empty stomach. The dose can be spread out, or two lots of 12 pills taken morning and evening. When used to augment another formula, 4-6 pills three times daily is usually sufficient.

Cautions and contraindications

Contraindicated during pregnancy, where there is continuing bleeding or open wounds and in patients taking warfarin (coumarin). Caution in patients using mild anticoagulants such as aspirin and fish oil, as clotting time can be reduced.

GMP

10.6 JUAN BI WAN

蠲痹丸

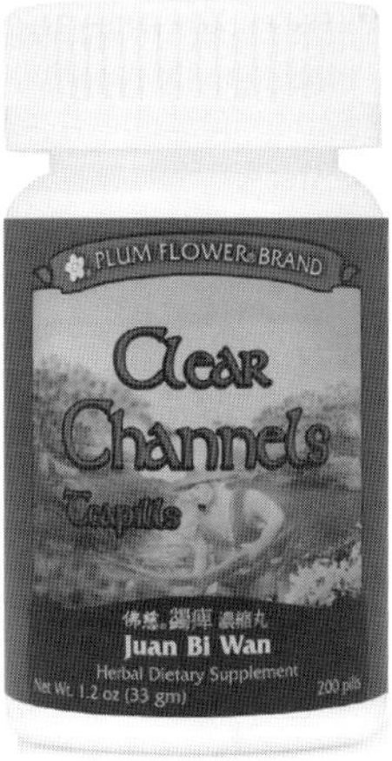

3+/12

Lanzhou Foci Pharmaceutical Factory (Gansu)
'Remove Painful Obstruction Pills'
Juan Bi Wan is packaged in bottles of 200 pills
Also available as: Notopterygium and Turmeric Combination (conc. extract)

Chinese medical action

Dispels wind cold damp, warms and unblocks the channels and collaterals, stops pain

Biomedical action

Analgesic, anti-arthritic, anti-inflammatory, enhances circulation

INDICATIONS

- Wind cold damp painful obstruction. Best for the early stages of a painful obstruction pattern, when pain and stiffness are intermittent, mild to moderate, and there is little or no underlying deficiency. Pain of this type is characterized by its responsiveness to changes in weather, being worse on wet, cold or humid days. It is also aggravated by lack of movement and alleviated by application of heat. Depending on the balance of wind and the other pathogens, pain may be fixed in location, or mobile, appearing in different parts of the body at different times. Generally considered best for painful obstruction affecting the upper body.
- With the appropriate identifying features, this formula can be used to treat osteoarthritis, bursitis, spondylosis, fibromyalgia and sciatic pain.

Composition

Morus alba (sang zhi, mulberry twig), *Piper futokadsura* (hai feng teng, kadsura stem), *Angelica sinensis* (dang gui, chinese angelica), *Notopterygium incisum* (qiang huo, notopterygium), *Angelica pubescens* (du huo, Tu-huo), *Gentiana macrophylla* (qin jiao, chin chiu), *Ligusticum wallichi* (chuan xiong, ligusticum), *Saussurea lappa* (mu xiang, saussurea), *Cinnamomum cassia* (gui zhi, cinnamon twigs), *Boswellia carteri* (ru xiang, frankincense), *Glycyrrhiza uralensis* (zhi gan cao, honey fried licorice)

Combine with

– **10.38 Plaster for Bruise and Analgesic** topically for localised pain
– **10.40 Porous Capsicum Plaster** for relatively severe pain with cold predominant

Pattern identifying features

- **wind cold damp painful obstruction**
- worse with changes of weather and lack of activity
- better for heat and movement
- relatively robust patient with little or no contributing deficiency

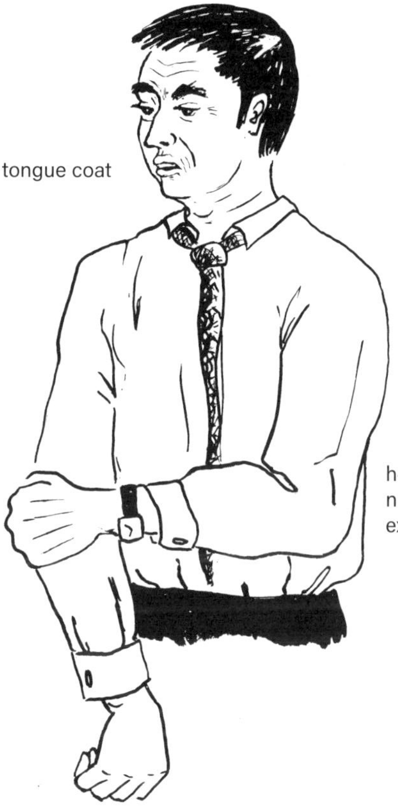

Dosage and method of administration

8-12 pills three times daily on an empty stomach. The dose can be spread out, or taken in two lots of 12-18 pills, morning and evening. In severe cases or during the early stages of treatment, a 50% increase in dose can be used, then reduced as treatment takes effect.

Cautions and contraindications

Contraindicated during pregnancy and for pain patterns with redness and heat in joints or muscles.

10.7 QU FENG ZHEN TONG CAPSULE

祛风镇痛丸

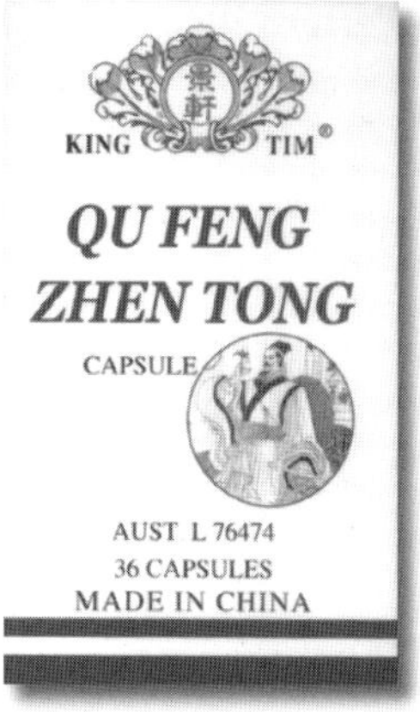

(*Qu Feng Zhen Tong Wan*)
Jing Xian Pharmaceutical Co. (Guangzhou)
'Expel Wind, Suppress Pain Pills'
Qu Feng Zhen Tong Capsules are packaged in bottles of 36 capsules

Chinese medical action

Dispels wind damp, warms and unblocks the channels and collaterals, stops pain

Biomedical action

Analgesic, anti-arthritic, enhances circulation

INDICATIONS

- Wind cold damp painful obstruction. Considered best for pain in the upper body, neck, shoulders, thoracic region and arms, but can be used for wind cold damp painful obstruction anywhere in the body. Quite dispersing and warm, this formula is best for cold damp patterns with localised pain and swelling in patients with little or no underlying deficiency.
- With the appropriate identifying features, this formula can assist in the treatment of pain from osteoarthritis, rheumatoid arthritis, fibromyalgia, osteophytes and spurs, cervical spondylosis, sciatica, migraine headache and tendinitis.

Composition (each capsule contains extracts equivalent to dry)

Notopterygium incisum (qiang huo, notopterygium) 500mg, *Angelica pubescens* (du huo, Tu-huo) 500mg, *Paeonia lactiflora* (bai shao, white peony) 500mg, *Chaenomeles speciosa* (mu gua, chinese quince) 500mg, *Spatholobus suberectus* (ji xue teng, spatholobus) 500mg, *Angelica polymorpha* (dang gui, chinese angelica) 500mg, *Morus alba* (sang zhi, mulberry twig) 400mg, *Clematis sinensis* (wei ling xian, chinese clematis) 400mg, *Curcuma longa* (jiang huang, turmeric rhizome) 400mg, *Gentiana macrophylla* (qin jiao, chin chiu) 400mg, *Achyranthes bidentata* (huai niu xi, achyranthes) 400mg

Dosage and method of administration

3-4 capsules, three times daily, on an empty stomach.

Pattern identifying features

- **wind cold damp painful obstruction**

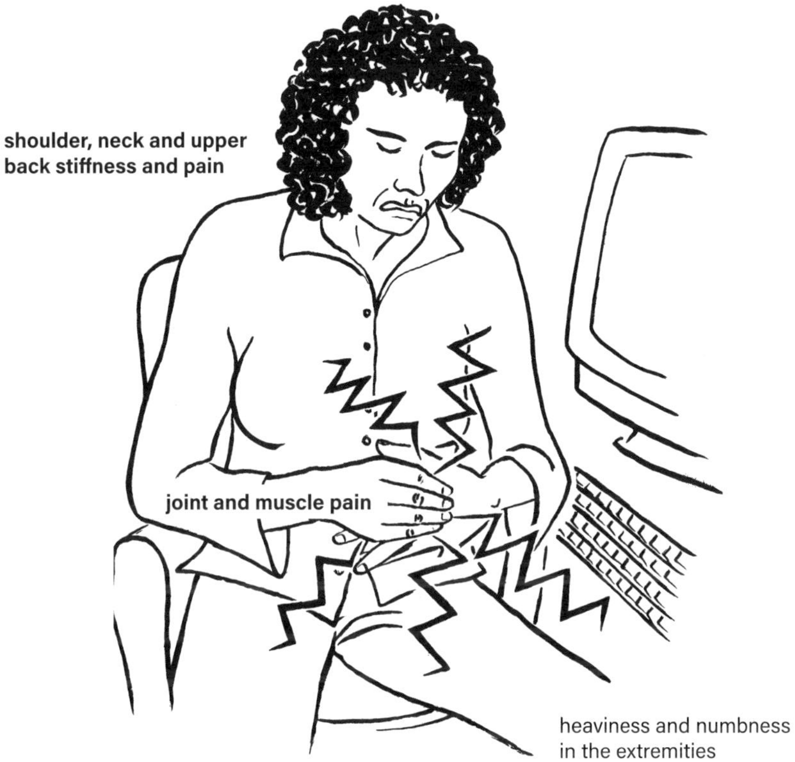

Cautions and contraindications

Contraindicated during pregnancy.

GMP

10.8 XIAO HUO LUO WAN

小活络丸

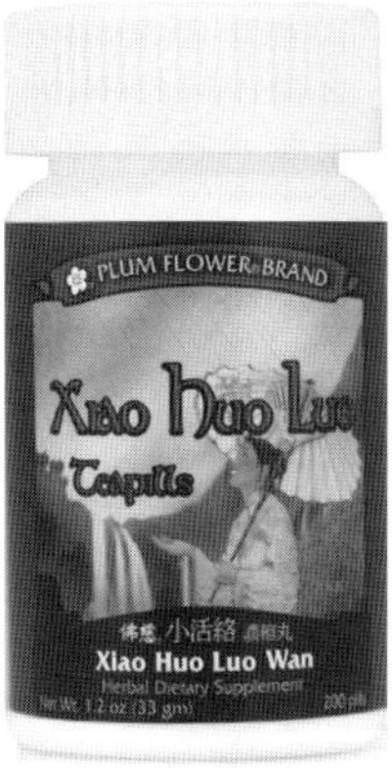

1-3/52

Lanzhou Foci Pharmaceutical Factory (Gansu)
'Minor Invigorate the Collaterals Pill'
Xiao Huo Luo Wan is packaged in bottles of 100 pills
Also available as: Myrrh and Aconite Formula (conc. extract)

Chinese medical action

Powerfully warms cold, dries damp, transforms phlegm and dispels static blood, unblocks the collaterals, stops pain

Biomedical action

Analgesic, anti-arthritic, enhances circulation

INDICATIONS

- Joint pain from chronic cold damp painful obstruction with phlegm and blood stasis. Pain is chronic, fixed in location, excruciating, markedly worse with cold and accompanied by stiffness, spasm, numbness and paresthesia in the extremities. An important and effective formula for chronic and recalcitrant pain, but must be used with caution and by experienced practitioners, as it is very hot, acrid and dispersing, and easily damages yin.
- Numbness and loss of function in the extremities following a wind-stroke in a patient tending to cold or yang deficiency. Also used for atrophy and muscular weakness syndrome from cold, phlegm and blood stasis in the channels.
- With the appropriate identifying features, this formula can assist in the treatment of conditions such as hemiplegia following a stroke, chronic rheumatoid or osteoarthritis, degenerative joint disease, sciatica, peripheral neuropathy, post herpetic neuralgia, cervical and lumbar spondylosis and numbness and wasting in the extremities.

Composition

Aconitium carmichaeli (chuan wu, aconite), *Aconitium kusnezoffii* (cao wu, wild aconite), *Arisaema consanguinum* (dan nan xing, bile treated arisaema), *Pheretima asiatica* (di long, earthworm), *Boswellia carterii* (ru xiang, frankincense), *Commiphora myrhha* (mo yao, myrhh)

Combine with

- **7.1.1 Liu Wei Di Huang Wan** for Kidney yang deficiency and cold painful obstruction
- **10.15 Du Huo Ji Sheng Wan** for chronic or stubborn wind damp painful obstruction
- **10.11 Shu Jin Huo Xue Wan** for chronic pain from blood and phlegm stagnation

Pattern identifying features

- **cold damp painful obstruction**
- **severe pain and stiffness pain, worse for cold, alleviated by heat**
- **no heat signs**
- cold intolerance

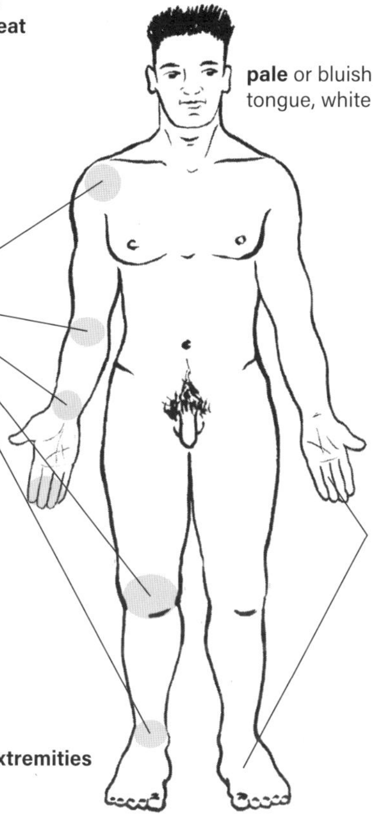

Dosage and method of administration

4 pills two or three times daily (maximum dose), on an empty stomach. Can be taken with a small shot of alcohol (vodka or sherry) to enhance the channel opening effect. Keeping to the recommended dose is important as it is very hot, can easily cause overheating and damage yin. Best to begin with a small dose (1-2 pills each time), see how the patient responds and then gradually increase the dose. Signs of overheating are usually flagged first by insomnia and restlessness, wild dreaming, facial flushing, sweats and thirst.

Cautions and contraindications

Contraindicated during pregnancy, in yin deficiency patterns and when there is any sign of heat at all (red tongue, warm joints, etc.). Should only be prescribed by experienced practitioners. Only suitable unmodified for patients with a relatively robust constitution or severe cold accumulation.

10.9 XUAN BI WAN

宣痹丸

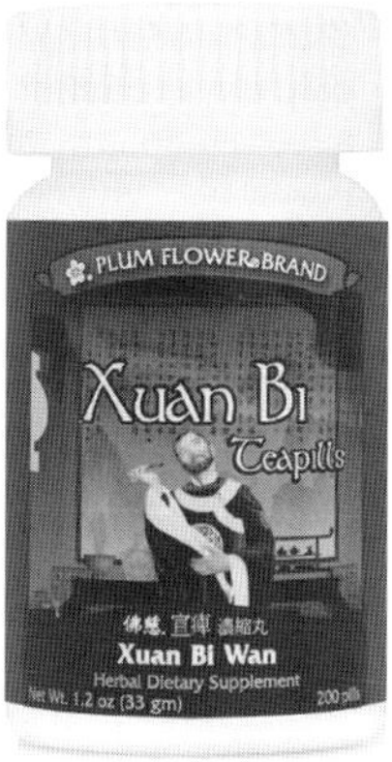

Lanzhou Foci Pharmaceutical Factory (Gansu)
'Drain Away Painful Obstruction Pills'
Xuan Bi Wan is packaged in bottles of 200 pills

Chinese medical action

Clears damp heat from the joints, unblocks the channels and collaterals, promotes urination and stops pain

Biomedical action

Analgesic, diuretic, anti-inflammatory, enhances circulation

INDICATIONS

- Heat or damp heat painful obstruction. Damp heat accumulation in joints characteristically causes palpable heat, swelling, redness and pain. Usually an acute disorder, or flare-up of a chronic disorder, but may be persistent in which case heat signs can be muted. Similar in action to **10.10 Guan Jie Yan Wan**, the main difference being that this formula is cooler and preferred for more acute damp heat painful obstruction.
- With the appropriate identifying features, this formula can assist in the treatment of conditions such as inflammatory joint disorders, inflammatory phase of osteoarthritis and rheumatoid arthritis, rheumatic fever, gouty arthritis, gout and connective tissue disorders.

Composition (each pill contains powdered)

Coix lachryma-jobi (yi yi ren, coix), *Stephania tetrandra* (han fang ji, stephania), *Prunus armeniaca* (xing ren, apricot seed), *Achyranthes bidentata* (huai niu xi, achyranthes), *Scutellaria baicalensis* (huang qin, scute), *Forsythia suspensa* (lian qiao, forsythia fruit), *Atractylodes lancea* (cang zhu, red atractylodes), *Gardenia florida* (shan zhi zi, gardenia fruit), *Pinellia ternata* (zhi ban xia, processed pinellia), *Akebia trifoliata* (mu tong, akebia)

Combine with

- **10.37 White Tiger Balm** topically for localised pain and inflammatory arthritis
- **14.1 Huang Lian Jie Du Wan** for acute gout

Dosage and method of administration

8-15 pills three times daily on an empty stomach. The dose can be spread out, or two lots of 12-22 pills taken morning and evening. In severe cases or during the early stages of treatment (the first two weeks), a 50% increase in dose can be used, then reduced as treatment takes effect.

Pattern identifying features

- **damp heat painful obstruction**
- heaviness and aching in the joints and limbs, worse during hot humid weather
- may be fever and chills

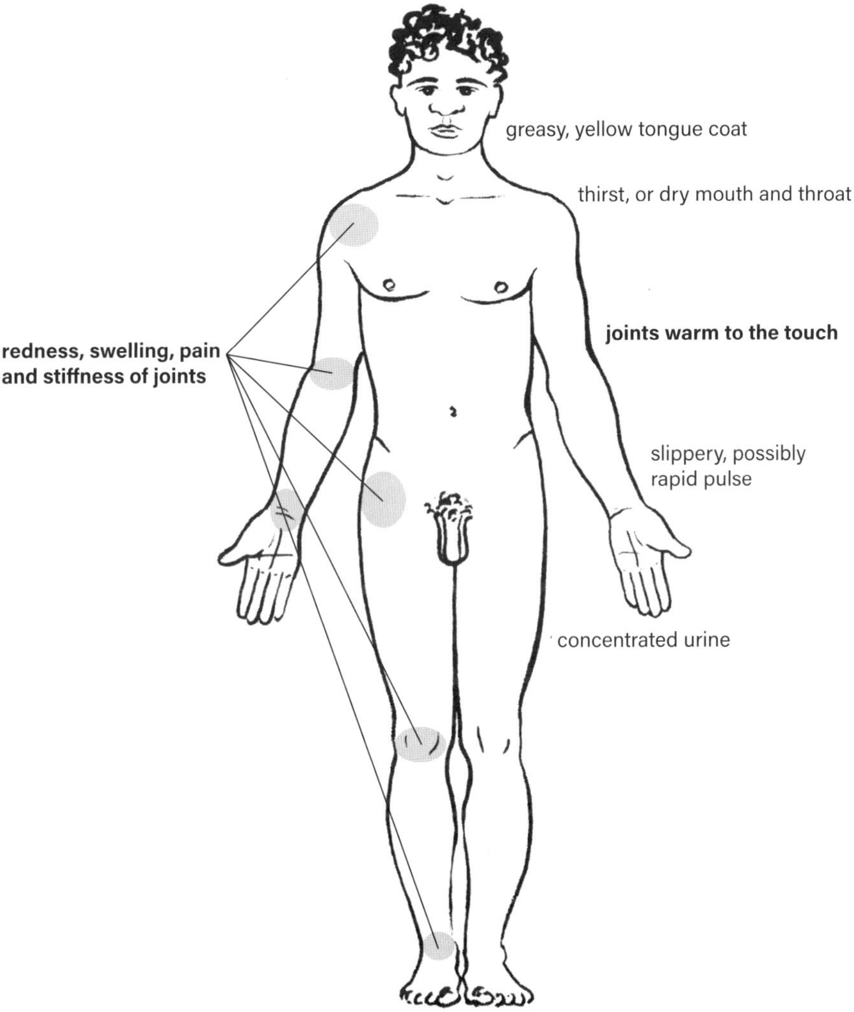

Cautions and contraindications

Contraindicated in wind cold painful obstruction patterns. Caution in patients with a tendency to mucus production or Spleen damp.

GMP

10.10 GUAN JIE YAN WAN

关节炎丸

3+/12

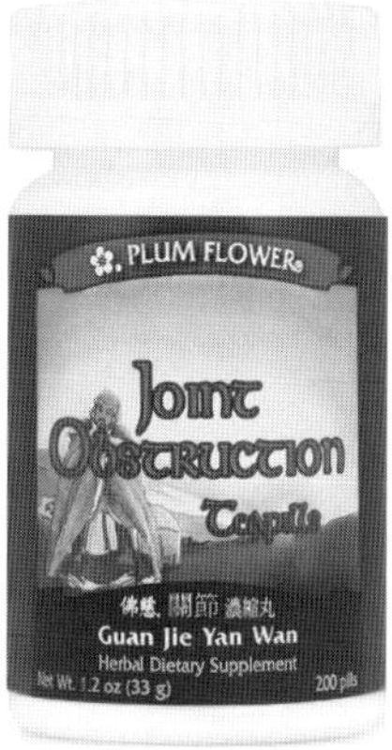

Lanzhou Foci Pharmaceutical Factory (Gansu)
'Joint Inflammation Pills'
Guan Jie Yan Wan is packaged in bottles of 200 pills

Chinese medical action

Clears damp heat from the joints, unblocks the channels and collaterals, stops pain

Biomedical action

Analgesic, diuretic, anti-inflammatory, enhances circulation

INDICATIONS

- Chronic joint and musculoskeletal pain and stiffness from damp heat. Best for damp heat affecting the lower body – hips, knees, ankles and toes. Even though the formula contains a few warming herbs, these serve to open up the channels to enable damp and heat to be dissipated. The thermal nature of the formula is cooling, although not quite as cooling as **10.9 Xuan Bi Wan**, which also varies from this formula by being preferred for more acute patterns of damp heat painful obstruction.
- With the appropriate identifying features, this formula can assist in the treatment of inflammatory joint disorders, inflammatory phase of osteoarthritis and rheumatoid arthritis, rheumatic fever, gouty arthritis and connective tissue disorders.

Composition

Coix lachryma-jobi (yi yi ren, coix), *Stephania tetrandra* (han fang ji, stephania), *Atractylodes lancea* (cang zhu, red atractylodes), *Erythrina variegata* (hai tong pi, erythrina bark), *Cinnamomum cassia* (gui zhi, cinnamon twigs), *Acanthopanax gracilistylus* (wu jia pi, acanthopanax), *Achyranthes bidentata* (huai niu xi, achyranthes), *Gentiana macrophylla* (qin jiao, chin chiu), *Evodia rutacarpae* (wu zhu yu, evodia), *Scutellaria baicalensis* (huang qin, scute), *Angelica pubescens* (du huo, Tu-huo), *Zingiber officinale* (sheng jiang, ginger)

Combine with

– **10.37 White Tiger Balm** topically for localised pain and inflammatory arthritis

Dosage and method of administration

8-15 pills three times daily on an empty stomach. The dose can be spread out, or two lots of 12-22 pills taken morning and evening. In severe cases or during the early stages of treatment (the first two weeks), a 50% increase in dose can be used, then reduced as treatment takes effect.

Pattern identifying features

- **damp heat painful obstruction**
- heaviness and aching in the joints and limbs, worse during hot humid weather

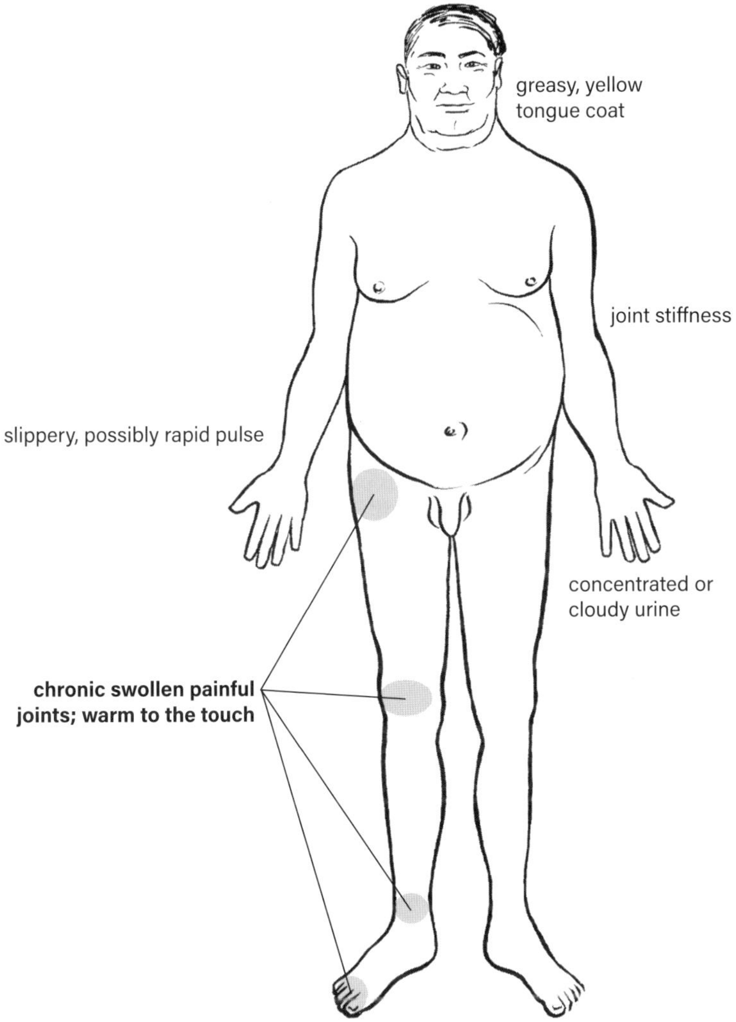

Cautions and contraindications

Contraindicated in wind cold painful obstruction patterns. Caution in patients with a tendency to mucus production or Spleen damp.

10.11 SHU JIN HUO XUE WAN
舒筋活血丸

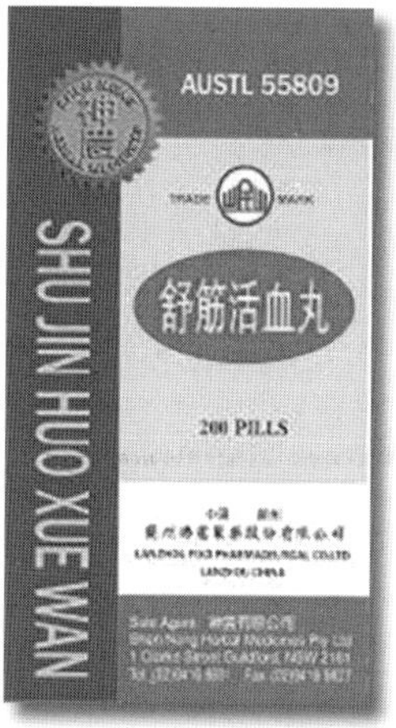

Lanzhou Foci Pharmaceutical Factory (Gansu)
'Soothe the Sinews and Invigorate Blood Pills'
Shu Jin Huo Xue Wan is packaged in bottles of 200 pills
A similar formula available as: Clematis and Stephania Combination (conc. extract)

Chinese medical action
Dispels wind damp, invigorates qi and blood, unblocks the channels and collaterals, transforms phlegm, stops pain

Biomedical action
Analgesic, anti-arthritic, anti-inflammatory, promotes circulation

INDICATIONS

- Wind cold damp painful obstruction with qi, blood and phlegm stagnation in the collaterals. This formula is used for chronic joint and muscle pain, spasm and paresthesia from predominantly excess pathology with little or no underlying deficiency. The main focus is on pain and stiffness in the lower body; lower back, hips, legs and knees, but it can be used for pain in any location. There may be a degree of bony deformity, osteophytes or tissue change, such as wasting, discoloration or distended or broken vessels over the affected tissues or joints.
- With the appropriate identifying features, this formula can assist in conditions such as cervical and lumbar spondylosis, osteoarthritis, arthritis following trauma, prolapsed intervertebral discs, sciatica, and slow healing of bone fractures.

Composition (each pill contains powdered)
Acanthopanax gracilistylus (wu jia pi, acanthopanax) 23.5mg, *Cinnamomun cassia* (gui zhi, cinnamon twig) 23.5mg, *Siegesbeckia orientalis* (xi xian cao, siegesbeckia) 15.7mg, *Angelica pubescens* (du huo, Tu-huo) 15.7mg, *Achyranthes bidentata* (niu xi, achyranthes) 15.7mg, *Angelica sinensis* (dang gui, chinese angelica) 15.7mg, *Chaenomeles speciosa* (mu gua, chinese quince) 15.7mg, *Clematis sinensis* (wei ling xian, chinese clematis) 15.7mg, *Notopterygium inscisum* (qiang huo, notopterygium) 15.7mg, *Angelica dahurica* (bai zhi, angelica) 7.8mg, *Illicium verum* (di feng pi, illicium bark) 7.8mg, *Pinellia ternata* (zhi ban xia, processed pinellia) 7.8mg

Combine with
- **5.8 Bu Yang Huan Wu Wan** for numbness, loss of sensation or other paresthesia in the limbs with discoloration
- **10.4 Chin Gu Tie Shang Wan** for slow knitting of bones
- **5.1 Xue Fu Zhu Yu Wan** for severe blood stasis
- **10.5 Huo Luo Xiao Ling Wan** for severe pain
- **10.23 Zheng Gu Shui** applied externally for chronic fixed joint pain

Pattern identifying features

- **wind cold damp painful obstruction with stagnation qi, blood and phlegm**
- slow healing of fractures

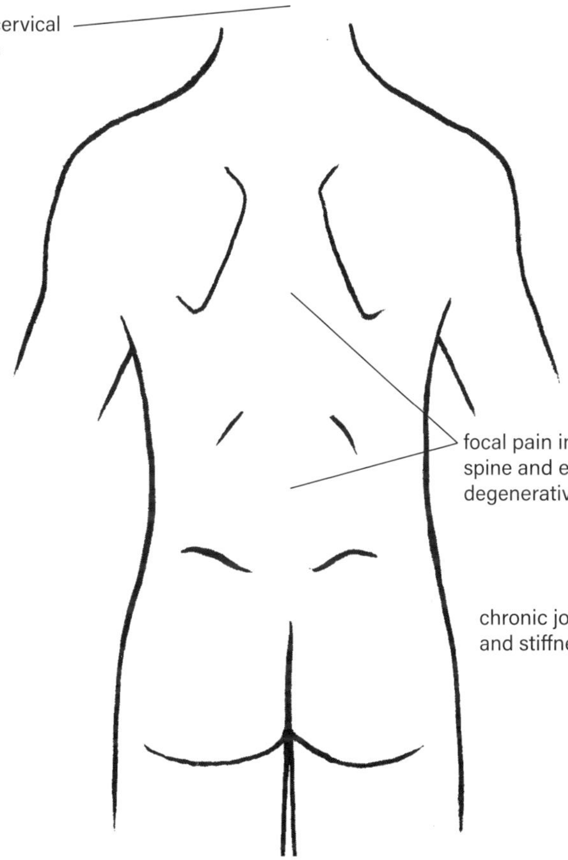

Dosage and method of administration

8-12 pills three times daily on an empty stomach. The dose can be spread out, or taken in two lots of 12-18 pills, morning and evening. In severe cases or during the early stages of treatment (the first few weeks), a 50% increase in dose can be used, then reduced as treatment takes effect.

Cautions and contraindications

Contraindicated during pregnancy. Not suitable for use in very deficient or run down patients without modification.

GMP

10.12 SHEN TONG ZHU YU WAN

身痛逐瘀丸

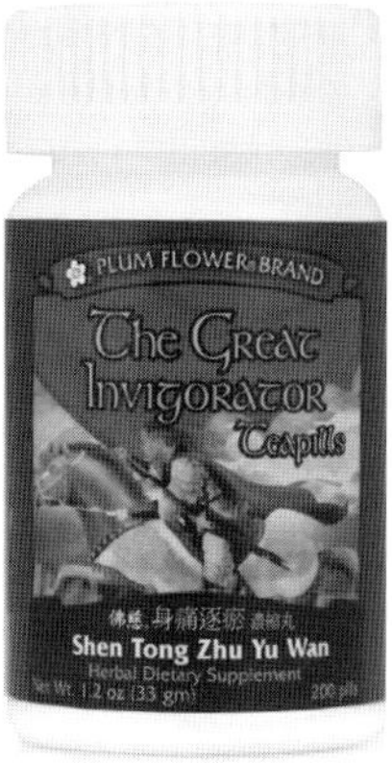

Lanzhou Foci Pharmaceutical Factory (Gansu)
'Remove Stagnant Blood from a Painful Body Pills'
Shen Tong Zhu Yu Wan is packaged in bottles of 200 pills
Also available as: Ligusticum and Notopterygium Combination (conc. extract)

Chinese medical action

Invigorates of qi and blood, breaks up and dispels static blood, unblocks the collaterals, stops pain

Biomedical action

Analgesic, antispasmodic, vasodilator, anti-platelet action

INDICATIONS

- Chronic, severe and persistent joint or muscular pain from blood stasis in the joints, channels and collaterals. This type of pain complicates long standing wind cold damp painful obstruction or trauma that has impeded the circulation of qi and blood. Pain is mostly fixed and focal, worse with pressure and deep seated, but can sometimes be diffuse and widely distributed. In some cases there may be associated bony deformity or tissue changes including wasting, discoloration or distended or broken vessels over the affected tissues or joints.
- With the appropriate identifying features, this formula can assist in treatment of conditions such as fibromyalgia, tendinitis, osteoarthritis and chronic rheumatoid arthritis, traumatic arthritis, pain following trauma, post surgical pain, sciatica, postherpetic neuralgia, phantom limb pain, dysmenorrhea and painful abdominal masses such as endometriosis.

Composition

Prunus persica (tao ren, peach seed), *Carthamus tinctorius* (hong hua, carthamus), *Angelica sinensis* (dang gui, chinese angelica), *Cyathula officinalis* (chuan niu xi, cyathula), *Ligusticum wallici* (chuan xiong, ligusticum), *Glycyrrhiza uralensis* (gan cao, licorice), *Commiphora myrrha* (mo yao, myrrh), *Pheretima asiatica* (di long, earthworm), *Gentiana macrophylla* (qin jiao, chin chiu), *Notopterygium incisum* (qiang huo, notopterygium), *Cyperus rotundus* (xiang fu, cyperus), *Boswellia carterii* (ru xiang*, frankincense) [*substituted for the restricted *Trogopterus xanthipes* (wu ling zhi, flying squirrel feces) of the original formula]

Combine with

- **10.23 Zheng Gu Shui** topically for chronic fixed joint pain
- **10.40 Porous Capsicum Plaster** topically for postherpetic neuralgia
- **5.4 Xin Mai Ling** or **5.2 Dan Shen Pill** for blood stasis painful obstruction with mild heat

Pattern identifying features

- **chronic painful obstruction with blood stasis**
- purple discoloration of face, lips, conjunctiva, nails
- chronic depression

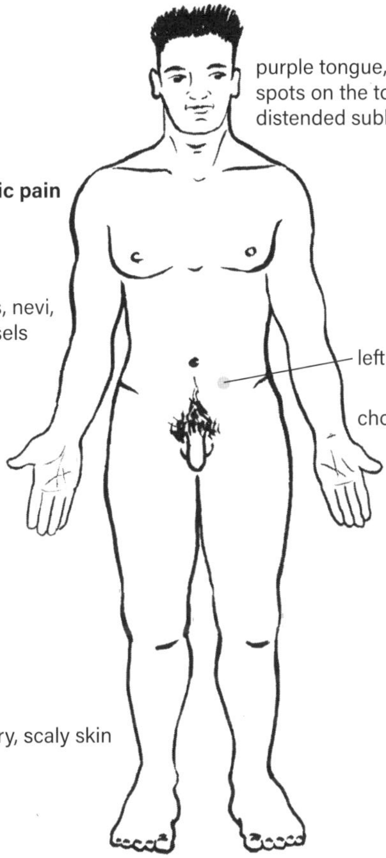

– A small dose of **10.8 Xiao Huo Luo Wan** for blood stasis with marked cold
– **10.41 Gou Pi Gao** plasters topically for severe pain and stiffness
– **1.16 Tao Hong Si Wu Wan** with a degree of blood deficiency

Dosage and method of administration

8-12 pills three times daily on an empty stomach. The dose can be spread out, or taken in two lots of 12-18 pills, morning and evening. In severe cases or during the early stages of treatment, a 50% increase in dose can be used, then reduced as treatment takes effect.

Cautions and contraindications

Contraindicated during pregnancy, in women with menorrhagia, and with bleeding disorders. Caution in patients on anticoagulant therapy. Watch for bruising or increased tendency to bleeding. Prolonged use may deplete qi and blood, so a break every 2-3 months, with a change to a simple qi and blood tonic formula for a few weeks, is recommended.

10.13 DA HUO LUO DAN

大活络丹

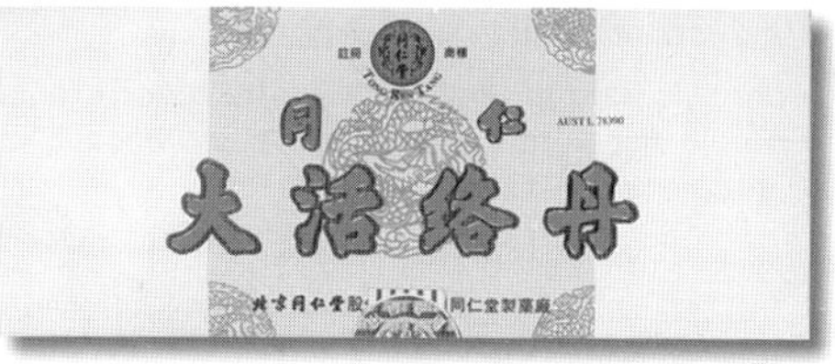

Tong Ren Tang (Beijing)
'Major Invigorate the Collaterals Special Pill'
Da Huo Luo Dan is packaged as 3.6 gram honey pills sealed inside a wax ball, ten balls per box

Chinese medical action

Dispels wind cold damp, eases the sinews, stops pain, tonifies qi and blood

Biomedical action

Analgesic, anti-arthritic, enhances circulation

INDICATIONS

- Wind cold damp painful obstruction with weakness of the Kidneys and qi and blood deficiency. This large and famous formula is used for chronic pain and paralysis patterns. Esteemed in China by the elderly for joint stiffness and pain, mobility disorders, general debility and the sequelae of wind-stroke causing hemiplegia, facial paralysis, aphasia and dysphagia.
- A general tonic for the elderly to promote vitality and protect against cerebrovascular disease.

Composition (each pill contains extracts equivalent to)

Panax ginseng (ren shen, ginseng) 30mg, *Siler divaricum* (fang feng, siler) 27mg, *Saussurea lappa* (mu xiang, saussurea) 27mg, *Agkistrodon acutus* (qi she*, tiger snake) 24mg, *Rehmannia glutinosa* (shu di, processed rehmannia) 19.5mg, *Cinnamomun cassia* (rou gui, cinnamon bark) 19.5mg, *Glycyrrhiza uralensis* (gan cao, licorice) 19.5mg, *Osmunda japonica* (guan zhong, shield fern) 19.5mg, *Agastache rugosa* (huo xiang, agastache) 19.5mg, *Rheum palmatum* (da huang, rhubarb root) 19.5mg, *Polygonum multiflorum* (he shou wu, polygonum root) 19.5mg, *Coptis chinensis* (huang lian, coptis) 19.5mg, *Gastrodia elata* (tian ma, gastrodia) 19.5mg, *Notopterygium forbesii* (qiang huo, notopterygium) 19.5mg, *Lindera strychnifolia* (wu yao, lindera) 19.5mg, *Clematis sinensis* (wei ling xian, chinese clematis) 19.5mg, *Angelica polymorpha* (dang gui, chinese angelica) 15mg, *Scrophularia ningpoensis* (xuan shen, scrophularia) 15mg, *Citrus reticulata* (qing pi, immature citrus) 10.5mg, *Zaocys dhumnades* (wu shao she*, black striped snake) 10.5mg, *Eugenia caryophyllata* (ding xiang, cloves) 10.5mg, *Asarum seiboldi* (xi xin*, asarum) 10.5mg, *Boswellia carteri* (ru xiang, frankincense) 10.5mg, *Commiphora myrrha* (mo yao, myrrh) 10.5mg, *Poria cocos* (fu ling, hoelen) 10.5mg, *Scutellaria baicalensis* (huang qin, scute) 10.5mg, *Paeonia veitchii* (chi shao, red peony) 10.5mg, *Atractylodes macrocephala* (bai zhu, atractylodes) 10.5mg, *Cyperus*

Pattern identifying features

- **chronic pain and hemiplegia, Kidney and qi and blood deficiency**

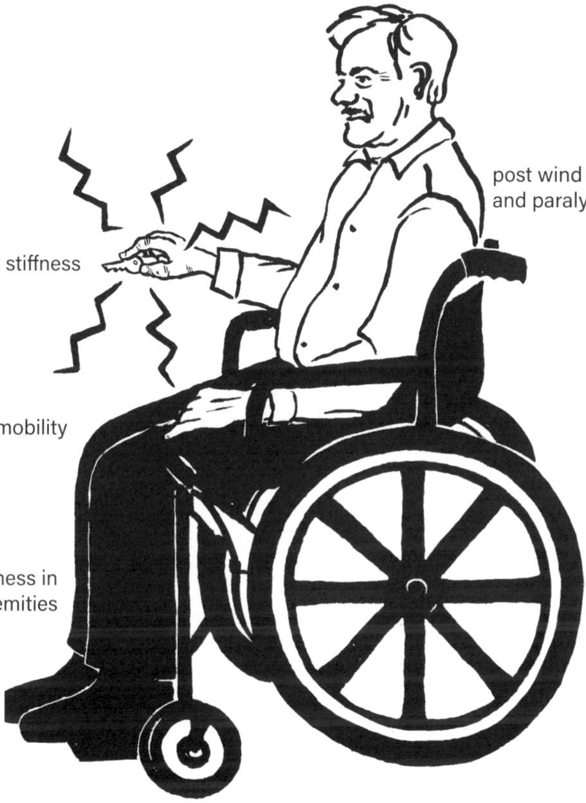

rotundus (xiang fu, cyperus) 10.5mg, *Styrax tonkinensis* (an xi xiang, benzoinum) 10.5mg, *Drynaria fortunei* (gu sui bu, drynaria) 10.5mg, *Elettaria cardamomum* (bai dou kou, amomum) 10.5mg, *Pueraria lobata* (ge gen, kudzu) 7.5mg, Bovine gallstone (niu huang*) 1.5mg, *Arisaema cosanguinium* (tian nan xing, arisaema) 1mg, honey. [**Restricted use in some jurisdictions; may be subject to substitution*]

Dosage and method of administration

One pill twice daily on an empty stomach. For patients with difficulty swallowing, the ball can be decocted and mashed into a slurry for ingestion.

Cautions and contraindications

Contraindicated during pregnancy.

GMP

10.14 SAN BI WAN

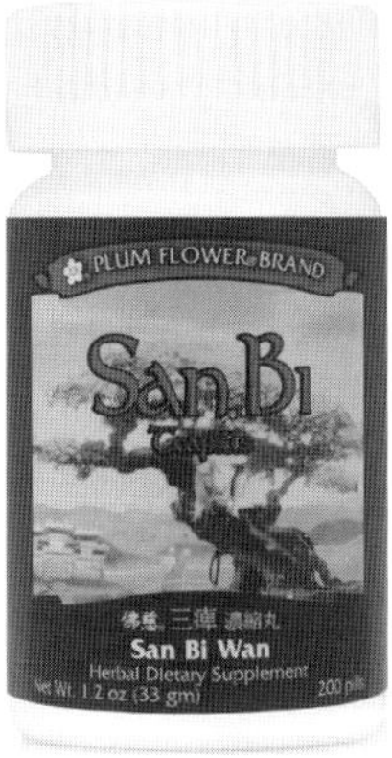

3+/12

三痹丸

Lanzhou Foci Pharmaceutical Factory (Gansu)
'Three Obstruction Pill'
San Bi Wan is packaged in bottles of 200 pills
Also available as: Tuhuo and Astragalus Combination (conc. extract)

Chinese medical action

Tonifies qi and blood, strengthens the Liver and Kidney, warms yang, dispels wind damp and stops pain

Biomedical action

Analgesic, anti-arthritic, anti-inflammatory, enhances circulation

INDICATIONS

- Chronic joint and muscle pain, stiffness, spasm, cramp, numbness and paresthesia from wind damp painful obstruction with underlying Kidney yang and Liver blood deficiency. Good for persistent pain in the lower body – lower back, hips, knees, ankles and feet. Similar in composition and action to **10.15 Du Huo Ji Sheng Wan**, the main difference being that **10.14 San Bi Wan** is more tonifying to qi.
- Mild tremors of the head, hands and feet from internal wind generated by qi and blood deficiency.
- With the appropriate identifying features, this formula can assist in the treatment of chronic arthritic conditions, osteoarthritis, rheumatism, joint pain in the elderly, debilitated and postpartum women, benign familial tremor and Parkinson's disease.

Composition

Dipsacus asper (xu duan, dipsacus), *Eucommia ulmoides* (du zhong, eucommia), *Ledebouriella divaricata* (fang feng, siler), *Cinnamomun cassia* (rou gui, cinnamon bark), *Panax ginseng* (ren shen, ginseng), *Poria cocos* (fu ling, hoelen) *Angelica sinensis* (dang gui, chinese angelica) *Paeonia lactiflora* (jiu chao bai shao, wine treated white peony), *Astragalus membranaceous* (huang qi, astragalus), *Achyranthes bidentata* (huai niu xi, achyranthes), *Glycyrrhiza uralensis* (zhi gan cao, honey fried licorice), *Gentiana macrophylla* (qin jiao, chin chiu), *Rehmannia glutinosa* (sheng di, raw rehmannia), *Angelica pubescens* (du huo, Tu-huo), *Ligusticum wallichi* (chuan xiong, ligusticum).

Combine with

- **7.9 Jin Gui Shen Qi Wan** for pain and spasm associated with cold, hypofunction and Kidney yang deficiency
- **10.16.1 Zhuang Yao Jian Shen** to enhance the general Kidney strengthening effect
- A small dose (1-2 pills twice daily) of **10.8 Xiao Huo Luo Wan** or **10.41 Gou Pi Gao** plaster topically for relatively severe cold symptoms with debilitating fixed pain
- **10.38 Plaster for Bruise and Analgesic** topically for localised pain

Pattern identifying features

- **wind cold damp painful obstruction with Kidney yang qi and Liver blood deficiency**
- pain worse in cold wet weather and with fatigue
- cold intolerance

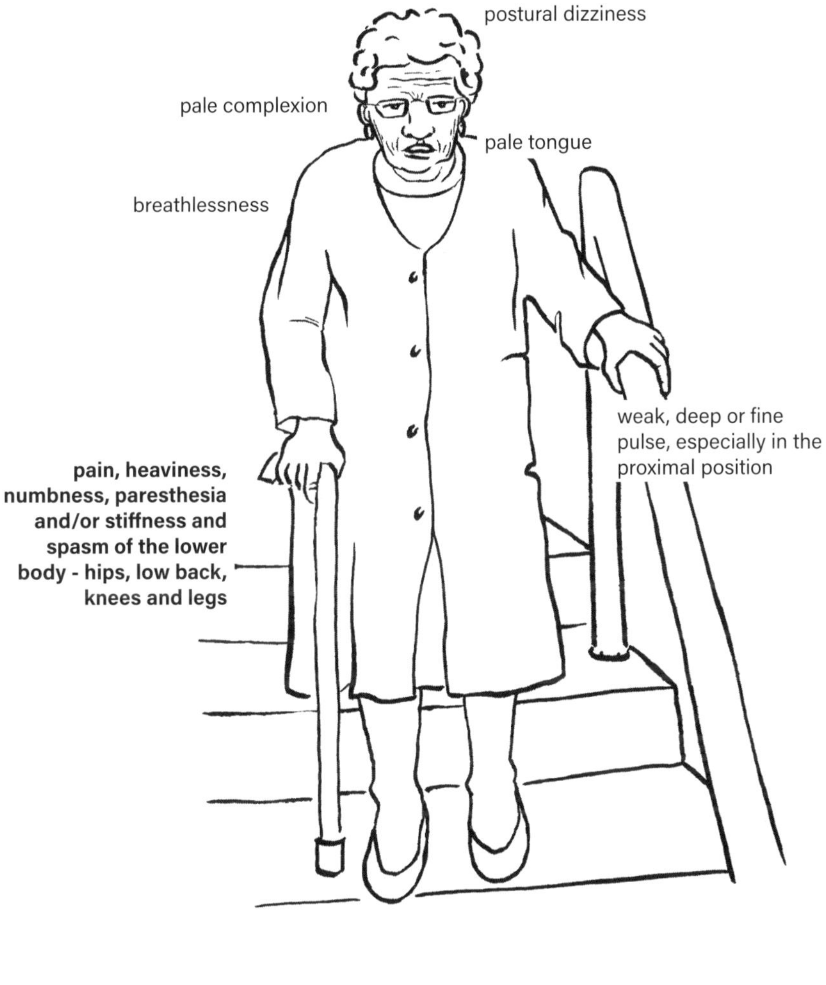

Dosage and method of administration

8-12 pills three times daily on an empty stomach. The dose can be spread out, or taken in two lots of 12-18 pills, morning and evening. In severe cases or during the early stages of treatment, a 50% increase in dose can be used, then reduced as treatment takes effect.

Cautions and contraindications

Contraindicated during the early stage of colds and flu, or other acute disorder.

10.15 DU HUO JI SHENG WAN

独活寄生丸

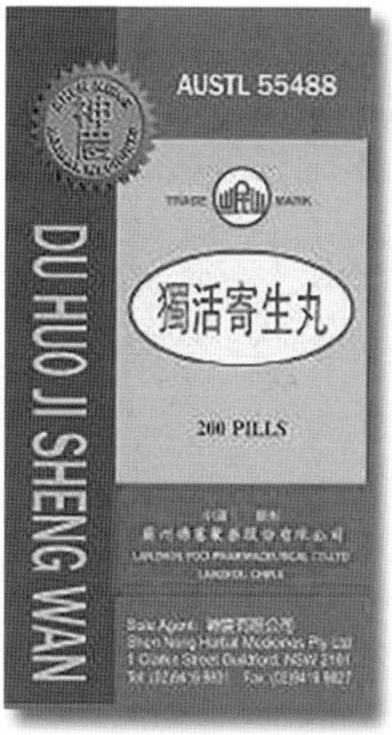

Lanzhou Foci Pharmaceutical Factory (Gansu)
'Angelica pubescens and Loranthus Pills'
Du Huo Ji Sheng Wan is packaged in bottles of 200 pills
Also available as: Solitary Hermit Teapills (PF), Tu Huo Ji Sheng Wan, Tuhuo and Loranthus Combination (conc. extract)

Chinese medical action

Dispels wind damp, tonifies qi and blood, strengthens the Liver and Kidneys, stops pain

Biomedical action

Analgesic, anti-arthritic, anti-inflammatory, enhances circulation

INDICATIONS

- Chronic joint and muscle pain, stiffness, spasm, cramp, numbness and paresthesia associated with osteoarthritis and/or sciatica in patients with wind damp, Kidney weakness and deficiency of qi and blood. Especially good for pain in the lower body – lower back, hips, knees, ankles and feet. Slightly more dispersing, yet similar in action to, and interchangeable with, **10.14 San Bi Wan**.
- With the appropriate identifying features, this formula can assist in the treatment of chronic arthritic conditions, osteoarthritis, degenerative joint disease, rheumatism, joint pain in the elderly and debilitated, chronic lower back ache and sciatica.

Composition (each pill contains powdered)

Angelica pubescens (du huo, Tu-huo) 15.8mg, *Viscum coloratum* (sang ji sheng, loranthus) 15.8mg, *Spatholobus suberectus* (ji xue teng, spatholobus) 10.3mg, *Gentiana macrophylla* (qin jiao, chin chiu) 10.3mg, *Ledebouriella divaricata* (fang feng, siler) 10.3mg, *Eucommia ulmoides* (du zhong, eucommia) 10.3mg, *Paeonia lactiflora* (bai shao, white peony) 10.3mg, *Angelica dahurica* (bai zhi, angelica) 10.3mg, *Rehmannia glutinosa* (shu di, prepared rehmannia) 10.3mg, *Angelica sinensis* (dang gui, chinese angelica) 10.3mg, *Cyathula officinalis* (chuan niu xi) 10.3mg, *Codonopsis pilosula* (dang shen, codonopsis) 10.3mg, *Poria cocos* (fu ling, hoelen) 10.3mg, *Glycyrrhiza uralensis* (gan cao, licorice) 10.3mg, *Zingiber officinalis* (sheng jiang, ginger), *Cinnamomun cassia* (rou gui, cinnamon bark) 10.3mg

Combine with

- **7.9 Jin Gui Shen Qi Wan** for pain and spasm associated with coldness, hypofunction and Kidney yang deficiency
- **10.16.1 Zhuang Yao Jian Shen** to enhance the Kidney strengthening effect
- A small dose (1-2 pills twice daily) of **10.8 Xiao Huo Luo Wan** or **10.41 Gou Pi Gao** plaster topically for relatively severe cold symptoms with debilitating fixed pain
- **10.38 Plaster for Bruise and Analgesic** topically for localised pain

Pattern identifying features

- **wind cold damp painful obstruction with Kidney yang qi and Liver blood deficiency**
- cold intolerance
- pain worse in cold wet weather
- fatigue and breathlessness

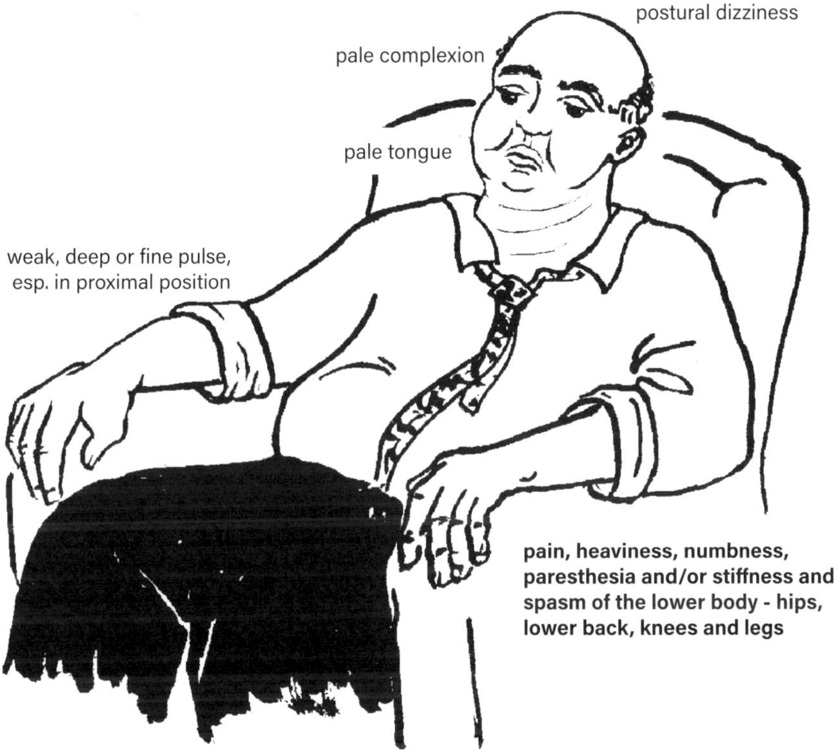

Dosage and method of administration

8-12 pills three times daily on an empty stomach. The dose can be spread out, or taken in two lots of 12-18 pills, morning and evening. In severe cases or during the early stages of treatment (the first two weeks), a 50% increase in dose can be used, then reduced as treatment takes effect.

Cautions and contraindications

Contraindicated during the early stage of colds and flu, or other acute disorder.

10.16.1 ZHUANG YAO JIAN SHEN

壮腰健肾

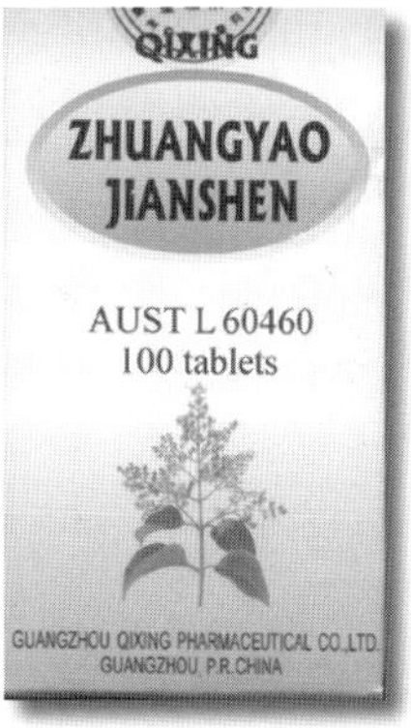

Guangzhou Qixing Pharmaceutical Co. (Guangzhou)
'Strengthen the Lower Back and Benefit the Kidney'
Zhuang Yao Jian Shen is packaged in bottles of 100 tablets

Chinese medical action

Tonifies, strengthens and warms the Kidneys, benefits and secures essence, dispels wind damp, stops pain

Biomedical action

Tonic, astringent, strengthens Kidney function

INDICATIONS

- Chronic wind damp painful obstruction with Kidney yang deficiency causing lower back, spine and lower limb pain, stiffness and heaviness. Good for weakness or pain in the hips, knees or ankles associated with osteoarthritis, sciatica, chronic lumbago, scoliosis and rheumatism. Although in general tending to be warm, this formula is mild enough to be used for patients with lower back pain tending to heat, cold or neither. It combines well with other more constitutional Kidney tonic formulas. Suitable for prolonged use to strengthen Kidney function.
- Urinary frequency, nocturia or incontinence from Kidney qi or yang deficiency.
- Kidney weakness and essence deficiency causing premature ejaculation and sperm disorders such as low sperm count, poor motility and poor sperm quality.

Composition (each pill contains extract equivalent to dry)

Cibotium barometz (gou ji, cibotium fern) 525.7mg, *Schizandra chinensis* (wu wei zi, schizandra) 280mg, *Spatholobus suberectus* (ji xue teng, spatholobus) 280mg, *Cuscuta hygropilae* (tu su zi, cuscuta) 208.6mg, *Viscum coloratum* (sang ji sheng, loranthus) 197.1mg, *Rosa laevigata* (jin ying zi, chinese rose fruit) 157.1mg, *Ligustrum lucidum* (nu zhen zi, privet fruit) 22.9mg

Combine with

- **7.9 Jin Gui Shen Qi Wan** for pain and spasm associated with more profound Kidney yang deficiency. This combination is also used for nocturia or urinary frequency from yang or qi deficiency
- **10.15 Du Huo Ji Sheng Wan** for chronic wind damp painful obstruction with Kidney qi and Liver blood deficiency
- **7.1.1 Liu Wei Di Huang Wan** for painful obstruction in those prone to Kidney yin deficiency
- **5.1 Xue Fu Zhu Yu Wan** or **10.11 Shu Jin Huo Xue Wan** for chronic stubborn fixed pain associated with blood stasis and Kidney yang deficiency

Pattern identifying features

- **Kidney qi and yang deficiency lower back and leg pain**
- aches and pains worse with cold wet weather

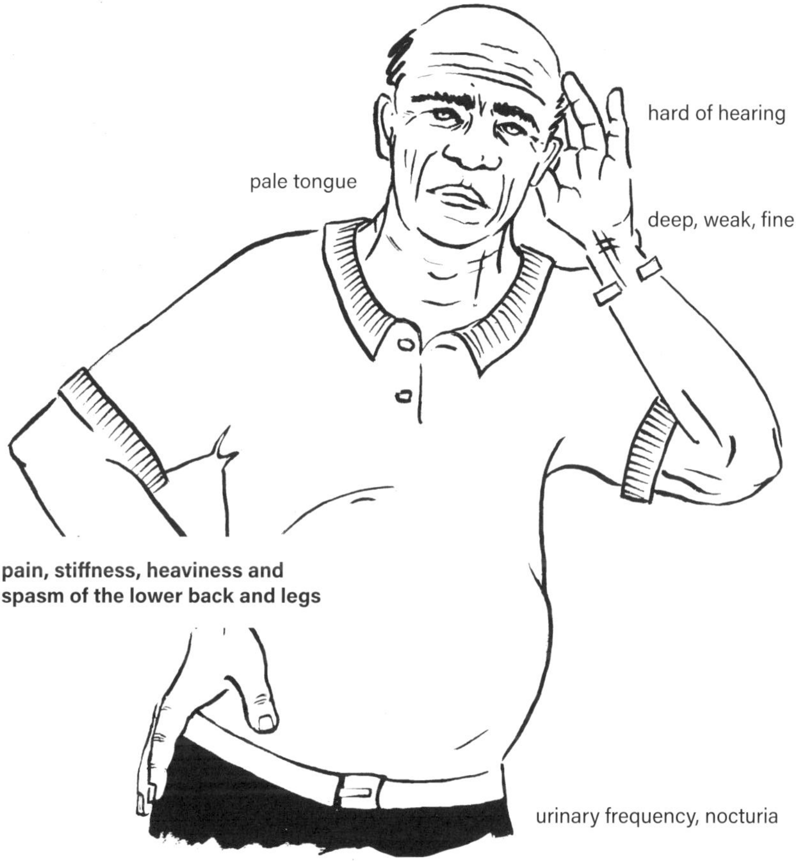

Dosage and method of administration

4 pills three times daily on an empty stomach; doubled in the early stages of treatment (first two weeks) then reduced as the treatment takes effect. When combined with a constitutional formula, four pills twice daily is usually sufficient.

Cautions and contraindications

Contraindicated during the early stage of colds and flu, or other acute disorder.

10.16.2 ZHUANG YAO JIAN SHEN TABLET

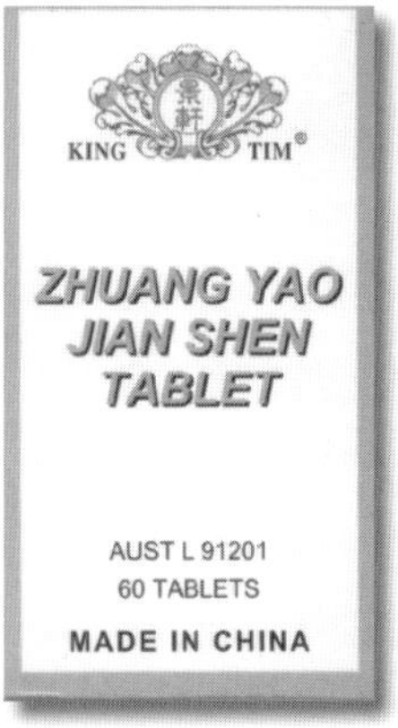

壮腰健肾片

(*Zhuang Yao Jian Shen Pian*)
Jing Xian Pharmaceutical Co. (Guangzhou)
'Strengthen the Lower Back and Kidney Tablets'
Zhuang Yao Jian Shen Tablet is packaged in bottles of 60 tablets

Chinese medical action

Tonifies, strengthens and warms the Kidneys, benefits and secures essence, dispels wind damp, stops pain

Biomedical action

Tonic, astringent, strengthens Kidney function

INDICATIONS

- As for **10.16.1 Zhuang Yao Jian Shen**. With basically the same action and indications, the only difference between these formulas is that this version has slightly more Kidney tonic activity with the inclusion of prepared rehmannia, solomon seal rhizome and polygonum root. Achyranthes is added to direct the action of the formula to the lower body.

Composition (each pill contains extract equivalent to dry)

Rehmannia glutinosa (shu di, prepared rehmannia) 333mg, *Spatholobus suberectus* (ji xue teng, spatholobus) 333mg, *Polygonum multiflorum* (he shou wu, polygonum root) 222mg, *Polygonatum sibiricum* (huang jing, solomon seal rhizome) 178mg, *Rosa laevigata* (jin ying zi, chinese rose fruit) 178mg, *Cibotium barometz* (gou ji, cibotium fern) 167mg, *Achyranthes bidentata* (niu xi, achyranthes) 114mg, *Dipsacus asper* (xu duan, dipsacus) 68mg, *Ligustrum lucidum* (nu zhen zi, privet fruit) 68mg

Dosage and method of administration

3-5 tablets, three times daily on an empty stomach; can be doubled during the early stages of treatment (first two weeks), then reduced as treatment takes effect.

Cautions and contraindications

Contraindicated during the early stage of colds and flu, or other acute disorder.

10.17 TONG LUO ZHI TONG TABLET

通络止痛片

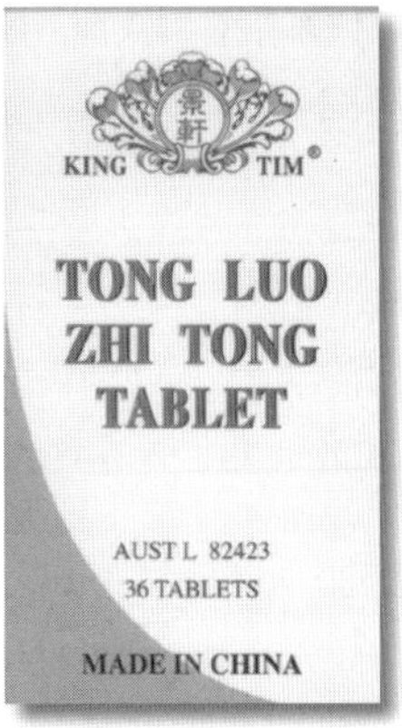

(*Tong Luo Zhi Tong Pian*)
Jing Xian Pharmaceutical Co. (Guangzhou)
'Collateral Opening, Analgesic Tablets'
Tong Luo Zhi Tong Tablets are packaged in bottles of 36 tablets

Chinese medical action

Invigorates and tonifies blood, stimulates circulation in the channels and collaterals, eases the sinews

Biomedical action

Analgesic, anti-inflammatory

INDICATIONS

- A modern formulation utilizing the channel opening and blood regulating effects of spatholobus with the hematinic and relaxing effects of B group vitamins.
- Can stimulate production of leukocytes in patients with low white blood cell counts and following chemotherapy or radiotherapy.
- Can assist in the treatment of neurological and vascular pain such as sciatica, trigeminal neuralgia, intercostal neuralgia and migraine headache, as well as facial paralysis, numbness and paresthesia in the extremities, hemiplegia following wind-stroke, dysmenorrhea, irregular menstruation and premenstrual syndrome.

Composition (each tablets contains)

Spatholobus suberectus (ji xue teng, spatholobus) 550mg, Thiamine hydrochloride (Vitamin B1) 100mg, Pyridoxine hydrochloride (Vitamin B6) 10mg, Cyanocobalamin (Vitamin B12) 50μg

Dosage and method of administration

1-2 tablets, three times daily on an empty stomach to a maximum of 5 tablets per day.

Cautions and contraindications

Contraindicated in patients with bleeding disorders or menorrhagia.

10.18 JIAN BU QIANG SHEN WAN

健步强身丸

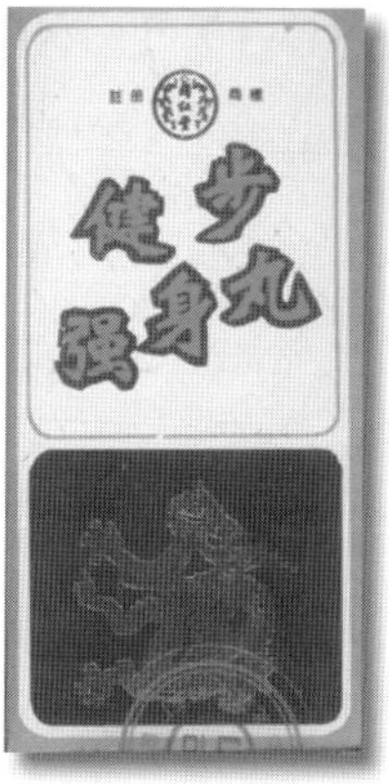

(Aches and Pains Relief Pill)
Tong Ren Tang (Beijing)
'Walk with Vigour, Body Strengthening Pills'
Jian Bu Qiang Shen Wan is packaged in bottles of 600 small pills

Chinese medical action

Dispels wind damp, tonifies qi and blood, strengthens the Liver and Kidneys, stops pain

Biomedical action

Analgesic, anti-arthritic, anti-inflammatory, enhances circulation

INDICATIONS

- Kidney qi or yang deficiency type lower back pain, general muscular aches, pains, stiffness, cramps, spasms and weakness, especially in the lower body and legs. Similar in action to **10.15 Du Huo Ji Sheng Wan.**
- Useful as a general Kidney tonic for chronic problems such as lack of vitality, infertility, low libido, sperm disorders or urinary disorders.
- With the appropriate identifying features, this formula can assist in the treatment of conditions such as chronic osteoarthritis and rheumatoid arthritis, weakness of the lower back and legs, sciatic pain, numbness and paresthesia of the legs and recurrent ankle sprain or low back pain.

Composition (each dose of 60 pills [6 grams] contains)

Lycium barbarum (gou qi zi, lycium fruit) 360mg, *Chaenomeles lagenaria* (mu gua, chinese quince) 360mg, *Achyranthes bidentata* (huai niu xi, achyranthes) 336mg, *Dipsacus asper* (xu duan, dipsacus) 270mg, *Ledebouriella divaricata* (fang feng, siler) 240mg, *Poria cocos* (fu ling, hoelen) 210mg, *Notopterygium incisum* (qiang huo, notopterygium) 168mg, *Paeonia lactiflora* (bai shao, white peony) 168mg, *Astragalus membranaceous* (huang qi, astragalus) 168mg, *Cynomorium songariorum* (suo yang, cynomorium) 168mg, *Angelica pubescens* (du huo, Tu-huo) 168mg, *Rehmannia glutinosa* (shu di, prepared rehmannia) 168mg, *Angelica polymorpha* (dang gui, chinese angelica) 168mg, *Schizandra chinensis* (wu wei zi, schizandra) 168mg, *Psoralea corylifolia* (bu gu zhi, psoralea) 168mg, *Gentiana macrophylla* (qin jiao, chin chiu) 168mg, *Anemarrhena aspheloides* (zhi mu, anemarrhena) 168mg, *Panax ginseng* (ren shen, ginseng) 42mg, *Eucommia ulmoides* (du zhong, eucommia) 42mg, honey

Combine with

- **7.9 Jin Gui Shen Qi Wan** for pain and spasm associated with cold, hypofunction and Kidney yang deficiency
- **10.41 Gou Pi Gao** plaster topically over the lower back for chronic back ache

Pattern identifying features

- **Kidney deficiency lower back and leg pain**

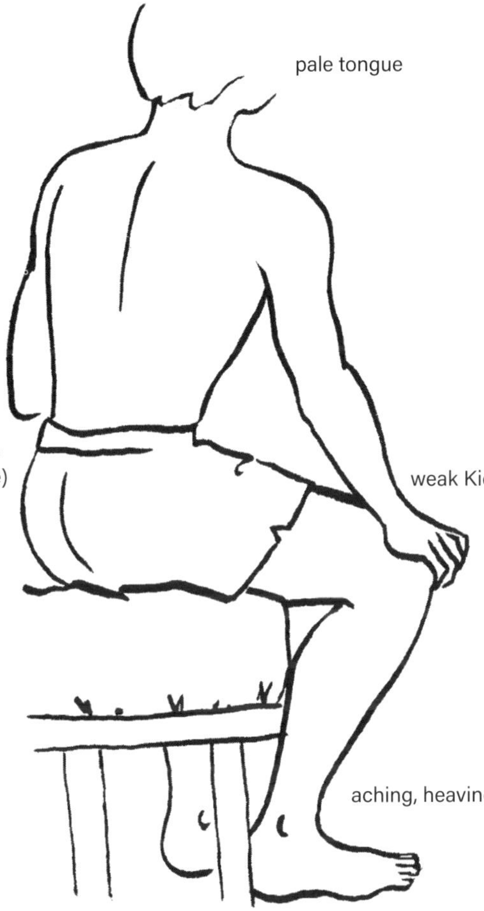

Dosage and method of administration

The recommended dose is 60 pills twice daily, before meals. In most cases, this is inconvenient as counting the right dose can be extremely tedious and lead to poor compliance. The best way to take it is not to worry about getting exactly the right dose each time, instead aim to finish a jar in 5 days. Patients can estimate the dose by taking as many pills as fit into the lid of the bottle, which is close enough to 60.

Cautions and contraindications

Contraindicated during the early stages of colds and flu, and other acute pathogenic invasion.

GMP

10.19 KANG GU ZENG SHENG PIAN

抗骨增生片

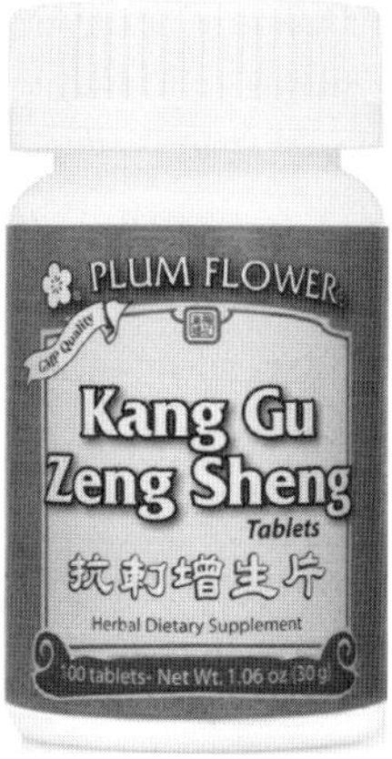

Guangzhou Qixing Pharmaceutical Co. (Guangzhou)
'Inhibit Bony Proliferation Pill'
Kang Gu Zeng Sheng Pian is packaged in bottles of 100 pills

Chinese medical action

Tonifies the Liver and Kidneys, strengthens sinews and bones, invigorates qi and blood, stops pain

Biomedical action

Analgesic, encourages bony matrix remodelling, enhances circulation

INDICATIONS

- Proliferative bone disorders such as osteophytosis, vertebral calcification, ankylosing spondylitis, vertebral and cervical spondylitis, heel spurs, bony deformity consequent upon chronic rheumatoid arthritis, Kashin-Beck disease, traumatic arthritis and Heberden's nodes.

Composition

Rehmannia glutinosa (shu di, processed rehmannia), *Spatholobus suberectus* (ji xue teng, spatholobus), *Pyrola rotundifolia* (lu xian cao, pyrola), *Cynomorium songariorum* (suo yang, cynomorium), *Drynaria fortunei* (gu sui bu, drynaria), *Epimedium brevicornu* (xian ling pi, epimedium), *Raphanus sativus* (chao lai fu zi, stir fried radish seed)

Dosage and method of administration

6-8 pills, three times daily, on an empty stomach.

Cautions and contraindications

Contraindicated during pregnancy.

10.20 TIAN MA TOU TONG CAPSULE

天麻头痛丸

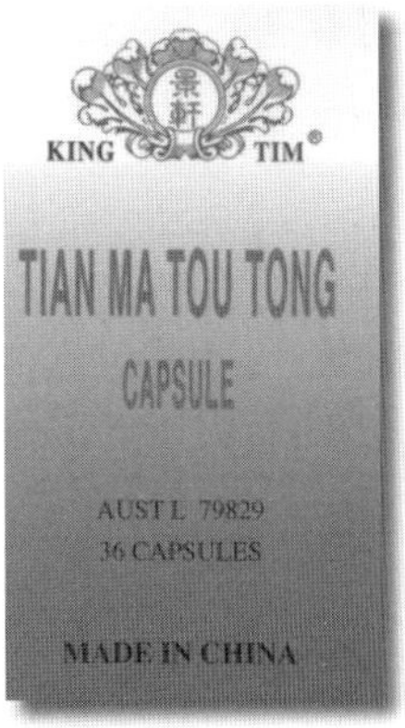

(*Tian Ma Tou Tong Wan*)
Jing Xian Pharmaceutical Co. (Guangzhou)
'Gastrodia Headache Pills'
Tian Ma Tou Tong Capsules are packaged in bottles of 36 capsules

Chinese medical action

Dispels external wind, extinguishes internal wind, restrains ascendant Liver yang

Biomedical action

Analgesic, enhances circulation

INDICATIONS

- Headache, including tension headache, cluster headache and migraine associated with the common cold, ascendant Liver yang, Liver wind or mild blood stasis.
- Dizziness or vertigo from ascendant Liver yang.

Composition (each capsule contains extracts equivalent to dry)

Gastrodia elata (tian ma, gastrodia) 540mg, *Angelica dahurica* (bai zhi, angelica) 540mg, *Ligusticum sinense* (gao ben, ligusticum) 540mg, *Schizonepeta tenuifolia* (jing jie, schizonepeta) 360mg, *Angelica polymorpha* (dang gui, chinese angelica) 360mg, *Boswellia carteri* (ru xiang, frankincense) 45mg

Combine with

– **15.4 Tian Ma Gou Teng Wan** for ascendant Liver yang
– **15.9 Headache and Dizziness Reliever** for occipital headache

Dosage and method of administration

3-4 capsules, three times daily, on an empty stomach.

Cautions and contraindications

None noted.

GMP

10.21 YAN HU SUO ZHI TONG WAN

延胡索止痛丸

1-3/12

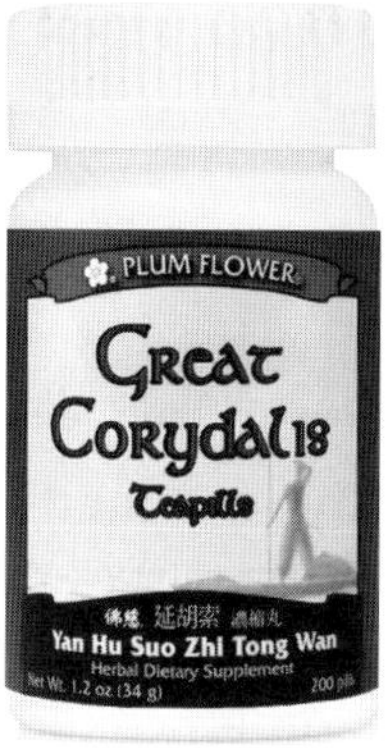

Lanzhou Foci Pharmaceutical Factory (Gansu)
'Corydalis Analgesic Pill'
Yan Hu Suo Zhi Tong Wan is packaged in bottles of 200 pills

Chinese medical action

Invigorates qi and blood, stops pain

Biomedical action

Analgesic

INDICATIONS

- A wide variety of pain problems associated with qi and/or blood stasis. Can be added to a constitutional or targeting formula when enhanced analgesia is desired. Generally considered best for pain associated with the Liver and Heart organ systems and channels.
- Because both herbs are quite dispersing, this formula can also be used for the generalized muscle aches that accompany a wind cold type common cold.

Composition

Corydalis turtschaninovii (yan hu suo, corydalis), *Angelica dahurica* (bai zhi, angelica)

Combine with

- **5.1 Xue Fu Zhu Yu Wan** for migraine headache, facial pain or postherpetic neuralgia from stagnant qi and blood
- **10.9 Xuan Bi Wan** for acute joint pain from damp heat painful obstruction
- **1.18 Shao Fu Zhu Yu Wan** for severe dysmenorrhea
- **10.5 Huo Luo Xiao Ling Wan** for severe pain from trauma
- **11.4 Tian Tai Wu Yao Wan** for testicular or inguinal pain from cold in the Liver channel
- **5.2 Dan Shen Pill** for angina

Dosage and method of administration

8-12 pills, three times daily used alone. When combined with a targeting formula, 4-8 pills, three times daily is usually sufficient.

Cautions and contraindications

Contraindicated during pregnancy.

GMP

3+/12

10.22 SHAO YAO GAN CAO WAN

芍药甘草丸

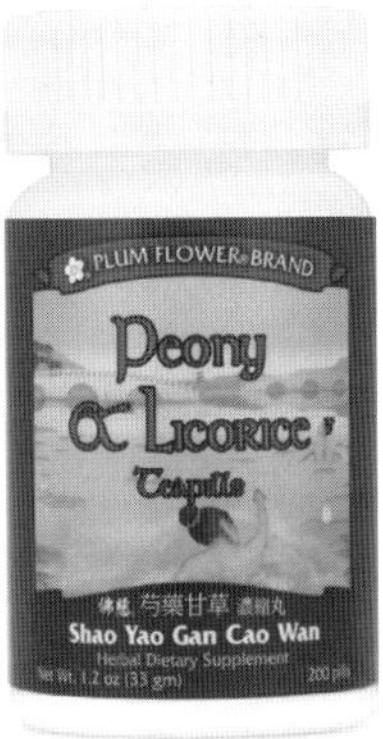

Lanzhou Foci Pharmaceutical Factory (Gansu)
'Peony and Licorice Pill'
Shao Yao Gan Cao Wan is packaged in bottles of 200 pills
Also available as: Peony and Licorice Combination (conc. extract)

Chinese medical action

Softens the Liver, benefits yin, eases cramps, stops pain

Biomedical action

Antispasmodic, analgesic

INDICATIONS

- Pain from spasm and cramping of smooth and skeletal muscle. Primarily used for muscle spasm from Liver yin or blood deficiency failing to moisten and nourish the sinews, it can be used for any pattern where smooth or skeletal muscle spasm is a problem. This includes spasmodic epigastric and abdominal pain from Liver invading the Spleen and Stomach, neck and upper back pain from qi constraint, calf cramps and restless leg syndrome, writers cramp, post febrile and dehydration muscle spasm, intercostal and trigeminal neuralgia, generalized muscle spasm, urinary bladder and gallbladder colic, spasm of the uterus and vasospasm.
- Polycystic ovarian disease. The combination of sour (peony) and sweet (licorice) helps creates physiological yin to replace pathological yin, seen here in the form of phlegm cysts on the ovaries.

Composition

Paeonia lactiflora (bai shao, white peony), *Glycyrrhiza uralensis* (zhi gan cao, honey fried licorice)

Combine with

- **6.3 Chai Hu Shu Gan Wan** for abdominal pain from Liver Spleen disharmony
- **7.1.1 Liu Wei Di Huang Wan** for nocturnal calf cramps and restless leg

Dosage and method of administration

8-12 pills, three times daily used alone. When combined with a targeting formula, 4-8 pills, three times daily is usually sufficient.

Cautions and contraindications

None noted.

10.23 ZHENG GU SHUI

正骨水

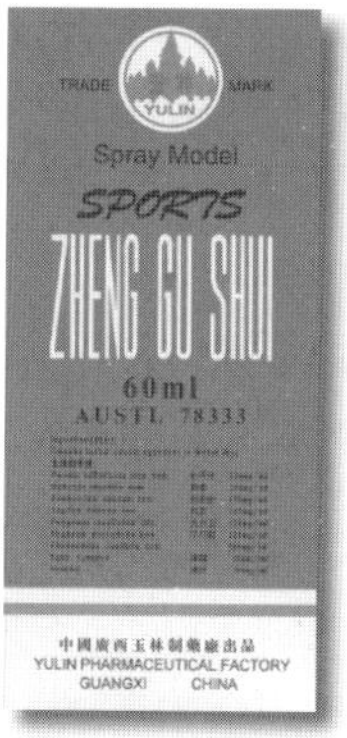

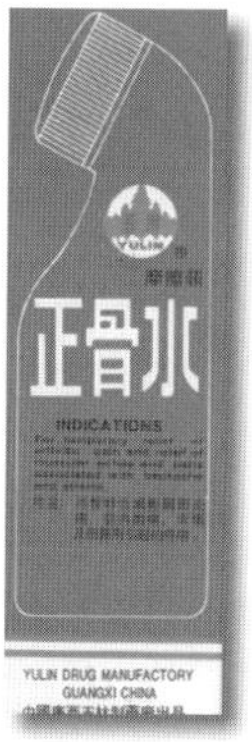

Yulin Drug Manufactory (Guangxi)
'Mend Bone Water'
Zheng Gu Shui is packaged in several forms with different applicators, including roll on (pictured), spray packs, aerosols and small and large bottles

Chinese medical action
Invigorates blood and disperses static blood, stops pain, promotes healing; warm and dispersing

Biomedical action
Anodyne, rubefacient

INDICATIONS

- Blood stasis pain and bruising from trauma, sprains, strains and uncomplicated fractures. Alcohol based and absorbed quickly. Stimulates local circulation and metabolism, accelerates osteoblast activity. Significantly reduces recovery time for all types of closed trauma.
- Used extensively to aid the healing of simple fractures (such as green-stick), or to encourage non-healing bones to knit.
- Relief of the chronic pain of wind damp painful obstruction, osteoarthritis or rheumatoid arthritis and old injuries.

Composition (each ml contains)
Cinnamomum camphora (zhang nao, camphor) 500mg, *Panax notoginseng* (tian qi, tianqi ginseng) 220mg, *Paeonia suffruticosa* (mu dan pi, moutan) 220mg, *Dalbergia odorifera* (jiang xiang, dalbergia wood) 209mg, *Zanthoxylum nitidum* (liang mian zhen, zanthoxylum root) 176mg, *Angelica dahurica* (bai zhi, angelica root) 143mg, *Polygonum cuspidatum* (hu zhang, bushy knotweed) 121mg, *Moghania macrophylla* (qian jin ba, moghania) 121mg, menthol 50mg

Combine with
- **10.4 Chin Gu Tie Shang Wan** or **1.30 Bu Gai Zhuang Gu Capsule** to encourage the healing of slow knitting fractures and broken bones
- **10.3 Die Da Zhi Tong Capsules** for pain and bruising from trauma

Dosage and method of administration
Rub liberally and firmly into the affected area as often as practical, or apply on cotton wool and bandage for up to 2 hours at a time.

Pattern identifying features

- **traumatic injury with bruising and simple fractures**
- chronic pain from static blood

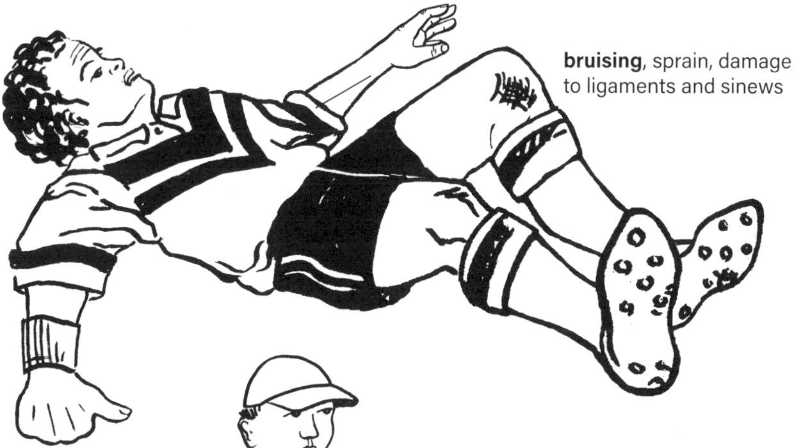

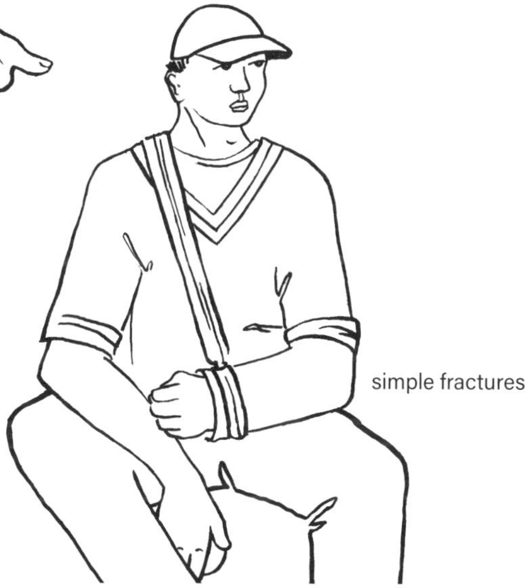

Cautions and contraindications

Contraindicated during pregnancy, for children under 5 years, when there is skin disease such as eczema, and for patients with acute inflammation where RICE (rest, ice, compression, elevation) is the appropriate treatment. Not suitable for use on broken skin. For external use only. Keep out of reach of children. May irritate the skin of some patients causing redness and itch, especially those with fair skin. Avoid contact with the eyes, mucous membranes and other sensitive areas.

10.24 ZHENG GU GING

正骨精

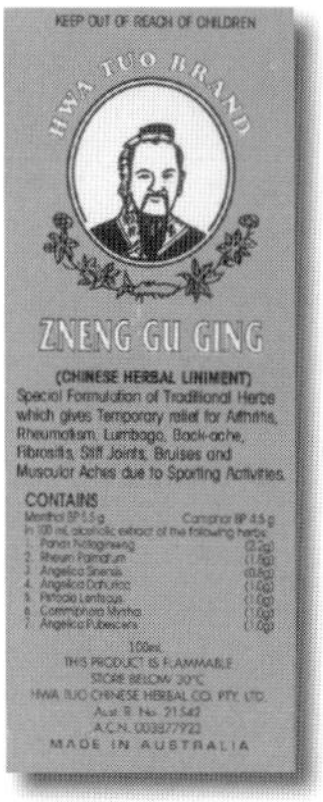

(*Zheng Gu Jing*)
Hua Tuo Chinese Herbal Co. (Australia)
'Mend Bone Essence'
Zheng Gu Ging is packaged in bottles of 100 ml

E

Chinese medical action

Invigorates blood and disperses stagnant blood, stops pain, promotes healing; warm and dispersing

Biomedical action

Anodyne, rubefacient

INDICATIONS

- Similar to **10.23 Zheng Gu Shui**. For blood stasis type pain from trauma, sprains, strains and uncomplicated fractures. Stimulates local circulation and metabolism, accelerates osteoblast activity.
- Wind damp painful obstruction or blood stasis type chronic joint pain, spasm and stiffness associated with arthritic conditions.

Composition (each bottle contains)

Menthol 5.5g, Camphor 4.5g, *Panax notoginseng* (tian qi, tianqi ginseng) 2.2g, *Rheum palmatum* (da huang, rhubarb root) 1.8g, *Angelica dahurica* (bai zhi, angelica) 1g, *Angelica pubescens* (du huo, Tu-huo) 1g, *Commiphora myrhha* (mo yao, myrhh) 1g, *Pistocia lentiscus* (mastic) 1g, *Angelica sinensis* (dang gui, chinese angelica) 0.8g, ethanol

Dosage and method of administration

Rub liberally and firmly into the affected area as often as practical, or apply on cotton wool and bandage for up to 2 hours at a time.

Cautions and contraindications

Contraindicated during pregnancy, for children under 5 years, when there is skin disease such as eczema, and for patients with acute inflammation where RICE (rest, ice, compression, elevation) is the appropriate treatment. Not suitable for use on broken skin. For external use only. Keep out of reach of children. May irritate the skin of some patients causing redness and itch, especially those with fair skin. Avoid contact with the eyes, mucous membranes and other sensitive areas.

10.25 DIE DA TIAN QI YAO JIU

跌打田七药酒

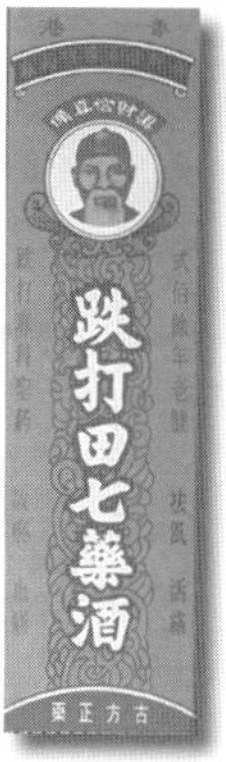

1-3/52

E

Wu Xiang Brand (Hong Kong)
'Pseudoginseng Alcohol Extract for Traumatic Injury'
Die Da Tian Qi Yao Jiu is packaged in bottles of 198 ml

Chinese medical action

Invigorates blood and disperses stagnant blood, stops pain, promotes healing; warm and dispersing

Biomedical action

Anodyne, rubefacient

INDICATIONS

- Similar to **10.23 Zheng Gu Shui**. For blood stasis type pain from trauma, sprains, strains and uncomplicated fractures. Stimulates local circulation and metabolism, accelerates osteoblast activity. This formula is particularly popular amongst martial arts enthusiasts.
- Wind damp painful obstruction or blood stasis type chronic joint pain, spasm and stiffness associated with arthritic conditions.

Composition

Panax notoginseng (tian qi, tianqi ginseng) 20%, *Angelica sinensis* (dang gui, chinese angelica) 20%, *Daemonorops draco* (xue jie, dragons blood) 15%, *Typhae augustifolia* (pu huang, bulrush pollen) 15%, *Carthamus tinctorius* (hong hua, carthamus) 10%, *Paeonia veitchii* (chi shao, red peony) 10%, *Boswellia carterii* (ru xiang, frankincense) 5%, *Commiphora myrhha* (mo yao, myrhh) 5%, ethanol

Dosage and method of administration

Rub liberally and firmly into the affected area as often as practical, or apply on cotton wool and bandage for up to 2 hours at a time.

Cautions and contraindications

Contraindicated during pregnancy, for children under 5 years, when there is skin disease such as eczema, and for patients with acute inflammation where RICE (rest, ice, compression, elevation) is the appropriate treatment. Not suitable for use on broken skin. For external use only. Keep out of reach of children. May irritate the skin of some patients causing redness and itch, especially those with fair skin. Avoid contact with the eyes, mucous membranes and other sensitive areas.

1-3/12

E

10.26 MINJAK GOSOK

莪术油

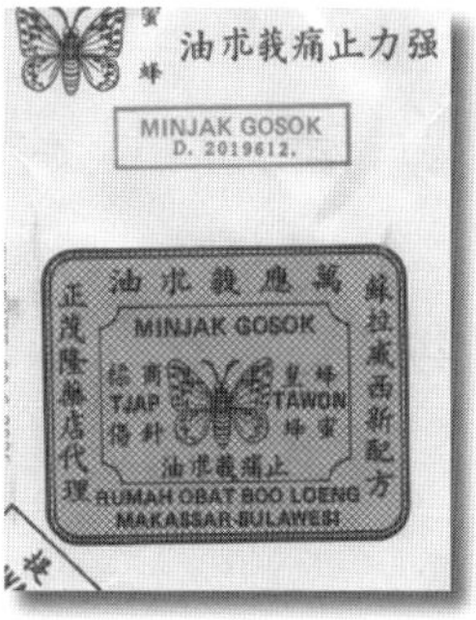

Wu Xiang Brand (Sulawesi)
'Curcuma Oil'
Min Jak Gosok is packaged in 50 ml bottles

Chinese medical action

Invigorates blood and disperses stagnant blood, dispels wind cold damp, stops pain, promotes healing; warm and dispersing

Biomedical action

Anodyne, rubefacient

INDICATIONS

- Chronic pain, stiffness, numbness and paresthesia from wind cold damp painful obstruction or blood stasis. Also for acute pain following trauma. This liniment is quite warming and best for cold type pain.
- Can also be applied to the lower abdomen for dysmenorrhea and for gynecological pain from blood stasis or masses.

Composition

Curcuma zeodoria (e zhu, curcuma ezhu)

Dosage and method of administration

Rub liberally and firmly into affected area as often as practical. Good as an invigorating and heating massage oil.

Cautions and contraindications

Contraindicated during pregnancy, for children under 5 years, when there is skin disease such as eczema, and for patients with acute inflammation where RICE (rest, ice, compression, elevation) is the appropriate treatment. Not suitable for use on broken skin. For external use only. Keep out of reach of children. May irritate the skin of some patients causing redness and itch, especially those with fair skin. Avoid contact with the eyes, mucous membranes and other sensitive areas.

10.27 ZHI TONG YOU

止痛油

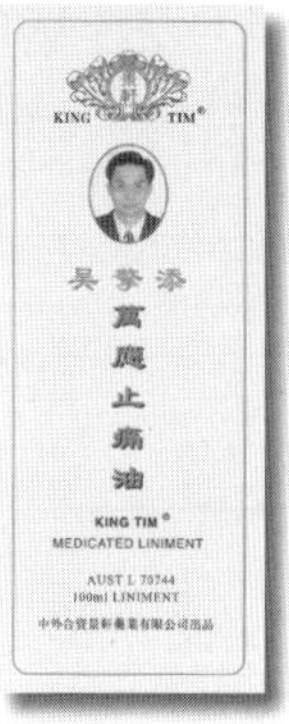

Jing Xian Pharmaceutical Co. (Guangzhou)
'Analgesic Oil'
Zhi Tong You is packaged in 198 ml bottles

Chinese medical action
Dispels wind cold damp, invigorates blood, disperses stagnant blood, stops pain; moderately warm and dispersing

Biomedical action
Anodyne, rubefacient

INDICATIONS
- Temporary relief of pain associated with rheumatic conditions, arthritis, sciatica, fibrositis, neuralgia, traumatic injury, sprains and bruising.
- Relief of muscular pain, spasm and cramp, tension headache.

Composition (each 100ml contains extracts equivalent to)
Gaultheria procumbens (wintergreen oil) 35g, *Pinus massoniana* (turpentine oil) 18g, *Cinnamomum cassia* (rou gui, cinnamon bark oil) 18g, *Mentha haplocalyx* (peppermint oil) 12.5g, *Panax notoginseng* (tian qi, tianqi ginseng) 250mg, *Angelica polymorpha* (dang gui, chinese angelica) 250mg

Dosage and method of administration
Massage 3-5 drops onto the affected area several times daily.

Cautions and contraindications
Contraindicated during pregnancy, for children under 5 years, when there is skin disease such as eczema, and for patients with acute inflammation where RICE (rest, ice, compression, elevation) is the appropriate treatment. Not suitable for use on broken skin. For external use only. Keep out of reach of children. May irritate the skin of some patients causing redness and itch, especially those with fair skin. Avoid contact with the eyes, mucous membranes and other sensitive areas.

10.28 WONG LOP KONG MEDICATED OIL

祛风止痛油

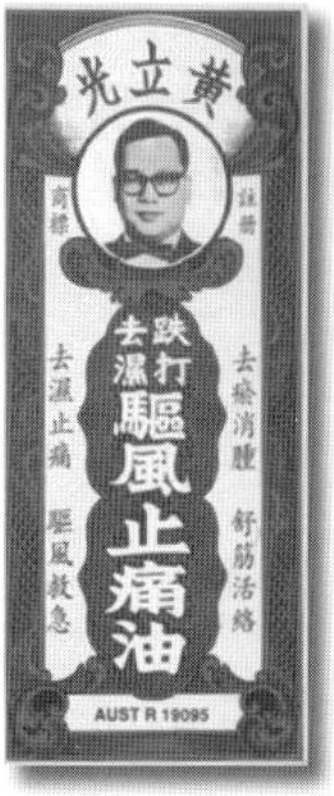

(*Qu Feng Zhi Tong You*)
Wong Lap Kwong Medicine Co. (Hong Kong)
'Expel wind Stop Pain Oil'
Wong Lop Kong Medicated Oil is packaged in 30 ml bottles

E

Chinese medical action

Invigorates qi and invigorates blood, disperses stagnant blood, dispels wind cold damp, stops pain; warm and dispersing

Biomedical action

Anodyne, rubefacient

INDICATIONS

- Used for a variety of minor muscular and joint aches and pains associated with simple backache, strains, bruising, trauma and overuse. Arthritic pain. As with all oils, this is slowly absorbed and long acting.
- Alleviates itching and irritation from insect bites and stings.

Composition (w/v)

Camphor oil 34%, *Camellia oleifera* (tea oil) 30%, *Pinus massoniana* (turpentine oil) 12%, *Daemonorops draco* (xue jie, dragons blood oil) 4%, *Mentha haplocalyx* (peppermint oil) 4%, *Angelica sinensis* (dang gui, chinese angelica) 4%, *Carthamus tinctorius* (hong hua, carthamus) 4%, *Commiphora myrrha* (mo yao, myrrh) 4%, *Boswellia carterii* (ru xiang, frankincense) 4%

Dosage and method of administration

Massage 3-5 drops into the affected area several times daily.

Cautions and contraindications

Contraindicated during pregnancy, for children under 5 years and for patients with acute inflammation where RICE (rest, ice, compression, elevation) is the appropriate treatment. Not suitable for use on broken skin. For external use only. Keep out of reach of children. May irritate the skin of some patients causing redness and itch, especially those with fair skin. Avoid contact with the eyes, mucous membranes and other sensitive areas.

10.29 WHITE FLOWER EMBROCATION

白花油

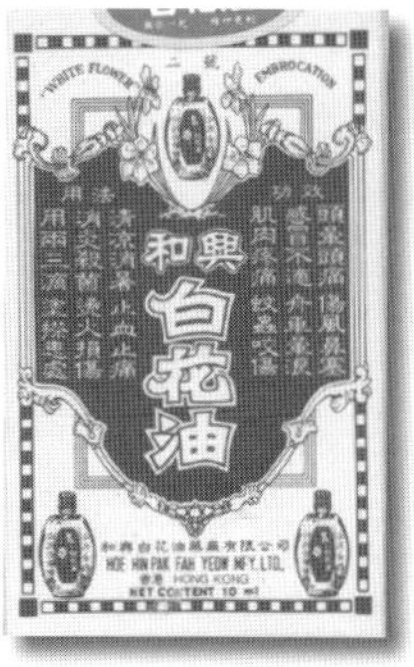

TGA

1-3/52

E

(*Bai Hua You*)
'White Flower Oil'
Hoe Hin Pak Fah Yeow Manufactory (Hong Kong)
White Flower Embrocation is packaged in bottles of 10 and 20ml

Chinese medical action

Stimulates and moves qi and eases the muscles, transforms and disperses phlegm and opens the orifices; cool and dispersing

Biomedical action

Anodyne, rubefacient

INDICATIONS

- Temporary relief of minor muscular aches and pains from fatigue and exertion, minor muscular strains and minor arthritic pain. Best when some degree of heat or inflammation is obvious.
- Useful for tension headaches and epigastric pain.
- Alleviates itching and irritation from insect bites and stings.
- Relieves chest, nasal and sinus congestion associated with colds and flu. Can also clear stuffiness in the head. May assist in alleviating motion sickness.

Composition (w/v)

Gaultheria procumbens (wintergreen oil) 40%, Menthol crystal 30%, Eucalyptus Oil 18%, Camphor 6%, Lavender Oil 6%

Dosage and method of administration

Rub a few drops into the affected area. If necessary, repeat every two hours. Can be mixed with a carrier oil if too strong. A few drops in hot water as a steam inhalation can relieve nasal and sinus congestion associated with colds and flu. Can also be rubbed on the chest for congestion and mucus accumulation. A few drops can be inhaled on a tissue to alleviate motion sickness.

Cautions and contraindications

Contraindicated during pregnancy. May cause skin irritation in some patients. Avoid contact with the eyes and mucous membranes. Not suitable for use on broken skin. Keep out of reach of children.

10.30 PO SUM ON MEDICATED OIL

保心安

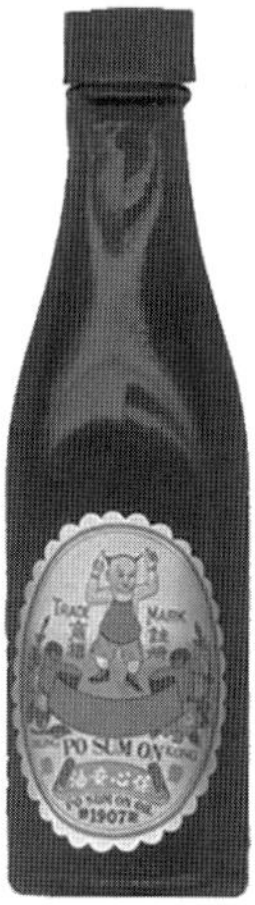

(*Bao Xin An*)
Po Sum On Medicine Factory (Hong Kong)
'Protect and Calm the Heart'
Po Sum On Medicated Oil is packaged in small bottles of 30ml

Chinese medical action

Stimulates movement of qi and invigorates blood, regulates Liver qi, eases the muscles and stops pain; cool and dispersing

Biomedical action

Relaxes muscles, anodyne, rubefacient

INDICATIONS

- Regulates and disperses stagnant qi. Used as a massage oil for tight muscles, especially good on the neck and shoulders. Good for tense, uptight patients and those with chronically constrained Liver qi, as it vigorously moves qi in the muscles of the Liver and Gallbladder channel pathways, easing and soothing muscular tension and stress.
- Nasal and sinus congestion and tension headaches. A little on a tissue can clear blocked sinuses and a dab rubbed on the temples can ease tension and stress headaches. Can assist in relieving chest congestion associated with colds and flu. Can also clear stuffiness in the head.

Composition

Mentha haplocalyx (peppermint oil) 57.3% v/v, *Camelia sinensis* (tea oil) 39.4% v/v, *Daemonorops draco* (xue jie, dragons blood) 2.07% w/v, *Scutellaria baicalensis* (huang qin, scute) 0.58% w/v, *Cinnamon cassia* (rou gui, cinnamon bark) 0.32% w/v, *Glycyrrhiza uralensis* (gan cao, licorice) 0.32% w/v

Combine with

- **6.4 Xiao Yao Wan** or **6.5 Jia Wei Xiao Yao Wan** for constitutionally stressed and uptight patients with chronic neck and upper back spasm and pain
- **15.4 Tian Ma Gou Teng Wan** for frontal or temporal headaches or migraines from Liver qi constraint with ascendant yang
- **3.9 Chuan Xiong Cha Tiao Wan** for headache from wind cold

Dosage and method of administration

Rub a few drops into the affected area and massage gently. If necessary, repeat every two hours. Can be mixed with a carrier oil if too strong. A few drops in hot water as a steam inhalation can relieve nasal and sinus congestion associated with colds and flu. Can also be rubbed on the chest for congestion and mucus accumulation. A few drops can be inhaled on a tissue to alleviate motion sickness.

Pattern identifying features

- muscle tightness and spasm from constrained Liver qi

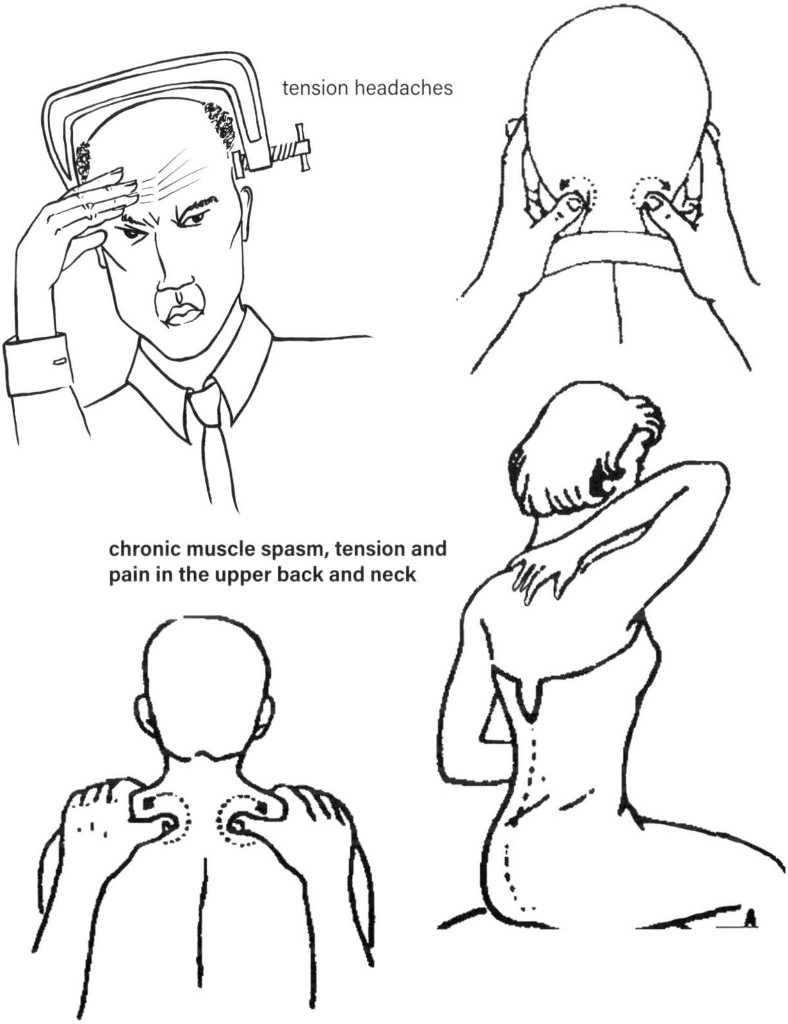

Cautions and contraindications

Contraindicated during pregnancy. Not recommended in very run down individuals, as the acrid, dispersing nature of the components can disperse qi and cause fatigue and dizziness. Keep out of reach of children. May irritate the skin in some patients, especially those with fair skin, causing redness and itch. Avoid contact with the eyes, mucous membranes and other sensitive areas.

10.31 TRANS WOOD LOCK LINIMENT

鸸鹋活络油

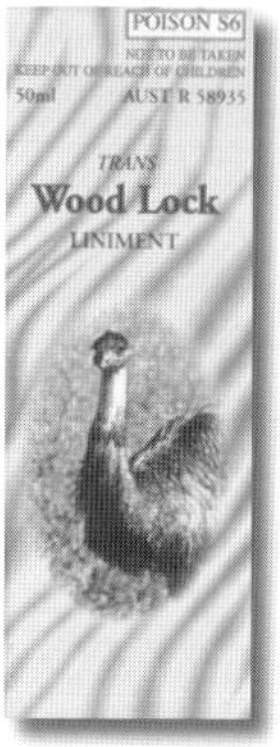

(*Er Miao Huo Luo You*)
Sunho Traditional Medicine Company (Australia)
'Emu Oil to Invigorate the Collaterals'
Trans Wood Lock Liniment is packaged in 50 ml bottles

Chinese medical action

Dispels wind cold damp, warms the channels, stops pain; warm to hot and dispersing

Biomedical action

Anodyne, rubefacient

INDICATIONS

- A very warming liniment for wind cold damp painful obstruction, rheumatic pain, musculoskeletal aches and pains, chronic heaviness, aching and pain of joints and muscles, stiffness and spasm of muscles and sinews. Emu oil is absorbed quite slowly, so **10.31 Trans Wood Lock Liniment** is useful for prolonged relief of the pain associated with osteoarthritis and rheumatoid arthritis, muscular and joint sprain, trauma and overuse, lumbago and sciatica.
- Itching and pain of insect bites and stings.

Composition (per 100ml)

Australian Emu Oil 20ml, Menthol 25g, Methyl Salicylate 25ml, Camphor 10g, Turpentine oil 15ml, Oleoresin Capsicum 0.5ml

Dosage and method of administration

Apply generously to the affected area and gently massage into the skin 1-2 times daily and before bed. Emu oil is absorbed slowly, warmth and analgesia increase gradually and last a relatively long time. It is wise to wait for 30-60 minutes before assuming that insufficient liniment was applied because the patient does not feel the effect. If too much is applied, it can become uncomfortably hot.

Cautions and contraindications

Contraindicated during pregnancy, for children under 5 years, when there is skin disease such as eczema, and for patients with acute inflammation where RICE (rest, ice, compression, elevation) is the appropriate treatment. Not suitable for use on broken skin. For external use only. Keep out of reach of children. May irritate the skin of some patients causing redness and itch, especially those with fair skin. Avoid contact with the eyes, mucous membranes and other sensitive areas.

10.32 DIE DA JIU

特效跌打酒

(*Te Xiao Die Da Jiu*)
Wu Min Pharmaceutical Co. (Guangzhou)
'Specially Effective Trauma [Alcohol based] Liniment'
Die Da Jiu is packaged in 100ml bottles

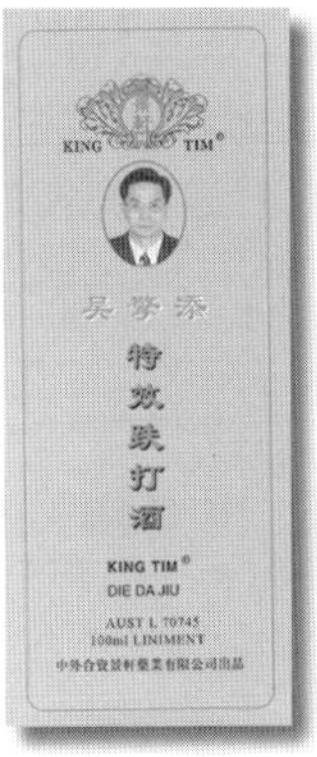

Chinese medical action

Invigorates blood and disperses stagnant blood, stops pain, promotes healing; moderately warm and dispersing

Biomedical action

Anodyne, rubefacient

INDICATIONS

- Similar to **10.23 Zheng Gu Shui**. For blood stasis type pain from sports injuries and trauma, sprains, strains and uncomplicated fractures. Stimulates local circulation and metabolism, accelerates osteoblast activity.
- Wind damp painful obstruction or blood stasis type chronic joint pain, spasm and stiffness associated with arthritic conditions.

Composition (per 100ml)

Panax notoginseng (tian qi, tianqi ginseng) 250mg, *Angelica dahurica* (bai zhi, angelica) 250mg, *Angelica pubescens* (du huo, Tu-huo) 250mg, *Ligusticum wallichi* (chuan xiong, ligusticum) 250mg, *Boswellia carterii* (ru xiang, frankincense) 250mg, *Angelica polymorpha* (dang gui, chinese angelica) 250mg, ethanol

Dosage and method of administration

Rub liberally and firmly into the affected area as often as practical, or apply on cotton wool and bandage for up to 2 hours at a time.

Cautions and contraindications

Contraindicated during pregnancy, for children under 5 years, when there is skin disease such as eczema, and for patients with acute inflammation where RICE (rest, ice, compression, elevation) is the appropriate treatment. Not suitable for use on broken skin. For external use only. Keep out of reach of children. May irritate the skin of some patients causing redness and itch, especially those with fair skin. Avoid contact with the eyes, mucous membranes and other sensitive areas.

10.33 WOOD LOCK MEDICATED BALM

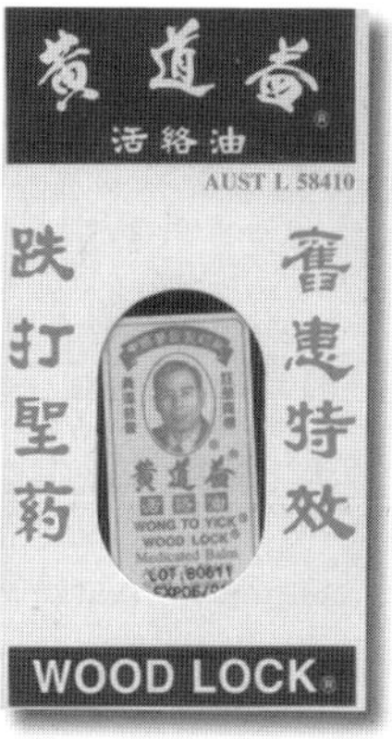

黄道益活络油

(*Huang Dao Yi Huo Luo You*)
China Medical Laboratory (Hong Kong)
'Huang Dao Yi's Invigorate (circulation in) the Collaterals Oil'
Wood Lock Medicated Balm is packaged in bottles of 50ml

E

Chinese medical action

Moves qi and eases the muscles, transforms and disperses phlegm and opens the orifices; cool and dispersing

Biomedical action

Anodyne, rubefacient

INDICATIONS

- Temporary relief of the pain of arthritis and rheumatism; relief of muscular aches and pains, cramps and spasms. Best when a degree of heat or inflammation is obvious.
- Symptoms of influenza, nasal, sinus and chest congestion.
- Can relieve tension headache and neuralgia. Good for tightness in the muscles of the neck and shoulders.

Composition (each gram contains)

Mentha haplocalyx (peppermint oil) 350mg, *Gaultheria procumbens* (wintergreen oil) 240mg, Turpentine oil 225mg, Lavender oil 130mg, Camphor oil 25mg; liquid extracts equivalent to dry *Angelica polymorpha* (dang gui, chinese angelica) 55mg, *Eucommia ulmoides* (du zhong, eucommia) 55mg

Dosage and method of administration

Rub a few drops into the affected area. If necessary, repeat every two hours. Can be mixed with a carrier oil if too strong. A few drops in hot water as a steam inhalation can relieve nasal and sinus congestion associated with colds and flu. Can also be rubbed on the chest for congestion and mucus accumulation. A few drops can be inhaled on a tissue to alleviate motion sickness.

Cautions and contraindications

Contraindicated during pregnancy. For external use only. Do not massage too vigorously or the skin may become irritated. Avoid contact with eyes and mucous membranes. Not suitable for use on open wounds or skin diseases. Not suitable for children under 3 years old.

10.34 IMADA RED FLOWER OIL

正红花油

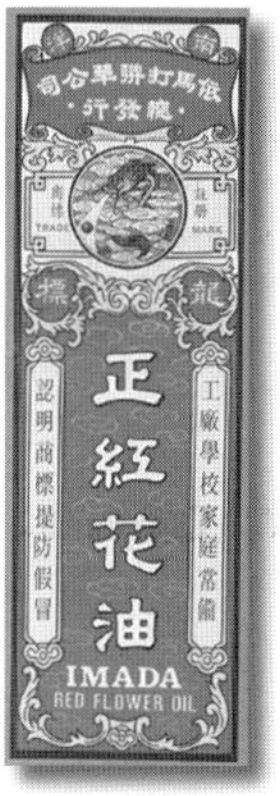

1-3/52

E

(*Zheng Hong Hua You*)
Imada Pharmaceutical Co. (Hong Kong)
'Authentic Carthamus Oil'
Imada Red Flower Oil is packaged in bottles of 50ml

Chinese medical action

Invigorates qi and invigorates blood, dispels cold, stops pain; moderately warm and dispersing

Biomedical action

Anodyne, rubefacient

INDICATIONS

- Temporary relief of pain associated with rheumatic conditions, arthritis, sciatica, fibrositis, neuralgia, traumatic injury, sprains and bruising.
- Relief of muscular pain, spasms and cramps.
- Insect bites and stings.

Composition

Methyl Salicylate, Cinnamon leaf oil, *Eugenia caryophyllata* (ding xiang, clove oil), Citronella oil, *Daemonorops draco* (xue jie, dragons blood), *Carthamus tinctorius* (hong hua, carthamus)

Dosage and method of administration

Apply to the affected area and massage gently. Repeat every four hours as necessary.

Cautions and contraindications

Contraindicated during pregnancy. For external use only. Do not massage too vigorously or the skin may become irritated. Avoid contact with eyes and mucous membranes. Not suitable for use on open wounds or skin diseases. Not suitable for children under 3 years old.

10.35 EAGLE BRAND MEDICATED OIL

德国风油精

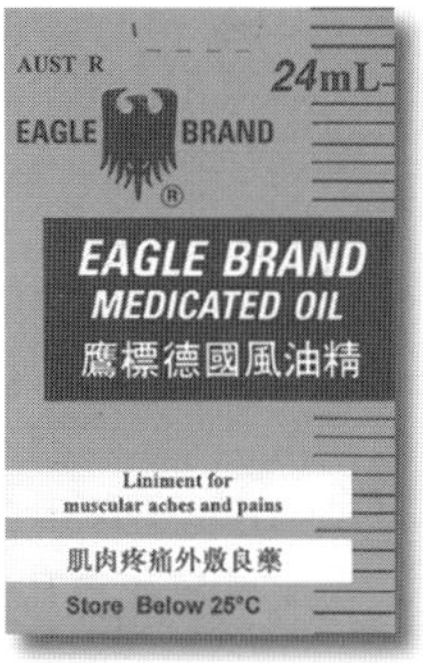

(*De Guo Feng You Jing*)
Borden Co. Pte Ltd (Singapore)
'German Wind Essential Oil'
Eagle Brand Medicated Oil is packaged in bottles of 24ml

Chinese medical action

Moves qi, eases the muscles, stops pain; cool and dispersing

Biomedical action

Relaxes muscles, anodyne, rubefacient

INDICATIONS

- Temporary relief of muscular aches and pains associated with simple backache, rheumatic conditions, osteoarthritis, strains and sprains. Best when a degree of heat or inflammation is obvious.
- Also used for stress and tension headaches. Especially good on the neck and upper back. The relatively high proportion of menthol makes this oil quite good for regulating and invigorating stagnant qi in the superficial muscles.

Composition

Menthol 28.5% w/w, Methyl Salicylate 18.6% w/w, Eucalyptus oil 1.56% w/w, ethanol

Dosage and method of administration

Rub a few drops into the affected area and massage gently. If necessary, repeat every two hours. Maximum application is four times daily. Can be mixed with a carrier oil if too strong.

Cautions and contraindications

Caution during pregnancy. For external use only. Do not massage too vigorously or the skin can become irritated. Avoid contact with eyes and mucous membranes. Not suitable for use on open wounds or skin diseases. Not suitable for children under 3 years old.

10.36 KUNG FU OIL

功夫油

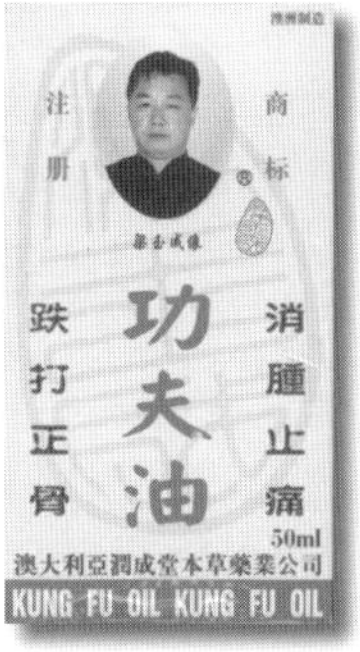

E

(*Gong Fu You*)
Run Cheng Tang Herbal Remedies Co. (Australia)
'Gong Fu [Martial Arts] Oil'
Kung Fu Oil is packaged in bottles of 50ml

Chinese medical action

Moves qi, eases the muscles, dispels wind cold damp, warms the channels, stops pain; moderately warm and dispersing

Biomedical action

Anodyne, rubefacient

INDICATIONS

- Temporary relief of chronic muscular aches and pains associated with sporting injuries, overuse syndromes, rheumatic conditions, osteoarthritis, strains and sprains.
- Particularly useful as an adjunct treatment for chronic wind cold damp painful obstruction due to the inclusion of the wind damp expelling Tu-huo, and the yang warming asarum and clove oil.

Composition (w/v)

Mentha haplocalyx (peppermint oil) 40%, *Eugenia caryophyllata* (ding xiang, clove oil) 6%, *Gaultheria procumbens* (wintergreen oil) 10%, Paraffin oil 24%, *Angelica pubescens* (du huo, Tu-huo) 1.5%, *Asarum seiboldi* (xi xin, asarum) 1.7%, ethanol 16.8%

Dosage and method of administration

Apply 3-6 drops to the affected area and massage gently. Maximum application is three times daily.

Cautions and contraindications

Contraindicated during pregnancy. For external use only. Do not massage too vigorously or the skin can become irritated. Avoid contact with eyes and mucous membranes. Not suitable for use on open wounds or skin diseases. Not suitable for children under 3 years old.

10.37 TIGER BALM

虎標万金油

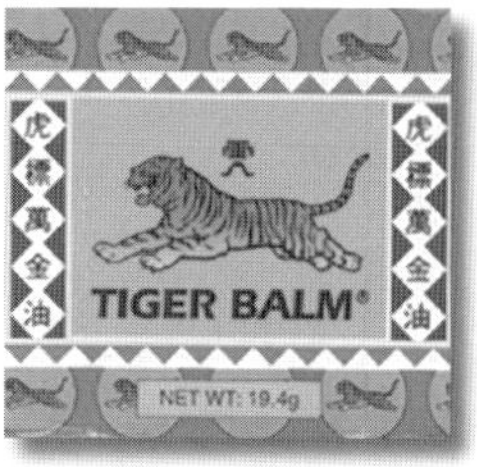

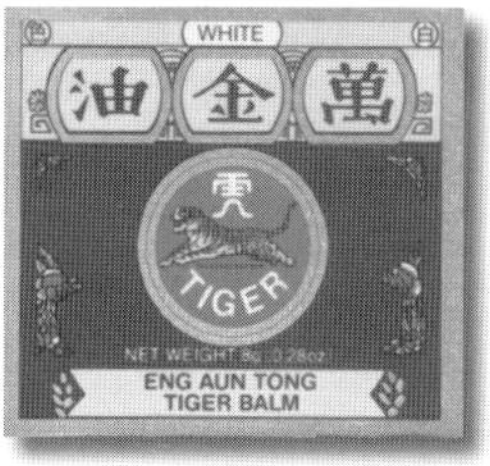

(*Hu Biao Wan Jin You*)
Haw Par Corporation (Singapore)
Tiger Balm is packaged in small jars or flat tins of ointment. There are two types, red and white.

Chinese medical action

Moves qi and eases the muscles, transforms and disperses phlegm and opens the orifices

Biomedical action

Relaxes muscles, improves local circulation, analgesic

INDICATIONS

- Temporary relief of muscular aches, pain and spasm, arthritic or rheumatic pain, sprains, headaches, nasal, sinus and chest congestion, insect bites, itch and flatulence. Useful for the pain of gout (White Tiger balm).
- Quick relief of cramps and spasms in the muscles.
- **Red Tiger Balm** contains cinnamon oil and thus is hotter and better for wind cold damp painful obstruction and pain associated with poor circulation or exposure to cold.
- **White Tiger Balm** is more cooling and better at moving stagnant qi locally–ideal for cramps and spasms, inflammatory pain and gout.

Composition

Tiger Balm Red

Camphor 25%, Menthol 10%, *Melaleuca cajuputi* (cajuput teatree oil) 7%, dementholised mint oil 6%, *Eugenia caryophyllata* (ding xiang, clove oil) 5%, *Cinnamon cassia* (rou gui, cinnamon bark oil) 5%, paraffin and petroleum jelly to 100%

Tiger Balm White

Camphor 25%, dementholised mint oil 16%, *Melaleuca cajuputi* (cajuput teatree oil) 13%, Menthol 8%, *Eugenia caryophyllata* (ding xiang, clove oil) 1.5%, yellow soft paraffin 10.5%, hard paraffin to 100%

Dosage and method of administration

Apply gently to the affected area.

Pattern identifying features

- temporary relief of aches and pains, spasms, cramps and congestion

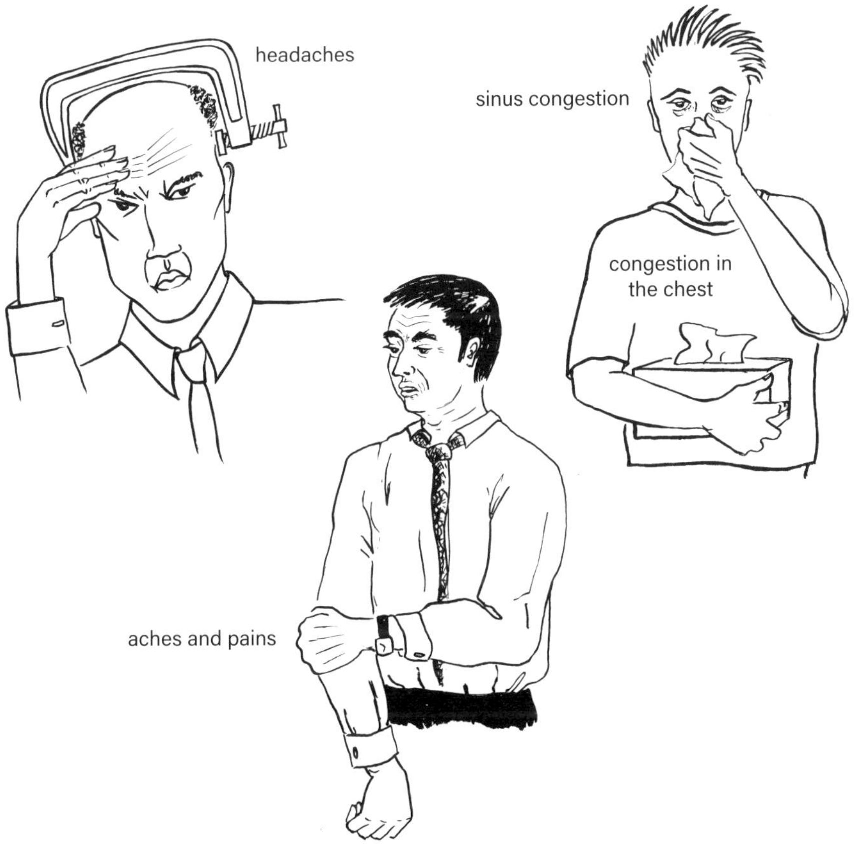

Cautions and contraindications

Contraindicated during pregnancy and for children under three years old. Keep out of reach of children. For external use only. Avoid contact with the eyes, mucous membranes and broken skin. May irritate the skin of some patients, especially those with fair skin, causing redness and itch. **Red Tiger Balm** can stain clothes.

10.38 PLASTER FOR BRUISE AND ANALGESIC

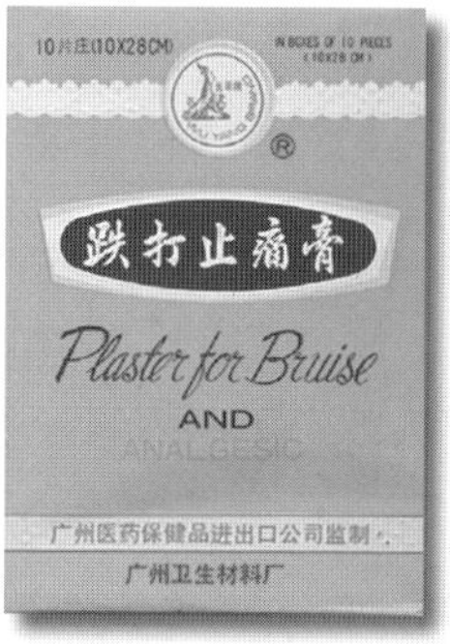

跌打止痛膏

(Die Da Zhi Tong Gao)
Guangzhou Medicine and Health Products Import Export Corp. (Guangzhou)
'Analgesic Trauma Plaster'
Plaster for Bruise and Analgesic is packaged as sticky herb lined cloth sheet, ten sheets per box

Chinese medical action

Invigorates blood, dispels stagnant blood, stops pain

Biomedical action

Invigorates local circulation, anti-inflammatory, anodyne

INDICATIONS

- Applied topically for acute injuries, including sprains and strains, bruising, and trauma where the skin is unbroken. Can significantly accelerate resolution of bruising and healing of damaged tissues.
- For chronic osteoarthritis, rheumatoid arthritic and other wind cold damp painful obstruction conditions. Especially good for chronic lower back ache.
- May also assist in the relief of neuralgic pain, such as intercostal and postherpetic neuralgia.

Composition

Lonicera japonica (jin yin hua, lonicera) 20%, *Os draconis* (long gu, dragon bone) 10.42%, *Eupolyphaga sinensis* (di bie chong, field cockroach) 10.42%, *Carthamus tinctorius* (hong hua, carthamus) 9.17%, *Rheum palmatum* (da huang, rhubarb) 8.33%, *Gardenia jasminoides* (shan zhi zi, gardenia) 8.32%, *Taraxacum mongolicum* (pu gong ying, dandelion) 8.33%, *Daemonorops draco* (xue jie, dragons blood) 4.17%, *Acacia catechu* (hai er cha, catechu) 6.25%, *Commiphora myrrha* (mo yao, myrrh) 6.25%, *Drynaria fortunei* (gu sui bu, drynaria) 4.17%, *Dipsacus asper* (xu duan, dipsacus) 4.17%

Combine with

- **10.1 Yunnan Paiyao** or **10.3 Die Da Zhi Tong Capsule** for pain and bruising from trauma
- **10.15 Du Huo Ji Sheng Wan** for Kidney deficiency aches and pains
- **7.9 Jin Gui Shen Qi Wan** for Kidney yang deficiency pain and stiffness
- **5.1 Xue Fu Zhu Yu Wan** for postherpetic neuralgia associated with static blood

Pattern identifying features

- **blood stasis**
- wind cold damp painful obstruction

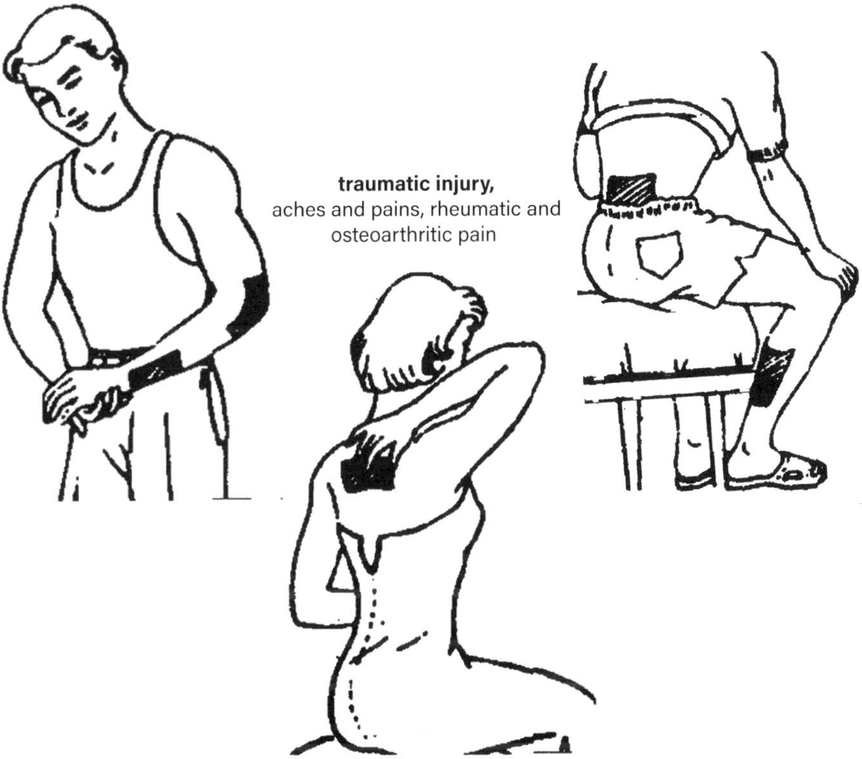

Dosage and method of administration

Cut a sheet to the desired size and apply to the affected area after removal of the transparent backing plastic. Mobile or hairy areas may need to be bound with a bandage or thermo skin to keep the plaster in place. Good at night when movement is less. Effective for 24 hours.

Cautions and Contraindications

Contraindicated during pregnancy, on skin disease and during acute inflammation following trauma where RICE (rest, ice, compression, elevation) is the appropriate treatment (usually the first 24-48 hours). Not suitable for use on broken skin and on young children. May cause skin irritation in some patients, usually those with fair skin. Any irritation usually subsides quickly once the patch is removed.

10.39 DIE DA FENG SHI PLASTER

跌打风湿膏

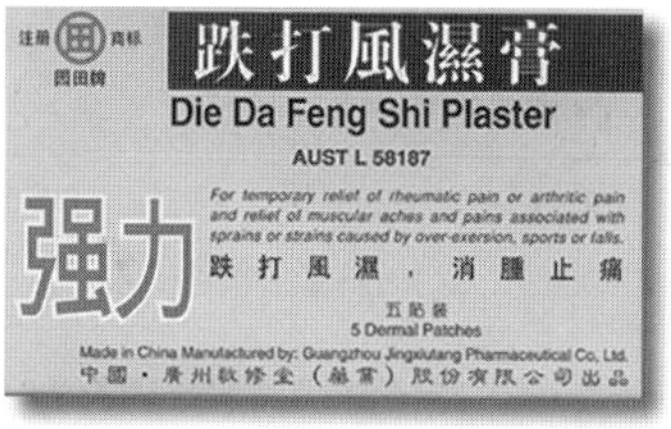

Guangzhou Jingxiutang Pharmaceutical Co. (Guangzhou)
'Trauma and Arthritis Plaster'
Die Da Feng Shi Plasters are packaged in boxes of five small sheets

E

Chinese medical action

Dispels wind damp, stops pain

Biomedical action

Invigorates local circulation, anti-inflammatory, anodyne

INDICATIONS

- Temporary relief of wind cold damp painful obstruction, osteoarthritic or rheumatic pain and musculoskeletal aches and pains associated with sprains and strains, sports injury, trauma and overexertion.

Composition (each plaster contains)

Dryobalanops aromatica (bing pian, borneol) 137mg, *Nardostachys chinensis* (gan song, nardostachys) 360mg, *Zanthoxylum nitidum* (liang mian zhen) 159mg, *Eucalyptus globus* (eucalyptus oil) 80mg, *Ilex chinensis* (chinese holly seed oil) 69mg, *Kaempferia galanga* 36mg, *Schizonepeta tenuifolia* (jing jie, schizonepeta) 32mg, *Impatiens balsamina* (ji xing zi, impatiens) 32mg, *Angelica dahurica* (bai zhi, angelica) 30mg, *Zingiber officinalis* (sheng jiang, ginger) 26mg, *Ledebouriella divaricata* (fang feng, siler) 24mg, *Drynaria fortunei* (gu sui bu, drynaria) 20mg, *Cinnamomum cassia* (rou gui, cinnamon oil) 20mg, *Syzygium aromaticum* (ding xiang, clove oil) 14mg

Dosage and method of administration

Applied to the affected area after removal of the transparent plastic backing. Mobile or hairy areas may need to be bound with a bandage or thermo skin to keep the plaster in place. Good at night when movement is less. Effective for 24 hours.

Pattern identifying features

- **wind cold damp painful obstruction**

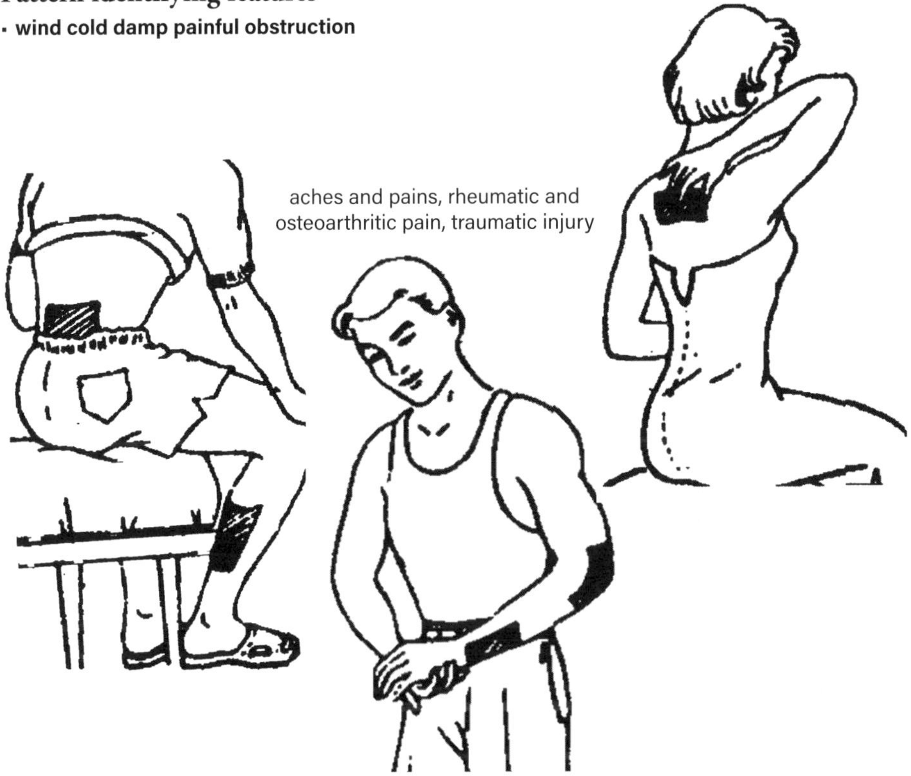

Cautions and Contraindications

Contraindicated over the lower abdomen and lower back during pregnancy, on skin disease and during acute inflammation following trauma where RICE (rest, ice, compression, elevation) is the appropriate treatment (usually the first 24-48 hours). Not suitable for use on broken skin and or on children under six years old. May cause skin irritation in some patients, usually those with fair skin. Any irritation usually subsides quickly once the patch is removed.

10.40 POROUS CAPSICUM PLASTER

辣椒膏

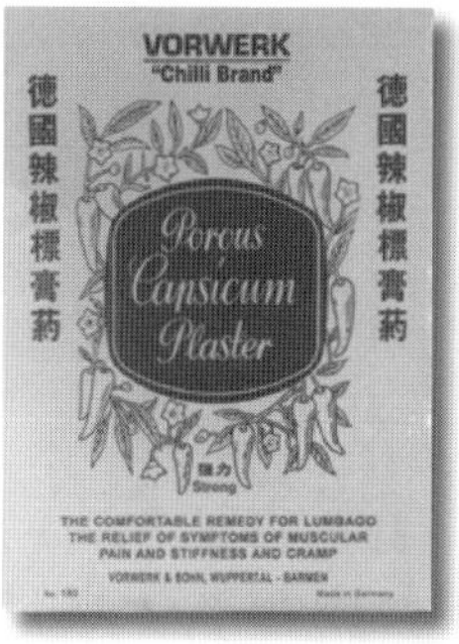

(*La Jiao Gao*)
Vorwerk and Sohn (Germany)
Porous Capsicum Plasters are packaged as large and small rubber backed sheets lined with the sticky herbal extract

Chinese medical action

Warms the channels and dispels cold, stops pain

Biomedical action

Invigorates local circulation, counter-irritant, dilates capillaries, anodyne

INDICATIONS

- A hot plaster for pain from cold and cold damp pathology. Widely used for wind cold damp painful obstruction, cold type dysmenorrhea, osteoarthritis and generalized musculoskeletal aches and pains that are worse in cold weather.

Composition

Pinus massoniana (turpentine oil) 27%, *Capsicum oleoresin* (la jiao, chilli) 3%, Zinc oxide 14%, Ferric oxide 1%, rubber 55%

Combine with

- **10.8 Xiao Huo Luo Wan** for severe cold painful obstruction
- **10.15 Du Huo Ji Sheng Wan** for Kidney deficiency aches and pains
- **7.9 Jin Gui Shen Qi Wan** for Kidney yang deficiency pain and stiffness
- **10.18 Jian Bu Qiang Shen Wan** for lower back ache from Kidney yang deficiency with wind damp

Dosage and method of administration

Wash the skin with soap and dry well. Apply the sticky side to the affected area after removal of the backing sheet. Mobile or hairy areas may need to be bound with a bandage or thermo skin to keep the plaster in place. Good at night when movement is less. Effective for 24-48 hours. Rest the area for a few days before applying another plaster. The large plasters are good for big areas, but can be cut to fit on small areas such as the fingers and toes. Any residue left after removal of the plaster can be removed with alcohol.

Pattern identifying features

- **cold painful obstruction**

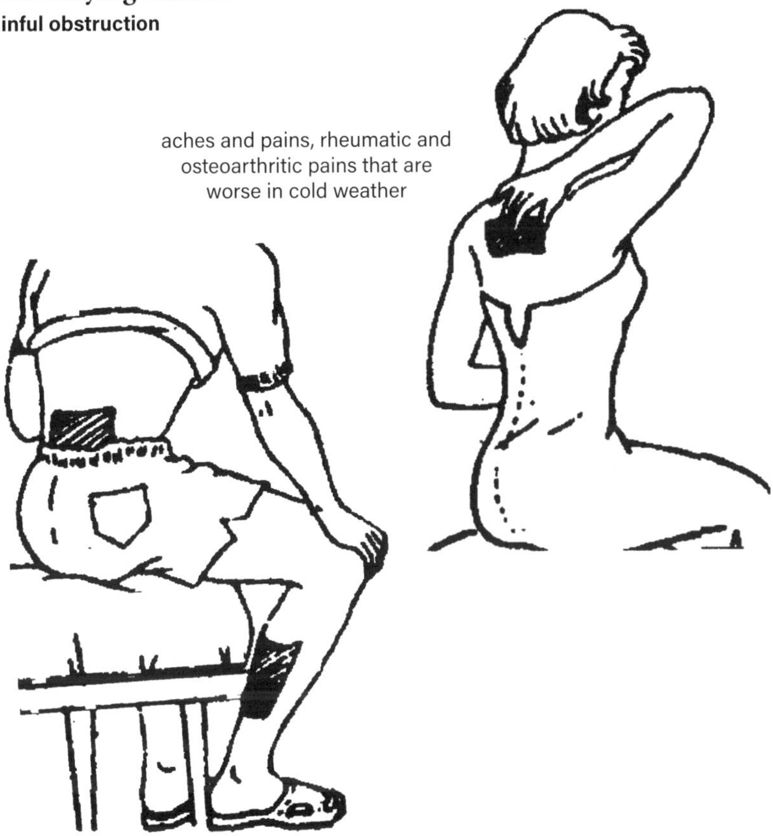

Cautions and Contraindications

Contraindicated over the lower abdomen and lower back during pregnancy, on skin diseases, and during acute inflammation where RICE (rest, ice, compression, elevation) is the appropriate treatment (usually the first 24-48 hours). Not suitable for use on broken skin or on young children. These plasters are very hot and will often cause skin irritation or blistering in fair skinned patients if left too long. Be careful with the elderly and with those who may have reduced sensation in the skin.

GMP

10.41 GOU PI GAO

狗皮膏

Tong Ren Tang (Beijing)
'Dog Skin Plaster'
Gou Pi Gou is packaged as a 15 gram mass of herbs on a cloth square

E

Chinese medical action

Warms the channels and collaterals, powerfully dispels cold, stops pain

Biomedical action

Invigorates local circulation, counter-irritant, dilates capillaries, anodyne

INDICATIONS

- A very hot plaster for localised joint or muscle pain, numbness, paresthesia or compromised circulation associated with chronic cold damp painful obstruction, arthritic conditions or trauma. The pain is fixed, worse with cold, damp weather and significantly improved with warmth.
- Used locally or on selected acupuncture points for yang deficient or cold type disorders such as dysmenorrhea, chronic lower back ache, impotence, lung disease with copious thin watery sputum (e.g. chronic bronchitis), and abdominal masses from cold accumulation.

Composition

Aconitium carmichaeli (chuan wu, aconite), *Aconitium kusnezoffii* (cao wu, wild aconite), *Angelica pubescens* (du huo, Tu-huo), *Notopterygium incisum* (qiang huo, notopterygium), *Periploca sepium* (xiang jia pi), *Clematis chinensis* (wei ling xian, chinese clematis), *Dipsacus asper* (xu duan, dipsacus), *Angelica sinensis* (dang gui, chinese angelica)

Combine with

- **10.8 Xiao Huo Luo Wan** for severe or chronic cold arthritic pain
- **1.13 Woo Garm Yuen Medical Pills**, **1.18 Shao Fu Zhu Yu Wan** or **1.14 Wen Jing Wan** for severe cold type dysmenorrhea
- **10.15 Du Huo Ji Sheng Wan** for Kidney deficiency aches and pains
- **7.9 Jin Gui Shen Qi Wan** for Kidney yang deficiency lower back and joint pain and stiffness

Dosage and method of administration

The mass of herbs is hard and need to be softened before use. To do this, place in an oven or microwave and gently warm, or steam over a boiling jug until soft. While still warm (not hot), apply to the affected area. If no irritation occurs it can be left in place for a several days at a time. The same plaster can be gently removed and reused a few times.

Pattern identifying features

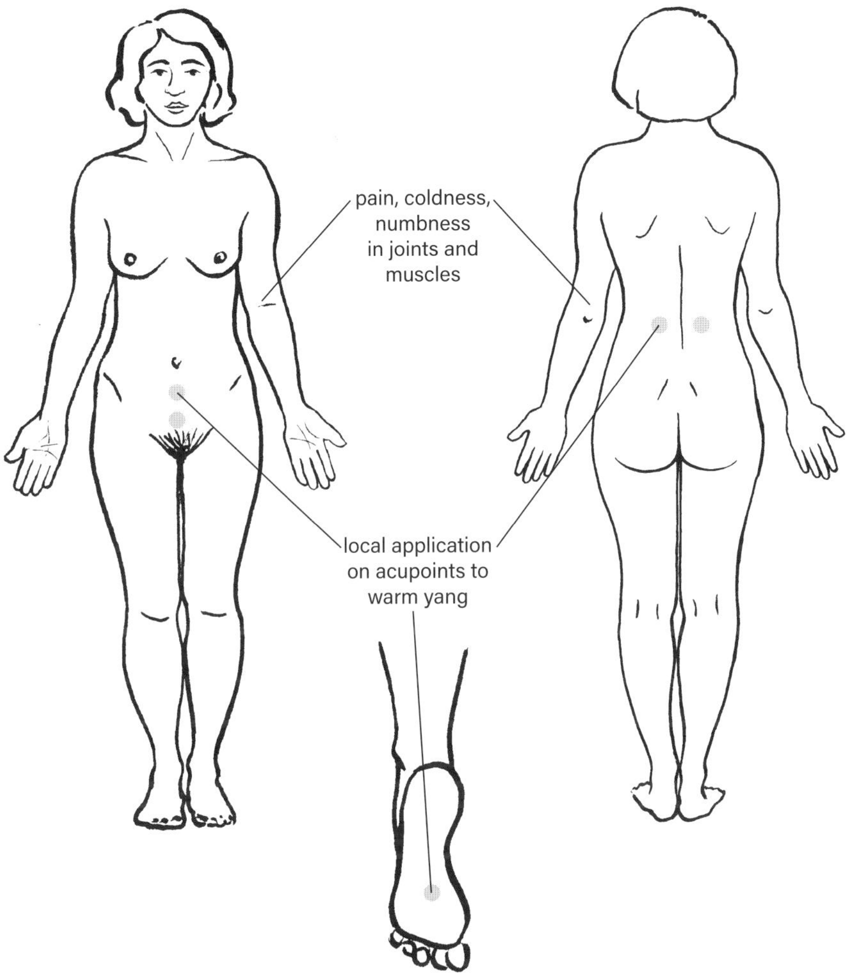

Cautions and Contraindications

Contraindicated during pregnancy, on skin diseases, and during acute inflammation where RICE (rest, ice, compression, elevation) is the appropriate treatment (usually the first 24-48 hours). Not suitable for use on broken skin or on young children. These plasters are very hot and will often cause skin irritation or blistering in fair skinned patients if left too long. Be careful with the elderly and those who may have reduced sensation in the skin.

男科 11

Men's Health

11.1 QIAN LIE XIAN CAPSULE

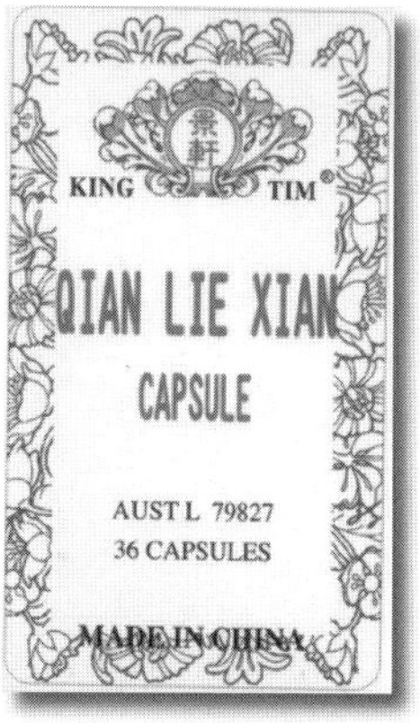

特效前列腺丸

(Te Xiao Qian Lie Xian Wan)
Jing Xian Pharmaceutical Co. (Guangzhou)
'Especially Effective Prostate Gland Pills'
Qian Lie Xian Capsules are packaged in bottles of 36 capsules

Chinese medical action

Clears damp and toxic heat from the prostate and lower burner, invigorates blood, transforms phlegm, warms Kidney yang, stops pain

Biomedical action

Conditions and improves the functional activity of the prostate gland, reduces inflammation and swelling, stops pain, improves fluid metabolism, diuretic

INDICATIONS

- Chronic prostatitis. Used for persistent damp heat and static blood in the prostate. Supports Kidney yang and the transformation and processing of pathological fluids that tend to accumulate in the prostate gland. The combination of vaccaria seed and astragalus assists in 'opening up' the prostate gland to facilitate access by herbs or drugs.
- Also used for prostatic hypertrophy, elevated prostate specific antigen (PSA), testicular swelling and pain, urinary tract infection, epididymitis, hematuria and inguinal pain due to chronic damp heat and/or blood stasis.

Composition (each capsule contains extracts equivalent to dry)

Phellodendron amurense (huang bai, phellodendron) 340mg, *Polygonum cuspidatum* (hu zhang, bushy knotweed) 306mg, *Raphanus sativus* (lai fu zi, radish seed) 306mg, *Cuscuta hygrophila* (tu su zi, cuscuta) 306mg, *Hedyotis diffusa* (bai hua she she cao, oldenlandia) 306mg, *Vaccaria segetalis* (wang bu liu xing, vaccaria seed) 306mg, *Epimedium brevicornu* (xian ling pi, epimedium) 306mg, *Poria cocos* (fu ling, hoelen) 306mg, *Plantago asiatica* (che qian zi, plantago) 230mg, *Lycium barbarum* (gou qi zi, lycium fruit) 230mg, *Astragalus membranaceous* (huang qi, astragalus) 230mg, *Schizandra chinensis* (wu wei zi, schizandra) 230mg, *Glycyrrhiza uralensis* (gan cao, licorice) 191mg

Combine with

- **4.10 Shi Lin Tong** for urinary calculi and to enhance the diuretic action of the formula
- **2.24 Shu Gan Wan** or **11.4 Tian Tai Wu Yao Wan** for Liver qi constraint type testicular pain or painful urination
- **1.35 Nei Xiao Luo Li Wan** or **11.3 Ji Sheng Ju He Wan** for persistent prostate swelling and elevated prostate specific antigen (PSA) from chronic damp heat or phlegm heat

Pattern identifying features

- **damp heat and blood stasis affecting the prostate gland**
- difficulty starting urination, broken or weak urinary stream, dribbling, nocturia

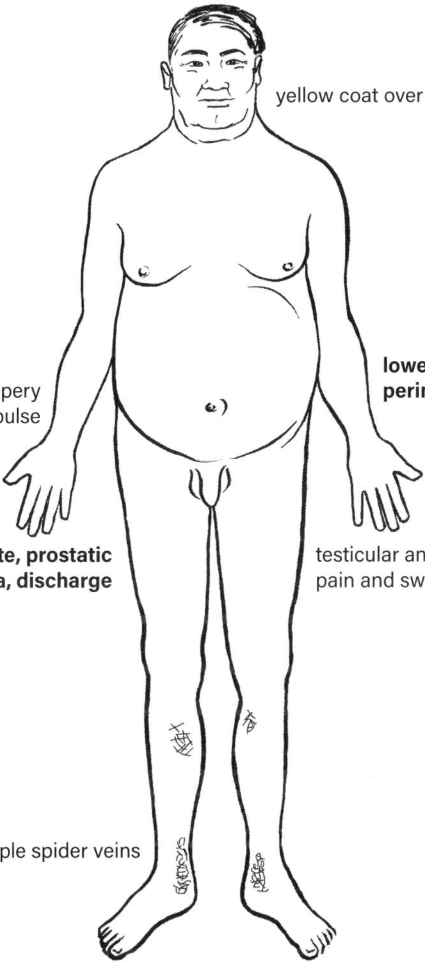

- **7.9 Jin Gui Shen Qi Wan** or **4.11 Ba Ji Yin Yang Wan** for patients with yang deficiency and prostate swelling
- **1.17 Gui Zhi Fu Ling Wan** (mild) or **1.18 Shao Fu Zhu Yu Wan** for sharp or stabbing prostatic or perineal pain

Dosage and method of administration

3-4 capsules, three times daily on an empty stomach. In severe cases, the dose can be increased by 50% until results are noted, then scaled back to the recommended dose. For best results, combine with prostate drainage massage.

Cautions and contraindications

None noted.

3+/12

11.2 PROSTATE GLAND PILLS

前列腺丸

(*Qian Lie Xian Wan*)
United Manufactory of Chinese Medicine (Guangzhou)
Prostate Gland Pills are packaged in bottles of 90 pills
A similar formula available as: Kai Kit Wan (PF)

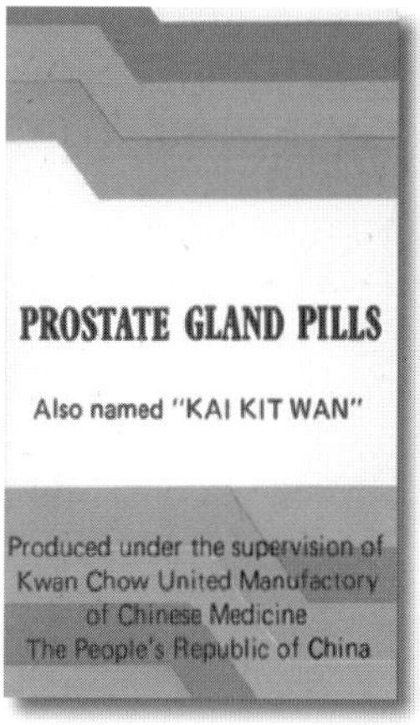

Chinese medical action

Clears persistent damp and toxic heat from the prostate and lower burner, invigorates blood, stops pain

Biomedical action

Conditions and improves the functional activity of the prostate gland, reduces inflammation and swelling, stops pain

INDICATIONS

- Chronic prostatitis. Similar in scope and action to **11.1 Qian Lie Xian Capsule**, the main difference being the absence of Kidney yang tonification in this formula, making it better for patients with underlying yin deficiency.
- Can also be used for prostatic hypertrophy, elevated prostate specific antigen (PSA), testicular swelling and pain, urinary tract infection, hematuria and inguinal pain due to chronic damp heat and/or blood stasis.

Composition

Vaccaria segetalis (wang bu liu xing, vaccaria seed), *Paeonia suffruticosa* (mu dan pi, moutan), *Paeonia rubra* (chi shao, red peony), *Astragalus membranaceous* (huang qi, astragalus), *Patrinia villosa* (bai jiang cao, patrinia), *Corydalis turtschaninovii* (yan hu suo, corydalis), *Codonopsis pilosula* (dang shen, codonopsis), *Glycyrrhiza uralensis* (gan cao, licorice), *Akebia trifoliata* (mu tong, akebia)

Combine with

- **4.10 Shi Lin Tong** for urinary calculi and to enhance the diuretic action of the formula
- **2.24 Shu Gan Wan** or **11.4 Tian Tai Wu Yao Wan** for Liver qi constraint type testicular pain or painful urination
- **1.35 Nei Xiao Luo Li Wan** or **11.3 Ji Sheng Ju He Wan** for persistent prostate swelling and elevated prostate specific antigen (PSA) arising from chronic damp heat or phlegm heat
- **7.9 Jin Gui Shen Qi Wan** or **4.11 Ba Ji Yin Yang Wan** for prostate swelling from yang deficiency
- **1.17 Gui Zhi Fu Ling Wan** (mild) or **1.18 Shao Fu Zhu Yu Wan** for sharp or stabbing prostatic or perineal pain
- **1.23 Zhi Bai Di Huang Wan** for yin deficiency with chronic damp heat in the lower burner

Pattern identifying features

- **damp heat and blood stasis affecting the prostate gland**

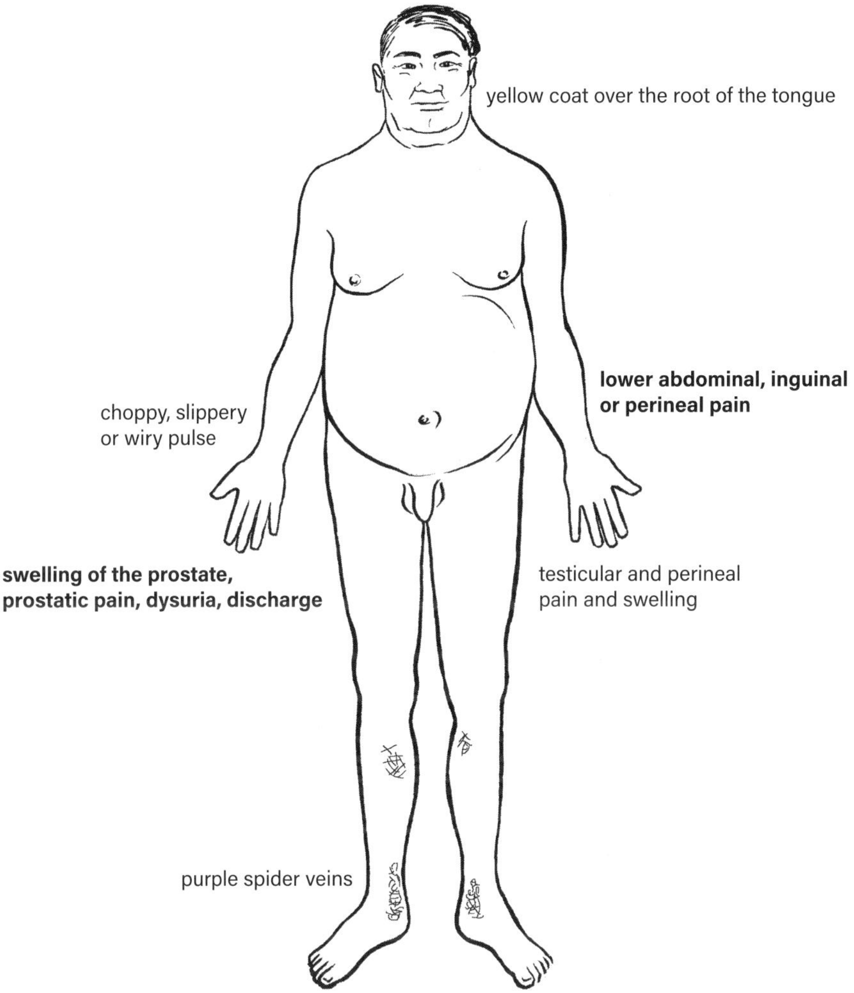

Dosage and method of administration

6 pills, three times daily on an empty stomach. **11.2 Prostate Gland Pills** need to be taken for some months to achieve a satisfactory result. For best results, combine with prostate drainage massage.

Cautions and contraindications

None noted.

GMP

11.3 JI SHENG JU HE WAN

济生橘核丸

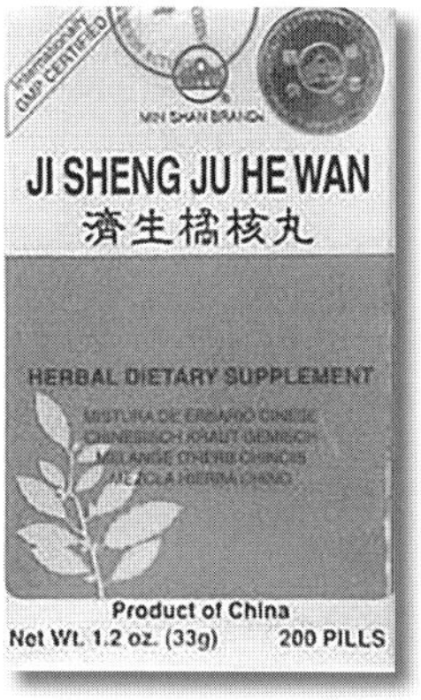

Lanzhou Foci Pharmaceutical Factory (Gansu)
'Tangerine Seed Pills [from Formulas to Aid the Living])'
Ji Sheng Ju He Wan is packaged in bottles of 200 pills
Also available as: Citrus Aurantium Compound Pills, Citrus Seed Pills, Vigorexin Extract, Citrus Seed Formula (conc. extract)

Chinese medical action

Regulates qi and blood, softens hardness, transforms phlegm, reduces swelling, dissipates nodules, stops pain

Biomedical action

Reduces swelling, stops pain

INDICATIONS

- Testicular swelling and lumps. These masses are firm and rubbery, and may or may not be tender. Usually associated with chronic accumulation of cold and damp in the Liver channel, compounded by Liver qi constraint with eventual congealing into phlegm and blood stasis.
- Phlegm and qi constraint type masses, such as thyroid nodules, breast, benign ovarian and uterine tumors, fibroids, ovarian cysts and other phlegm type swellings.
- With the appropriate identifying features, this formula can assist in the treatment of conditions such as varicocele, hydrocele, chronic orchitis, epididymitis, uterine fibroids, breast and ovarian cysts and thyroid swellings.

Composition

Citrus reticulata (ju he, citrus seed), *Melia toosendan* (chuan lian zi, melia fruit), *Ecklonia kurome* (kun bu, kelp), *Laminaria japonica* (hai dai, laminaria), *Sargassum pallidum* (hai zao, sargassum seaweed), *Prunus persica* (tao ren, peach seed), *Corydalis turtschaninovii* (yan hu suo, corydalis), *Cinnamomum cassia* (rou gui, cinnamon bark), *Magnolia officinalis* (hou po, magnolia bark), *Saussurea lappa* (mu xiang, saussurea), *Akebia trifoliata* (mu tong, akebia), *Citrus aurantium* (zhi shi, aurantium)

Combine with

– **6.6 Long Dan Xie Gan Wan** for nodules and masses with warmth and redness

Dosage and method of administration

8-12 pills three times daily on an empty stomach. The dose can be spread out, or taken in two lots of 12-18 pills, morning and evening. In severe cases or during the early stages of treatment (the first few weeks), a 50% increase in dose can be used, then reduced as treatment takes effect.

Pattern identifying features

- **cold damp, phlegm and qi constraint in the Liver channel and testicles**
- phlegm nodules and masses

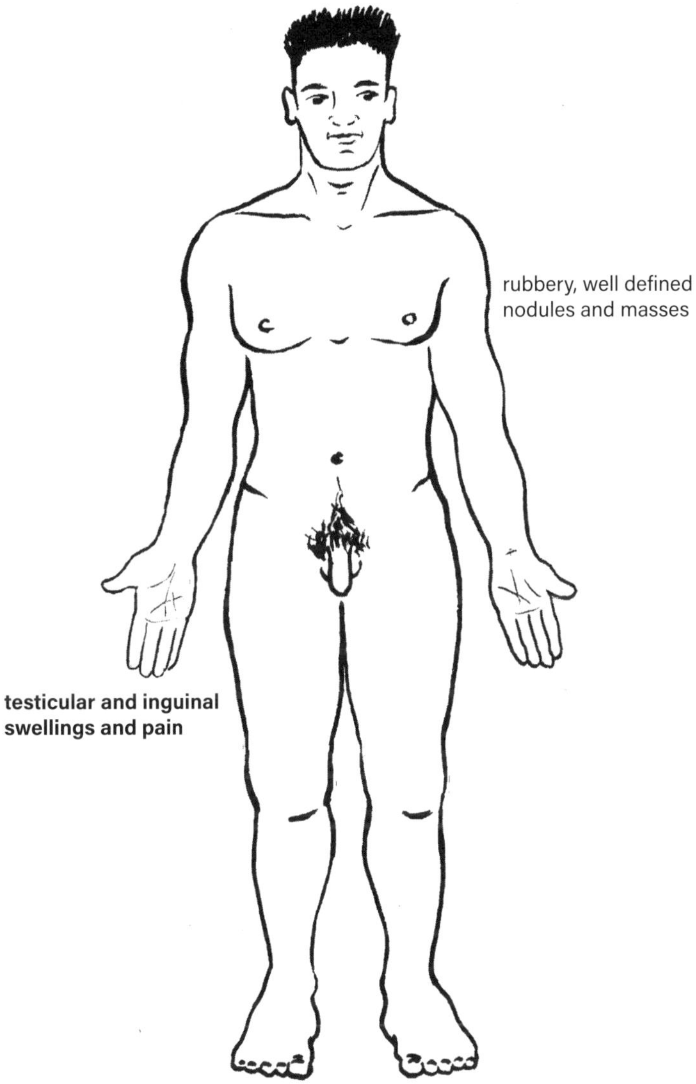

Cautions and contraindications

Contraindicated during pregnancy.

GMP

11.4 TIAN TAI WU YAO WAN

天台乌药丸

3+/12

Lanzhou Foci Pharmaceutical Factory (Gansu)
'Top Quality Lindera Pills'
Tian Tai Wu Yao Wan is packaged in bottles of 200 pills

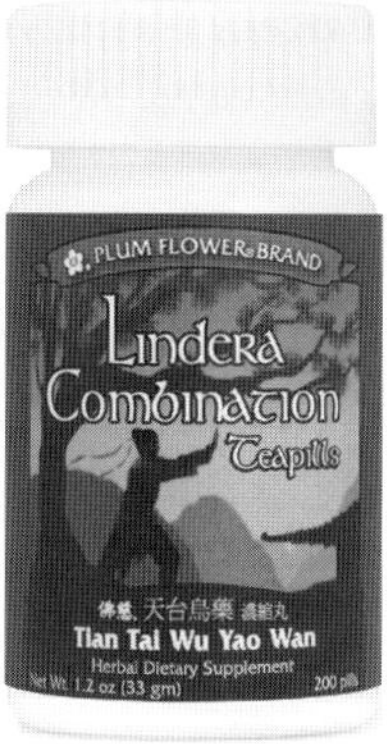

Chinese medical action

Regulates and invigorates Liver qi, warms and dispels cold from the Liver channel, stops pain

Biomedical action

Analgesic, improves circulation

INDICATIONS

- Liver qi constraint and/or cold accumulation in the Liver channel causing pain in the lower abdomen, inguinal region or testicles, with testicular swelling, contracture or cold. When affected, the scrotum is bilaterally or unilaterally swollen and distended, with distension or pain radiating from or to the lower abdomen and/or the lumbar region; the condition is aggravated or initiated by anger, stress and exposure to cold, and is alleviated by relaxation and warmth.
- For dysmenorrhea associated with cold and qi constraint in the Liver channel, and epigastric and abdominal pain from cold and qi stagnation in the Spleen and Intestines.
- With the appropriate identifying features this formula can assist in treatment of conditions such as the discomfort and pain of inguinal hernia, orchitis, epididymitis and dysmenorrhea.

Composition

Lindera strychnifolia (wu yao, lindera), *Foeniculum vulgarae* (xiao hui xiang, fennel seed), *Alpinia officinarum* (gao liang jiang, galangal), *Saussurea lappa* (mu xiang, saussurea), *Citrus reticulata* (qing pi, immature citrus), *Melia toosendan* (chuan lian zi, melia fruit), *Areca catechu* (bing lang, betel nut), *Evodia rutacarpae* (wu zhu yu, evodia)

Combine with

- **11.3 Ji Sheng Ju He Wan** for hard painful swellings of the testicles
- **1.2 Si Wu Wan** or **1.14 Wen Jing Wan** for cold type dysmenorrhea

Dosage and method of administration

8-12 pills three times daily, on an empty stomach or with a warm drink (a little warm red wine or ginger tea is ideal). The dose can be spread out, or taken in two lots of 12-18 pills, morning and evening. In severe cases or during the early stages of treatment (the first few weeks), a 50% increase in dose can be used, then reduced as treatment takes effect.

Pattern identifying features

- **cold and qi constraint in the Liver channel**
- pain aggravated by stress and exposure to cold

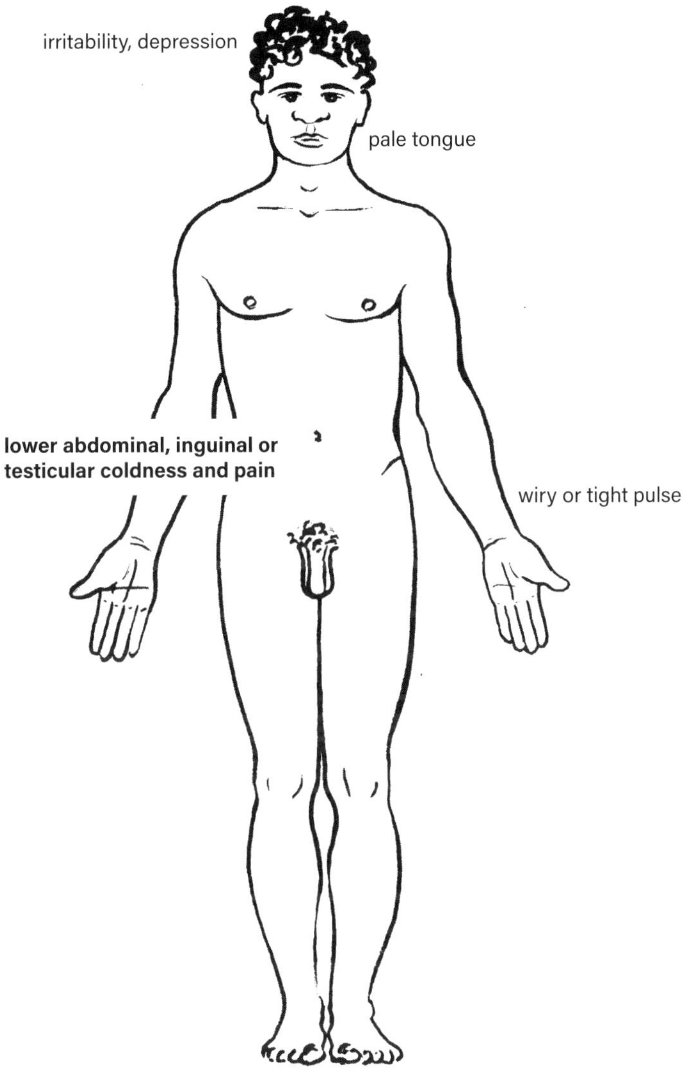

Cautions and contraindications

None noted.

11.5 WU ZI YAN ZONG WAN

五子衍宗丸

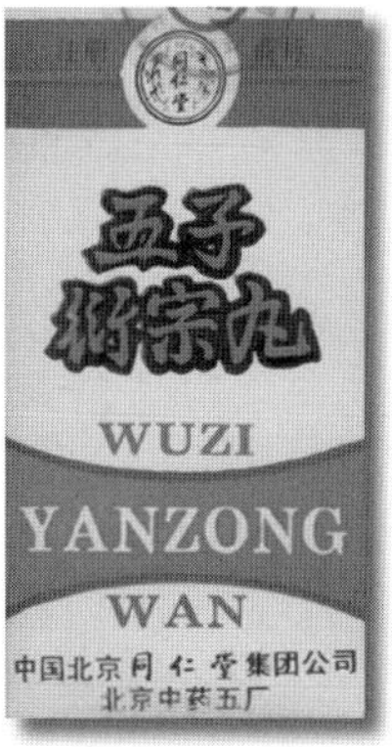

Tong Ren Tang (Beijing)
'Pills of Five Seeds to Bring Forth Offspring'
Wu Zi Yan Zong Wan is packaged in bottles of 600 small pills
Also available as: Five Ancestors Teapills (PF)

Chinese medical action

Strengthens and benefits the Liver and Kidneys, nourishes essence and yin, benefits the eyes

Biomedical action

Improves sperm quality and motility, tonic, may aid in counteracting antisperm antibody formation, antioxidant

INDICATIONS

- Essence deficiency sperm disorders, including motility disorders, oligospermia, poor sperm quality, seminal abnormalities, sperm viscosity and liquefaction disorders. Used as preparation for, and convalescence from, vasectomy reversal to help prevent antibody production.
- Visual disorders, including problems such as floaters, loss of visual acuity and weakening vision associated with Liver or Kidney weakness.
- Used to assist in Kidney deficient conditions such as premature ejaculation, impotence and lower back ache.
- Neutral in temperature and therefore often combined with another formula aimed at correcting the primary constitutional imbalance.

Composition

Lycium chinensis (gou qi zi, lycium), *Cuscuta chinensis* (tu su zi, cuscuta), *Rubus chingii* (fu pen zi, rubus), *Plantago asiatica* (che qian zi, plantago), *Schizandra chinensis* (wu wei zi, schizandra), honey

Combine with

- **7.9 Jin Gui Shen Qi Wan** or **7.10 You Gui Wan** for patients tending to yang deficiency; add **7.11 Deer Velvet** or **7.12 Lu Rong Jiao** for severe cases
- **2.11 Bu Zhong Yi Qi Wan** for patients with qi deficiency
- **1.9 Gui Pi Wan** for patients prone to anxiety and nervousness
- **1.23 Zhi Bai Di Huang Wan**, **7.1.1 Liu Wei Di Huang Wan** or **7.3 Zuo Gui Wan** for patients tending to yin deficiency. These combinations are also used for problems with sperm liquefaction and agglutination
- **7.8 Shou Wu Chih** for blood deficiency
- **1.2 Si Wu Wan** for visual disorders from Liver blood deficiency
- **7.2.2 Qi Ju Di Huang Wan** or **9.23 Ming Mu Capsule** for visual disorders from Liver yin deficiency

Pattern identifying features

- **Liver and Kidney deficiency, insufficient essence**

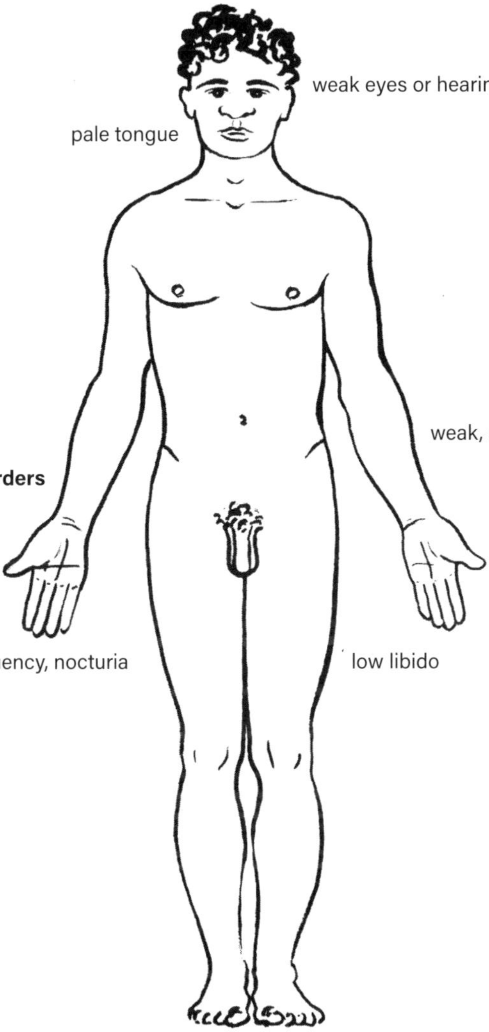

Dosage and method of administration

The recommended dose is rather large at 30-40 (very small) pills three times daily before meals. The pills may be soaked in boiling water first, but are best just eaten by the handful. For practical purposes, one jar should be consumed every 4-5 days.

Cautions and contraindications

Contraindicated during the early phase of acute illness such as colds and flu, and in patients with sperm disorders associated with lingering damp heat (*see* **11.1 Qian Lie Xian Capsule** or **1.37 Bi Xie Sheng Shi Wan**).

11.6 GU BEN FU ZHENG CAPSULE

TGA

3+/12

固本扶正丹

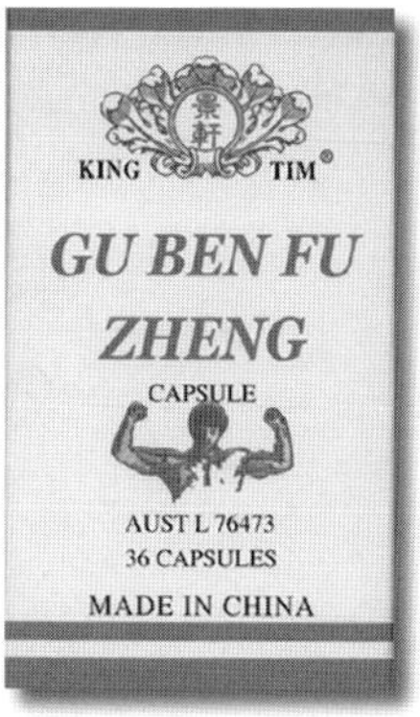

(*Gu Ben Fu Zheng Dan*)
'Secure the Root and Support Normal [Qi] Special Pill'
Gu Ben Fu Zheng Capsule is packaged in bottles of 36 capsules

Chinese medical action

Strengthens and warms Kidney yang, nourishes blood, tonifies qi

Biomedical action

Stimulant, tonic, adaptogen, warms the body and stimulates libido

INDICATIONS

- Erectile dysfunction, impotence, loss of libido, premature ejaculation, infertility associated with poor sperm motility from Kidney yang deficiency. This formula is quite warming and stimulating, and so is also good for the general lack of yang motivation typical of yang deficiency and cold accumulation, such as is found in elderly patients.
- Lack of energy, vitality and motivation; tendency to sleep too much or desire to sleep too much, cold intolerance, patient feels cold to the touch, urinary frequency or nocturia, lower back ache.
- Warms yang and augments essence to treat male infertility and sperm disorders, such as low sperm count and poor sperm motility.

Composition (each capsule contains extracts equivalent to dry)

Epimedium brevicornu (xian ling pi, epimedium) 455mg, *Angelica polymorpha* (dang gui, chinese angelica) 455mg, *Curculigo orchioides* (xian mao, curculigo) 364mg, *Allium odorum* (jiu zi, chinese chive seed) 364mg, *Paeonia lactiflora* (bai shao, white peony) 364mg, *Panax ginseng* (ren shen, ginseng) 364mg, *Psoralea corylifolia* (bu gu zhi, psoralea) 364mg, *Eucommia ulmoides* (du zhong, eucommia) 364mg, *Cynomorium songaricum* (suo yang, cynomorium) 364mg, *Lycium barbarum* (gou qi zi, lycium fruit) 364mg, *Morinda officinalis* (ba ji tian, morinda) 364mg, *Glycyrrhiza uralensis* (gan cao, licorice) 364mg

Combine with

– **4.14 Chin So Ku Ching Wan** for nocturia or urinary frequency
– **11.5 Wu Zi Yan Zong Wan** for sperm disorders from Kidney yang deficiency

Pattern identifying features
- **Kidney yang deficiency**
- erectile dysfunction, loss of libido
- lethargy, lack of vitality

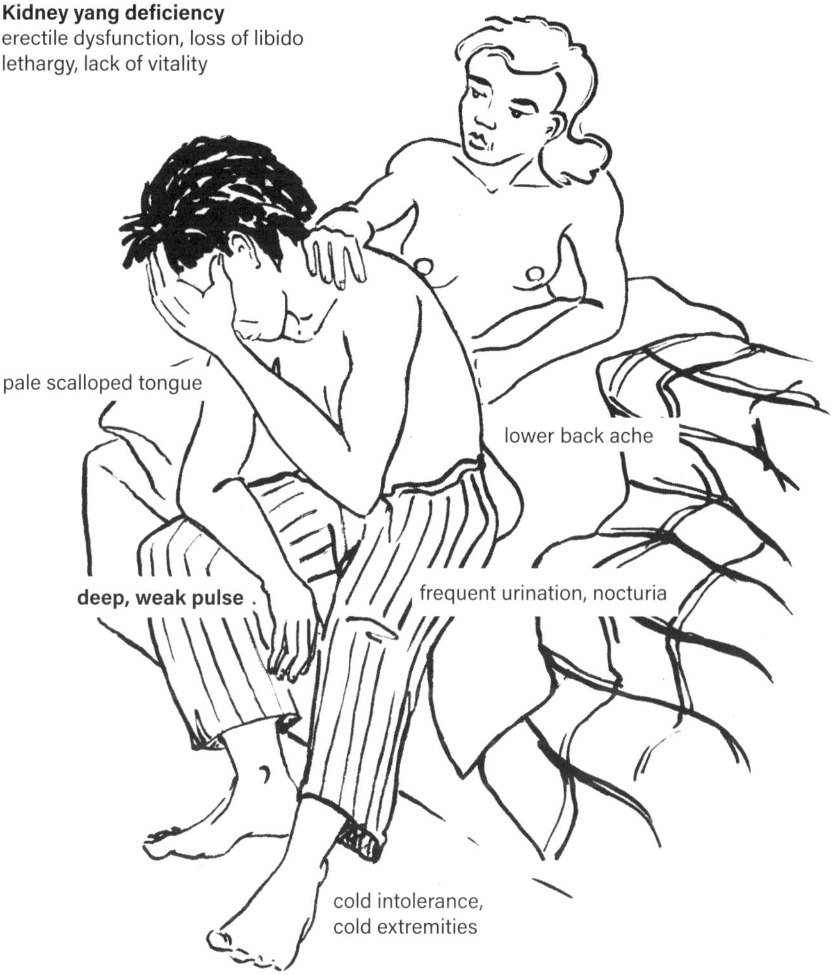

Dosage and method of administration
3-4 capsules, three times daily, on an empty stomach.

Cautions and contraindications
Contraindicated during the early phase of acute illness such as colds and flu, and in yin deficiency or internal excess heat patterns.

11.7 NAN BAO CAPSULES

男宝

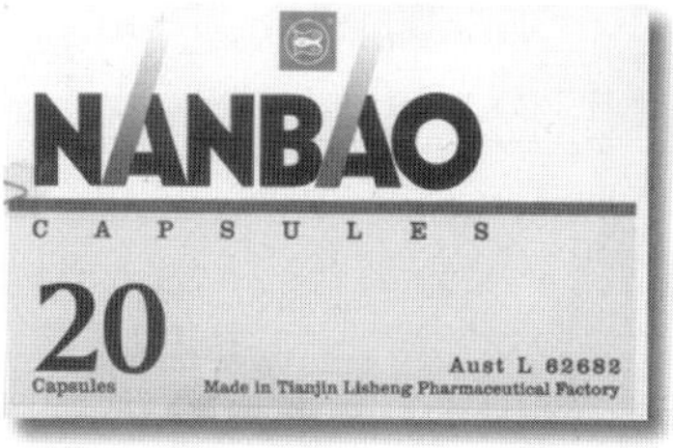

(*Nan Bao*)
Tianjin Lisheng Pharmaceutical Factory (Shandong)
'Male Treasure'
Nan Bao Capsules are packaged on blister sheets of ten capsules, two sheets per box

Chinese medical action

Strengthens and tones the Kidneys, warms and supports yang

Biomedical action

Stimulant, tonic, adaptogen, warms the body and stimulates the libido

INDICATIONS

- Sexual dysfunction, impotence, loss of libido, premature ejaculation from Kidney yang qi deficiency. A general and broad acting formula with almost every yang warming and tonic herb in the materia medica, at quite low doses.
- Kidney yang weakness patterns with lack of vitality and drive, fatigue, lower back ache, weakness in the legs, fearfulness and timidity and cold intolerance.

Composition (each capsule contains)

Panax ginseng (ren shen, ginseng) 33.25mg, *Angelica sinensis* (dang gui, chinese angelica) 33.25mg, *Astragalus membranaceous* (huang qi, astragalus) 33.25mg, *Rehmannia glutinosa* (shu di, processed rehmannia) 33.25mg, *Epimedium brevicornu* (xian ling pi, epimedium) 33.25mg, *Lycium barbarum* (gou qi zi, lycium fruit) 33.25mg, *Poria cocos* (fu ling, hoelen) 33.25mg, *Eucommia ulmoides* (du zhong, eucommia) 16.75mg, *Psoralea corylifolia* (bu gu zhi, psoralea) 16.75mg, *Morinda officinalis* (ba ji tian, morinda) 16.75mg, *Cistanches deserticola* (rou cong rong, cistanches) 16.75mg, *Cuscuta chinensis* (tu su zi, cuscuta) 16.75mg, *Cornus officinalis* (shan zhu yu, cornus) 16.75mg, *Atractylodes macrocephala* (bai zhu, atractylodes) 16.75mg, *Rubus chingii* (fu pen zi, rubus) 16.75mg, *Trigonella foenum-graecum* (hu lu ba, fenugreek seed) 16.75mg, *Ophiopogon japonicum* (mai dong, ophiopogon) 16.75mg, *Cynomorium songaricum* (suo yang, cynomorium) 16.75mg, *Scrophularia ningpoensis* (xuan shen, scrophularia) 16.75mg, *Cinnamomum cassia* (rou gui, cinnamon bark) 13.25mg, *Paeonia suffruticosa* (mu dan pi, peony root bark) 8.25mg, *Dipsacus asper* (xu duan, dipsacus) 8.25mg, *Achyranthes bidentata* (huai niu xi, achyranthes) 8.25mg

Combine with

- **7.9 Jin Gui Shen Qi Wan** or **7.10 You Gui Wan** for patients tending to yang deficiency; add **7.12 Lu Rong Jiao** for severe cases
- **2.11 Bu Zhong Yi Qi Wan** or **7.22 Shen Qi Da Bu Wan** for severe qi deficiency
- **1.9 Gui Pi Wan** for those with Spleen and Heart deficiency and a tendency to anxiety and nervousness

Pattern identifying features

- **Kidney yang qi deficiency**
- inability to maintain an erection
- low libido
- premature ejaculation
- fatigue, lack of vitality
- cold intolerance

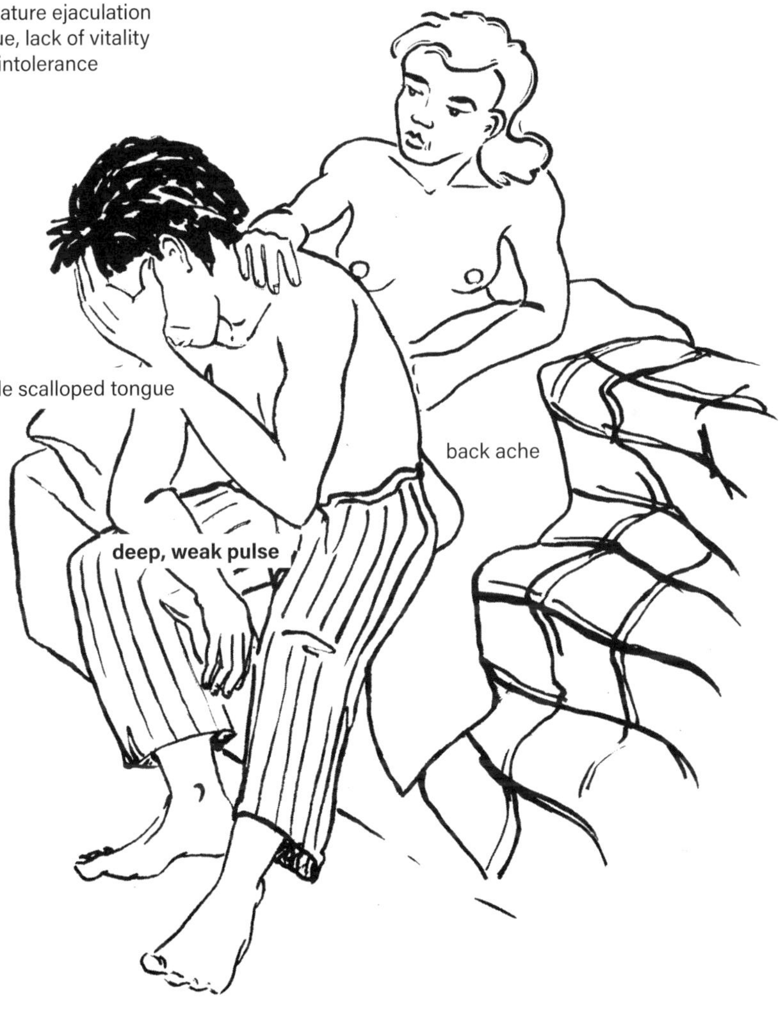

Dosage and method of administration

2 capsules twice daily, on an empty stomach.

Cautions and contraindications

Contraindicated during the early phase of acute illness such as colds and flu.

11.8 KANG WEI LING WAN

亢痿灵

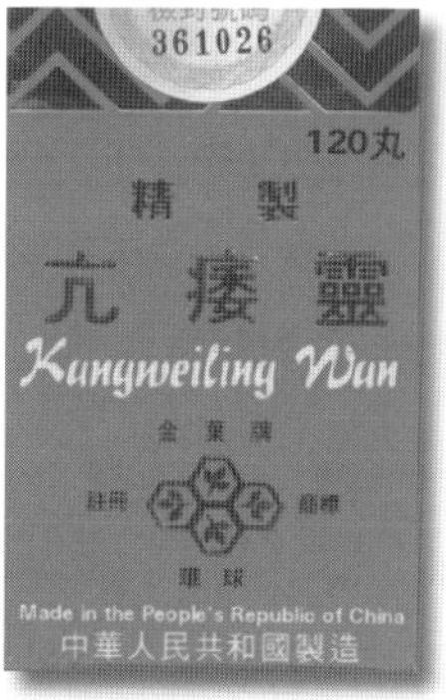

Kuan Chiu Medical Company (Hong Kong)
'Marvellous Pills to Combat Impotence'
Kang Wei Ling Wan is packaged in bottles of 120 pills

Chinese medical action

Regulates blood and disperses static blood to open up circulation through the channels to nourish and revitalize the sinews, in particular the ancestral sinew of the Liver, tonifies qi, blood and yang

Biomedical action

Improves circulation, hematinic, stimulant

INDICATIONS

- Erectile dysfunction from blood stasis, with a degree of yang and blood deficiency. This formula contains a powerful blood invigorating substance and works by improving the circulation to the penis, while at the same time strengthening yang. Useful in impotence associated with reduced blood circulation to the penis, chronic prostatitis or other genital blood stasis syndromes.
- The main ingredient, scolopendra centipede, is a strong substance used to 'burrow' through obstruction and extinguish wind, so this formula can be useful as an adjunct treatment for facial paralysis or Bell's palsy, hemiplegia, facial pain and neuralgia, severe chronic migraines or trigeminal neuralgia.

Composition

Paeonia alba (bai shao, white peony) 30%, *Cervus nippon* (lu jiao, deer antler cartilage) 16%, *Panax ginseng* (ren shen, ginseng) 15%, *Angelica sinensis* (dang gui) 15%, *Scolopendra subspinipes* (wu gong, centipede) 12%, *Glycyrrhiza uralensis* (gan cao, licorice) 12%

Combine with

- **7.9 Jin Gui Shen Qi Wan** or **7.10 You Gui Wan** for patients tending to yang deficiency
- **5.1 Xue Fu Zhu Yu Wan** for patients with systemic signs of qi and blood stasis
- **6.4 Xiao Yao Wan** or **6.5 Jia Wei Xiao Yao Wan** for stressed patients with performance anxiety
- **3.9 Chuan Xiong Cha Tiao Wan** for marked migraine headache associated with exposure to cold
- **5.8 Bu Yang Huan Wu Wan** for chronic facial paralysis

Pattern identifying features

- **blood stasis** with qi, blood and yang deficiency
- **inability to achieve or maintain erection; no nocturnal erection**

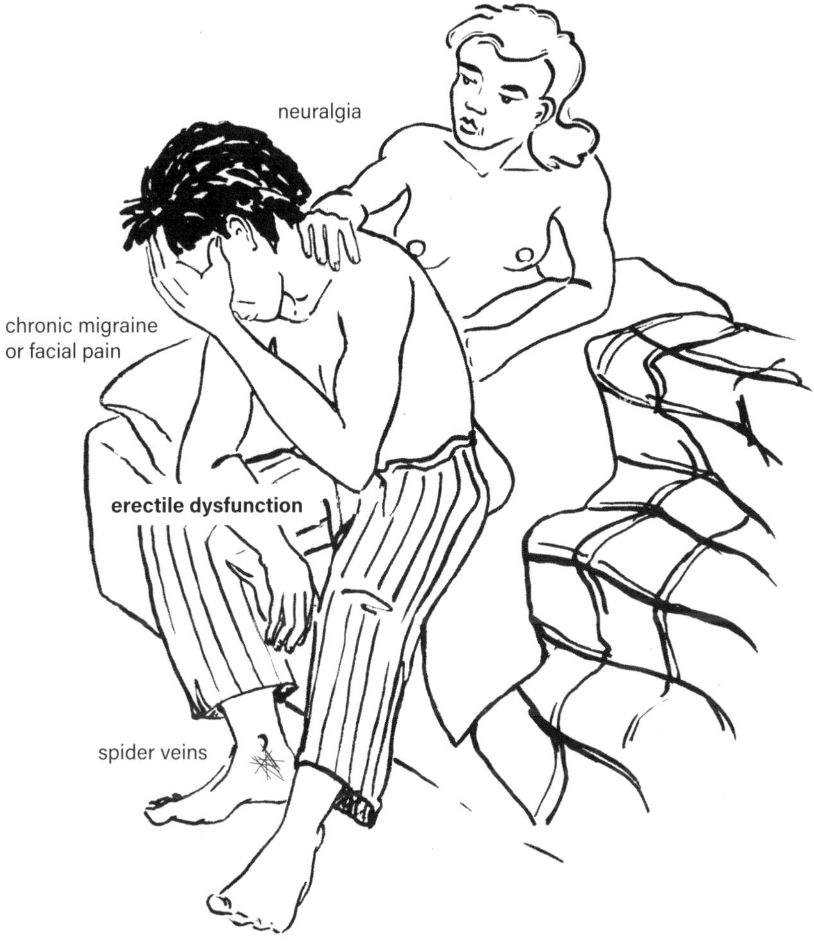

Dosage and method of administration

The recommended dose is 10-15 pills twice daily for fifteen to thirty days, ideally with a small shot of vodka or sherry to open the vessels and promote circulation. Usually given in two courses of 15 days each, with a break of a few days in between courses.

Cautions and contraindications

Contraindicated during pregnancy. Not suitable for prolonged use, usually no more than 2-3 courses.

小儿科 12

Children

See also

2.1 Xing Jun San
2.12 Shen Ling Bai Zhu Wan
2.15 Xiao Jian Zhong Wan
4.15 Sang Piao Xiao Wan

GMP

12.1 BO YING COMPOUND

保婴丹

1-3/12

(*Bao Ying Dan*)
Eu Yan Sang (Hong Kong)
'Protect Children Special Pills'
Bo Ying Compound is packaged as a fine powder in small vials of 0.33g powder, six vials to a box

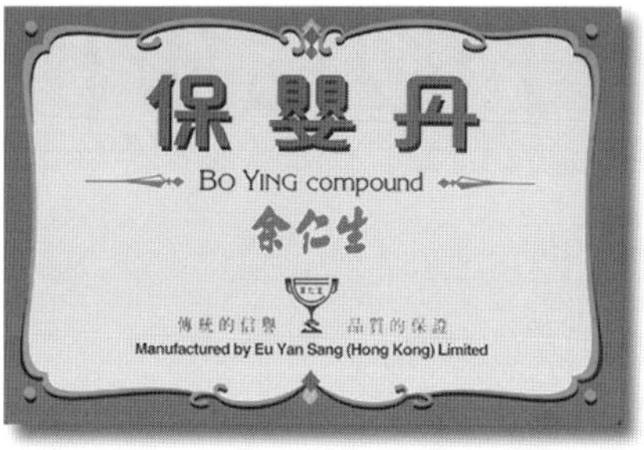

Chinese medical action

Strengthens the Spleen, transforms phlegm, extinguishes wind, clears heat

Biomedical action

Strengthens digestion and immunity, mucolytic

INDICATIONS

- Accumulation disorder (*see* glossary). A popular formula for childhood fever and restlessness, mucus congestion and digestive problems from accumulation. Only used for children up to 5 years old.
- For children with a tendency to mucus production, digestive weakness and poor appetite. This includes so called 'colicky babies', problems such as 'glue ear', chronic productive cough, tummy ache, tendency to reflux, vomiting or diarrhea, constant dribbling in toddlers, chronic or recurrent tonsillitis, and children prone to frequent colds or other upper respiratory tract or ear infections.
- Skin disease associated with accumulation disorder, such as childhood eczema, dermatitis and nappy (diaper) rash.
- Useful for dispelling lingering pathogens introduced by vaccination, causing chronic swollen tonsils, low grade fever, swelling at the site of the vaccination, and general malaise persisting some weeks after vaccination.

Composition

Bambusa textillis (tian zhu huang, bamboo sap) 7%, *Bombyx mori* (jiang can, silkworm) 8%, Borax (peng sha) 4%, Bovine gallstone (niu huang) 3%, Borneol (bing pian) 4%, *Cryptotympana atrata* (chan tui, cicada shell) 7%, *Fritillaria cirrhosa* (chuan bei mu, fritillaria) 7%, Mica (meng shi) 5%, *Uncaria rhynchophylla* (gou teng, gambir) 8%, Pearl (zhen zhu) 4%, *Mentha haplocalycis* (bo he, mint) 6%, *Curcuma longa* (yu jin, curcuma) 3%, *Gastrodia elata* (tian ma, gastrodia) 4%, *Buthus martensi* (quan xie, scorpion) 8%, *Siler divaricum* (fang feng, siler) 8%, Amber (hu po) 3%, *Zingiber officinale* (sheng jiang, ginger) 2%

Dosage and method of administration

In the early stages of treatment ¼-1 vial can be given daily mixed in with food such as apple sauce, or a fluid until the appetite improves or the mucus starts to clear. The dose is then tapered off over a couple of weeks to a maintenance dose. Very mucus prone children may need longer treatment (up to three months).

Pattern identifying features

- **accumulation disorder, food stagnation**
- **poor appetite, picky eater**
- **tendency to mucus production,** constantly runny or snotty nose, post nasal drip
- irritability, bad temper
- generally robust, cries loudly and with vigor
- insomnia and restlessness, heat and sweating at night
- eczema along Stomach channel
- chronic, swollen, pea like lymph nodes
- sweet cravings
- fevers
- snoring

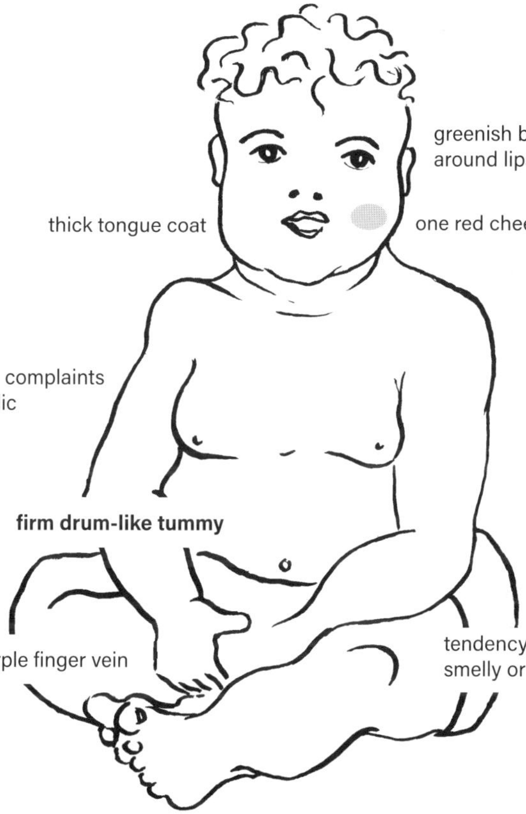

Maintenance dose

- Infants to one month ....½-1 vial per week dissolved in hot water and administered by an eye-dropper or a warm bottle of liquid
- 1 month to 2 years ....1-2 vials per week
- 2-5 years...........................2-3 vials per week

Cautions and contraindications

While dispensing this formula, parents or carers should eliminate or minimize mucus producing foods from the child's diet. These include raw or greasy foods, peanut butter, excess sugar and dairy products. Avoid overfeeding the child. **12.1 Bo Ying Compound** is a reliable formula with a long history of safe usage, suitable for prolonged use in children with a constitutional tendency to mucus production.

12.2 KING FUNG POWDER

惊风散

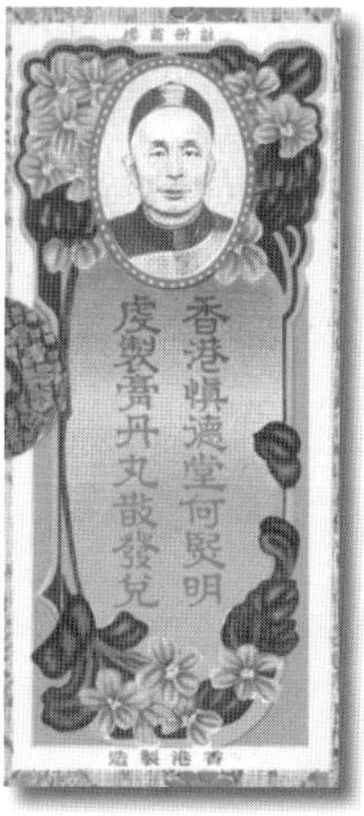

(*Jing Feng San*)
Ho Hei Ming Pharmaceutical Company (Hong Kong)
'Convulsion Powder'
King Fung Powder is packaged as a fine powder in small plastic jars, ten jars to a box

Chinese medical action

Dispels and extinguishes wind, stops spasms, clears heat, transforms phlegm

Biomedical action

Antipyretic, febrifuge, antispasmodic, mucolytic

INDICATIONS

- Childhood fevers from heat or phlegm heat. The fever may be moderate or high, associated with common childhood infections such as upper respiratory tract infection (with yellow sputum) and cystitis, or may have no obvious cause. Also used for febrile convulsions or mild seizures associated with phlegm heat.
- Red, itchy skin diseases, such as eczema and dermatitis in infants.
- Restlessness, difficulty settling babies at night (night crying), easy fright and frequent waking associated with accumulation of heat and phlegm.
- For children with a tendency to poor appetite, chronic productive cough, tummy ache, tendency to vomiting, diarrhea or constipation, reflux, colic, mucus production and digestive weakness associated with accumulation disorder (*see* glossary).

Composition

Tribulus terrestris (bai ji li, tribulus) 15%, *Cryptotympana atrata* (chan tui, cicada shell) 15%, *Bambusa textillis* (tian zhu huang, bamboo sap) 15%, *Buthus martensi* (quan xie, scorpion) 15%, *Bombyx mori* (jiang can, silkworm) 15%, *Uncaria rhynchophylla* (gou teng, gambir) 10%, *Glycyrrhiza uralensis* (gan cao, licorice) 5%, Borneol (bing pian) 4%, *Fritillaria cirrhosa* (chuan bei mu, fritillaria) 3%, *Trichosanthes kirilowii* (tian hua fen, trichosanthes root) 3%

Dosage and method of administration

- Infants to 1 year ..... 1 jar per day in small doses (about every 4 hours) dissolved in warm water and administered by an eye-dropper or bottle
- 1-3 years................. 1 jar three times daily, with water, breast milk or apple sauce
- 3-6 years................. 2 jars three times daily, with water or apple sauce

Pattern identifying features

- **phlegm, phlegm heat**
- **fevers, convulsions**
- accumulation disorder with heat
- restlessness, night crying
- easy fright, nightmares, night terrors

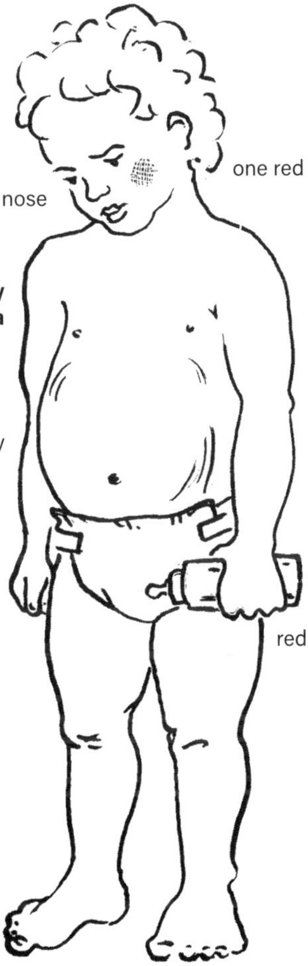

Cautions and contraindications

While dispensing this formula, parents or carers should eliminate or minimize mucus producing foods from the child's diet. These include raw or greasy foods, peanut butter, excess sugar and dairy products. Avoid overfeeding the child.

1-3/52

12.3 BABY FAT POWDER

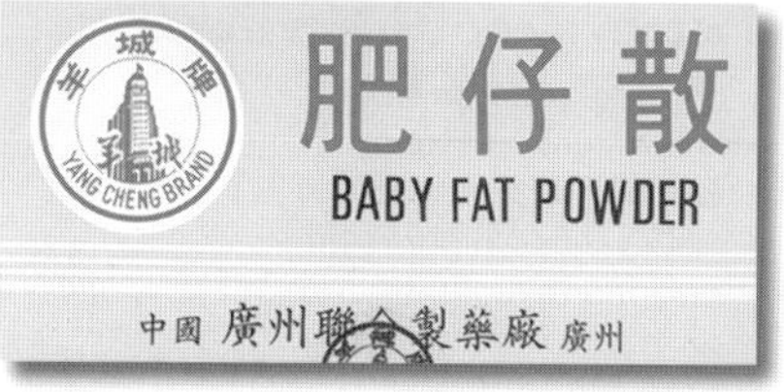

肥仔散

(*Fei Zi San*)
United Pharmaceutical Manufactory (Guangzhou)
'Fat Baby Powder'
Baby Fat Powder is packaged as a fine powder in plastic vials, six vials to a box

Chinese medical action

Kills intestinal parasites

Biomedical action

Broad spectrum antihelminthic

INDICATIONS

- Intestinal parasites, such as thread worm, tapeworm and roundworm. A broad spectrum antiparasitic agent, which can assist in conditions such as *gu* syndrome (*see* glossary) in combination with appropriate constitutional formulas. The name of this formula derives from the fact that children with parasites are likely to be thin or emaciated, thus its use will 'fatten up the baby'.

Composition

Quisqualis indica (shi jun zi, rangoon creeper fruit) 14.8%, *Areca catechu* (bing lang, betel nut) 14.8%, *Osmunda japonica* (guan zhong) 13.4%, *Poria cocos* (fu ling, hoelen) 9%, *Pharbitis nil* (qian niu zi, morning glory seed) 9%, *Glycyrrhiza uralensis* (gan cao, licorice) 7.5%, *Omphalia lapidescens* (lei wan, omphalia puffball) 7.5%, *Punica granatum* (shi liu pi, pomegranate skin) 6%, *Dioscorea opposita* (shan yao, dioscorea) 6%, *Saussurea lappa* (mu xiang, saussurea) 6%, *Stemona sessilifolia* (bai bu, stemona) 6%

Dosage and method of administration

3 months–2 years old .... ¼ jar twice daily
3–5 years old .... ½ jar twice daily
6–10 years old .... 1 jar twice daily
10–14 years old .... 1-3 jars twice daily
Adults...................................... 4 jars daily

Pattern identifying features

- **intestinal parasites**
- loss of appetite or ravenous appetite, eating unusual things (dirt, sand etc.), craving for unusual foods
- restless sleep, easy fright
- fatigue, malaise, restlessness
- dull, lifeless hair
- dark rings under the eyes

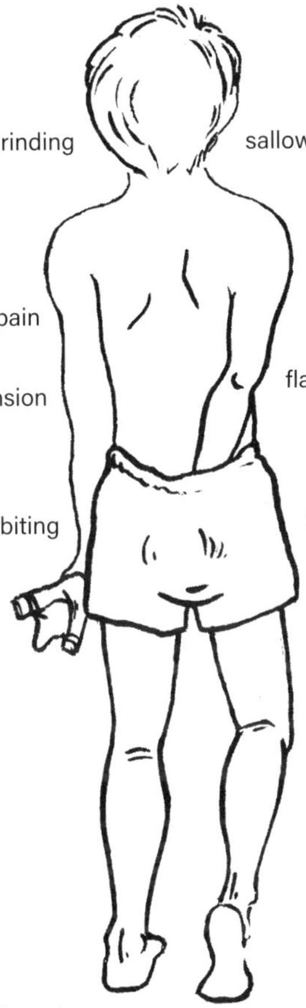

Cautions and contraindications

None noted. Generally only used for short periods of time (~2 weeks), then followed by a formula to strengthen the digestive system, such as **2.9 Xiang Sha Liu Jun Wan** for older children or adults, or **12.6 Healthy Child Tea** for children under three years old.

12.4 HUA JI XIAO ZHI ORAL LIQUID

TGA

1-3/52

小儿化积消滞口服液

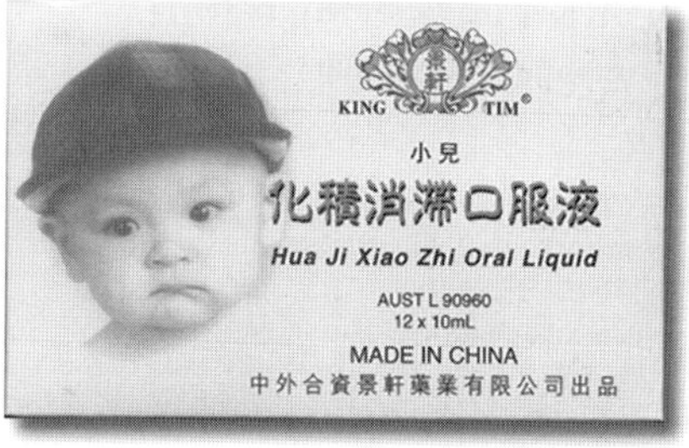

(*Xiao Er Hua Ji Xiao Zhi Kou Fu Ye*)
Jing Xian Pharmaceutical Co. (Guangzhou)
'Children's Digestive Accumulation Drink'
Hua Ji Xiao Zhi Oral Liquid is packaged in vials of 10ml, 10 vials per box

Chinese medical action

Strengthens the Spleen and harmonizes the Stomach, kills intestinal parasites

Biomedical action

Antihelminthic, strengthens digestion

INDICATIONS

- Childhood accumulation disorder, indigestion and gastrointestinal weakness associated with parasitic infestation by thread worm, tapeworm or roundworm. Similar to **12.3 Baby Fat Powder**, with a larger proportion of the Spleen strengthening hoelen, this formula is more strengthening to the digestion, with fewer antiparasitic herbs. The indications are much the same, although milder.

Composition (each 10ml dose contains extracts equivalent to dry)

Poria cocos (fu ling, hoelen) 2.33g, *Crategus pinnatifida* (shan zha, crategus) 830mg, *Carthamus tinctorius* (hong hua, carthamus) 632mg, *Carpesium abrotanoides* (he shi, carpesium fruit) 500mg, *Quisqualis indica* (shi jun zi, rangoon creeper fruit) 500mg, *Areca catechu* (bing lang, betel nut) 500mg, *Sparganium stoloniferum* (san leng, sparganium) 500mg, *Omphalia lapidescens* (lei wan, omphalia puffball) 500mg, *Raphanus sativus* (lai fu zi, radish seed) 500mg

Dosage and method of administration

Infants to 2 years.......5ml, twice daily
2-5 years....................10ml, twice daily
5 years + ...10ml three times daily

Cautions and contraindications

None noted.

12.5 GAN MAO TEA

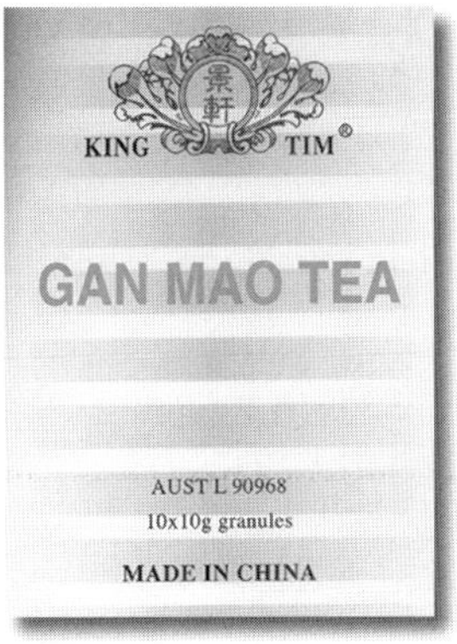

小儿感冒退热冲剂

(*Xiao Er Gan Mao Liang Re Chong Ji*)
Jing Xian Pharmaceutical Co. (Guangzhou)
'Children's Cold and Fever Relieving Soluble Granules'
Gan Mao Tea is packaged in 10 gram sachets of granules, ten sachets per box

Chinese medical action
Dispels wind heat, stops cough, supports yin

Biomedical action
Antipyretic, diaphoretic, antiviral

INDICATIONS

- Wind heat common cold and upper respiratory tract infections with fever, sore throat, headache, stomach upset, nausea, vomiting and productive cough with yellow sputum. Similar in composition and action to **12.7 Xiao Er Gan Mao Chong Ji**.

Composition (each sachet contains extracts equivalent to dry)
Platycodon grandiflorum (jie geng, platycodon) 1.25g, *Morus alba* (sang ye, mulberry leaf) 1.25g, *Agastache rugosa* (huo xiang, agastache) 752mg, *Chrysanthemum sinense* (ju hua, chrysanthemum flower) 752mg, *Forsythia suspensa* (lian qiao, forsythia) 752mg, *Rehmannia glutinosa* (sheng di, raw rehmannia) 752mg, *Lycium chinensis* (di gu pi, lycium root bark) 752mg, *Scutellaria baicalensis* (huang qin, scute) 752mg, *Cynanchum atratum* (bai wei, cynanchum) 752mg, *Mentha haplocalycis* (bo he, mint) 504mg

Dosage and method of administration
Dissolve the granules in a little hot water. For infants, the resulting warm liquid can be delivered by eye-dropper.
1-2 years....................¼-½ sachet twice daily
2-3 years....................½-1 sachet twice daily
4-7 years....................1 sachet 2-3 times daily

Cautions and contraindications
None noted.

12.6 HEALTHY CHILD TEA

肥仔散*

3+ 12

(*Fei Zi San*)
Jing Xian Pharmaceutical Co. (Guangzhou)
'Fat Baby Powder'
*Note: The Chinese name of this formula is the same as that of **12.3 Baby Fat Powder**, however their composition and mode of action are quite different
Healthy Child Tea is packaged in 10 gram sachets of soluble granules, ten sachets per box

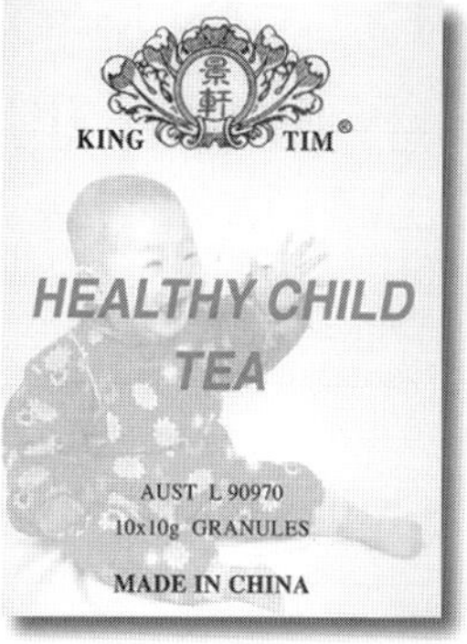

Chinese medical action

Strengthens the Spleen and Stomach, tonifies qi, improves digestion

Biomedical action

Digestive stimulant

INDICATIONS

- Digestive weakness and indigestion from Spleen and Stomach qi deficiency. In contrast to the pathology treated by **12.1 Bo Ying Compound** and **12.8 Qi Xing Tea**, where a robust child suffers from food accumulation from overfeeding or inappropriate feeding, the main problem here is the underlying weakness of the Spleen and Stomach which fail to process food and extract sufficient nutrition from it. Children with digestive weakness of this type lack the vitality of childhood, tend to be thin, picky eaters or lacking in appetite, look pale and wan, and lack the sparkle of *shén* in their eyes.
- Constitutionally weak children and premature babies who fail to thrive.
- To rebuild a child's Spleen qi following a protracted or severe illness.

Composition (each sachet contains extracts equivalent to dry)

Coicis lachryma-jobi (yi yi ren, coix) 1.5g, *Paeonia lactiflora* (bai shao, white peony) 1.5g, *Nelumbus speciosum* (lian zi, lotus seed) 1.5g, *Hordeum vulgare* (mai ya, sprouted barley) 1.5g, *Prunus mume* (wu mei, black plum) 1.5g, *Poria cocos* (fu ling, hoelen) 1.5g, *Dioscorea opposita* (shan yao, dioscorea) 1.25g, *Atractylodes macrocephala* (bai zhu, atractylodes) 1.25g, *Pseudostellaria heterophylla* (tai zi shen, pseudostellaria) 1g

Combine with

– Nutritious rice porridge for children with very weak digestions
– **3.41 Xu Han Ting** for spontaneous sweating and weakened immunity

Pattern identifying features

- **Spleen and Stomach qi deficiency**
- weak, thin child
- listlessness, lack of vitality
- lack of hair and nail growth
- spontaneous sweating, night sweats
- restless sleep
- teeth grinding
- poor appetite, picky eater
- tends to be clingy and shy

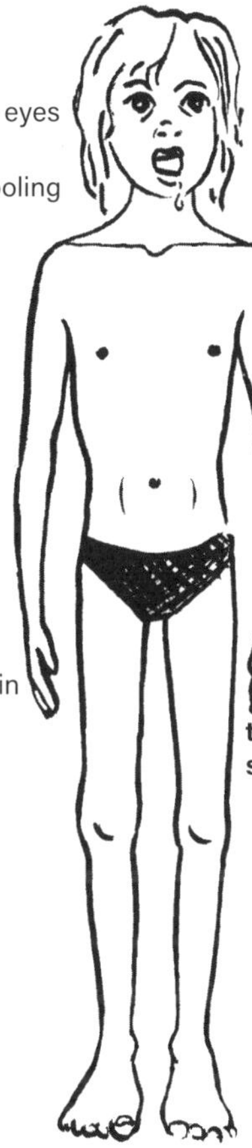

Dosage and method of administration

Dissolve the granules in a little hot water. For infants, the resulting warm liquid can be delivered by eye-dropper

1-2 years....................¼-½ sachet twice daily
2-3 years....................½-1 sachet twice daily
4-7 years....................1 sachet 2-3 times daily

Cautions and contraindications

None noted. In addition to any herbal therapy, an appropriate diet is essential for success, in particular avoidance of raw whole foods, juices, sweets and dairy products.

12.7 XIAO ER GAN MAO CHONG JI

小儿感冒冲剂

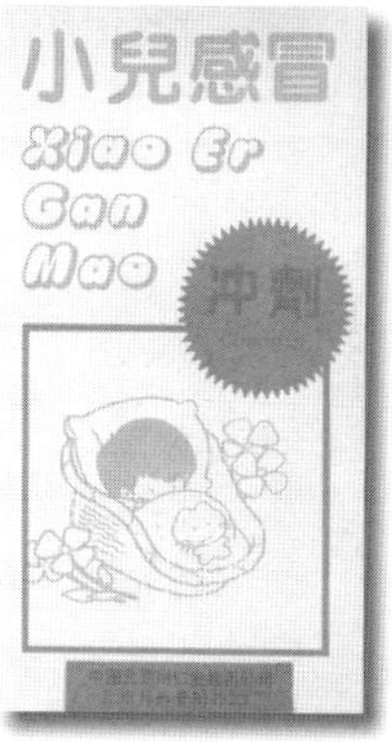

Tong Ren Tang (Beijing)
'Children's Common Cold Soluble Granules'
Xiao Er Gan Mao Chong Ji is packaged as soluble granules in single dose sachets of 12 grams, ten sachets per box

Chinese medical action

Dispels wind heat, clears toxic heat, benefits the throat

Biomedical action

Antipyretic, diaphoretic, anti-inflammatory, antiviral

INDICATIONS

- Wind heat common cold with fever, sore throat, and cough. Used for colds, influenza, tonsillitis and early stage of upper respiratory tract infection in children. Especially good for sore throat.
- Wind or toxic heat patterns affecting the ears and eyes of small children, causing disorders such as otitis media and conjunctivitis.
- For acute inflammatory rashes and eczema in small children, including impetigo and hand, foot and mouth disease.

Composition (each sachet contains extracts equivalent to dry)

Isatis tinctoria (da qing ye, isatis leaf) 1.6g, *Rehmannia glutinosa* (sheng di, raw rehmannia) 986mg, *Cynanchum atratum* (bai wei, cynanchum) 986mg, *Lycium chinensis* (di gu pi, lycium root bark) 986mg, *Chrysanthemum chinensis* (ju hua, chrysanthemum flower) 986mg, *Isatis tinctoria* (ban lan gen, isatis root) 986mg, *Forsythia suspensa* (lian qiao, forsythia essential oil) 4.4mg, *Pogostemon cablin* (huo xiang, agastache essential oil) 2.95mg, *Mentha haplocalycis* (bo he, mint essential oil) 2.63mg, sugar 5.3g

Combine with

- **9.10 Sanjin Watermelon Frost** for mouth ulcers or gum inflammation
- **9.9 Superior Sore Throat Powder** for acute tonsillitis and otitis
- pear juice for cough

Dosage and method of administration

Dissolve the granules in a little hot water. Allow to cool before use. For small children, the resulting liquid can be delivered by eye-dropper.

1-2 years....................½ sachet 2-3 times daily
2-3 years....................1-1½ sachets 2-3 times daily
4-7 years....................1-1½ sachets every 2-4 hours
7-10 years..................2 sachets every 2-4 hours

Pattern identifying features

- **wind heat common cold**
- **acute colds and flu**
- early upper respiratory tract infection
- fever

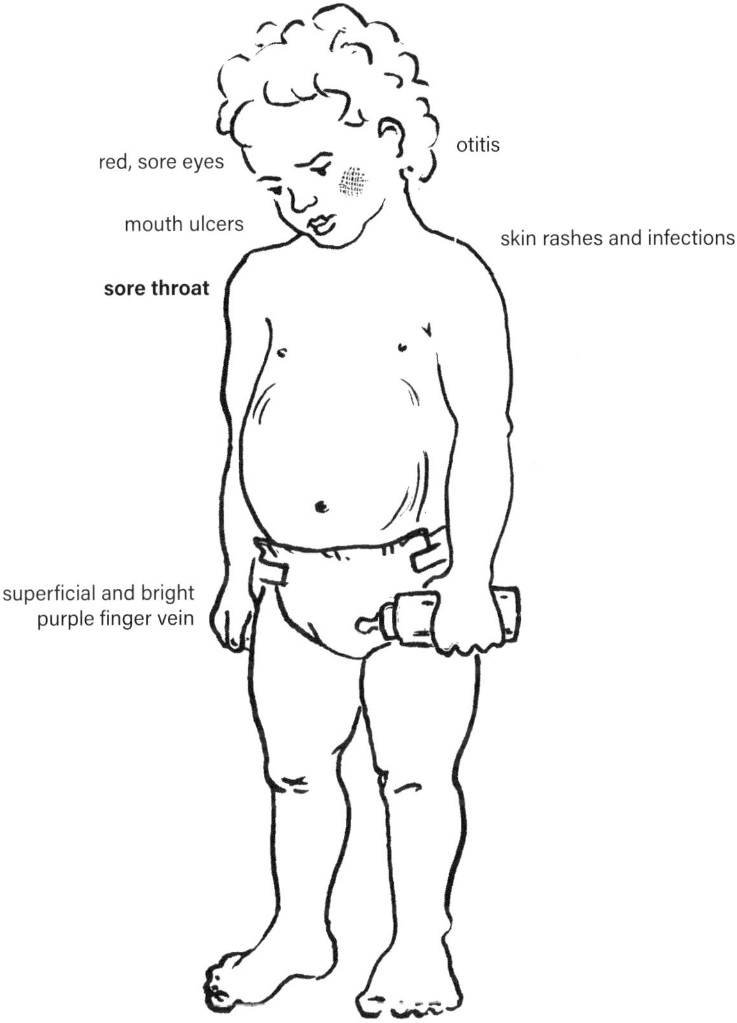

Cautions and contraindications

None noted.

12.8 QI XING TEA

七星茶

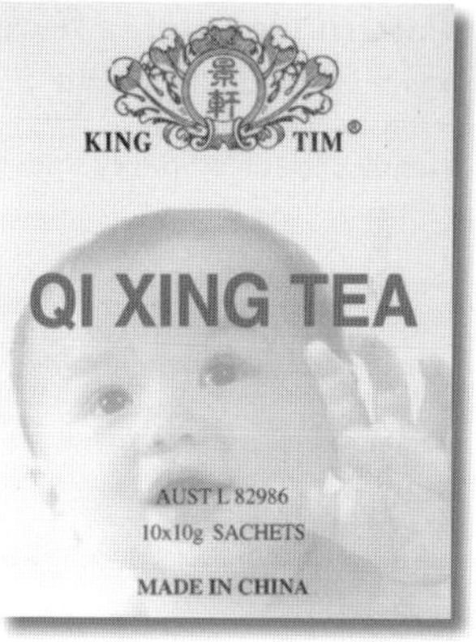

(*Qi Xing Cha*)
Jing Xian Pharmaceutical Co. (Guangzhou)
'Seven Star Tea'
Qi Xing Tea is packaged in 10 gram sachets of soluble granules, ten sachets per box

Chinese medical action

Alleviates food stagnation, strengthens the Spleen, clears heat and damp heat, extinguishes internal wind and calms the *shén*

Biomedical action

Digestive, tonic, calmative

INDICATIONS

- Indigestion, poor feeding, colic and accumulation disorder in babies and small children. In contrast to **12.1 Bo Ying Compound**, used for accumulation disorder causing phlegm buildup, this formula is for accumulation disorder leading to heat. The main focus of the formula is in clearing out accumulation in the digestive system. Can be used for infants having difficulty digesting milk, or suffering repeated reflux.
- Restlessness, insomnia, gum pain and diaper rash associated with teething.
- Urinary tract infection, mouth ulcers or other infection from heat or Heart fire; acute gastroenteritis.
- General restlessness, night crying, insomnia or restless sleep, fearfulness and irritability associated with heat or accumulation disorder. In some cases there may be mild convulsions, muscular spasms or seizures.
- Useful for acute rashes and eczema in small children, especially those associated with food intolerance, poor diet or overeating.

Composition (each sachet contains extracts equivalent to dry)

Crategus pinnatifida (shan zha, crategus) 5.4g, *Uncaria rhynchophylla* (gou teng, gambir) 5.4g, *Setaria italica* (gu ya, sprouted rice) 4.8g, *Hordeum vulgare* (mai ya, sprouted barley) 4.8g, *Lophatherum elatum* (dan zhu ye, bamboo leaves) 3.2g, *Coicis lachryma-jobi* (yi yi ren, coix) 3.2g, *Juncus effusus* (deng xin cao, juncus) 3.2g, *Glycyrrhiza uralensis* (gan cao, licorice) 1.9g, sucrose

Combine with

– **9.10 Sanjin Watermelon Frost** for mouth ulcers, teething or gum pain and inflammation

Pattern identifying features

- **accumulation disorder**
- **infantile colic**
- **insomnia, night crying**, restlessness, fractiousness
- the child is generally robust and will cry loudly and with vigor
- clammy, night sweats
- bad breath
- reflux

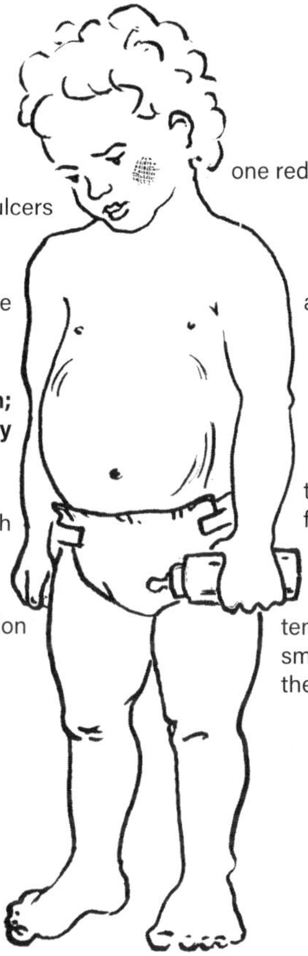

Dosage and method of administration

Dissolve the granules in a little hot water. For infants, the resulting warm liquid can be delivered by eye-dropper

1-2 years....................¼-½ sachet twice daily
2-3 years....................½-1 sachet twice daily
4-7 years....................1 sachet 2-3 times daily

Cautions and contraindications

None noted.

GMP

12.9 XIAO'ER QI XING CHA CHONG JI

1/52

小儿七星茶冲剂

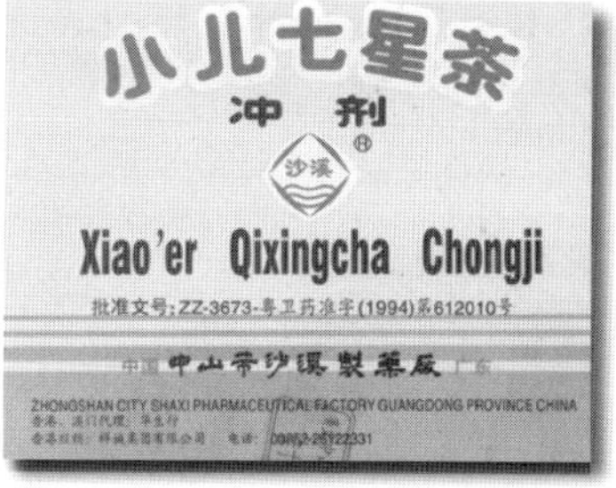

Zhongshan City Pharmaceutical Factory (Guangdong)
'Children's Seven Star Soluble Granules'
Xiao'er Qi Xing Cha Chong Ji is packaged as soluble granules in plastic jars shaped like panda bears. Seven grams per jar, 12 jars to a box

Chinese medical action

Alleviates food stagnation, strengthens the Spleen, clears heat and damp heat, extinguishes internal wind, calms the *shén*

Biomedical action

Digestive, tonic, calmative

INDICATIONS

- Similar to **12.8 Qi Xing Tea**, with less emphasis on accumulation disorder and more on internal wind resulting from heat.
- Allergic eczema that occurs in the child that eats too much sugar and starts scratching.
- Used as a mild digestive stimulant for children that lack appetite or pick at food, or who complain of abdominal pain after eating.

Composition

Coicis lachryma-jobi (yi yi ren, coix), *Uncaria rhynchophylla* (gou teng, gambir), *Lophatherum elatum* (dan zhu ye, bamboo leaves), *Cryptotympana atrata* (chan tui, cicada shell), *Crategus pinnatifida* (shan zha, crategus), *Glycyrrhiza uralensis* (gan cao, licorice), *Oryza sativa* (dao ya, sprouted rice)

Dosage and method of administration

Dissolve the granules in a little hot water. For infants, the resulting warm liquid can be delivered by eye-dropper

1-2 years....................1 jar twice daily
2-3 years....................1 jar three times daily
4-7 years....................1-2 jars three times daily

Cautions and contraindications

None noted.

皮肤病 13

Skin

13.1 LIEN CHIAO PAI TU PIEN

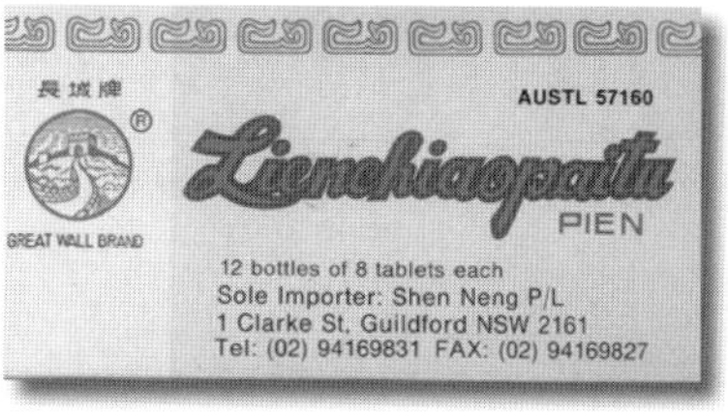

连翘败毒片

(*Lian Qiao Bai Du Pian*)
Tianjin Drug Manufactory (Shandong)
'Forsythia Antitoxic Pills'
Lien Chiao Pai Tu Pien is packaged in vials of eight uncoated pills, twelve vials per box

Chinese medical action
Dispels wind heat, clears toxic heat, relieves itch

Biomedical action
Diaphoretic, antibiotic, detoxicant, antipruritic, laxative

INDICATIONS

- Toxic heat and wind heat type skin disorders, including –
  – early stage of suppurative skin disorders, such as boils, carbuncles, acne, folliculitis, abscess, paronychia, cellulitis, erysipelas, mastitis, shingles, lymphangitis, lymphadenitis, impetigo and hand foot and mouth disease
  – acute or chronic itchy inflamed skin disorders such as eczema, dermatitis, psoriasis, pityriasis rosea and lichen sclerosis
  – allergic skin eruptions such as contact dermatitis, urticaria and poison ivy
  – viral skin disorders and rashes, such as herpes zoster and simplex, measles and chicken pox
- Severe wind heat type common cold or warm disease.

Composition (each pill contains)
Lonicera japonica (jin yin hua, lonicera) 1.03g, *Forsythia suspensa* (lian qiao, forsythia) 1.03g, *Gardenia jasminoides* (shan zhi zi, gardenia) 739mg, *Cryptotympana atrata* (chan tui, cicada shell) 739mg, *Lophatherum gracile* (dan zhu ye, bamboo leaves) 517mg, *Scutellaria baicalensis* (huang qin, scute) 455mg, *Dictamnus desycarpus* (bai xian pi, dictamnus) 455mg, *Rheum palmatum* (da huang, rhubarb root) 83mg, *Paeonia lac* (bai shao, white peony) 65mg

Combine with
– **1.2 Si Wu Wan** for chronic or stubborn skin diseases with a degree of blood deficiency
– **13.13 Fu Yin Tai Liniment** topically for dermatitis and eczema
– **14.5 Chuan Xin Lian Antiphlogistic Tablets** for lymphangitis or pityriasis
– **9.9 Superior Sore Throat Powder** for suppurative tonsillitis or pharyngeal abscess
– **6.1 Xiao Chai Hu Wan** for acute mastitis

Pattern identifying features

- **wind heat and toxic heat in the skin**
- **acute and chronic red, itchy skin lesions**
- fever, headache, sore, dry throat
- red tipped tongue, yellow coat

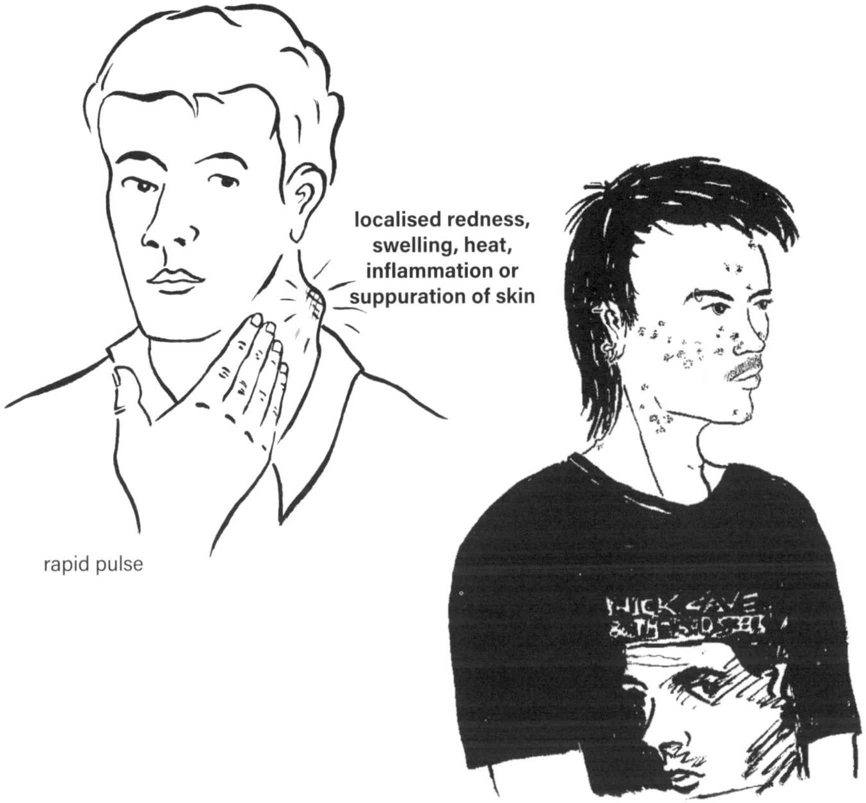

Dosage and method of administration

The recommended dose is 2-4 pills twice daily on an empty stomach. In acute or severe cases, take one vial every 2-3 hours for a few days. When used for chronic disorders the recommended dose, or less, can be taken over several months. Patient should be advised that diarrhea may occur initially; the dose should be adjusted until diarrhea is alleviated.

Cautions and contraindications

Contraindicated during pregnancy. Avoid all drying, greasy or heating food or substances, especially seafood and shellfish, coffee, alcohol, spicy foods and tobacco.

13.2 XIAO FENG WAN

消风丸

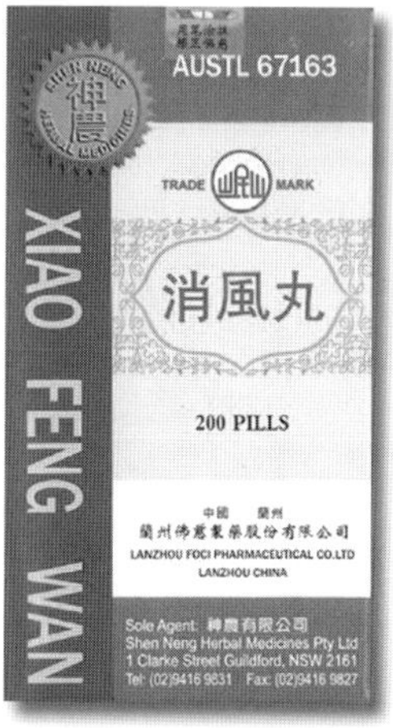

Lanzhou Foci Pharmaceutical Factory (Gansu)
'Disperse Wind Pills'
Xiao Feng Wan is packaged in bottles of 200 pills.
Also available as: Great Windkeeper Teapills (PF), Tangkuei and Arctium Formula (conc. extract)

Chinese medical action

Dispels wind, clears damp and heat, nourishes blood, stops itch

Biomedical action

Anti-inflammatory, diaphoretic, antipruritic

INDICATIONS

- Itchy, red skin diseases from wind heat or wind damp in the skin. Used for the itch and inflammation of acute and chronic skin diseases. Can be used for both wet and dry skin disorders.
- With the appropriate identifying features, this formula can assist in the treatment of conditions such as eczema, contact dermatitis, neurodermatitis, psoriasis, tinea infection, lichen simplex, nappy (diaper) rash, urticaria and generalized idiopathic pruritus.

Composition

Ledebouriella divaricata (fang feng, siler), *Sophora angustifolia* (ku shen, sophora), *Gypsum fibrosum* (shi gao, gypsum), *Rehmannia glutinosa* (sheng di, raw rehmannia), *Schizonepeta tenuifolia* (jing jie, schizonepeta), *Cryptotympana atrata* (chan tui, cicada shell), *Arctium lappa* (niu bang zi, arctium), *Sesamum indicum* (hei zhi ma, sesame seed), *Anemarrhena aspheloides* (zhi mu, anemarrhena), *Angelica sinensis* (dang gui, chinese angelica), *Atractylodes lancea* (cang zhu, red atractylodes), *Akebia trifoliata* (mu tong, akebia), *Glycyrrhiza uralensis* (gan cao, licorice)

Combine with

- **1.2 Si Wu Wan** for chronic eczema, dermatitis or other itchy dry skin disorder arising from blood deficiency. This combination is also used for dry skin disorders that are worse in cold or dry weather
- **13.19 Pearl Powder** topically (mixed in a little sorbolene) for moist eczema or other weeping itchy lesions
- **5.1 Xue Fu Zhu Yu Wan** or **13.11 Dan Shen Huo Xue Wan** for chronic purplish lesions with itchy, dry, scaly skin, the itch worse at night
- **13.4 Ke Yin Wan** for severe itch, weeping lesions, or very stubborn cases. This combination is useful for psoriasis and nummular dermatitis
- **6.5 Jia Wei Xiao Yao Wan** for dermatitis or eczema that is worse when the patient is stressed

Pattern identifying features
- **wind heat or wind damp in the skin**

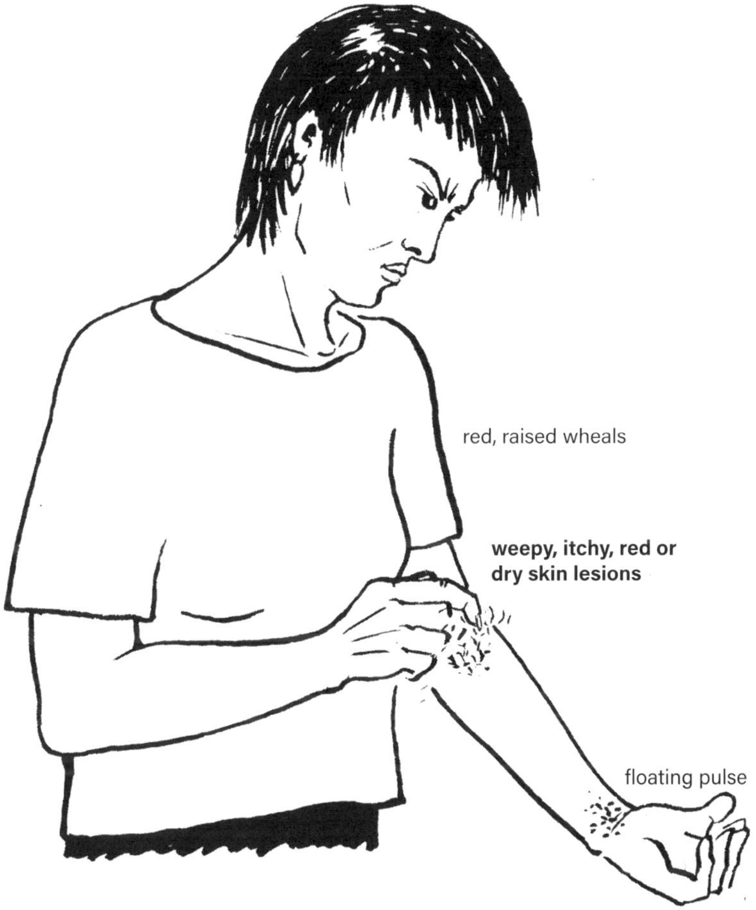

Dosage and method of administration
12-15 pills three times daily on an empty stomach. The dose can be spread out, or taken in two lots of about 20 pills, morning and evening. In severe cases or during the early stages of treatment (the first few weeks), a 50% increase in dose can be used, then reduced as treatment takes effect.

Cautions and contraindications
Not suitable alone for patients with significant blood deficiency. Avoid all drying, greasy or heating food and substances, especially seafood and shellfish, coffee, alcohol, spicy foods and tobacco.

GMP

13.3 DANG GUI YIN ZI WAN

当归饮子丸

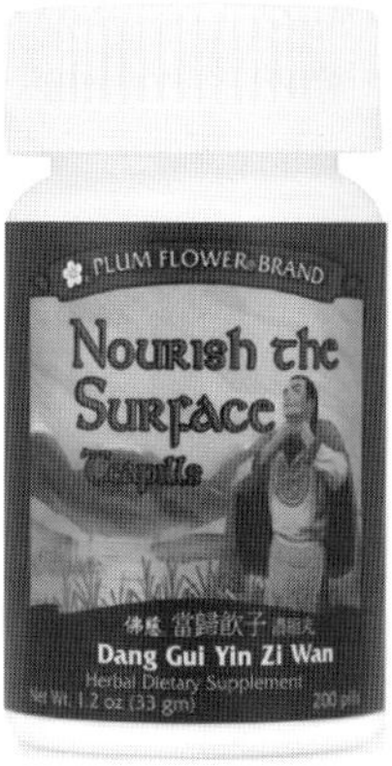

Lanzhou Foci Pharmaceutical Factory (Gansu)
'Chinese Angelica Decoction Pills'
Dang Gui Yin Zi Wan is packaged in bottles of 200 pills
Also available as: Tangkuei and Tribulus Combination (conc. extract)

Chinese medical action

Nourishes and cools blood, tonifies qi, fortifies defensive qi, dispels wind, stops itch

Biomedical action

Hematinic, diaphoretic, antipruritic

INDICATIONS

- Chronic skin diseases from blood deficiency with wind in the skin. A variation **1.2 Si Wu Wan**, with the addition of herbs to dispel wind and tonify qi. The main focus of the formula is to replenish blood to nourish the skin – when blood is abundant in the skin, any existing wind is expelled and new pathogens cannot get a foothold. The main features of this pathology are dryness, itch and the duration of the condition. Skin is thickened due to chronic irritation and relentless scratching. Itching and irritation are worse following menstruation, when fatigued and during dry or windy weather. The upper body, especially chest, neck and face are most affected.
- With the appropriate identifying features, this formula can assist in treatment of conditions such as chronic eczema or dermatitis, neurodermatitis, psoriasis, idiopathic pruritus, winter itch and senile pruritus.

Composition

Angelica sinensis (dang gui, chinese angelica), *Rehmannia glutinosa* (sheng di, raw rehmannia), *Ligusticum wallichi* (chuan xiong, ligusticum), *Ledebouriella divaricata* (fang feng, siler), *Paeonia lactiflora* (bai shao, peony root), *Tribulus terrestris* (bai ji li, tribulus), *Polygonum multiflorum* (he shou wu, polygonum root), *Astragalus membranaceous* (huang qi, astragalus), *Schizonepeta tenuifolia* (jing jie, schizonepeta), *Glycyrrhiza uralensis* (gan cao, licorice)

Combine with

- **3.6 Gui Zhi Wan** for itch and skin rashes that are worse in cold weather
- **1.16 Tao Hong Si Wu Wan** for patients with a greater degree of blood deficiency, mild blood stasis and dull purple lesions
- **6.4 Xiao Yao Wan** or **6.5 Jia Wei Xiao Yao Wan** for chronic dermatitis or eczema that is worse when the patient is stressed

Pattern identifying features

- **blood deficiency with chronic wind in the skin**
- scanty menstruation
- spots before eyes, blurring vision, dry eyes

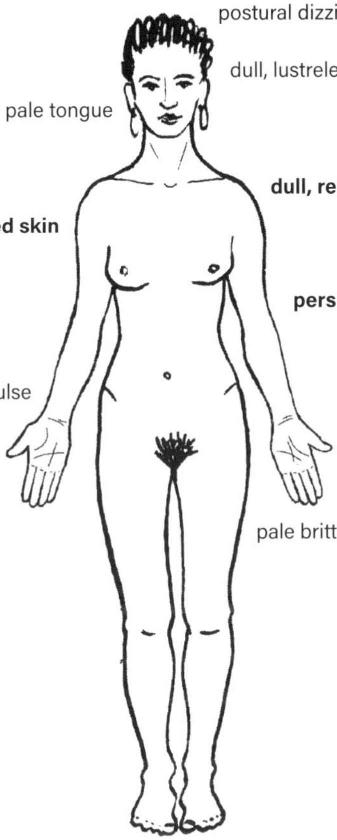

Dosage and method of administration

8-12 pills three times daily on an empty stomach. The dose can be spread out, or taken in two lots of 12-18 pills, morning and evening. In severe cases or during the early stages of treatment (the first few weeks), a 50% increase in dose can be used, then reduced as treatment takes effect.

Cautions and contraindications

Care should be taken in patients with a tendency to abdominal distension, loose stools or general digestive weakness. Some patients may find **13.3 Dang Gui Yin Zi Wan** aggravates these symptoms. This can usually be alleviated by taking it with a small dose (3-6 pills at the same time) of **2.18 Bao He Wan** or **2.9 Xiang Sha Liu Jun Wan**.

13.4 KE YIN WAN

克银丸

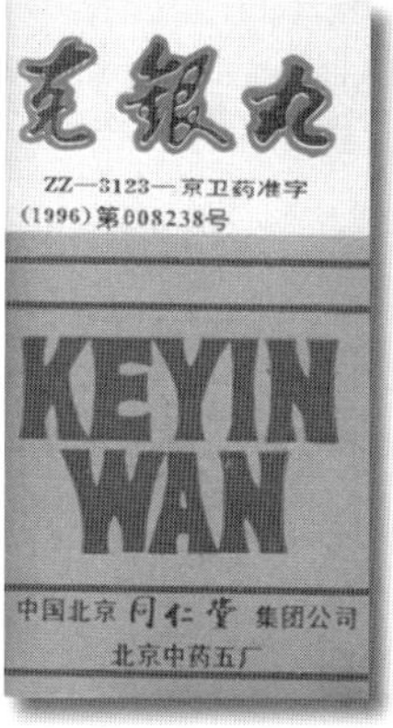

Tong Ren Tang (Beijing)
'Overcome Psoriasis Pills'
Ke Yin Wan is packaged in bottles of 300 small pills.

Chinese medical action

Clears toxic heat and drains damp, dispels wind, promotes urination, stops itch

Biomedical action

Anti-inflammatory, diaphoretic, diuretic, antipruritic

INDICATIONS

- Stubborn toxic heat or damp heat skin conditions. Mainly used for psoriasis, but also useful for eczema, dermatitis and other difficult and persistent wet or dry, itchy skin diseases. The main herb, smilax root, is traditionally used for syphilitic skin lesions. Often added to a targeting formula when enhanced toxic and damp heat clearing action is desired.
- Used to clear damp heat from the lower burner to treat conditions such as acute urinary tract infection, cystitis, urethritis, heat or damp heat painful urination, vaginal pruritus and vulvitis.

Composition

Smilax glabra (tu fu ling, smilax root), *Dictamnus desycarpus* (bai xian pi, dictamnus)

Combine with

- **5.1 Xue Fu Zhu Yu Wan** for chronic, purplish, thickened lesions from blood stasis
- **13.1 Lien Chiao Pai Tu Pien** for chronic psoriasis with heat
- **1.2 Si Wu Wan** with blood deficiency
- **4.8 Tao Chih Pien**, **6.6 Long Dan Xie Gan Wan** or **14.5 Chuan Xin Lian Antiphlogistic Tablets** for urinary tract infection
- **14.1 Huang Lian Jie Du Wan** for recurrent boils and sores
- **6.5 Jia Wei Xiao Yao Wan** for psoriasis, neurodermatitis or lichen simplex worse with stress
- **1.37 Bi Xie Sheng Shi Wan** for acute vulvitis and moist, itchy skin lesions of the lower limbs
- **1.39 Chien Chin Chih Tai Wan** for chronic or recurrent pelvic infections

Pattern identifying features
- chronic damp heat
- stubborn, chronic, itchy skin diseases

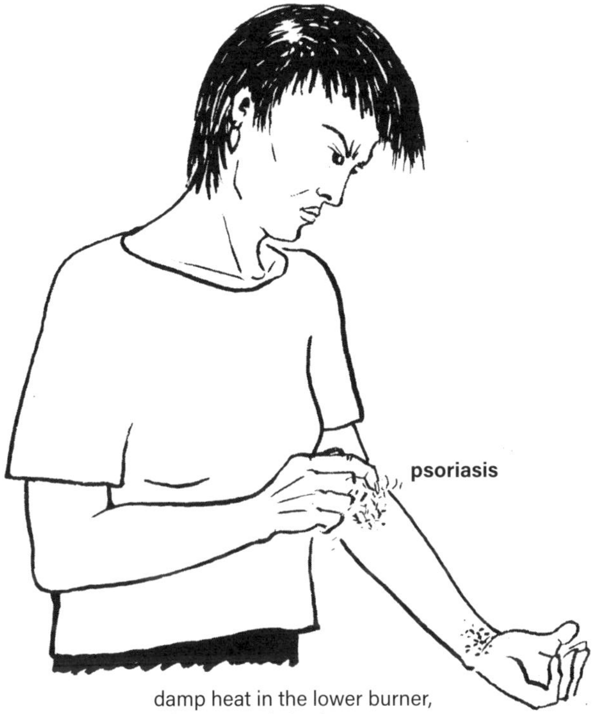

Dosage and method of administration
The recommended dose is 100 pills twice daily, but this is impractical for all but the most fastidious patient. The practical way to use the formula is to consume two bottles every 2-3 days without regard for how many pills are taken at any one time. This may appear to be a huge dose, but a large quantity of these herbs is required for a satisfactory result.

Cautions and contraindications
None noted.

13.5 SHI DU QING CAPSULE

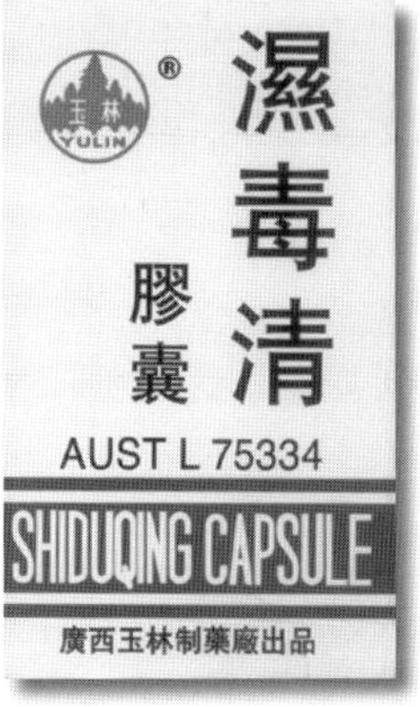

湿毒清胶囊

(*Shi Du Qing Jiao Nang*)
Yulin Drug Manufactory (Guangxi)
'Capsules to Clear Damp Toxin'
Shi Du Qing Capsules are packaged in bottles of 30 capsules

Chinese medical action

Clears damp and dispels wind from the skin, nourishes yin and blood, stops itch

Biomedical action

Anti-inflammatory, antipruritic

INDICATIONS

- Itchy skin conditions. A general antipruritic formula suitable for skin conditions with itch the main feature, including idiopathic pruritus, eczema, psoriasis and dermatitis. Most beneficial for lesions that weep and itch intolerably. Essentially a symptomatic formula, it is best when added to a more complete constitutional formula where enhanced antipruritic action is desired.

Composition (each capsule contains)

Rehmannia glutinosa (sheng di, raw rehmannia) 150mg, *Sophora angustifolia* (ku shen, sophora) 95mg, *Xanthium sibiricum* (cang er zi, xanthium) 95mg, *Paeonia veitchii* (chi shao, red peony) 85mg, *Dictamnus desycarpus* (bai xian pi, dictamnus) 75mg

Combine with

– **13.2 Xiao Feng Wan** for severe itch in eczema
– **1.2 Si Wu Wan** with blood deficiency

Dosage and method of administration

3 capsules three times daily, on an empty stomach.

Cautions and contraindications

This formula is quite drying and excessive use can dry the skin and mucous membranes. May occasionally cause headache or nausea as xanthium is slightly toxic and strongly dispersing to both wind and normal qi.

13.6 SHI DU QING

湿毒清

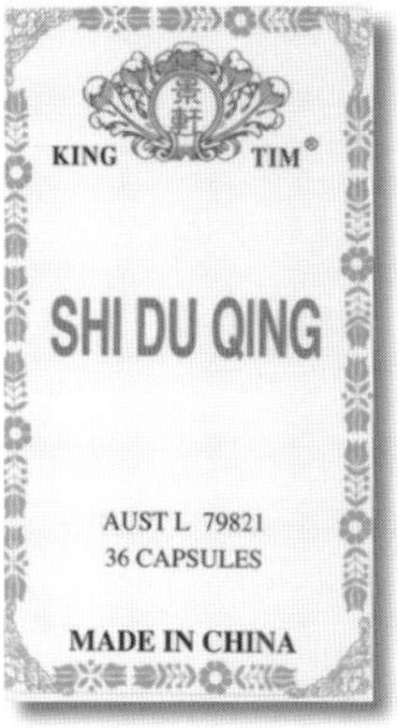

Jing Xian Pharmaceutical Co. (Guangzhou)
'Clear Damp Toxin'
Shi Du Qing is packaged in bottles of 36 capsules

Chinese medical action

Nourishes yin and blood, cools and invigorates the blood, dispels wind, clears heat and damp from the skin, stops itch

Biomedical action

Anti-inflammatory, antipruritic

INDICATIONS

- Stubborn, itchy, dry skin conditions associated with blood deficiency, blood stasis and chronic wind damp in the skin. Even though the name of this formula is similar to **13.5 Shi Du Qing Capsule**, it's composition and actions are quite different. This formula has more yin and blood tonic activity, and a stronger heat clearing action. The combination of salvia to regulate the blood and smilax to leach damp and clear stubborn heat, makes this especially good for difficult and chronic conditions such as psoriasis, eczema and allergic dermatitis. Also used for acne, nettle rash, urticaria, tinea and vulvitis.

Composition (each capsule contains extracts equivalent to dry)

Smilax glabra (tu fu ling, smilax) 630mg, *Dictamnus desycarpus* (bai xian pi, dictamnus) 490mg, *Rehmannia glutinosa* (di huang, rehmannia) 378mg, *Sophora angustifolia* (ku shen, sophora) 350mg, *Glycyrrhiza uralensis* (gan cao, licorice) 315mg, *Angelica polymorpha* (dang gui, chinese angelica) 252mg, *Salvia miltiorrhiza* (dan shen, salvia) 252mg, *Scutellaria baicalensis* (huang qin, scute) 252mg

Dosage and method of administration

3-4 capsules three times daily, on an empty stomach.

Cautions and contraindications

Contraindicated during pregnancy and in patients taking warfarin (coumarin). Caution when taking other anticoagulants such as aspirin and fish oil as clotting time can be reduced.

13.7 ECZEMA HERBAL FORMULA

皮肤病血毒丸

(Pi Fu Bing Xue Du Wan)
Tong Ren Tang (Beijing)
'Skin Disease Toxic Blood Pills'
Eczema Herbal Formula is packaged in bottles of 200 pills

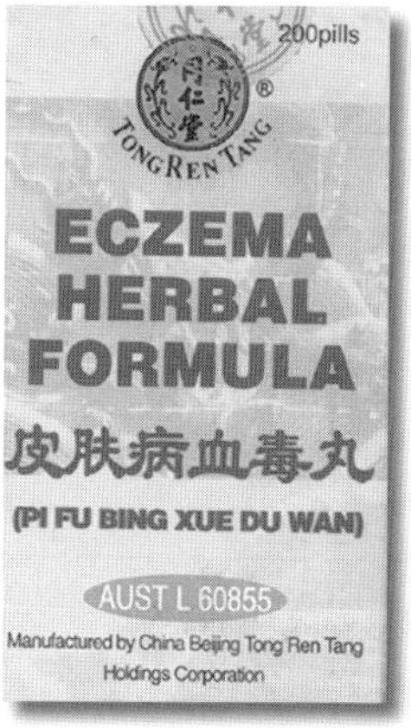

Chinese medical action

Clears toxic heat and damp heat from the skin, nourishes, invigorates and cools the blood, dispels wind, drains dampness and stops itch

Biomedical action

Anti-inflammatory, diaphoretic, antipruritic

INDICATIONS

- Chronic eczema, neurodermatitis, contact dermatitis and psoriasis. Also used for pustular and cystic acne. This is a broad acting 'shotgun' formula with just about every herb you could think of for the skin combined with herbs to invigorate stagnant blood, nourish blood, clear toxic heat and stop itch.

Composition (10 pills contain powdered)

Paeonia lactiflora (bai shao, peony root) 129mg, *Imperata cylindrica* (bai mao gen, imperata) 88mg, *Rehmannia glutinosa* (sheng di, raw rehmannia) 83mg, *Paeonia veitchii* (chi shao, red peony) 63mg, *Ledebouriella divaricata* (fang feng, siler) 63mg, *Arctium lappa* (niu bang zi, arctium) 63mg, *Ligusticum wallici* (chuan xiong, ligusticum) 63mg, *Rubia cordifolia* (qian cao gen, rubia) 41mg, *Juglans regia* (hu tao ren, walnut) 41mg, *Schizonepeta tenuifolia* (jing jie, schizonepeta) 41mg, *Angelica sinensis* (dang gui, chinese angelica) 41mg, *Kochia scoparia* (di fu zi, kochia) 41mg, *Xanthium sibiricum* (cang er zi, xanthium) 41mg, *Lonicera japonica* (jin yin hua, lonicera flower) 41mg, *Lonicera japonica* (ren dong teng, lonicera stem) 41mg, *Forsythia suspensa* (lian qiao, forsythia) 41mg, *Smilax glabra* (tu fu ling, smilax) 41mg, *Gleditsia australis* (zao jiao ci, gleditsia thorn) 41mg, *Platycodon grandiflorum* (jie geng, platycodon) 41mg, *Leonurus sibiricus* (yi mu cao, motherwort) 41mg, *Paeonia suffruticosa* (mu dan pi, moutan) 41mg, *Dictamnus desycarpus* (bai xian pi, dictamnus) 41mg, *Rheum palmatum* (da huang, rhubarb root) 41mg, *Glycyrrhiza uralensis* (gan cao, licorice) 41mg, *Angelica dahurica* (bai zhi, angelica) 41mg, *Spatholobus suberectus* (ji xue teng, spatholobus) 41mg, *Sempervivum tectorum* 41mg, *Arnebia euchroma* 21mg, *Carthamus tinctorius* (hong hua, carthamus) 21mg, *Spiroldela polyrrhiza* (fu ping, duckweed) 21mg

Combine with

- **13.4 Ke Yin Wan** for stubborn skin diseases
- **13.5 Shi Du Qing Capsule** for severe itch

Pattern identifying features

- toxic heat or damp heat in the skin

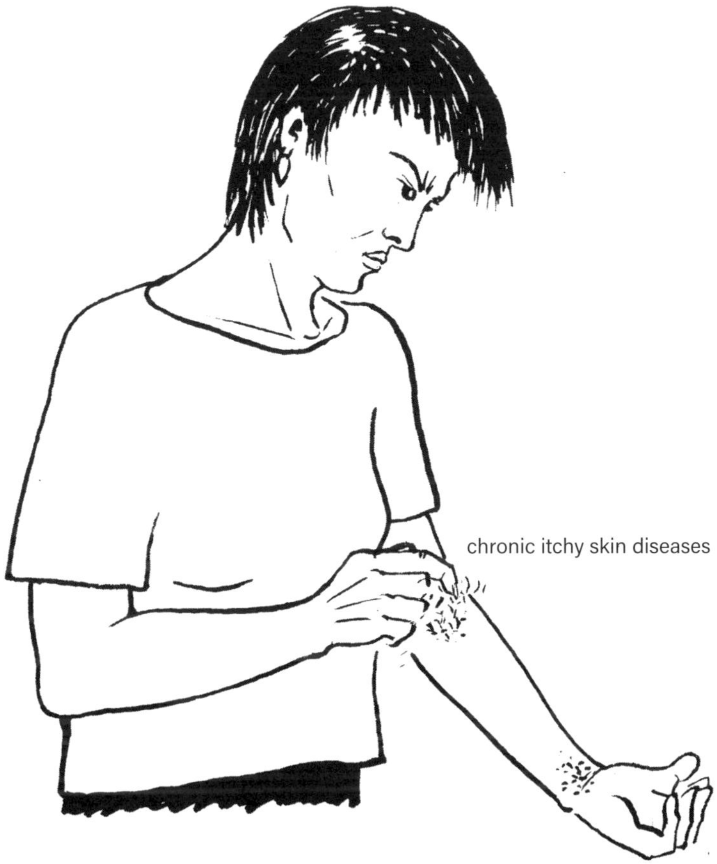

Dosage and method of administration

The recommended dose is 10-20 pills twice daily. The dose can be reduced to a maintenance dose (~50-75% of recommended dose) after about one month or when the patient sees obvious improvement.

Cautions and contraindications

Contraindicated during pregnancy.

13.8 FANG FENG TONG SHENG WAN

防风通圣丸

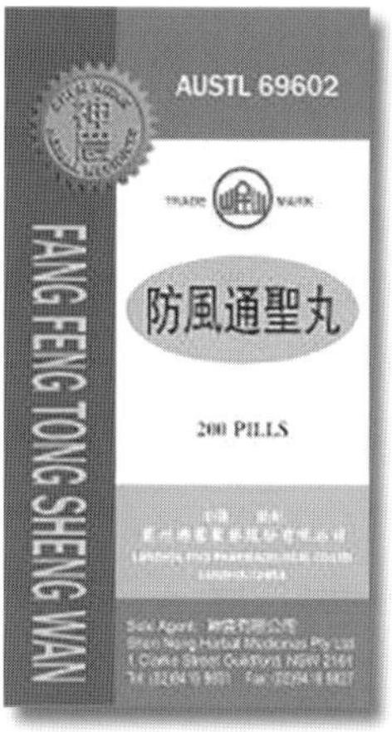

Lanzhou Foci Pharmaceutical Factory (Gansu)
'Ledebouriella Pills to Sagely Unblock'
Fang Feng Tong Sheng Wan is packaged in bottles of 200 pills
Also available as: Ledebouriella Sagely Unblocks Teapills (PF), Siler and Platycodon Formula (conc. extract)

Chinese medical action

Clears external and internal heat, dispels wind, promotes downward movement of qi and opens the bowels

Biomedical action

Anti-inflammatory, detoxicant, laxative

INDICATIONS

- Skin disease, rashes, contact dermatitis, hypersensitive or allergic dermatitis, urticaria, recurrent boils and sores, otitis externa or eczema from a combination of internal and external heat. Most commonly used in young or robust patients with these features. Internal heat is usually derived from the diet and located in the Stomach and Intestines, affecting the skin through the Intestines' relationship with the Lungs.
- Acute wind heat common cold in a patient with preexisting internal heat. Features include strong fever and chills, headache, dizziness, red, sore eyes, nasal congestion with thick, colored mucus, thirst, constipation, concentrated urine and a slippery rapid pulse. Similar to a *tài yáng – yáng míng* simultaneous pattern.
- Obesity in a robust or otherwise excess patient with a strong constitution and tendency to heat and constipation. These patients are yang in nature, and may suffer from disorders such as arteriosclerosis, gallbladder disease, hypertension or gout. **13.8 Fang Feng Tong Sheng Wan** is used by some practitioners as an adjunct 'clearing' formula in such patients trying to lose weight as they modify their diets and increase exercise.
- Chronic painful obstruction of a heat type, characterized by pain, redness, heat and swelling of joints, the pain worse in warm weather or with heat.

Composition

Ledebouriella divaricata (fang feng, siler) 9.1mg, *Glycyrrhiza uralensis* (gan cao, licorice) 36.6mg, *Scutellaria baicalensis* (huang qin, scute) 18.3mg, *Platycodon grandiflorum* (jie geng, platycodon) 18.3mg, *Schizonepeta tenuifolia* (jing jie, schizonepeta) 13.7mg, *Paeonia lactiflora* (bai shao, white peony) 9.1mg, *Rheum palmatum* (da huang, rhubarb) 9.1mg, *Ligusticum wallichi* (chuan xiong, ligusticum) 9.1mg, *Mentha haplocalycis* (bo he, mint) 9.1mg, *Angelica sinensis* (dang gui, chinese angelica) 9.1mg, *Forsythia suspensa* (lian qiao, forsythia) 9.1mg, *Gardenia jasminoides* (shan zhi zi, gardenia) 4.6mg, *Atractylodes macrocephala* (bai zhu, atractylodes) 4.6mg

Pattern identifying features

- **simultaneous internal and external excess heat**
- robust, overweight, large frame
- general tendency to heat

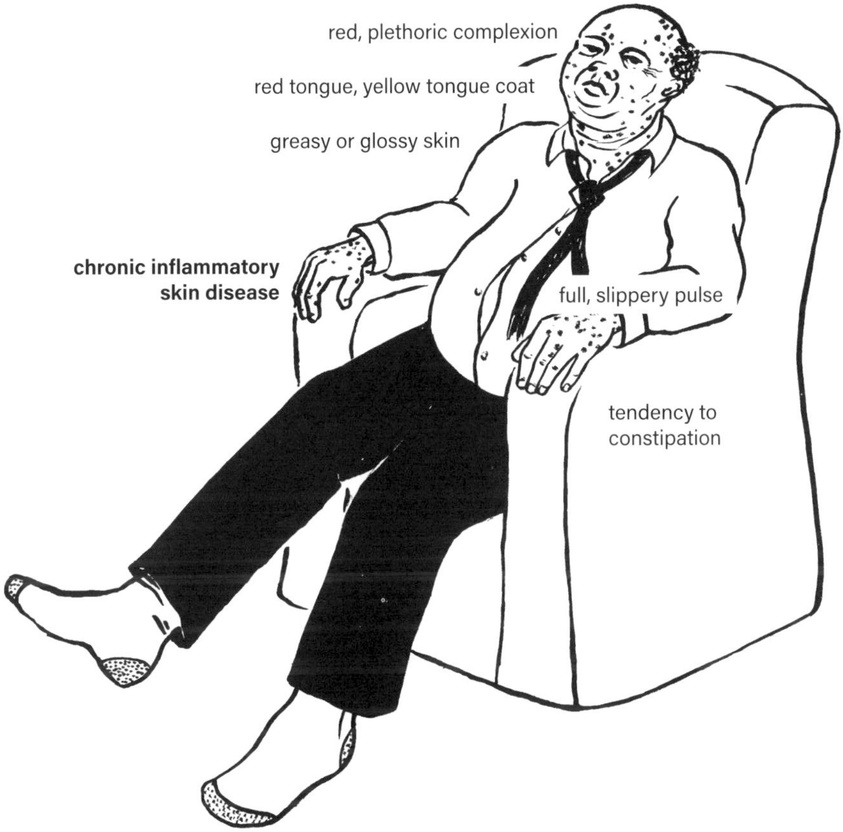

Combine with

– **13.4 Ke Yin Wan** for stubborn skin diseases

Dosage and method of administration

8-12 pills three times daily on an empty stomach. The dose can be spread out, or taken in two lots of 12-18 pills, morning and evening. In severe cases or during the early stages of treatment (the first few weeks), a 50% increase in dose can be used, then reduced as treatment takes effect.

Cautions and contraindications

Contraindicated during pregnancy.

13.9 QING RE AN CHUANG PIAN

清热暗疮片

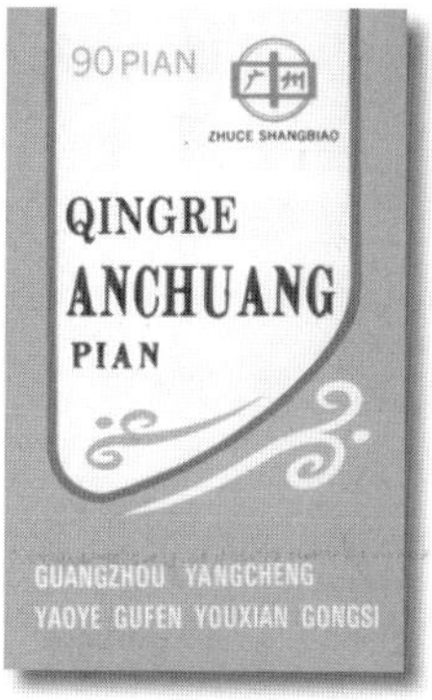

Yang Cheng Pharmaceutical Stock Co. (Guangzhou)
'Heat Clearing Acne Tablets'
Qing Re An Chuang Pian is packaged in bottles of 90 pills

Chinese medical action

Cools the blood, clears toxic heat from the skin, Lungs and Stomach

Biomedical action

Anti-inflammatory, antibiotic, detoxicant

INDICATIONS

- Toxic heat and hot blood type skin lesions. Used for a variety of suppurative skin infections, but in particular conditions such as teenage acne, acne vulgaris, abscesses, boils and sores, folliculitis and impetigo herpetiformis. The lesions are pustular, inflamed, angry and may be painful.

Composition

Andrographis paniculata (chuan xin lian, andrographis), *Taraxacum mongolicum* (pu gong ying, dandelion), *Lonicera japonica* (jin yin hua, lonicera), *Rheum palmatum* (da huang, rhubarb root), *Gardenia jasminoides* (shan zhi zi, gardenia), *Sophora tonkinensis* (shan dou gen, sophora), Synthetic Bovine Gallstone (ren gong niu huang), pearl powder (zhen zhu)

Combine with

- **14.5 Chuan Xin Lian Antiphlogistic Tablets**, **14.6 Fu Fang Nan Ban Lan Gen** or **14.1 Huang Lian Jie Du Wan** for severe or resistant cases
- **6.5 Jia Wei Xiao Yao Wan** for premenstrual acne

Dosage and method of administration

2-4 pills three times daily on an empty stomach. One course of treatment is 15 days, and usually 1-2 courses are needed to see a reasonable result. Refrain from greasy, spicy and excessively sweet foods, in particular junk food and soda. In addition, alcohol should be avoided. May cause diarrhea.

Cautions and contraindications

Contraindicated during pregnancy.

13.10 ZHEN ZHU AN CHUANG TABLET

珍珠暗疮片

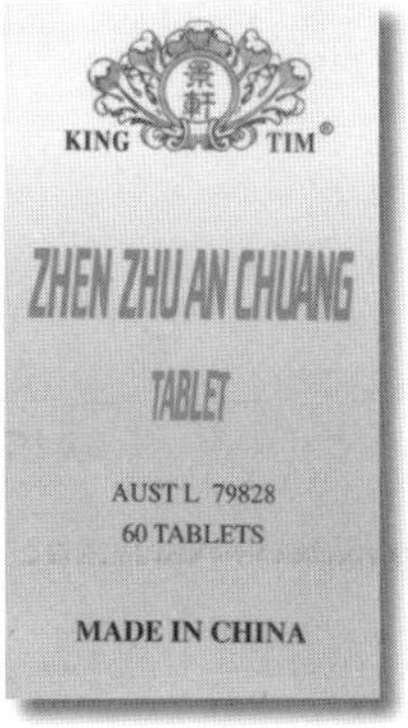

(*Zhen Zhu An Chuang Pian*)
Jing Xian Pharmaceutical Co. (Guangzhou)
'Pearl Acne Tablets'
Zhen Zhu An Chuang Tablets are packaged in bottles of 60 tablets. A similar formula available as: Margarite Acne Pills

Chinese medical action

Cools the blood, clears toxic heat from the skin, Lungs and Stomach

Biomedical action

Anti-inflammatory, antibiotic, detoxicant

INDICATIONS

- Toxic heat and damp heat in the skin. Used for acne, both cystic acne and with whiteheads. The characteristic feature is small red or white lumps and pimples on the skin of the face, neck and upper back that may or may not be painful. Suitable for teenage acne, acne vulgaris, boils and sores and folliculitis.

Composition (each tablet contains extracts equivalent to dry)

Lonicera japonica (jin yin hua, lonicera) 864mg, *Taraxacum mongolicum* (pu gong ying, dandelion) 864mg, *Gardenia florida* (shan zhi zi, gardenia) 864mg, *Sophora japonica* (huai hua, sophora flower bud) 648mg, *Rheum officinale* (da huang, rhubarb root), *Ostrea gigas* (mu li, oyster shell) 30mg, sucrose

Combine with

- **14.5 Chuan Xin Lian Antiphlogistic Tablets**, **14.6 Fu Fang Nan Ban Lan Gen** or **14.1 Huang Lian Jie Du Wan** for severe or resistant cases
- **6.5 Jia Wei Xiao Yao Wan** for premenstrual acne

Dosage and method of administration

3-5 tablets, three times daily on an empty stomach. Refrain from greasy, spicy and excessively sweet foods, in particular junk food and soda. In addition, alcohol should be avoided. This formula may cause diarrhea.

Cautions and contraindications

Contraindicated during pregnancy.

GMP

13.11 DAN SHEN HUO XUE WAN

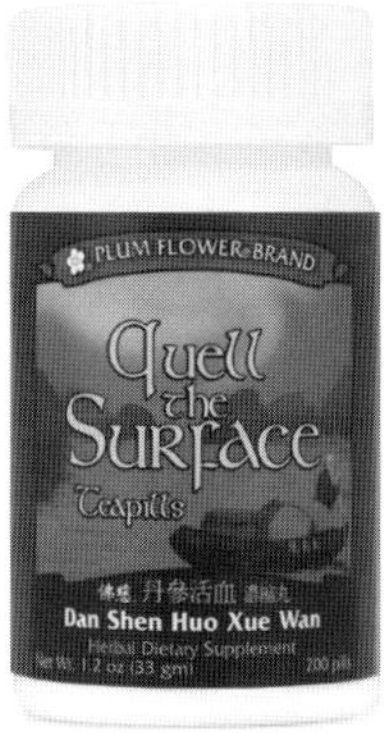

丹参活血丸

3+/12

Lanzhou Foci Pharmaceutical Factory (Gansu)
'Salvia Pills to Invigorate Blood'
Dan Shen Huo Xue Wan is packaged in bottles of 200 pills

Chinese medical action

Invigorates, cools and nourishes blood, regulates qi, clears heat, stops itch

Biomedical action

Anti-inflammatory, vasodilator, antipruritic

INDICATIONS

- Skin disorders from blood and qi stasis with heat in the blood. These are chronic and stubborn, characterized by persistent dull red or purplish lesions. Lesions tends to be fixed in location or recur in the same place, often along the course of the upper Liver channel – face, neck, chest – and are extremely itchy. An emotional component is common, with aggravation of skin brought on by stress. The genesis of this pattern is typically in the Liver, as prolonged Liver qi constraint is the precursor to heat in the blood (via heat from constraint) and blood stasis. In some cases there will be a dietary component as well – alcohol and heating spicy food in particular. Salvia serves a dual purpose here–not only does it cool and regulate the blood, it also calms the *shén* to assist in moderating the patients response to the intense itching.
- With the appropriate identifying features, this formula can assist in the treatment of conditions such as psoriasis, psoriatic arthritis, chronic eczema, systemic lupus erythematosus, rosacea and pityriasis rosea.

Composition

Salvia miltiorrhiza (dan shen, salvia), *Rehmannia glutinosa* (sheng di, raw rehmannia), *Rubia cordifolia* (qian cao gen, rubia), *Paeonia veitchii* (chi shao, red peony), *Carthamus tinctorius* (hong hua, carthamus), *Lycopus lucidus* (ze lan, bugleweed), *Dictamnus desycarpus* (bai xian pi, dictamnus), *Angelica sinensis* (dang gui wei, tail of chinese angelica), *Tribulus terrestris* (bai ji li, tribulus), *Paris polyphylla* (cao he che, paris), *Sophora subprostrata* (shan dou gen, sophora), *Citrus reticulata* (qing pi, immature citrus)

Combine with

- **13.4 Ke Yin Wan** for stubborn psoriasis
- **13.5 Shi Du Qing Capsule** for relentless itching

Pattern identifying features

- **blood stasis with heat in the blood**
- chronic skin rash or disease with a stress component
- itch worse at night
- thickened, dry, scaly skin

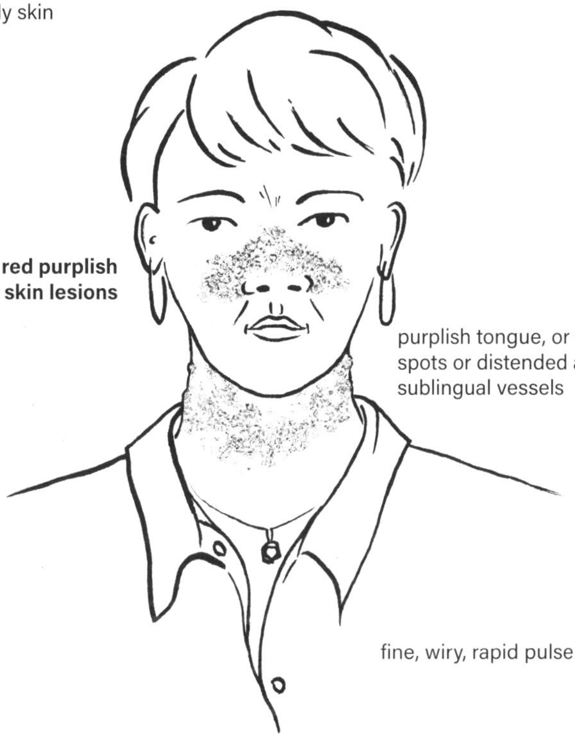

Dosage and method of administration

8-12 pills three times daily on an empty stomach. The dose can be spread out, or taken in two lots of 12-18 pills, morning and evening. In severe cases or during the early stages of treatment (the first few weeks), a 50% increase in dose can be used, then reduced as treatment takes effect.

Cautions and contraindications

Contraindicated during pregnancy, for women with menorrhagia, patients with bleeding disorders those taking warfarin (coumarin). Caution in patients on mild anticoagulants such as aspirin and fish oil. Watch for bruising or increased tendency to bleeding. Prolonged use can deplete qi and blood, so a break every 2-3 months, perhaps with a change to a simple clearing or wind expelling formula for a few weeks, is recommended.

13.12 CHUAN XIN LIAN CREAM

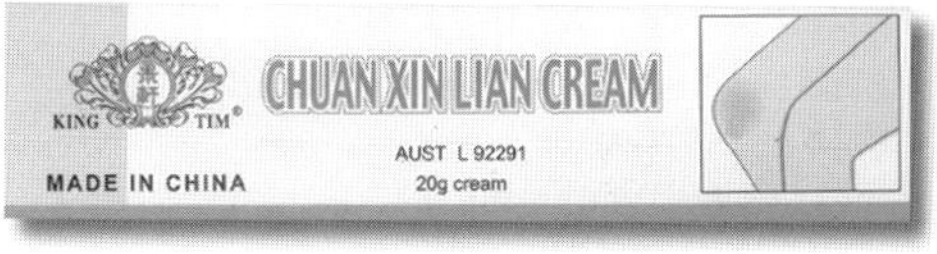

穿心莲消炎膏

(*Chuan Xin Lian Xiao Yan Gao*)
Jing Xian Pharmaceutical Co. (Guangzhou)
'Andrographis Anti-inflammatory Ointment'
Chuan Xin Lian Cream is packaged in tubes of 20 grams of ointment

Chinese medical action

Clears toxic heat and damp heat from the skin, reduces swelling

Biomedical action

Anti-inflammatory, antibiotic, detoxicant

INDICATIONS

- Damp heat and toxic heat in the skin. Used topically for inflammatory and suppurative skin disorders with redness, swelling and pain such as abscesses and boils, carbuncles and furuncles, acne, cellulitis, erysipelas, Bartholin's cyst, impetigo, eczema, dermatitis and other inflamed or infected skin conditions.
- Can be used to treat warts.

Composition (each 1 gram contains extracts equivalent to dry)

Andrographis paniculata (chuan xin lian, andrographis) 600mg, *Scutellaria baicalensis* (huang qin, scute) 300mg, *Coptis chinensis* (huang lian, coptis) 300mg

Combine with

- **14.1 Huang Lian Jie Du Wan** or **14.8 Wu Wei Xiao Du Wan** for abscesses, boils and paronychia from damp or toxic heat
- **13.1 Lien Chiao Pai Tu Pien** for cellulitis and erysipelas
- **6.6 Long Dan Xie Gan Wan** for Bartholin's cyst from damp heat from the Liver sinking into the lower burner
- **2.38 Hua Zhi Ling Tablet** for inflamed hemorrhoids

Dosage and method of administration

External use only. Apply locally to affected area 3-4 times daily.

Cautions and Contraindications

Avoid contact with the eyes and broken skin. For external use only.

13.13 FU YIN TAI LINIMENT

肤阴泰

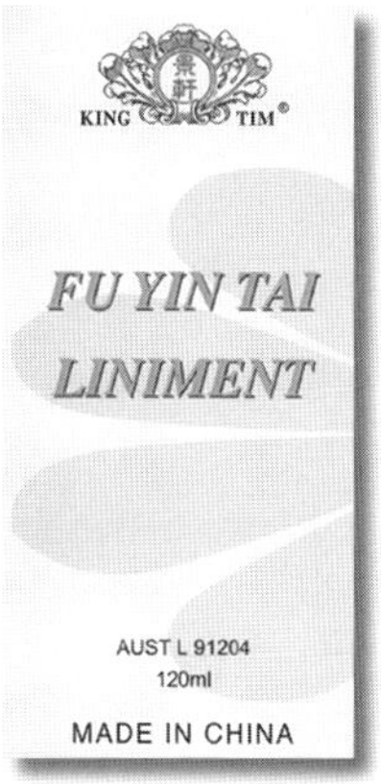

(*Fu Yin Tai*)
Jing Xian Pharmaceutical Co. (Guangzhou)
'Protect the Skin of the External Yin [Vulva]'
Fu Yin Tai Liniment is packaged in bottles of 120ml

Chinese medical action

Clears toxic heat, dispels wind, dries dampness, kills parasites, stops itch

Biomedical action

Anti-inflammatory, antipruritic, antifungal, detoxicant

INDICATIONS

- Applied topically for a variety of itchy skin conditions, including bacterial, viral, and fungal infections, and pruritic skin diseases.
- Vulval and vaginal infections by pathogens such as *Trichomonas*, cervical inflammation, vulval eczema and pruritus, yellow malodorous leukorrhea.
- Useful for painful and itching hemorrhoids, anal itch, stubborn itchy eczema and dermatitis, fungal infections of the skin, tinea, onychomycosis, tinea versicolour and prickly heat.

Composition (each 1 ml dose contains extracts equivalent to dry)

Cnidium monneri (she chuang zi, cnidium seed) 1.1g, *Eucalyptus globus* (an you, eucalyptus oil) 720mg, *Pinus massoniana* (song you, turpentine oil) 720mg, *Kochia scoparia* (di fu zi, kochia) 540mg, *Cinnamomum camphora* (zhang nao, camphor) 624mg, *Coptis chinensis* (huang lian, coptis) 72mg

Dosage and method of administration

External use only. Apply 1ml of liniment to the affected areas, or dilute 15ml of liniment in 1 litre of water and wash the affected area, once or twice daily.

Cautions and contraindications

Avoid contact with the eyes and broken skin. For external use only.

GMP

13.14 CHING WAN HUNG

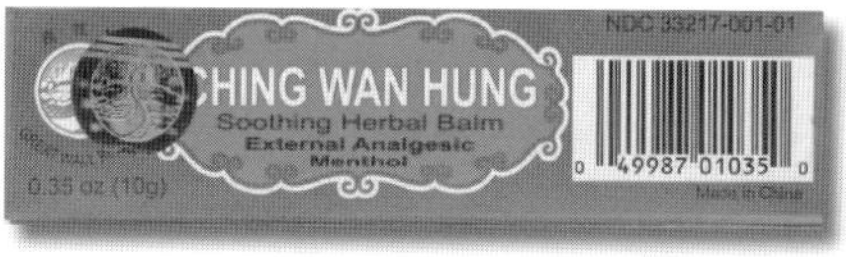

京万红

1-3/12

(Jing Wan Hong)

E

Tianjin Drug Manufactory (Shandong)
'Capital Ten Thousand Reds'
Ching Wan Hung is packaged in tubes of red ointment and in large tubs

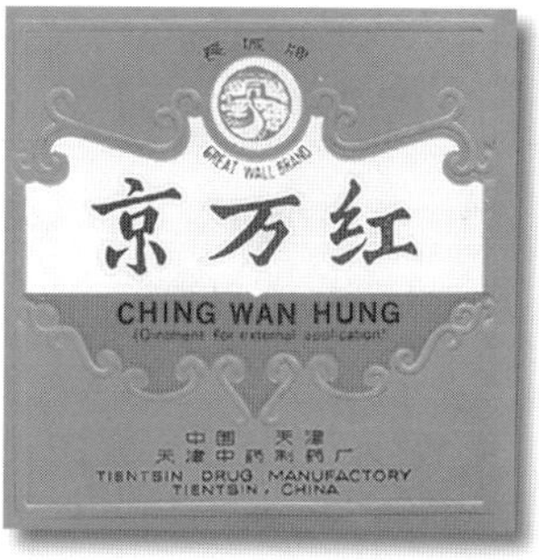

Chinese medical action

Stops pain, clears heat, invigorates blood, disperses static blood, promotes healing

Biomedical action

Anodyne, anti-inflammatory, bacteriocidal, vulnerary

INDICATIONS

- Topical ointment for burns and scalds, including electrical, chemical, solar and radiation. Can be used to relieve mild burns such as sunburn, and encourage the repair of tissues subject to severe burns or scalding, with blistering, redness, necrosis and pain.
- Applied to ulcerated or open skin lesions to accelerate granulation and healing, including painful, thrombosed or inflamed hemorrhoids, anal fissure, chronic diabetic or tropical ulcers and bedsores. Also used to alleviate and repair eczema, psoriasis and dermatitis.
- Essential for the acupuncturist who uses lots of moxa, for dabbing under rice grain moxa pellets to hold them on and prevent blistering.

Composition

Lobelia chinensis (ban bian lian, lobelia) 28%, *Commiphora myrrha* (mo yao, myrrh) 18%, *Angelica sinensis* (dang gui, chinese angelica) 12%, *Dryobalanops camphora* (bing pian, borneol) 12%, *Chaenomelas sinensis* (mu gua, chinese quince) 9%, *Sanguisorba officinalis* (di yu, sanguisorba) 9%, *Boswellia carteri* (ru xiang, frankincense) 6%, *Carthamus tinctorius* (hong hua, carthamus) 6%,

Combine with

- **1.1 Ba Zhen Wan** or **7.16.1 Shi Quan Da Bu Wan** for chronic ulcers and bed sores
- **2.38 Hua Zhi Ling Tablet** or **2.39 Fargelin for Piles** for inflamed or painful hemorrhoids or anal fissure
- **2.11 Bu Zhong Yi Qi Wan** for hemorrhoids from Spleen qi deficiency
- **5.1 Xue Fu Zhu Yu Wan** for inflamed venous or tropical ulcers; this combination is also useful for chronic blood stasis type anal fissures that refuse to heal

Pattern identifying features

- **burns and scalds**
- non-healing ulcers and sores

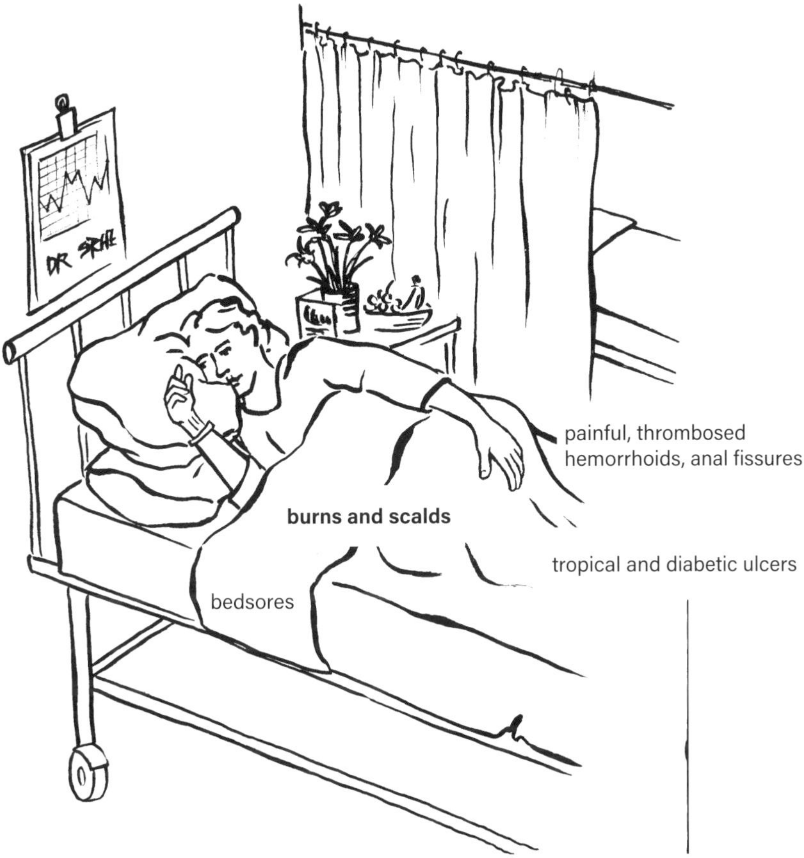

Dosage and method of administration

For mild scalds and burns, **13.14 Ching Wan Hung** is applied directly to the affected area after the wound is cleaned. The area can be covered with a piece of sterile gauze, changed daily. For deep wounds and full thickness burns, a thick layer is applied daily and covered with sterile gauze. The wound should be cleaned and debrided daily, as necessary. Apply locally for hemorrhoids and anal lesions.

Cautions and contraindications

For external use only. Avoid contact with the eyes. Can stain clothes.

1-3/52

13.15 TUJIN LINIMENT

E

土槿皮丁

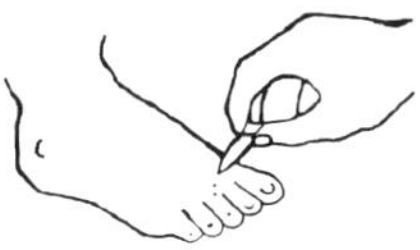

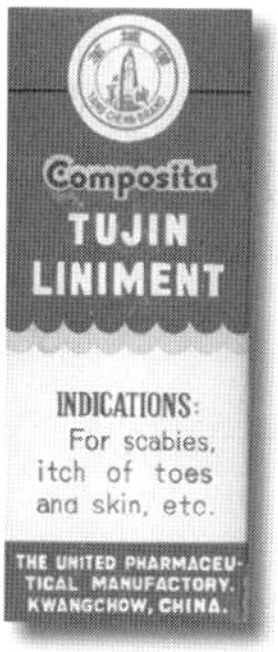

(*Tu Jin Pi Ding*)
The United Pharmaceutical Manufactory (Guangzhou)
'Hibiscus Bark Extract'
Tujin Liniment is packaged as a liquid extract in small plastic bottles

Chinese medical action
Dries damp, stops itching

Biomedical action
Antiparasitic, antifungal, disinfectant, antipruritic

INDICATIONS

- Localised fungal infections, including various manifestations of tinea (corporis, pedis, unguium, capitis etc.), jock itch, and scabies.
- Can be used for small areas of psoriasis and stubborn dermatitis.

Composition
Hibiscus syricus (mu jin pi, hibiscus bark), benzoic acid, salicylic acid, ethanol

Combine with
– **2.23 Ping Wei San**, **1.39 Chien Chin Chih Tai Wan** or **1.37 Bi Xie Sheng Shi Wan** for damp or damp heat accumulation in the lower body affecting the feet
– **14.1 Huang Lian Jie Du Wan** for damp heat pouring downwards
– **2.9 Xiang Sha Liu Jun Wan** for patients with Spleen damp

Dosage and method of administration
Rub a few drops on the affected area as often as practical. Good if left overnight beneath a covering bandage.

Cautions and Contraindications
For external use only. Avoid contact with the eyes. Can stain clothes.

13.16 HUA TUO GAO

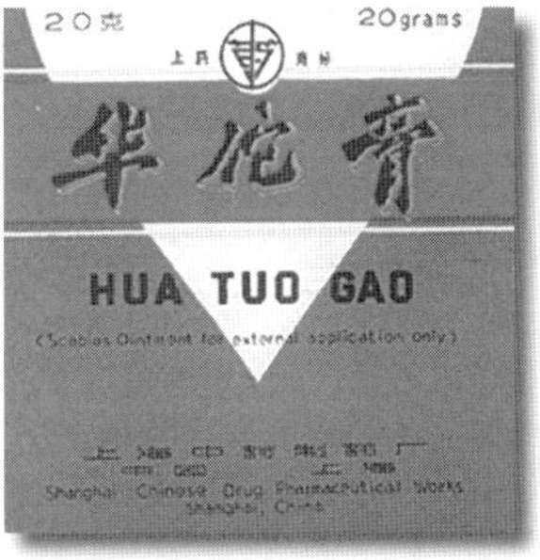

1-3/52

E

华佗膏

Shanghai Chinese Drug Pharmaceutical Works
'Hua Tuo's (famous doctor) Ointment'
Hua Tuo Gao is packaged in 20 gram jars of ointment

Chinese medical action

Dries damp, stops itching

Biomedical action

Antiparasitic, antifungal, disinfectant, antipruritic

INDICATIONS

- Scabies.
- Localised fungal infections, including various manifestations of tinea (corporis, pedis, unguium, capitis etc.), jock itch, Hong Kong foot, ringworm.
- Moist eczema, dermatitis with vesicles, crusting and itch, including pompholyx.

Composition

Benzoic acid 10%, Salicylic acid 5%, *Cera chinensis* 2%, Camphor 2%, *Chimonanthus praecox* (la mei) 1%, in a vaseline base

Combine with

- **2.23 Ping Wei San**, **1.39 Chien Chin Chih Tai Wan** or **1.37 Bi Xie Sheng Shi Wan** for damp or damp heat accumulation in the lower body affecting the feet
- **14.1 Huang Lian Jie Du Wan** for damp heat pouring downwards
- **2.9 Xiang Sha Liu Jun Wan** for patients with Spleen damp

Dosage and method of administration

Wash the affected area with warm water and apply twice daily. In areas where the skin is thickened, soak in warm water to soften it first. Useful applied at night on a cotton ball wedged between the toes. Do not use soap, alcohol, hydrogen peroxide, iodine or sulphur compounds on the skin while using this product.

Cautions and Contraindications

For external use only. Avoid contact with the eyes.

13.17 XIAO YAN TANG SHANG CREAM

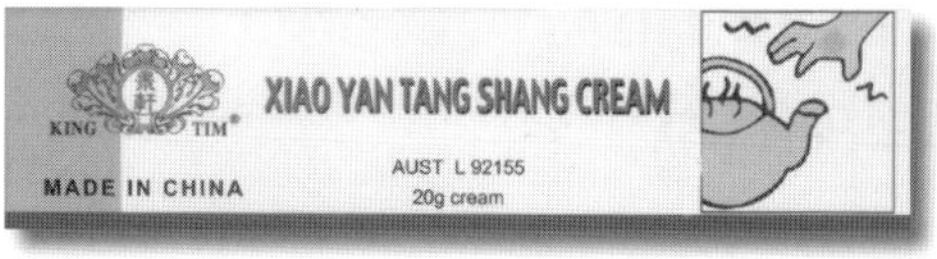

消炎清热烫伤膏

(*Xiao Yan Qing Re Tang Shang Gao*)
Jing Xian Pharmaceutical Co. (Guangzhou)
'Anti-inflammatory, Detoxifying, Burns Ointment'
Xiao Yan Tang Shang Cream is packaged in tubes of 20 grams ointment

Chinese medical action

Clears toxic heat and damp heat from the skin, invigorates and cools blood, reduces swelling and stops itch

Biomedical action

Anti-inflammatory, antibiotic, detoxicant

INDICATIONS

- Inflamed and itchy skin diseases, such as acute and chronic dermatitis, eczema, psoriasis, rosacea, urticaria and allergic eruptions, as well as superficial suppurative swellings, boils and sores.
- Painful, inflamed or itchy hemorrhoids and anal fissure.
- Fungal skin infections such as tinea and ringworm.
- Alleviates the pain and swelling of burns and scalds, and accelerates healing. Can be used on all types of burns including those from therapeutic radiation, electricity and sunburn.

Composition (each 1 gram contains extracts equivalent to dry)

Phellodendron amurense (huang bai, phellodendron) 924mg, *Scutellaria baicalensis* (huang qin, scute) 924mg, *Rheum palmatum* (da huang, rhubarb root) 924mg, *Sanguisorba officinalis* (di yu, sanguisorba) 924mg, *Paeonia suffruticosa* (mu dan pi, moutan) 924mg, *Arnebia euchroma* (zi cao, arnebia) 924mg, *Paeonia veitchii* (chi shao, red peony) 154mg, *Sophora angustifolia* (ku shen, sophora) 154mg, *Stemona sessifolia* (bai bu, stemona) 154mg

Dosage and method of administration

Apply locally to affected area 3-4 times daily.

Cautions and Contraindications

For external use only. Avoid contact with the eyes.

E

13.18 JI YAN GAO

鸡眼膏

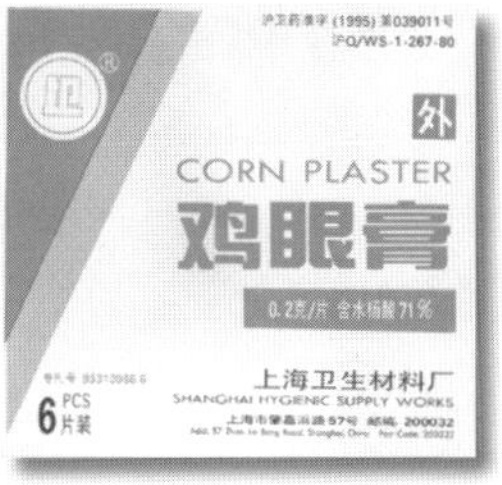

Shanghai Hygienic Supply Factory (Shanghai)
'Chicken Eye Plaster'
Ji Yan Gao is packaged in boxes of six plasters

Chinese medical action

Softens hardness, stops pain and removes warts and corns

INDICATIONS

- Corns, calluses and warts (including plantar warts) on the feet.

Composition

Salicylic Acid 70%, ointment 2g.

Combine with

– **14.5 Chuan Xin Lian Antiphlogistic Tablets** and **13.12 Chuan Xin Lian Cream** for recurrent warts

Dosage and method of administration

Bathe the feet in warm water for ten minutes and dry thoroughly. Gently tear off the thin plastic strip covering the plaster and apply to the corn, callus or wart, making sure the red ointment is firmly in position against the lesion. After three days, the skin beneath the plaster should become soft and white and may be gently removed before applying another plaster. If the skin is not soft and white, keep the plaster in place for another couple of days. After the plaster has been changed three times, wait a week before applying another. The treatment can be repeated as often as necessary to remove the lesion.

Cautions and contraindications

For external use only.

13.19 PEARL POWDER

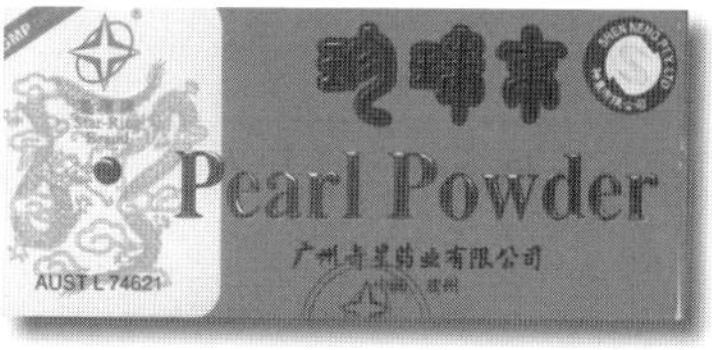

珍珠末

(*Zhen Zhu Mo*)

Guangzhou Qixing Pharmaceutical Co. (Guangzhou)

Pearl Powder is packaged in vials of 0.3 grams, twelve vials per box

Chinese medical action

Promotes healing, soothes inflamed tissues, brightens the eyes, calms the *shén*, extinguishes wind

Biomedical action

Anti-inflammatory, detoxicant, anodyne

INDICATIONS

- Applied topically to ease inflammation and promote healing. Used for redness and irritation of the skin in conditions such as diaper rash, moist eczema, and other wet skin conditions. Can be mixed with an emollient for dry or flaky skin conditions.
- Applied to minor open wounds to accelerate healing. Used topically for chronic non-healing ulcers and sores.
- Used internally for *shén* disturbances and tremors or spasms from internal wind. Also treats easy fright, fearfulness, anxiety, palpitations and insomnia in children.
- For visual weakness, inflammation of the eyes or growths over the eye, such as cataracts or pterygia.

Composition (each vial contains)

Pteria martensii (zhen zhu fen, pearl powder) 0.3g

Combine with

- **13.2 Xiao Feng Wan** for moist eczema or dermatitis
- **8.1 Tian Wang Bu Xin Dan**, **8.2 Bai Zi Yang Xin Wan** or **1.9 Gui Pi Wan** for severe insomnia, anxiety, panic attacks or palpitations
- **9.21 Ming Mu Shang Ching Pien** for sore eyes or visual disturbances from Liver heat
- **9.22 Ming Mu Di Huang Wan** or **7.2.2 Qi Ju Di Huang Wan** for visual weakness and cataracts from Liver and Kidney yin deficiency
- **7.16.1 Shi Quan Da Bu Wan** for chronic non-healing ulcers and sores

Pattern identifying features

- inflammation of the skin
- minor wounds
- moist eczema

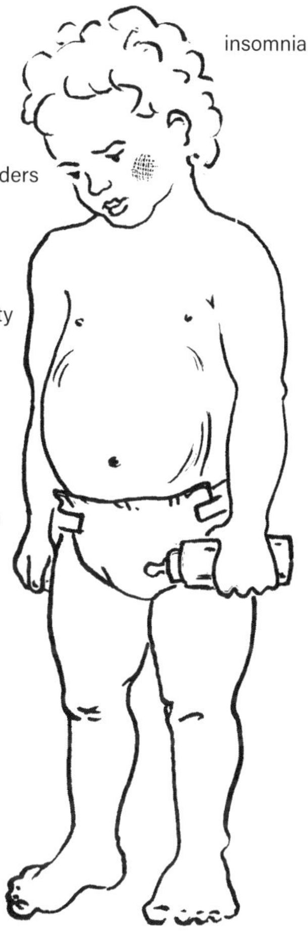

Dosage and method of administration

Apply pearl powder directly to red, itchy, moist eczema, 2-3 times daily. For dry flaking eczema or dermatitis, combine one vial of pearl powder with a half teaspoon of sorbolene and apply to the affected area. For diaper rash, sprinkle the powder directly onto the affected area after bathing.

Used internally the adult dose is 1-2 vials, twice daily, washed down with warm water. For children the dose is ½-1 vial twice daily. Can be used alone, but more commonly in combination with a constitutional formula. Pearl powder can also be made into eye-drops with saline for topical application.

Cautions and contraindications

Avoid soap while using pearl powder.

1-3/52

E

13.20 MOPIKO

无比膏

(*Wu Bi Gao*)
Ikeda Mohando Co. (Japan)
'Incomparable Ointment'
MOPIKO is packaged in 20 gram tubes of ointment

Chinese medical action
Stops pain and itching

Biomedical action
Analgesic, antipruritic

INDICATIONS
- Localised itching from eczema and other skin conditions.
- Itch and inflammation from insect bites and stings.

Composition (w/v)
Menthol crystals 3.92%, Camphor 5.83%, Methyl salicylate 3.75%

Dosage and method of administration
Apply locally to affected area 3-4 times daily.

Cautions and Contraindications
For external use only. Avoid contact with the eyes and broken skin.

热毒发炎 14

Infection and Inflammation

See also

14.1 HUANG LIAN JIE DU WAN

黄连解毒丸

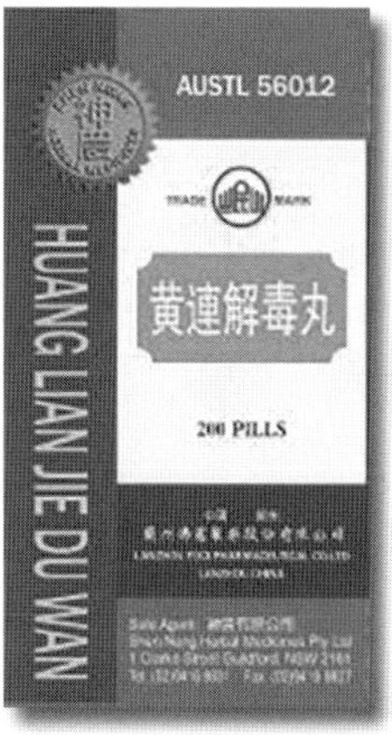

Lanzhou Foci Pharmaceutical Factory (Gansu)
'Coptis Pill to Eliminate Toxin'
Huang Lian Jie Du Wan is packaged in bottles of 200 pills
Also available as: Huang Lian Jie Du Teapills (PF), Coptis and Scute Combination (conc. extract)

Chinese medical action

Clears toxic heat and damp heat from the Triple Burner, purges fire, cools blood

Biomedical action

Antipyretic, antibiotic, anti-inflammatory

INDICATIONS

- Damp heat, toxic heat or fire affecting all three burners. An important antibiotic formula with wide application in both systemic and localised patterns of damp heat, toxic heat or fire, characterized by fever, redness, suppuration, swelling and other signs of excess heat. In severe cases, febrile rash, bleeding and disturbances of consciousness may occur. Especially good for damp or toxic heat in the gastrointestinal system (in particular dysenteric disorder), Lungs and skin.
- Bleeding disorders from the reckless movement of hot blood.
- With the appropriate identifying features, this formula can assist in the treatment of a wide variety of conditions, including:
  - **Systemic**: acute bacterial infections, septicemia, encephalitis, Beçhet's syndrome, fever of unknown origin, lymphangitis, hypertension
  - **Skin**: pyogenic skin infections, carbuncles, acne, boils, mastitis, erysipelas
  - **Upper burner**: acute bronchitis, pneumonia, gingivitis, stomatitis, acute conjunctivitis, acute sinusitis, acute otitis
  - **Middle burner**: acute hepatitis, cholecystitis, jaundice, *Helicobacter pylori*, gastritis
  - **Lower burner**: colitis, bacterial dysentery, amoebic dysentery, acute intestinal infections including those associated with *Giardia* and *Shigella*, urinary tract infection, acute pelvic inflammatory disease, acute appendicitis, acute gout

Composition (each pill contains powdered)

Coptis chinensis (huang lian, coptis) 30mg, *Gardenia jasminoides* (shan zhi zi, gardenia) 30mg, *Scutellaria baicalensis* (huang qin, scute) 20mg, *Phellodendron chinensis* (huang bai, phellodendron) 20mg

Combine with

- **1.2 Si Wu Wan** for chronic menstrual bleeding from blood deficiency and heat in the blood. This combination is also effective for stubborn skin diseases, such as psoriasis and dermatitis, from the same etiology
- **2.26 Xiang Lian Wan** for epigastric pain and reflux from Stomach heat and infection by *Helicobacter pylori*

Pattern identifying features

- **damp heat, toxic heat, fire**
- **fever**
- bleeding, especially from the upper body (nose, sclera, mouth)
- insomnia, restlessness and irritability
- thirst, dry mouth, voracious appetite

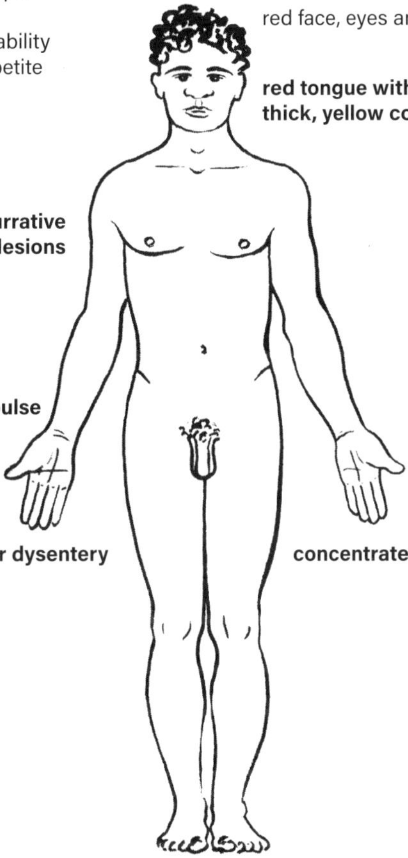

- **14.5 Chuan Xin Lian Antiphlogistic Tablets** for acute bacterial dysentery or appendicitis (Intestinal abscess)
- **14.6 Fu Fang Nan Ban Lan Gen** for encephalitis

Dosage and method of administration

10 pills every two or three hours for acute disorders. When used long term (for constitutional damp heat or fire), 6-8 pills three times daily is usually sufficient.

Cautions and contraindications

Contraindicated in patients (usually infants) with G6PD (Glucose-6-Phospate dehydrogenase) deficiency. Very bitter and cold, prolonged use can potentially damage Spleen yang, and deplete yin. Should only be used for the duration of the acute excess heat pattern, usually no longer than a few weeks. In circumstances where prolonged use is indicated (for example, when treating hypertension from a constitutional tendency to fire), pay close attention to the patient's digestive function. Overdose can cause dizziness and vomiting.

14.2 HUANG LIAN SU TABLETS

黄连素片

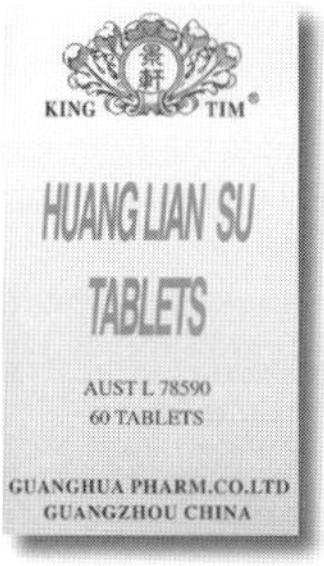

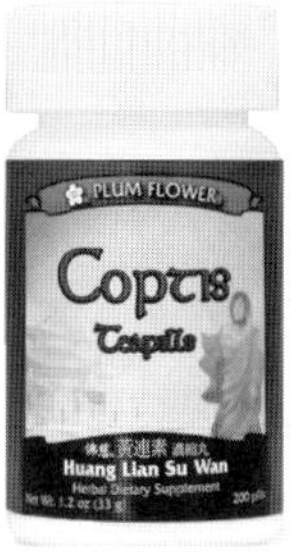

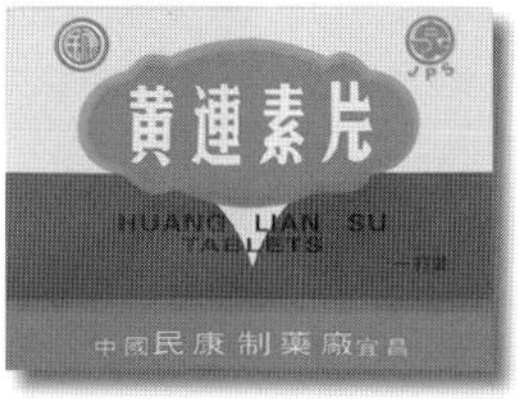

(*Huang Lian Su Pian*)
Jing Xian Pharmaceutical Co. (Guangzhou), Lanzhou Foci Pharmaceutical Factory (Gansu), Hubei Yichang Minkang Pharmaceutical Co.
'Coptis Extract Tablets'
Huang Lian Su Tablets are packaged in bottles of 60 tablets

Chinese medical action
Clears damp heat and toxic heat

Biomedical action
Antipyretic, antibiotic, anti-inflammatory

INDICATIONS

- Damp heat and toxic heat disorders, especially those affecting the gastrointestinal system, Lungs and skin. Effective against bacterial dysentery (*Shigella sp.*). Berberine, the main alkaloid, has a broad spectrum antibiotic activity, and inhibits the growth of other common parasites, including *Giardia lamblia*, *Trichomonas vaginalis* and *Entamoeba histolytica*. Also effective against *Helicobacter pylori*.
- Suppurative sores and localised infections.
- Fungal infections and as an adjunct treatment for pulmonary tuberculosis.
- **14.2 Huang Lian Su Tablets** can be combined with other formulas when an enhanced toxic heat clearing action is desired.
- With the appropriate identifying features, this single herb formula can assist in the treatment of a wide variety of infectious conditions, including bacterial and amoebic dysentery, acute colitis, appendicitis, acute infectious diarrhea, food poisoning, pyogenic skin infections, gout, cholecystitis, stomatitis, gingivitis, urinary tract infection, septicaemia and lymphangitis.

Composition
Coptis japonica (huang lian, coptis)

Combine with
- **6.6 Long Dan Xie Gan Wan** for acute cystitis, urethritis, orchitis, prostatitis or pelvic inflammatory disease from damp heat in the genitourinary system
- **6.1 Xiao Chai Hu Wan** for acute mastitis or otitis of a *shào yáng* type
- **2.3 So Hup Yuen Medical Pills** for *gu* syndrome
- **8.8 Wen Dan Wan** for strong phlegm heat patterns
- **4.6 Ba Zheng San Wan** for relatively severe urinary tract infection or pyelonephritis

Pattern identifying features

- **toxic heat and damp heat pathology, especially of the gastrointestinal system, Lung and skin**
- **suppurative infections**
- fever
- malaise

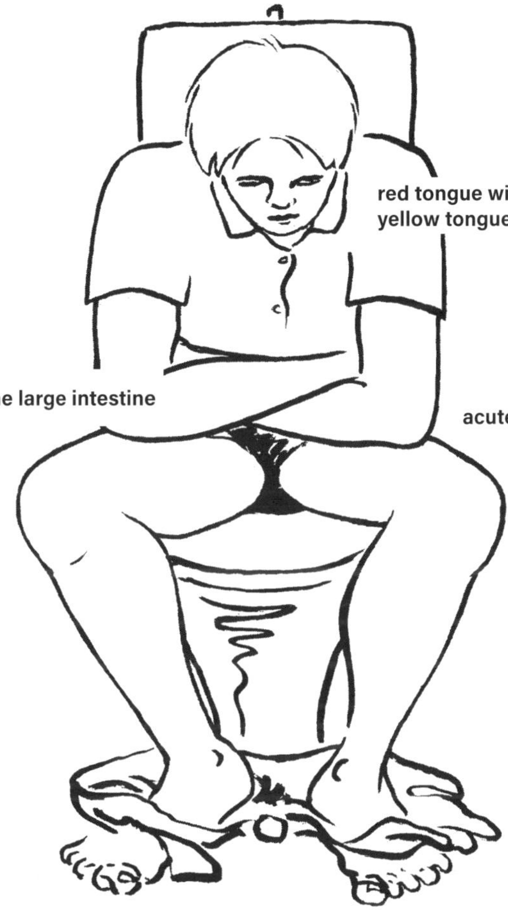

Dosage and method of administration

2-4 tablets three times daily on an empty stomach. For children the dose is ½-1 tablet three times daily.

Cautions and contraindications

Coptis is very bitter and cold and can easily damage Spleen yang, and deplete yin. It should only be used for the duration of the acute excess heat pattern, usually no longer than a few weeks. Contraindicated in patients (usually infants) with G6PD (Glucose-6-Phospate dehydrogenase) deficiency.

1-3/52

14.3 TABELLAE BERBERINI

黄连素片

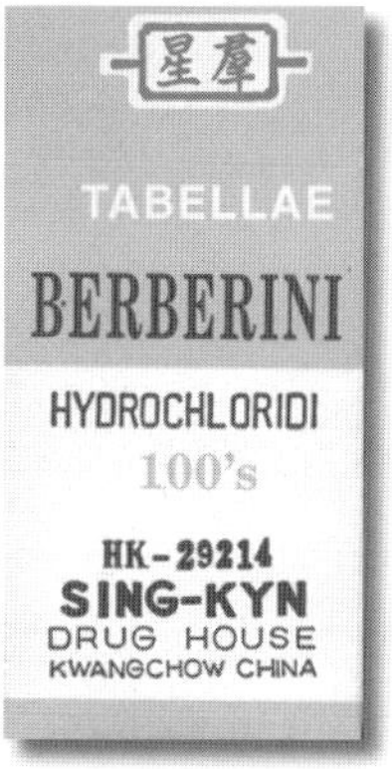

(*Huang Lian Su Pian*)
Sing-Kyn Drug House (Guangzhou)
'Coptis Extract Tablets'
Tabellae Berberini is packaged in bottles of 100 small pills

Chinese medical action

Clears damp heat and toxic heat

Biomedical action

Antipyretic, antibiotic, anti-inflammatory

INDICATIONS

- As for **14.2 Huang Lian Su Tablets**

Composition (each pill contains)

Berberine hydrochloride 50mg (extracted from *Coptis japonica* [huang lian and *Phellodendron chinensis* [huang bai])

Dosage and method of administration

1-3 tablets three times daily on an empty stomach. For children the dose is ½-1 tablet three times daily.

Cautions and contraindications

As for **14.2 Huang Lian Su Tablets**.

14.4 CHUAN XIN LIAN

穿心莲

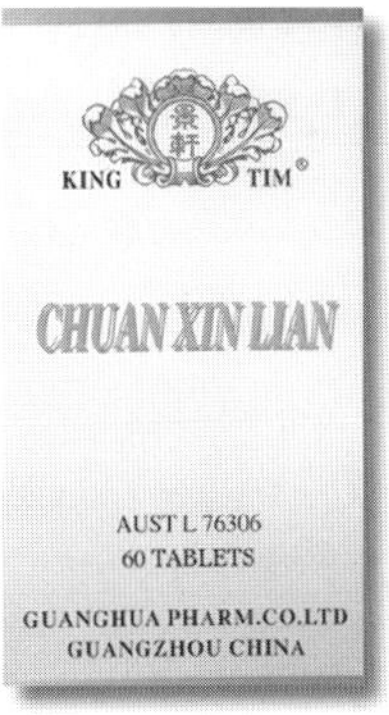

Guanghua Pharmaceutical Co. (Guangzhou)
'*Andrographis panicuata*'
Chuan Xin Lian is packaged in bottles of 60 sugar coated tablets

Chinese medical action

Clears toxic heat, cools the blood

Biomedical action

General antibiotic action–antiviral and antibacterial; hypoglycemic, antithrombotic, antipyretic

INDICATIONS

- As for **14.5 Chuan Xin Lian Antiphogistic Tablets**

Composition (each tablet contains extract equivalent to dry)

Andrographis paniculata (chuan xin lian, andrographis) 1050mg

Dosage and method of administration

3-5 tablets, three times daily on an empty stomach.

Cautions and contraindications

Contraindicated during pregnancy. **14.4 Chuan Xin Lian** is exceptionally bitter and quite cold – it easily damages Spleen qi so should only be used for a short time (i.e. the acute phase of an infection), except when used in small doses with an appropriate constitutional formula. Avoid chewing the tablets.

14.5 CHUAN XIN LIAN ANTIPHLOGISTIC TABLETS

穿心莲抗炎片

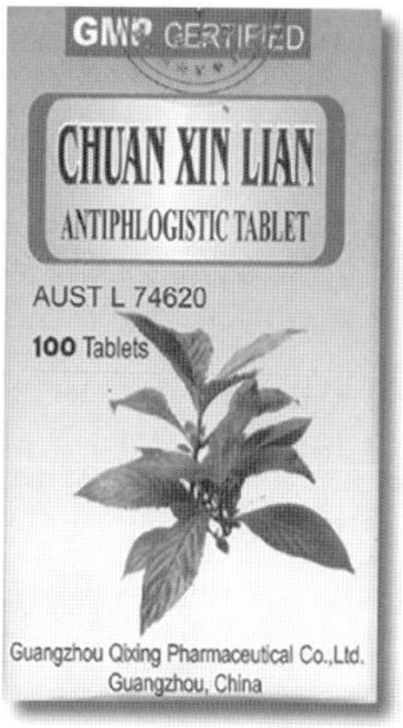

(*Chuan Xin Lian Kang Yan Pian*)
Guangzhou Qixing Pharmaceutical Factory (Guangzhou)
'Andrographis Anti-inflammatory Pills'
Chuan Xin Lian Antiphlogistic Tablets are packaged in bottles of 100 pills

Chinese medical action
Clears toxic heat, cools the blood

Biomedical action
General antibiotic action–antiviral and antibacterial; hypoglycemic, antithrombotic, antipyretic

INDICATIONS

- Toxic heat disorders and the early stage of warm diseases. Usually combined with a 'targeting' formula (such as **6.6 Long Dan Xie Gan Wan** to target the Liver, or **3.15 Qing Qi Hua Tan Wan** to target the Lungs) when enhanced toxic heat clearing action is desired. Useful against both bacterial and viral pathogens. The action and popularity of andrographis products lies in the ability of andrographis to stimulate the immune response. It operates by stimulating both antigen-specific (where antibodies are made to counteract an invading microorganism), and nonspecific immune responses (where the body's macrophage cells scavenge and destroy intruders).
- With the appropriate identifying features, this formula can assist in the treatment of conditions such as acute tonsillitis, pharyngitis, bronchitis and pneumonia, acute pyelonephritis, cystitis, urethritis and prostatitis, shingles, herpes, hepatitis, cholecystitis, genital infections, ear infections, bacterial and amoebic dysentery, suppurative sores, mastitis, erysipelas, pityriasis, mumps, systemic infections and encephalitis.

Composition (each tablet contains)
Andrographis paniculata (chuan xin lian, andrographis) 120mg, *Taraxacum mongolicum* (pu gong ying, dandelion) 60mg, *Isatis tinctora* (ban lan gen, isatis root) 60mg

Combine with
- **6.6 Long Dan Xie Gan Wan** for damp heat or toxic heat in the genitourinary system–acute cystitis, urethritis, prostatitis, pelvic inflammatory disease, hepatitis and shingles
- **9.3 Peking Niu Huang Jie Du Pian** for respiratory or skin infection–tonsillitis, erysipelas, boils and sores
- **6.1 Xiao Chai Hu Wan** for acute mastitis and otitis of a *shào yáng* type; this combination (with ¼-½ dose of **14.5 Chuan Xin Lian Antiphlogistic Tablets**) is also used for chronic low grade tonsillitis or salivary gland infection

Pattern identifying features

- **toxic heat**
- **acute viral or bacterial infection**
- **tonsillitis**
- **dysentery, diarrhea**
- **urinary tract infection**
- warm diseases (*wēn bìng* 温病)
- mastitis
- bronchitis
- suppurative sores

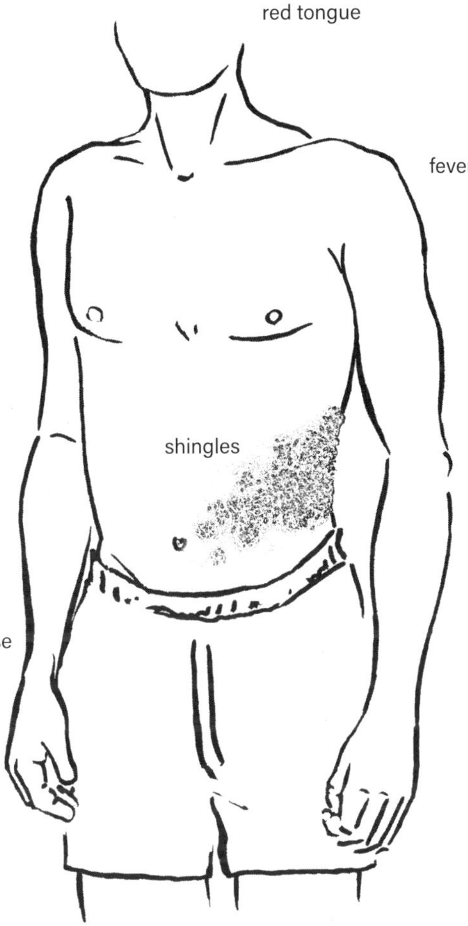

– **14.1 Huang Lian Jie Du Wan** for a variety of infections with fever including bacterial and amoebic dysentery and acute cholecystitis, damp heat acne and suppurative sores
– **6.5 Jia Wei Xiao Yao Wan** for severe premenstrual acne or boils

Dosage and method of administration

3 pills three times daily on an empty stomach. In severe cases, 5 pills every 2 hours can be used.

Cautions and contraindications

Contraindicated during pregnancy. **14.5 Chuan Xin Lian Antiphlogistic Tablets** are bitter and cold, and can easily damage Spleen qi so should only be used for a short time (i.e. the acute phase of an infection), except when used in small doses with an appropriate constitutional formula. Avoid chewing the tablets.

14.6 FU FANG NAN BAN LAN GEN

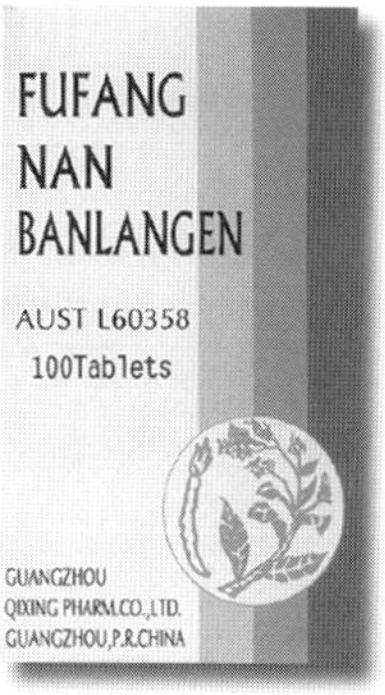

复方南板蓝根丸

(*Fu Fang Nan Ban Lan Gen Wan*)
Guangzhou Qixing Pharmaceutical Co. (Guangzhou)
'Southern Isatis Pills'
Fu Fang Nan Ban Lan Gen is packaged in bottles of 100 tablets

Chinese medical action
Clears toxic heat, cools the blood

Biomedical action
General antibiotic action–antiviral and antibacterial

INDICATIONS

- Toxic heat disorders. Similar in scope and action to **14.5 Chuan Xin Lian Antiphlogistic Tablets**, and may be combined in the same way with an appropriate targeting formula.
- Inflammatory skin disorders, such as acute eczema, psoriasis, dermatitis and pityriasis. Also used for various types of purpura (such as allergic and Henoch Schönlein) when associated with heat.

Composition (each pill contains)
Isatis tinctora (ban lan gen, isatis) 814.4mg, *Viola yedoensis* (zi hua di ding, viola) 814.4mg, *Taraxacum mongolicum* (pu gong ying, dandelion) 814.4mg

Combine with
– **1.23 Zhi Bai Di Huang Wan** for purpura associated with yin deficiency

Dosage and method of administration
4 tablets three times daily. In severe cases 5 pills every 2 hours can be used.

Cautions and contraindications
This formula is bitter and cold and can damage Spleen qi. It should only be used for a short time (i.e. the acute phase of an infection), except when used in small doses with an appropriate constitutional formula.

14.7 NIU HUANG QING HUO WAN

GMP

牛黄清火丸

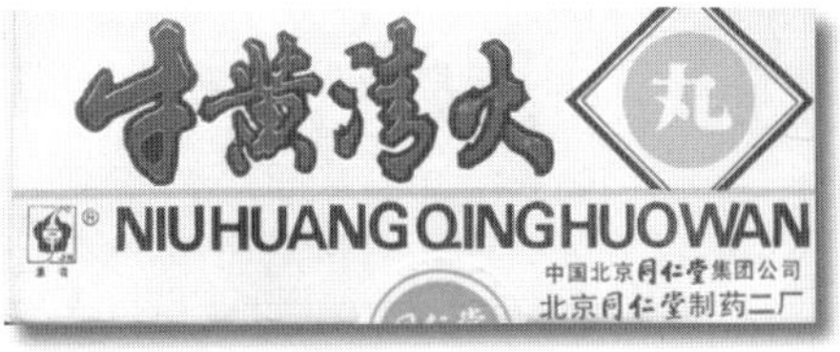

Tong Ren Tang (Beijing)
'Bovine Gallstone Fire Clearing Pills'
Niu Huang Qing Huo Wan is packaged as three gram honey pills sealed in small wax balls

Chinese medical action

Clears toxic heat, purges heat through *yáng míng*

Biomedical action

Anti-inflammatory, antibiotic, purgative

INDICATIONS

- Excess heat patterns of the Liver, Lungs and Stomach, including toothache from wind fire, gingivitis, dental abscess, abscessed gum, acute otitis media and externa, mouth ulcers, acute boils and sores, tonsillitis and mumps.
- Used in *yáng míng* organ system excess heat patterns, with high fever, thirst, sweating, big flooding pulse and constipation.
- Intestinal abscess (e.g. appendicitis, diverticulitis), with focal abdominal pain and difficult bowel movements.
- To quickly clear heat through the 'big exit' (i.e. the bowel) in cases of Liver fire, Liver wind or phlegm heat rushing up to the head. This occurs in wind-stroke or pre-stroke conditions.

Composition

Synthetic Bovine Gallstone (ren gong niu huang), *Rheum palmatum* (da huang, rhubarb root), *Platycodon grandiflorum* (jie geng, platycodon), *Dryobalanops aromatica* (bing pian, borneol)

Dosage and method of administration

2 pills twice daily. The patient should expect loose stools or diarrhea.

Cautions and contraindications

Contraindicated during pregnancy.

14.8 WU WEI XIAO DU WAN

TGA

五味消毒丸

1-3/52

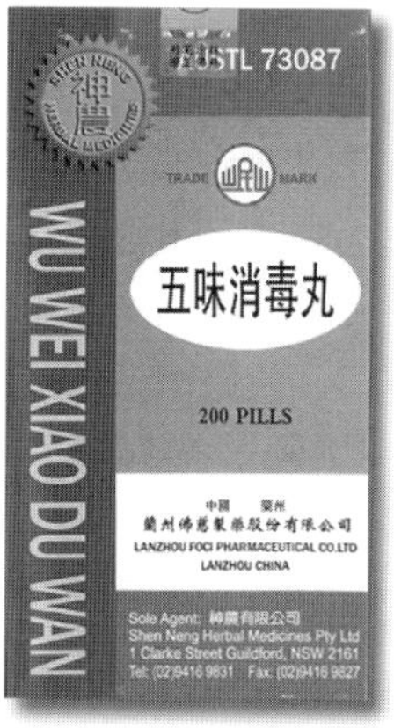

Lanzhou Foci Pharmaceutical Factory (Gansu)
'Five Ingredient Detoxifying Pills'
Wu Wei Xiao Du Wan is packaged in bottles of 200 pills
Also available as: Five Flavor Teapills (PF), Dandelion and Wild Chrysanthemum Combination (conc extract)

Chinese medical action

Clears toxic heat, reduces toxic swellings

Biomedical action

Broad spectrum antibacterial agent, anti-inflammatory, antipyretic, disinfectant

INDICATIONS

- Pyogenic and inflammatory focal skin lesions such as abscesses, boils, carbuncles and furuncles from toxic heat. Particularly good for hard, painful, deep rooted lesions. Generally considered best for bacterial infections. Most commonly applied to superficial lesions, but can be used for toxic heat and damp heat internal pathology as well.
- With the appropriate identifying features, this formula can be used as a general anti-toxic agent (or as an addition to a targeting formula) for localised toxic heat disorders such as erysipelas, cellulitis, paronychia, mastitis, otitis, tonsillitis and lymphangitis, acute urinary tract infections, pelvic inflammatory disease, orchitis and appendicitis.

Composition (each tablet contains powdered)

Lonicera japonica (jin yin hua, lonicera) 36.4mg, *Taraxacum mongolicum* (pu gong ying, dandelion) 36.7mg, *Chrysanthemum indicum* (ye ju hua, wild chrysanthemum) 36.7mg, *Viola yedoensis* (zi hua di ding, viola) 36.7mg, *Begonia fimbristipulata* (zi bei tian kui, begonia) 14.5mg

Combine with

- **14.1 Huang Lian Jie Du Wan** for severe infections with high fever
- **6.1 Xiao Chai Hu Wan** for acute mastitis, cystitis, or other acute infection characterized by distinct episodes of fever and chills
- **14.5 Chuan Xin Lian Antiphlogistic Tablets** for lymphangitis, bacteremia and impetigo
- **1.38 Yu Dai Wan** or **1.36 Fu Yan Qing Tablet** for toxic heat in the lower burner causing leukorrhea or pelvic inflammatory disease
- **11.1 Qian Lie Xian Capsule** for acute prostatitis

Pattern identifying features

- **toxic heat focal lesions**
- localised suppurative infections
- redness, swelling, inflammation, pain, pus
- may be fever and chills

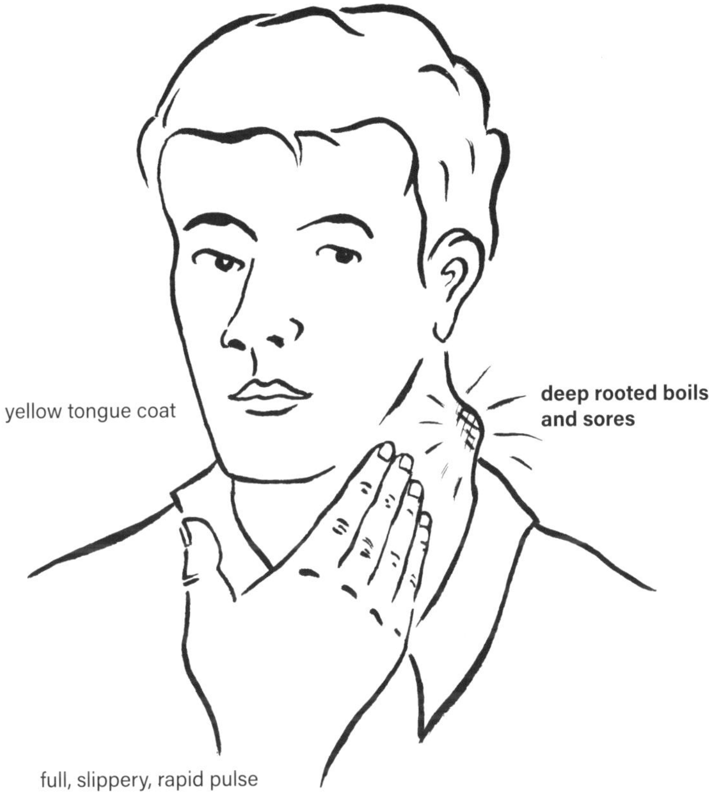

Dosage and method of administration

The recommended dose is 8-12 pills three times daily, however, in acute or severe disorders a higher dose is required to be effective, in general, 16-24 pills three times daily (or about 12 pills every two hours), on an empty stomach.

Cautions and contraindications

Contraindicated for yin type boils and swellings. Caution in patients with Spleen deficiency.

GMP

14.9 BAI HU WAN

白虎丸

1-3/7

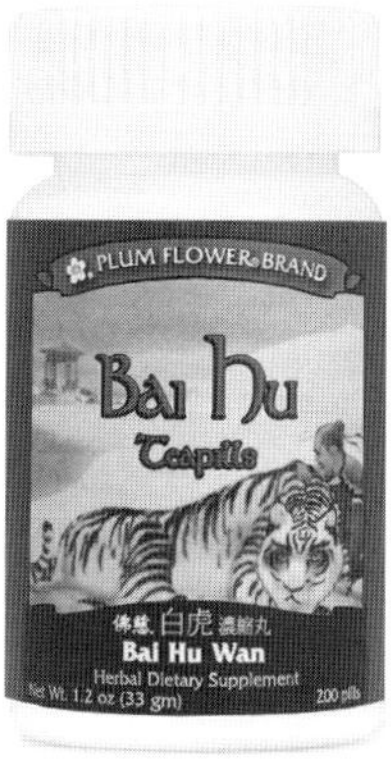

Lanzhou Foci Pharmaceutical Factory (Gansu)
'White Tiger Pills'
Bai Hu Wan is packaged in bottles of 200 pills
Also available as: Gypsum Combination (conc. extract)

Chinese medical action

Clears heat from the Lungs and Stomach (*yáng míng* or qi level)

Biomedical action

Antipyretic

INDICATIONS

- Acute fever associated with heat accumulation in the *yáng míng* channels. This pattern is classically attributed to the progress of a cold pathogen through the superficial layers (*tài yáng* and *shào yáng*) into the interior of the body, where, confronted by strong resistance from normal qi, it transforms from cold to heat. The *yáng míng* level (corresponding to the gastrointestinal system and Lungs) is the first point of contact between an invading pathogen and the internal organ systems, and as such represents a serious disorder. *Yáng míng* channel syndrome is so called because at this stage of the invasion, the heat is 'formless', and the *yáng míng* organ (here the Large Intestine) is not yet obstructed by constipation. The main features of *yáng míng* channel syndrome are quite specific and characterized by the 'four bigs' – fever, thirst, sweating and pulse. The intensity of the symptoms is the result of the clash between a strong pathogen and the normal qi of an otherwise robust patient.
- With the appropriate identifying features, this formula can assist in the treatment of conditions such as the fever of pneumonia, epidemic hemorrhagic fever, encephalitis, meningitis, heat stroke and childhood fevers such as measles.

Composition

Gypsum fibrosum (shi gao, gypsum), *Dioscorea opposita* (shan yao, dioscorea), *Anemarrhena aspheloides* (zhi mu, anemarrhena), *Glycyrrhiza uralensis* (gan cao, licorice)

Dosage and method of administration

The recommended dose for adults is 8-12 pills three times daily, however, in acute or severe disorders a higher dose is required to be effective, in general, 16-24 pills three times daily (or about 12 pills every two hours), on an empty stomach. For infants and small children, the pills should be ground up and decocted, and 5-10ml of the resulting lukewarm liquid delivered with an eye-dropper or teaspoon (3-5 squirts or 2 teaspoons), every 2-3 hours.

Pattern identifying features

- ***yáng míng* channel syndrome (heat accumulation in the Lungs and Intestines <u>without</u> constipation)**
- irritability
- frontal headache
- bleeding gums, mouth ulcers

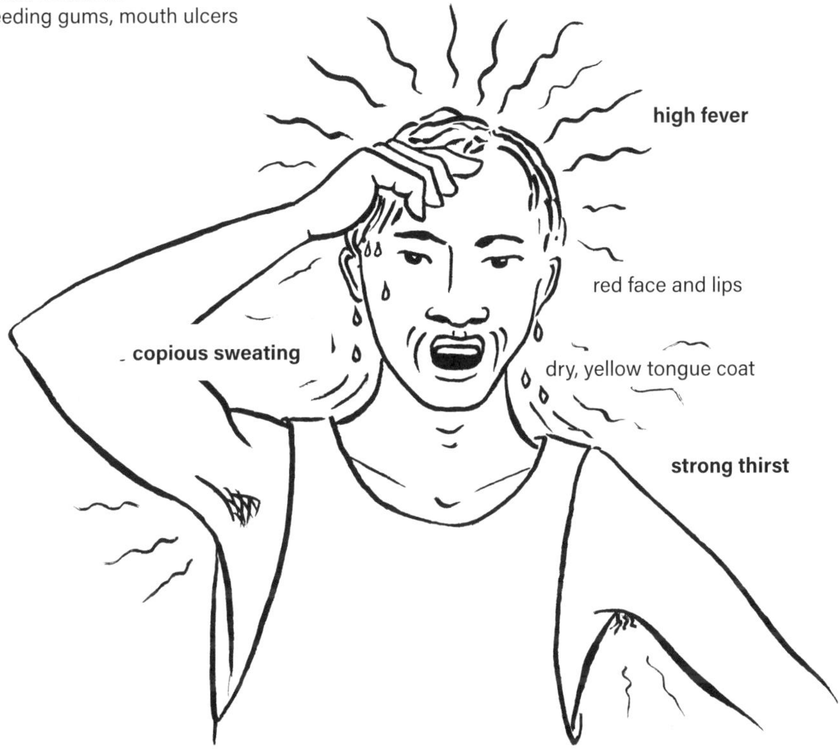

Cautions and contraindications

Contraindicated in any other fever type other than the *yáng míng* channel pattern described. Be careful with diagnosis because inappropriate usage can be dangerous. Watch for signs of over cooling, such as cold extremities and subjective feelings of cold, and stop the formula immediately if these symptoms occur.

14.9 Bai Hu Wan is designed to be used for a maximum of a few days. If the fever has not subsided within 2-3 days, the patient must be reassessed. Excessive use of gypsum can damage Spleen yang and lead to iatrogenic complication. Not suitable for the same presentation with constipation (*see* **3.16 Ching Fei Yi Huo Pien**, **14.10 Liang Ge Wan** or **14.7 Niu Huang Qing Huo Wan**).

GMP

14.10 LIANG GE WAN

凉膈丸

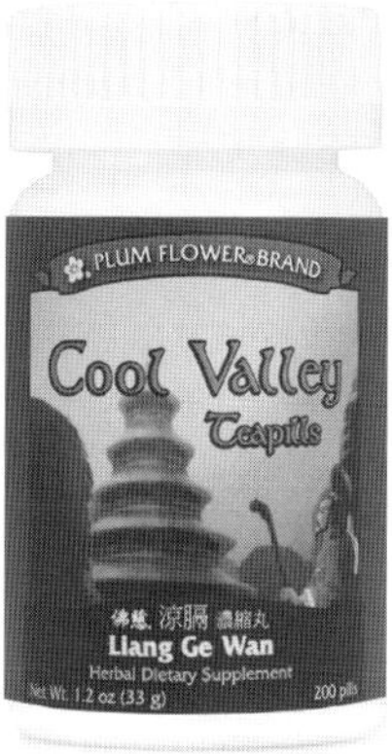

1/52

Lanzhou Foci Pharmaceutical Factory (Gansu)
'Pills for Cooling the Diaphragm'
Liang Ge Wan is packaged in bottles of 200 pills
Also available as: Forsythia and Rhubarb Combination (conc. extract)

Chinese medical action

Clears and purges toxic heat and fire from the qi (*yáng míng*) level, benefits the throat, opens the bowels

Biomedical action

Antipyretic, antibiotic, purgative

INDICATIONS

- Heat and fire in the upper and middle burner, (Lungs, Stomach and Intestines) with constipation. This pattern is a variation of the *yáng míng* heat pattern treated by **14.9 Bai Hu Wan**, in which heat has dried fluids and caused the complication of constipation. This formula simultaneously cools heat and provides an outlet for heat through the Large Intestine.
- Heat type skin rashes on the upper body. Rashes such as these are often associated with heat in the Stomach and have a dietary component, being aggravated by heating food and alcohol.
- With the appropriate identifying features, this formula can assist in the treatment of conditions such as acute tonsillitis and laryngitis, stomatitis, gingivitis, conjunctivitis, suppurative and inflammatory skin lesions, pneumonia, cholecystitis, acute appendicitis, meningitis, encephalitis, acute infectious hepatitis, erysipelas and measles.

Composition

Lophatherum gracile (dan zhu ye, bamboo leaves), *Forsythia suspensa* (lian qiao, forsythia), *Rheum palmatum* (da huang, rhubarb), Mirabilitum (mang xiao, sodium sulphate), *Glycyrrhiza uralensis* (gan cao, licorice), *Gardenia jasminoides* (shan zhi zi, gardenia), *Scutellaria baicalensis* (huang qin, scute), *Mentha haplocalycis* (bo he, mint)

Combine with

- **14.2 Huang Lian Su Tablets** or **14.5 Chuan Xin Lian Antiphlogistic Tablets** for severe infections with high fever
- **14.6 Fu Fang Nan Ban Lan Gen** for infectious encephalitis
- **9.10 Sanjin Watermelon Frost** for mouth ulcers from Heart fire
- **9.9 Superior Sore Throat Powder** for tonsillitis and toxic heat in the throat

Pattern identifying features

- **heat and fire accumulation in the middle and upper burner**
- **fever**
- irritability
- toothache, red, swollen gums
- mouth ulcers
- nosebleeds

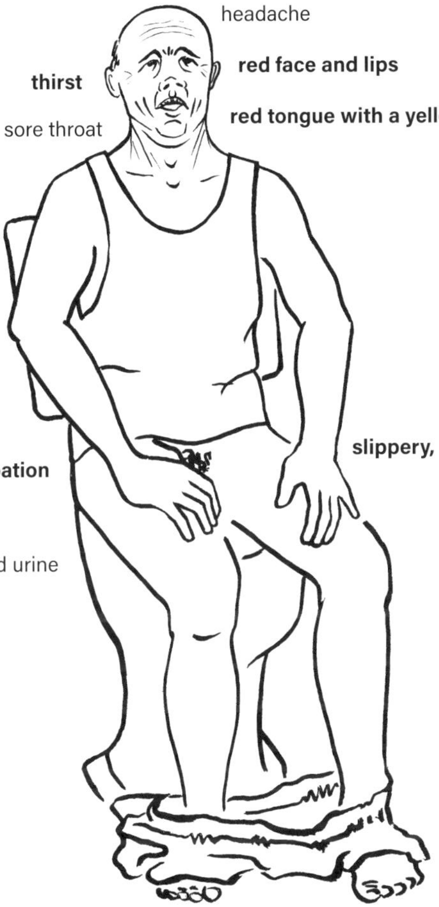

Dosage and method of administration

The recommended dose is 8-12 pills three times daily, however, in acute or severe disorders a higher dose is required to be effective, in general, 16-24 pills three times daily (or about 12 pills every two hours), on an empty stomach. The patient should be advised that diarrhea may occur.

Cautions and contraindications

Contraindicated during pregnancy and in the absence of excess heat patterns with constipation.

内风肝阳 15

Internal Wind and Ascendant Yang

GMP

15.1 PO LUNG YUEN MEDICAL PILLS

琥珀抱龙丸

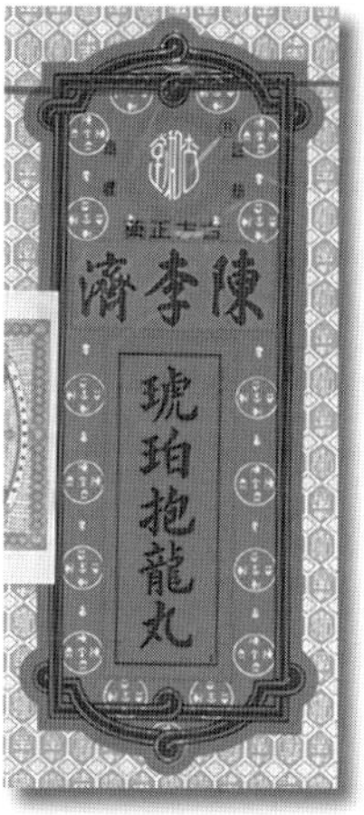

(*Hu Po Bao Long Wan*)
Chan Li Chai Medical Factory (Hong Kong)
'Amber Pills to Embrace the Dragon'
Po Lung Yuen Medical Pills are packaged as large honey pills sealed in wax balls, ten pills per box

Chinese medical action

Extinguishes Liver wind, clears and transforms phlegm heat, stops spasms and convulsions

Biomedical action

Calmative, sedative, antispasmodic

INDICATIONS

- Tics, tremor, spasms and involuntary movements from Liver wind and phlegm heat.
- Acute or chronic seizure patterns, as in epilepsy (particularly the mild forms, such as Jacksonian, or absences), associated with heat.
- *Shén* disturbance such as frequent anxiety, easily startled, excess timidity, phobias, inappropriate emotional responses, sleep disturbances and nightmares from Phlegm heat.
- Fever, impaired consciousness, febrile convulsions, irritability and restlessness from heat or phlegm heat affecting the Heart and Pericardium. This tends to occur in children. There may also be wheezing, cough and vomiting.

Composition

Gastrodia elata (tian ma, gastrodia) 16.5%, *Glycyrrhiza uralensis* (gan cao, licorice) 15%, *Arisaema cosnaguinium* (dan nan xing, bile treated arisaema) 11%, *Santalum album* (tan xiang, sandalwood) 11%, *Poria cocos* (fu ling, hoelen) 11%, *Mentha arvensis* (bo he, mint) 11%, *Atractylodes lancea* (cang zhu, red atractylodes) 11%, *Uncaria rhynchophylla* (gou teng, gambir) 5.5%, *Typhonium giganteum* (bai fu zi, typhonium) 5.5%, *Dryobalanops camphora* (bing pian, borneol) 1.5%, Amber (hu po) 1%

Combine with

- **8.8 Wen Dan Wan** for *shén* disturbance from severe phlegm heat
- **6.6 Long Dan Xie Gan Wan** for irrational anger, spasms and tic from phlegm heat with Liver fire

Pattern identifying features

- **Liver wind and phlegm heat**
- spasms, convulsions, seizures
- febrile convulsions
- disturbances of consciousness, extreme emotional fragility
- tics, tremors

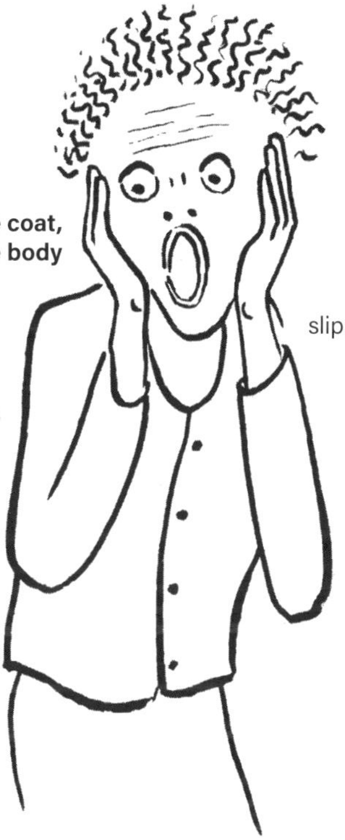

Dosage and method of administration

The recommended dose is one to two pills per day, with warm water or ginger tea. One third to half dose for children. These pills are hard and can be softened in boiling water for 10 minutes before ingestion.

Cautions and contraindications

Contraindicated during pregnancy. Not suitable for timidity, anxiety states or emotional fragility due to blood or yin deficiency.

15.2 NIU HUANG QING XIN WAN

同仁牛黄清心丸

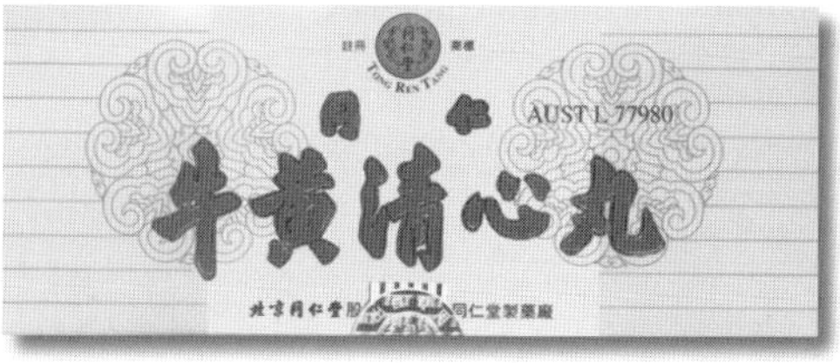

(*Tong Ren Niu Huang Qing Xin Wan*)
Tong Ren Tang Pharmaceutical Factory (Beijing)
'Bovine Gallstone Heart Cooling Pills from Tong Ren Tang'
Niu Huang Qing Xin Wan is packaged as 3 gram honey pills sealed inside a wax ball, ten balls per box

Chinese medical action

Clears heat from the Heart and Pericardium, transforms phlegm heat, extinguishes wind, regulates qi and blood, nourishes yin, opens the sensory orifices, calms the *shén*

Biomedical action

Sedative, tranquilizer, tonic, expectorant

INDICATIONS

- Internal wind type movement disorders, in patients with underlying deficiency. Used to treat tremor, spastic or flaccid paralysis, disturbances of consciousness, syncope, dizziness, muscular weakness, facial paralysis, aphasia, slurred speech and atrophy and muscular weakness syndrome. The original composition of this formula contained animal products aimed at calming the Liver, clearing heat and extinguishing wind. Some elements of this still remain, however, this is a toned down version. This large and complex formula is more focused on the underlying deficiency that has allowed generation of the wind. It addresses multiple aspects of what are usually complicated mixtures of pathology including excess heat, phlegm, stagnation of qi and blood and various deficiencies.
- With the appropriate identifying features, this formula can assist in the treatment of conditions such as Parkinson's disease, benign familial tremor, post wind-stroke hemiplegia, paralysis or numbness, multiple sclerosis and peripheral neuropathy.

Composition (each pill contains extracts equivalent to)

Dioscorea officinalis (shan yao, dioscorea) 111mg, *Equus asinus* (e jiao, gelatin) 79.5mg, *Glycyrrhiza uralensis* (gan cao, licorice) 73.5mg, *Siler divaricum* (fang feng, siler) 46.5mg, *Atractylodes macrocephala* (bai zhu, atractylodes) 45mg, *Panax ginseng* (ren shen, ginseng) 37.5mg, *Paeonia lactiflora* (bai shao, white peony) 37.5mg, *Poria cocos* (fu ling, hoelen) 37.5mg, *Cinnamomun cassia* (rou gui, cinnamon bark) 27mg, Massa Fermentata (shen qu) 27mg, *Angelica polymorpha* (dang gui, chinese angelica) 22.5mg, *Platycodon grandiflorum* (jie geng, platycodon) 22.5mg, *Astragalus membranaceous* (huang qi, astragalus) 22.5mg, *Zingiber officinale* (gan jiang, dry ginger) 22.5mg, *Ligusticum wallichi* (chuan xiong, ligusticum) 19.5mg, *Bupleurum falcatum* (chai hu, bupleurum) 19.5mg, Bovine gallstone (niu huang) 12mg, *Prunus armenica* (xing ren, apricot seed) 9.5mg, *Typhae angustifolia* (pu huang, bulrush pollen) 7.5mg, *Ophiopogon japonicus* (mai dong, ophiopogon) 7.5mg, *Ampelopsis japonica* (bai lian, ampelopsis) 3mg, honey

Pattern identifying features

- **phlegm heat, internal wind;** qi and blood deficiency with mild stasis
- atrophy and muscular weakness syndromes
- seizure disorders
- sequelae of wind stroke
- flaccid or spastic paralysis

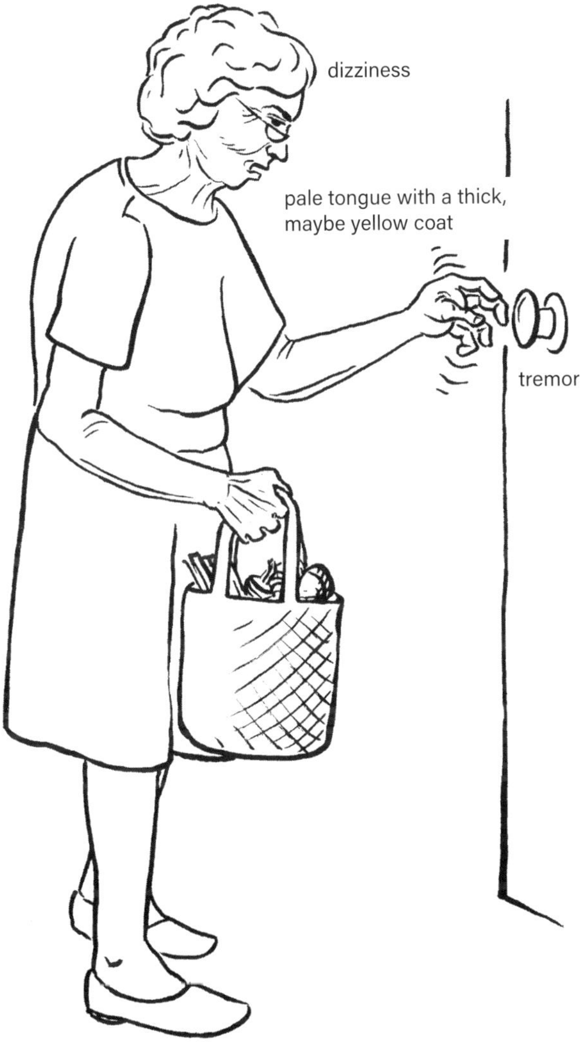

Dosage and method of administration

One pill chewed twice daily on an empty stomach.

Cautions and contraindications

Contraindicated during pregnancy. Not suitable for children.

GMP

15.3 BAN XIA BAI ZHU TIAN MA WAN

半夏白术天麻丸

1-3/12

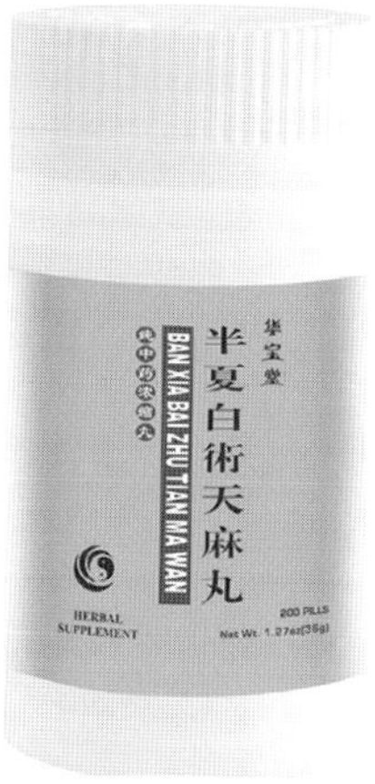

Hwa Bao Tang (Liaoning)
'Pinellia, Atractylodes and Gastrodia Pills'
Ban Xia Bai Zhu Tian Ma Wan is packaged in bottles of 200 pills
Also available as: Head Clear Pill (BE), Vertigoff (GCT), Pinellia and Gastrodia Combination (conc. extract)

Chinese medical action

Strengthens the Spleen, dries damp, transforms phlegm and extinguishes wind

Biomedical action

Sedative, calmative

INDICATIONS

- Wind phlegm giving rise to sudden episodes of dizziness and vertigo accompanied by nausea, vomiting and tinnitus. May also be frontal headaches, generalized heaviness and somnolence. The genesis of this pattern is twofold – Spleen deficiency allowing accumulation of phlegm damp, and Liver qi constraint that weakens the Spleen and creates the conditions for the generation of internal wind that carries the phlegm to the head. The vertigo of this pattern is distinctive. It is usually quite severe, even to the point of falling over and may occur when the patient is prone in bed. The sensation is sometimes likened to being on a ship or having the world spin around. Some people are even woken with vertigo, and it may be triggered by stress or exposure to strong penetrating smells such as perfume and gasoline.
- With the appropriate identifying features, this formula can assist in the treatment of conditions such as Ménière's disease, aural vertigo, benign positional vertigo and hypertension.

Composition

Pinellia ternata (zhi ban xia, processed pinellia), *Atractylodes macrocephala* (bai zhu, atractylodes), *Gastrodia elata* (tian ma, gastrodia), *Poria cocos* (fu ling, hoelen), *Citrus reticulata* (chen pi, citrus), *Zingiber officinale* (sheng jiang, ginger), *Zizyphus jujuba* (da zao, chinese dates), *Glycyrrhiza uralensis* (gan cao, licorice)

Combine with

- **7.22 Shen Qi Da Bu Wan** or **2.8 Liu Jun Zi Wan** for significant qi deficiency
- **4.2 Wu Ling Wan** for severe damp and fluid metabolism dysfunction
- **8.8 Wen Dan Wan** for severe vertigo from phlegm heat

Dosage and method of administration

8-12 pills three times daily, before meals. The dose can be spread out, or taken in two lots of 12-18 pills, morning and evening. In severe cases or during the early stages of treatment (the first two weeks), a 50% increase in dose can be used, then reduced as treatment takes effect.

Pattern identifying features

- **wind phlegm**
- increased desire to sleep
- heavy sensations in the body
- poor appetite
- foggy head

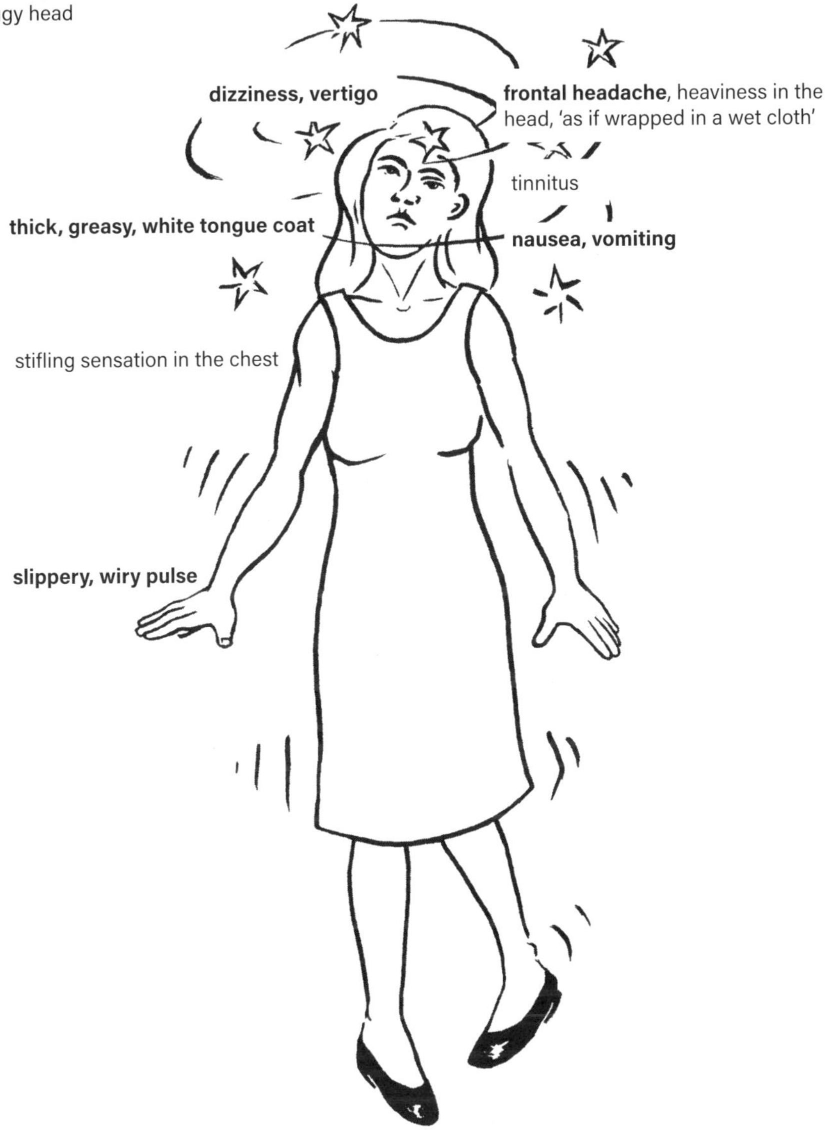

Cautions and contraindications

Contraindicated in dizziness and vertigo patterns associated with Liver fire or blood deficiency.

15.4 TIAN MA GOU TENG WAN

天麻钩藤丸

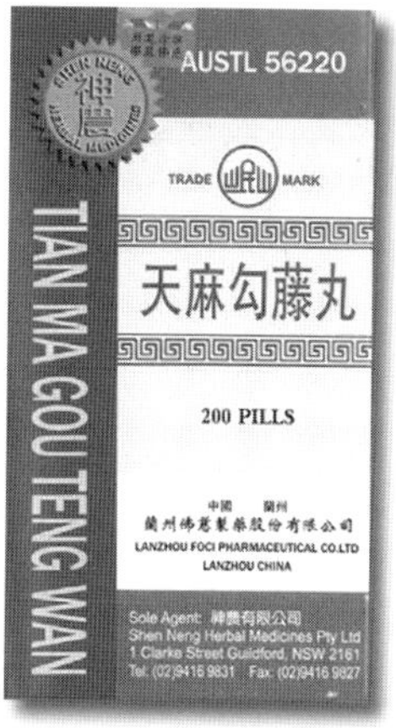

Lanzhou Foci Pharmaceutical Factory (Gansu)
'Gastrodia and Uncaria Pills'
Tian Ma Gou Teng Wan is packaged in bottles of 200 pills
Also available as: Tian Ma Gou Teng Teapills (PF), Gastodia and Gambir Combination (conc. extract)

Chinese medical action

Calms the Liver, extinguishes wind, clears heat and pacifies ascendant Liver yang

Biomedical action

Anti-hypertensive, sedative to the nervous system, calmative

INDICATIONS

- Headache and dizziness from ascendant Liver yang and Liver wind. The ascendant yang is usually the result of prolonged Liver qi constraint.
- Liver wind patterns with numbness and paresthesia of the extremities, tics, tremors and spasms. This formula is used for conditions that are predominantly excess, more commonly seen in younger, stressed, yet relatively robust individuals (for internal wind and vigorous ascendant yang from marked yin deficiency in older patients, a potentially dangerous situation contributing to wind stroke, see **15.6 Zhen Gan Xi Feng Wan**).
- With the appropriate identifying features, this formula can assist in the treatment of disorders such as chronic headache and migraine, essential hypertension, renal hypertension, transient ischaemic attacks, autonomic nervous system imbalance, preeclampsia and epilepsy.

Composition (each pill contains powdered)

Viscum coloratum (sang ji sheng, vaecium) 22mg, calcium sulphate (substitute for conch shell, shi jue ming) 22mg, *Uncaria rhyncophylla* (gou teng, gambir) 14mg, *Polygonum multiflorum* (ye jiao teng, polygonum stem) 14mg, *Poria cocos* (fu ling, hoelen) 14mg, *Achyranthes bidentata* (niu xi, achyranthes) 11mg, *Leonurus sibirica* (yi mu cao, motherwort) 11mg, *Gastrodia elata* (tian ma, gastrodia) 8mg, *Gardenia florida* (shan zhi zi, gardenia) 8mg, *Eucommia ulmoides* (du zhong, eucommia) 8mg

Combine with

- **7.1.1 Liu Wei Di Huang Wan** with underlying Liver and Kidney yin deficiency
- **6.6 Long Dan Xie Gan Wan** with Liver fire headaches and vertigo
- **8.8 Wen Dan Wan** for phlegm heat in the head

Pattern identifying features

- **Ascendant Liver yang and Liver wind (with little underlying deficiency)**
- stiffness and pain in the neck and shoulders
- sleep disturbances
- irritability, irascibility, anger
- tics, tremors, muscles spasm
- hypertension

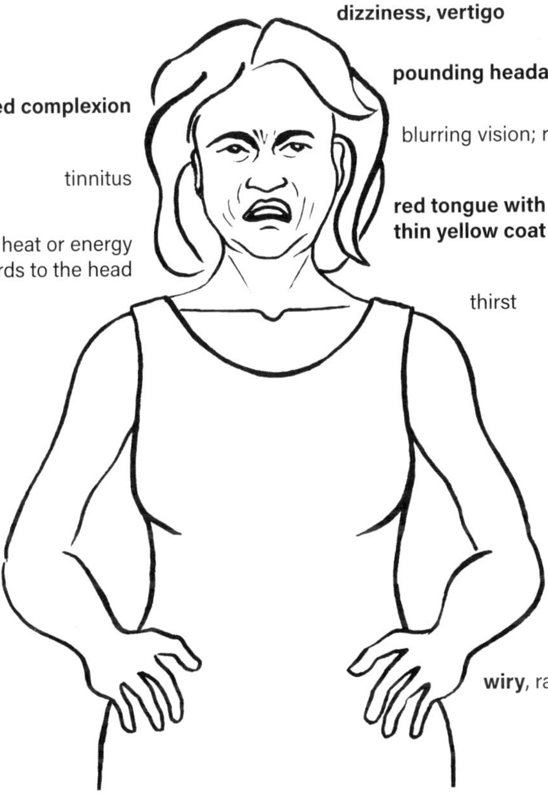

Dosage and method of administration

8-12 pills three times daily on an empty stomach. The dose can be spread out, or taken in two lots of 12-18 pills, morning and evening. In severe cases or during the early stages of treatment (the first few weeks), a 50% increase in dose can be used, then reduced to a maintenance dose as treatment takes effect.

Cautions and contraindications

Contraindicated for patients without ascendant Liver yang, and for patients with dizziness and headaches from blood deficiency.

GMP

15.5 TIAN MA WAN

天麻丸

3+ 12

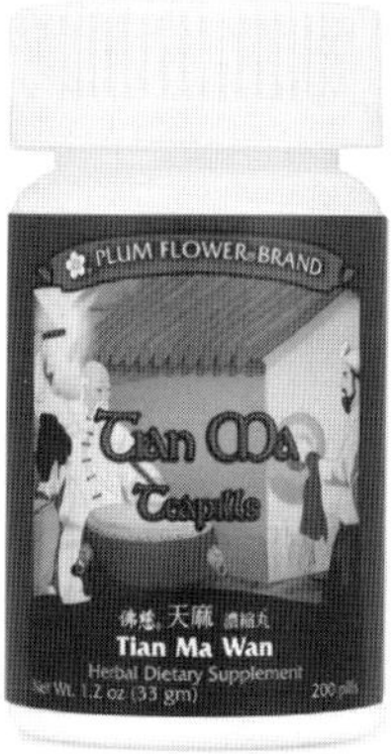

Lanzhou Foci Pharmaceutical Factory (Gansu)
'Gastrodia Pills'
Tian Ma Wan is packaged in bottles of 200 pills

Chinese medical action

Dispels wind cold damp from the channels and opens up qi flow, regulates blood, extinguishes internal wind, pacifies yang, stops pain, tonifies the Liver and Kidneys

Biomedical action

Analgesic, stimulant

INDICATIONS

- Wind damp painful obstruction with underlying Liver and Kidney deficiency. For chronic aching and stiffness in the joints, especially those of the lower back, hips and legs, making walking difficult. A well balanced and thermally neutral formula suitable for older patients with a mix of yin and yang deficiency.
- Post stroke hemiplegia, numbness and spasm of the extremities from residual internal wind with Liver and Kidney deficiency (cf. **5.8 Bu Yang Huan Wu Wan**).
- Mild to moderate high blood pressure from yin deficiency with intermittent ascendant yang. While the formula focuses on tonifying yin to restrain yang, the inclusion of a small proportion of processed aconite assists in 'returning yang to its source' (i.e. the Kidneys) as well as encouraging yang transformation to help rebuild yin and movement of yang qi through the channel network.
- With the appropriate identifying features, this formula can assist in treatment of chronic pain from osteoarthritis and rheumatoid arthritis, sequelae of stroke and hypertension.

Composition

Gastrodia elata (tian ma, gastrodia), *Achyranthes bidentata* (huai niu xi, achyranthes), *Rehmannia glutinosa* (shu di, prepared rehmannia), *Scrophularia ningpoensis* (xuan shen, scrophularia), *Angelica polymorpha* (dang gui, chinese angelica), *Eucommia ulmoides* (du zhong, eucommia), *Dioscorea hypoglauca* (bi xie, fish poison yam), *Angelica pubescens* (du huo, Tu-huo), *Notopterygium incisum* (qiang huo, notopterygium), *Aconitum carmichaeli* (zhi fu zi, processed aconite)

Combine with

- **7.1.1 Liu Wei Di Huang Wan** with pronounced yin deficiency
- **10.38 Plaster for Analgesic and Bruise** for chronic joint pain

Pattern identifying features

- **Liver and Kidney deficiency, wind damp in the channels, ascendant yang**
- **mild to moderate, or intermittent hypertension**
- **sequelae of wind stroke; hemiplegia, poor mobility**
- **weakness; easy fatigue**

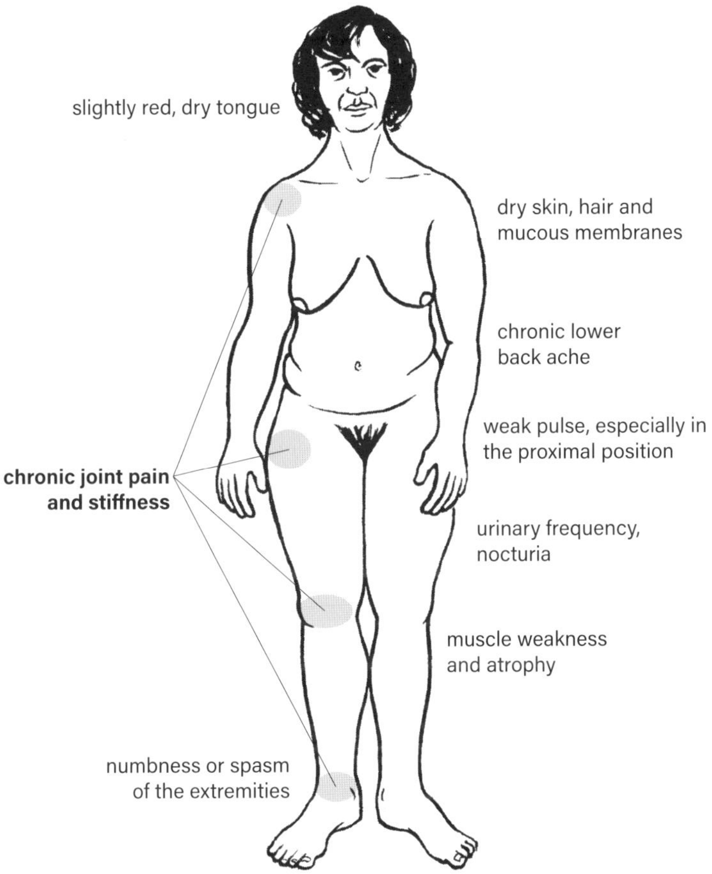

Dosage and method of administration

8-12 pills three times daily, before meals. The dose can be spread out, or taken in two lots of 12-18 pills, morning and evening. In severe cases or during the early stages of treatment (the first two weeks), a 50% increase in dose can be used, then reduced as treatment takes effect.

Cautions and contraindications

Contraindicated during pregnancy.

GMP

15.6 ZHEN GAN XI FENG WAN

镇肝熄风丸

1-3/12

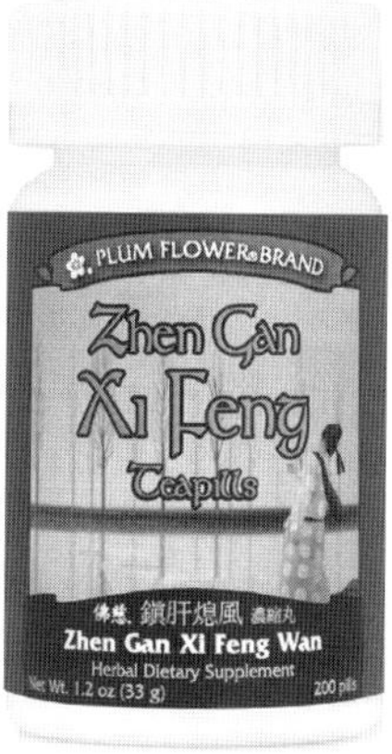

Lanzhou Foci Pharmaceutical Factory (Gansu)
'Pills to Sedate the Liver and Extinguish Wind'
Zhen Gan Xi Feng Wan is packaged in bottles of 200 pills
Also available as: Hematite and Scrophularia Combination (conc. extract)

Chinese medical action

Sedates ascendant Liver yang, regulates qi, extinguishes wind, nourishes Liver and Kidney yin, anchors yang

Biomedical action

Anti-hypertensive, sedative to the nervous system, calmative

INDICATIONS

- Ascendant Liver yang and Liver wind with underlying Liver and Kidney yin deficiency. Used for symptoms of yang excess and internal wind in the upper body, including pain (migraine headache, facial pain), high blood pressure, visual disturbances, vertigo, facial paralysis and hemiplegia. While both the root and branch are addressed, the main strategy of the formula is to swiftly subdue the ascendant yang and extinguish wind.
- With the appropriate identifying features, this formula can assist in the treatment of conditions such as transient ischaemic attacks (TIAs), cerebral arteriosclerosis, cerebrovascular accident, essential hypertension, renal hypertension, arteriosclerosis, vascular and migraine headaches, trigeminal neuralgia, post concussion syndrome, intractable hiccuping, prevention of stroke in patients at risk and post stroke recovery when the patient continues to exhibit signs of ascendant Liver yang (but *see also* **5.8 Bu Yang Huan Wu Wan** for those with qi deficiency and blood stasis sequelae).

Composition

Achyranthes bidentata (niu xi, achyranthes), *Hematitum* (dai zhe shi, hematite), *Chinemys reevesii* (gui ban, turtle shell), *Scrophularia ningpoensis* (xuan shen, scrophularia), *Paeonia lactiflora* (bai shao, white peony), *Asparagus lucidius* (tian dong, asparagus), *Os draconis* (long gu, dragon bone), *Ostrea gigas* (mu li, oyster shell), *Melia toosendan* (chuan lian zi, melia fruit), *Hordeum vulgare* (mai ya, sprouted barley), *Artemesia capillaris* (yin chen, capillaris), *Glycyrrhiza uralensis* (gan cao, licorice)

Combine with

- **15.9 Headache and Dizziness Reliever** to enhance to anti-hypertensive aspects of the formula
- **2.18 Bao He Wan** or **2.17 Jian Pi Wan** to protect the Spleen and Stomach in patients with a tendency to digestive weakness

Pattern identifying features

- **ascendant Liver yang, Liver wind with underlying yin deficiency**
- pre wind stroke conditions, transient ischaemic attacks (TIAs), hypertension
- in severe cases, confusion, disturbances of consciousness or sudden collapse
- maybe weak and sore low back and legs, urinary disturbances, sleeplessness and sweats

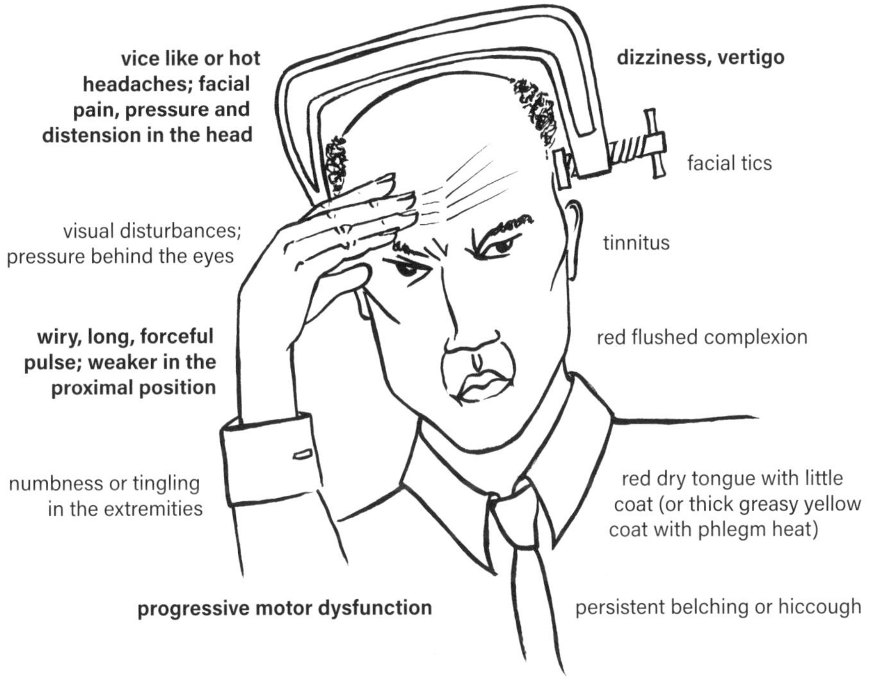

Dosage and method of administration

8-12 pills three times daily on an empty stomach. The dose can be spread out, or taken in two lots of 12-18 pills, morning and evening. In severe cases or during the early stages of treatment (the first few weeks), a 50% increase in dose can be used, then reduced to a maintenance dose as treatment takes effect. Not suitable for prolonged use. Once ascendant yang is better managed, a more yin nourishing strategy should be phased in.

Cautions and contraindications

Contraindicated during pregnancy and in patients without rising yang. The mineral substances can be hard on the Spleen and Stomach, so caution in patients with Spleen qi deficiency.

15.7 YANG YIN JIANG YA WAN

养阴降压丸

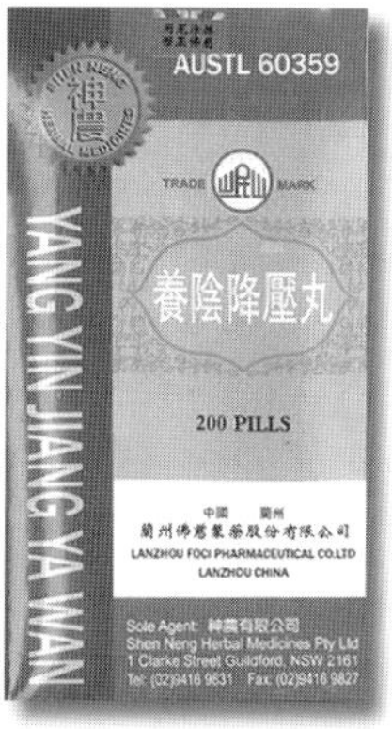

Lanzhou Foci Pharmaceutical Factory (Gansu)
'Yin Nourishing, Blood Pressure Lowering Pills'
Yang Yin Jiang Ya Wan is packaged in bottles of 200 pills

Chinese medical action

Nourishes yin, calms the Liver, restrains and anchors the yang, promotes urination

Biomedical action

Anti-hypertensive, sedative, calmative

INDICATIONS

- Hypertension associated with ascendant Liver yang. This formula is designed specifically for hypertension and contains numerous herbs with well documented anti-hypertensive action.
- Can be used for a variety of symptoms attributed to yang rising patterns, including headaches, dizziness, tinnitus, transient ischaemic attacks, anger outbursts and sore eyes.

Composition (each pill contains powdered)

Polygonatum multiflorum (he shou wu, polygonum root) 21.6mg, *Cassia tora* (jue ming zi, cassia seed) 20.7mg, *Paeonia lactiflora* (bai shao, white peony) 18mg, *Poria cocos* (fu ling, hoelen) 16.2mg, *Eucommia ulmoides* (du zhong, eucommia) 14.4mg, *Alisma orientale* (ze xie, alisma) 14.4mg, *Achyranthes bidentata* (huai niu xi, achyranthes) 12.6mg, *Dendrobium nobile* (shi hu, dendrobium) 12.6mg, *Uncaria rhyncophylla* (gou teng, gambir) 9mg; and extracts equivalent to dry: *Zea mays* (yu mi xu, corn silk) 109mg, *Polygonatum sibirica* (yuan zhi, polygala) 76.4mg, *Chysanthemum sinensis* (ju hua, chrysanthemum flower) 54.6mg

Combine with

- **6.6 Long Dan Xie Gan Wan** for heat in the Liver
- **7.2.2 Qi Ju Di Huang Wan** for significant yin deficiency

Dosage and method of administration

8-12 pills three times daily, before meals. The dose can be spread out, or taken in two lots of 12-18 pills, morning and evening. In severe cases or during the early stages of treatment (the first two weeks), a 50% increase in dose can be used, then reduced as treatment takes effect.

Pattern identifying features

- **ascendant Liver yang**
- **hypertension**

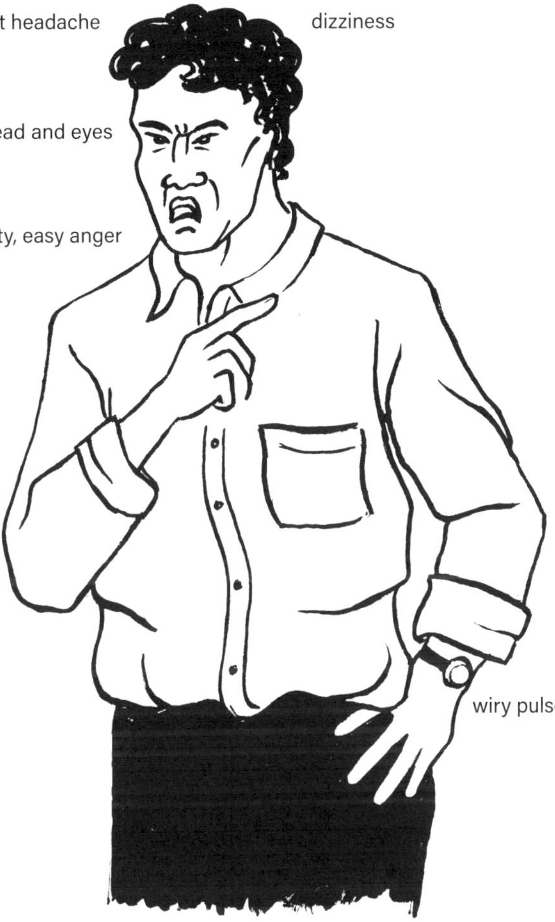

Cautions and contraindications

Contraindicated in patients without rising yang and with dizziness and headaches from blood deficiency.

15.8 FU FANG JIANG YA CAPSULE

复方降压丸

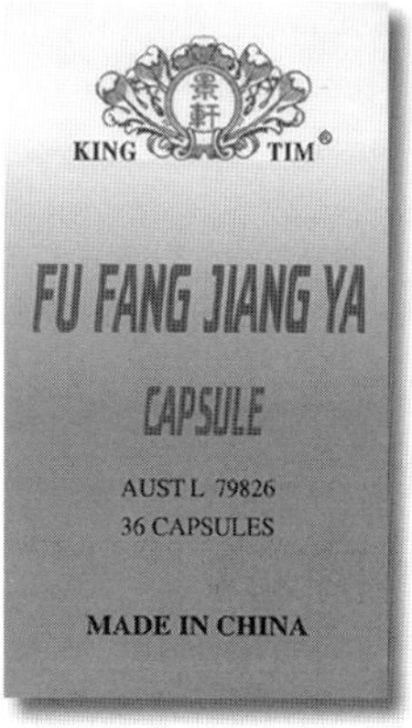

(*Fu Fang Jiang Ya Wan*)
Jing Xian Pharmaceutical Co. (Guangzhou)
'Compound Anti-hypertensive Pills'
Fu Fang Jiang Ya Capsules are packaged in bottles of 36 capsules

Chinese medical action

Calms the Liver and *shén*, extinguishes wind, restrains yang, promotes urination

Biomedical action

Antihypertensive, diuretic, sedative

INDICATIONS

- Hypertension associated with ascendant Liver yang or Liver wind patterns. Similar to **15.7 Yang Yin Jiang Ya Wan**, with a focus on herbs with a known anti-hypertensive effect. Although this formula is best for hypertension associated with Liver yang or Liver wind, it is broad enough to be useful in any type of hypertension when combined with an appropriate constitutional formula.

Composition (each capsule contains extracts equivalent to dry)

Alisma orientale (ze xie, alisma) 378mg, *Crategus pinnatifida* (shan zha, crategus) 378mg, *Prunella vulgaris* (xia ku cao, prunella) 378mg, *Chysanthemum sinensis* (ju hua, chrysanthemum flower) 315mg, *Uncaria rhyncophylla* (gou teng, gambir) 315mg, *Eucommia ulmoides* (du zhong, eucommia) 252mg, *Achyranthes bidentata* (huai niu xi, achyranthes) 252mg, *Ostrea gigas* (mu li, oyster shell) 54mg

Dosage and method of administration

3-4 capsules, three times daily on an empty stomach.

Cautions and contraindications

Contraindicated in patients without rising yang and with dizziness and headaches from blood deficiency. Caution during pregnancy.

15.9 HEADACHE AND DIZZINESS RELIEVER

愈风宁心片

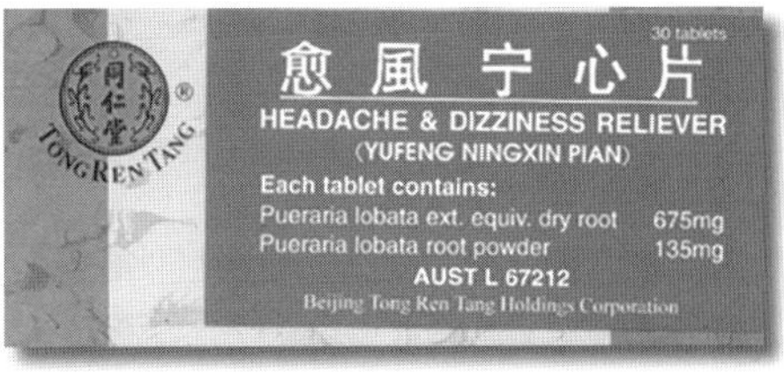

(*Yu Feng Ning Xin Pian*)
Tong Ren Tang (Beijing)
'Cure Wind and Calm the Heart Pills'
Headache and Dizziness Reliever is packaged in boxes of 30 blister packed tablets

Chinese medical action

Dispels wind heat, generates fluids, stops thirst, alleviates diarrhea, eases the muscles

Biomedical action

Anti-hypertensive, diaphoretic, antispasmodic

INDICATIONS

- Temporary relief of stiff neck and shoulders, headaches, dizziness and paresthesia associated with external pathogenic invasion, hypertension or ascendant Liver yang.
- Diarrhea. Can be used for a variety of types of diarrhea and dysenteric disorder, depending on the formula with which it is combined.
- Recently researched for effects on reducing craving for alcohol. May be useful as an adjunct treatment for patients recovering from alcohol addiction.

Composition (each tablet contains)

Pueraria lobata (ge gen, pueraria) 810mg

Combine with

– **14.1 Huang Lian Jie Du Wan** or **14.2 Huang Lian Su Tablets** for acute damp heat diarrhea

Dosage and method of administration

5 tablets three times daily, on an empty stomach. In severe cases or during the early stages of treatment (the first two weeks), a 50% increase in dose can be used, then reduced as treatment takes effect.

Cautions and contraindications

None noted.

Potential Herb Drug Interactions

Many, if not most, patients presenting in Chinese medicine clinics are taking one or more therapeutic substances of some description. These substances may include pharmaceuticals, herbal remedies, vitamins and minerals, either professionally prescribed or purchased over the counter. When wishing to prescribe a Chinese herbal formula, it is essential to have some idea of the potential for herb-drug or herb-herb interactions. In some cases, the patients existing medications will preclude the use of certain formulae, or warrant special monitoring of the patient when additional medications are prescribed.

Interaction refers to the possibility that one substance may alter the effectiveness or availability of another substance. The information following is based on both known interactions, and theoretical interactions based on an understanding of the pharmacology of the substances involved.

Drug	Herb	Mechanism	Interaction	Advice
Antiplatelet and anticoagulant drugs (Warfarin, Aspirin, Heparin	*Salvia miltiorrhizae* (dan shen[1])	components may inhibit platelet aggregation	increased prothrombin time and INR[3], increased tendency to bleed	Avoid concurrent use or monitor for bruising and bleeding and stop herb if increased. Have INR values monitored during initial therapy until stabilized, then routinely thereafter
	Angelica sinensis (dang gui[2])	unknown		
	Panax ginseng (ren shen)	unknown	may decrease the effectiveness of warfarin, decreased INR	
	Gingko biloba (yin xing)	ginkoside B may inhibit platelet activating factor		

1. Common and well documented
2. Uncommon
3. International Normalisation Ratio: A corrected measure of prothrombin time (the time it takes blood to clot) established against a pre-medication baseline. Usual values are in the range of 2-4.5 over baseline

Potassium retaining diuretics (Aldactone, Spironolactone)	*Glycyrrhiza uralensis* (gan cao)	glycyrrhizic acid prevents conversion of deoxycorticosterone into active glucocorticoids, cortisol and corticosterone	Na+ retention, K+ loss, edema, hypertension	avoid concurrent use
Potassium losing diuretics, loop diuretics (Lasix)	*Glycyrrhiza uralensis* (gan cao) *Desmodium styracifolium (jin qian cao)*	aggravate K+ loss	hypokalemia, numbness, muscle weakness, cramps, palpitations	monitor patient carefully or avoid concurrent use
Theophylline	Ephedra sinica (ma huang)	ephedrine can cause stimulation	increases sympathetic and stimulatory effects, insomnia, tachycardia, tremor	monitor changes in blood pressure, heart rate, insomnia, tremor and headache or avoid concurrent use
Decongestants (Actifed, Sudafed)	*Ephedra sinica* (ma huang)	aggregate action with pseudoephedrine		
Hypoglycemic agents (Insulin, Glyburide, Tolbutamide, Metformin)	*Glycyrrhiza uralensis* (gan cao)	glycyrrhizic acid prevents conversion of deoxycorticosterone	reduced hypoglycemic action	avoid concurrent use
	Panax ginseng (ren shen)	unknown	decreased blood glucose levels	monitor blood glucose levels, watch for signs of hypoglcemia
Antihypertensive agents(beta blockers)	*Ephedra sinica* (ma huang)	ephedrine may oppose the effects of beta blockers	hypertension	monitor changes in blood pressure and heart rate or avoid concurrent use
	Glycyrrhiza uralensis (gan cao)	increase Na+ and water retention	counter the effects of medication and increased blood pressure	

Chloramphenicol	*Artemesia scoparia* (yin chen hao)	antagonize each other	reduced efficacy	allow some time between administration
Codeine	Prunus persica (xing ren) *Gingko biloba* (yin xing)	amygdaline suppresses the respiratory center	respiratory center depression	avoid concurrent use
Corticosteroids	*Glycyrrhiza uralensis* (gan cao)	glycyrrhizic acid prevents conversion of deoxycorticosterone into active glucocorticoids, cortisol and corticosterone	potentiation of both oral and topical steroids	monitor use carefully
Cardiac glycosides (Digoxin, Lanoxin)	*Panax ginseng* (ren shen)	unknown	may falsely elevate digoxin levels; difficulty in monitoring drug response	avoid concurrent use
	Aconite spp. (fu zi, wu tou, chuan wu)	additive effects of aconitine		avoid concurrent use
	Glycyrrhiza uralensis (gan cao)	deoxycorticosterone like action causes retention of Na+, loss of K+ and increases cardiac muscle sensitivity to digoxin		avoid long term concurrent use

MAO inhibitors (Phenelzine, Nardil)	*Ephedra sinica* (ma huang)	ephedrine can cause stimulation	increases sympathetic and stimulatory effects, insomnia, tachycardia, tremor	monitor changes in blood pressure, heart rate, insomnia, tremor and headache or avoid concurrent use
	Panax ginseng (ren shen)	inhibits cAMP phosphodieserase activity	increases psychoactive stimulation and may induce mania in depressed patients	avoid concurrent use
Immunosuppressive drugs (Cyclosporine, Azathioprine)	*Astragalus membranaceous* (huang qi)	stimulates T cell activity	decreases immunosuppressive effect	avoid concurrent use
Interferon	6.1 Xiao Chai Hu Tang Wan (formula)	unknown	may induce interstitial pneumonitis in susceptible patients	avoid concurrent use
Osmotic laxatives, bulking agents (psyllium)	all herbs	binding of herbs in insoluble matrix, increases transit time	active ingredients carried out through the bowel	allow some time between administration
Niacin (vitamin B6)	warming herbs and yang tonics	compounds heat	can cause patient to overheat	avoid concurrent use

Comparison between selected medicines

ACUTE COMMON COLD AND INFECTION	
3.1.1 Yin Chiao Chieh Tu Pien	Formula of choice for wind heat common cold patterns, especially those characterized by sore throat or acute itchy skin rashes
3.2 Gan Mao Zhi Ke Chong Ji	For cough or wind heat type common cold that has been dragging on for a few days, or has begun to creep into the *shào yáng* level
3.3 Sang Ju Wan	Mild or early stage wind heat type common cold with cough
3.4 Gan Mao Ling	A general medicine for non specific common cold from wind invasion. Although it leans towards wind heat, it can be used for non specific colds and flu, or those that are vague and without any clear heat or cold tendency
3.5 Ma Huang Wan	Wind cold type common cold with wheezing and dyspnea, absence of sweating and cough. The classical formula for 'exterior excess', that is, tightly locked pores preventing the cold pathogen from being expelled
3. 6 Gui Zhi Wan	Wind invasion type common cold with exterior deficiency, that is, weak defensive qi that allows the lingering presence of an invading pathogen
3.8 Xiao Qing Long Wan	Wind cold type common cold with watery sputum causing productive cough, wheezing and dyspnea or runny nose and sinuses. Also used for acute hay fever
3.9 Chuan Xiong Cha Tiao Wan	Wind cold type common cold, especially when headache is a major features. Also used for headaches and facial pain triggered by exposure to cold or sudden temperature change
3.10 Jing Fang Bai Du Wan	Wind cold damp type common cold, or wind cold common cold that is beginning to transform into heat
3.11 Ge Gen Wan	Wind cold type common cold with neck and upper back stiffness and pain
3.12 Gan Mao Qing Re Chong Ji	Wind cold type common cold with muscle aches as a prominent feature. Good for those who find pills hard to take

ACUTE COMMON COLD AND INFECTION (cont.)	
2.1 Xing Jun San	A powerful and fragrant powder for acute summerdamp invasion and gastric upsets with nausea and vomiting. Strong tasting and fast acting
2.2.1 Huo Hsiang Cheng Chi Pien	Similar to 2.1 Xing Jun San but not as strong. Also for wind cold type common cold with internal damp and for lingering or hidden damp patterns of the Spleen and Stomach
2.4 Fu Ke An 2.5 Bao Ji Pills 2.6 Po Chai Pills	Acute damp heat invasion of the Intestines causing diarrhea. These medicines, while different in composition, are quite similar in effect
2.13 Li Zhong Wan	While not usually considered for acute exterior disorders, this medicine can be used for acute patterns of vomiting and diarrhea from cold invasion into *tài yīn*
9.3 Peking Niu Huang Jie Du Pian	Acute wind and toxic heat patterns of the upper body, including superficial infections, sore throat, conjunctivitis, abscess and otitis
9.5 Pu Ji Xiao Du Wan	Toxic heat in the head and throat; tonsillitis, strep throat, erysipelas
9.6 Ban Lan Gen Chong Ji	Popular as treatment and preventative for acute wind heat and toxic heat patterns, especially sore throat
14.5 Chuan Xin Lian Antiphlogistic Tablets	A good all round antibiotic and antiviral agent for a range of acute exterior disorders and infectious processes. Especially good for infection of the throat and intestines
14.9 Bai Hu Wan	Acute heat in *yáng míng* channels. This pattern is often quite severe and may equate to biomedical conditions such as encephalitis, meningitis and pncumonia
14.10 Liang Ge Wan	Acute heat in *tài yáng* and *yáng míng* organs. This pattern is similar to that in 14.9 Bai Hu Wan, with the added complication of constipation

QI CONSTRAINT AND QI STAGNATION	
6.2 Si Ni Wan	The base formula for Liver qi constraint and the fundamental unit from which all other Liver qi regulating formulas are built. Good added to another constitutional medicine when a degree of qi regulating activity is required
6.3 Chai Hu Shu Gan Wan	Similar to 6.2 Si Ni Wan with additional qi regulating herbs. Especially good for Liver Spleen disharmony, this formula has no tonic activity and is best for qi constraint patterns without deficiency. Most commonly used in young, robust, stressed individuals
2.24 Shu Gan Wan	Strong qi moving formula with a focus on pain, especially hypochondriac, epigastric and abdominal
6.3 Xiao Yao Wan	Liver qi constraint with Spleen weakness and blood deficiency. A good all round and gentle qi moving formula suitable for long term use. Particularly good for Liver qi constraint patterns in women causing menstrual disorders and premenstrual syndrome
6.4 Jia Wei Xiao Yao Wan	Similar to 6.3 Xiao Yao Wan with the addition of cooling herbs to clear heat generated by chronic qi constraint
6.8 Yi Guan Jian Wan	Liver qi constraint with Liver yin deficiency
2.25 Tong Xie Yao Fang Wan	Liver qi invading the Spleen causing diarrhea preceded by spasmodic abdominal pain. An important formula for irritable bowel syndrome
8.7 An Shen Jie Yu Capsule	Liver qi constraint causing shen disturbances and sleep disorders
2.10 Xiang Sha Yang Wei Wan	Middle burner qi and damp stagnation. Good for upper abdominal qi stagnation causing distension, epigastric discomfort, heartburn, reflux and belching
2.29 Mu Xiang Shun Qi Wan	Middle burner qi stagnation, with disruption of the qi dynamic causing abdominal distension and constipation

BLOOD STASIS	
5.1 Xue Fu Zhu Yu Wan	Qi and blood stasis. All purpose blood stasis dispelling formula. Particularly good for blood stasis complicated by, or resulting from Liver qi constraint. Best for blood stasis patterns of the upper body, chest and head
1.18 Shao Fu Zhu Yu Wan	Blood stasis and cold in the lower burner. Used for gynecological and urogenital pain, and masses in the pelvic basin
6.12 Ge Xia Zhu Yu Wan	Blood stasis masses. The strongest of the Zhu Yu formulas, designed for abdominal masses, especially those below the diaphragm, i.e. swelling and pathology of the liver and spleen
10.12 Shen Tong Zhu Yu Wan	Blood stasis pain disorders. A powerful blood moving formula for chronic pain and stiffness patterns in the joints and muscles. Used for chronic arthritis and fibromyalgia
9.2 Tong Qiao Huo Xue Wan	Blood stasis in the head, affecting the sense organs; post traumatic memory problems; post concussion syndrome
5.2 Dan Shen Pill	Blood stasis affecting the Heart. For angina and chest pain
5.3 Dan Shen Wan	Blood stasis affecting the Heart, chest or Stomach
5.7 Sunho Multi Ginseng Tablets	Mild blood stasis in the chest, stomach and periphery. Lowers cholesterol
5.4 Xin Mai Ling	Blood stasis affecting the Heart and periphery. For angina and peripheral vascular disease
1.16 Tao Hong Si Wu Wan	Blood stasis with blood deficiency. Especially good for gynecological disorders. Good for prolonged use
1.15 Tong Jing Wan	Relatively severe blood stasis in the uterus causing dysmenorrhea
1.17 Gui Zhi Fu Ling Wan	Mild blood stasis patterns or the uterus, genitourinary system and pelvic basin with small benign masses. Suitable for prolonged use
1.13 Woo Garm Yuen Medical Pills	Relatively severe cold accumulation and blood stasis in the uterus and pelvic basin with a degree of qi and blood deficiency
1.14 Wen Jing Wan	Blood stasis and cold in the Uterus with deficiency of qi, blood and yang

BLOOD STASIS (cont.)	
10.21 Yan Hu Suo Wan	General analgesic formula for all types of pain from qi and blood stasis
1.12 Shi Xiao Wan	Simple formula for blood stasis pain, especially of the Stomach and Uterus. Usually added to another formula to enhance the analgesic effect
5.8 Bu Yang Huan Wu Wan	Blood stasis and qi deficiency type hemiplegia and paralysis. Used in peripheral neuropathy and following wind-stroke
5.9 Dang Gui Si Ni Wan	Blood stasis and cold in the channels of the periphery and extremities causing numbness, cold and pain
10.1 Yun Nan Bai Yao	Blood stasis with bleeding
10.2 Raw Tienchi Tablets	Blood stasis with bleeding; blood stasis in the cardiovascular and hepatic systems; lowers blood cholesterol
10.3 Die Da Zhi Tong Capsule	Acute traumatic blood stasis with bruising and pain
10.4 Chin Gu Tie Shang Wan	Acute traumatic blood stasis with bruising and pain. Assists in accelerating slow healing of fractures
10.5 Huo Luo Xiao Ling Wan	Traumatic blood stasis; blood stasis pain, skin disease and inflammatory masses
10.11 Shu Jin Huo Xue Wan	Chronic painful obstruction with blood stasis causing joint and muscle pain and stiffness
10.23 Zheng Gu Shui	Topical application for acute traumatic blood stasis with bruising and pain. Assists in healing of bone fractures
10.38 Plaster for Bruise and Analgesic	Similar to 10.23 Zheng Gu Shui on a sticky plaster. Good for overnight use
11.1 Qian Lie Xian Capsule 11.2 Prostate Gland Pills	Blood stasis and damp heat accumulation in the prostate gland. For chronic prostatitis
11.3 Ji Sheng Ju He Wan	Blood stasis and phlegm masses in the testicles
11.8 Kang Wei Ling Wan	Erectile dysfunction from blood stasis. Combines a powerful blood invigorating substance with qi, blood and yang tonics to assist in moving blood in the penis
12.11 Dan Shen Huo Xue Wan	Blood stasis with heat in the blood type chronic skin disorders

DAMPNESS AND PHLEGM	
2.1 Xing Jun San	A powerful and fragrant powder for acute gastrointestinal summerdamp with nausea and vomiting
2.2 Huo Hsiang Cheng Chi Pien	Similar to 2.1 Xing Jun San but not as strong. Also for wind cold type common cold with internal damp and for lingering or hidden damp patterns of the Spleen and Stomach
2.22 Er Chen Wan	The base formula for phlegm damp and the fundamental unit from which all phlegm transforming formulas are built. Good added to an appropriate constitutional formula when a degree of phlegm transformation is desired. Used for phlegm anywhere in the body, but especially good for phlegm in the Lung system and nausea
2.23 Ping Wei San	Cold damp accumulation in the Spleen and Stomach
3.7 Su Zi Jiang Qi Wan	Wheezing, cough and asthma from thin phlegm accumulation in the Lungs
3.8 Xiao Qing Long Wan	Wheezing, cough and hay fever from wind cold type common cold with accumulation of thin phlegm in the Lungs
3.21 She Dan Chuan Bei Ye	Phlegm accumulation in the Lungs. Good for resolving residual and persistent phlegm in the aftermath of an upper respiratory tract infection
3.22 Orange Peel Powder	Phlegm accumulation in the Lungs
4.5 Bi Xie Fen Qing Wan	Damp accumulation in the lower burner and reproductive system causing discharge and vesicular eruptions
1.33 Ru Jie Xiao Tablets	Phlegm and qi constraint type breast lumps
1.34 Hai Zao Jing Wan	Phlegm type swellings, masses and nodules
1.35 Nei Xiao Luo Li Wan	Hard phlegm type masses, lumps and nodules
11.3 Ji Sheng Ju He Wan	Cold damp, phlegm and blood stasis masses in the testicles
6.10 Qing Gan Li Dan Tablets	Damp with mild heat in the Liver and Gallbladder causing sludge accumulation and gall stones
8.10 Cerebral Tonic Pills	Phlegm in the head, misting the senses and mind
8.11 Jian Nao Yi Zhi Capsule	Phlegm in the head causing poor memory and concentration
9.12 Ban Xia Hou Po Wan	Phlegm and qi constraint in the throat; 'plum pit qi'

DAMPNESS AND PHLEGM (cont.)	
9.18 Xin Yi San	Phlegm damp accumulating in the sinuses
10.8 Xiao Huo Luo Dan	Severe cold damp accumulation in the joints
12.1 Bo Ying Compound	Phlegm accumulation in infants, accumulation disorder
13.2 Xiao Feng Wan	Damp and wind accumulation in the skin
13.5 Shi Du Qing Capsule	Damp accumulation in the skin causing intense itching and weeping rashes
13.15 Tujin Liniment	Damp accumulation between the toes
15.3 Ban Xia Bai Zhu Tian Ma Wan	Wind phlegm in the head causing vertigo, nausea and tinnitus
2.8 Liu Jun Zi Wan	Spleen qi deficiency with phlegm damp
2.9 Xiang Sha Liu Jun Wan	Spleen qi deficiency with phlegm damp and qi stagnation disrupting the qi dynamic
2.12 Shen Ling Bai Zhu Wan	Spleen qi deficiency with damp pouring downwards as diarrhea

DAMP HEAT, PHLEGM HEAT, TOXIC HEAT, FIRE	
2.4 Fu Ke An 2.5 Bao Ji Pills 2.6 Po Chai Pills	Acute damp heat invasion of the Intestines causing diarrhea. These medicines, while different in composition, are quite similar in effect
14.1 Huang Lian Jie Du Wan	General formula for systemic or focal damp or toxic heat patterns. Also for heat in the blood
14.5 Chuan Xin Lian Antiphlogistic Tablets	All round antibiotic and antiviral agent for a range of acute infectious disorders. Especially good for infection of the throat and intestines
14.6 Fu Fang Nan Ban Lan Gen	Toxic heat and hot blood patterns with sores and boils, skin disorders, purpura and acute infections
14.8 Wu Wei Xiao Du Wan	Toxic heat in the skin causing deep rooted boils and sores, as well as infections such as mastitis, appendicitis and tonsillitis
13.1 Lien Chiao Pai Tu Pien	Wind heat and toxic heat type skin disorders
9.6 Ban Lan Gen Chong Ji	Popular both as treatment and preventative for acute wind heat and toxic heat patterns, especially sore throat
9.5 Pu Ji Xiao Du Wan	Toxic heat in the head and throat; tonsillitis, strep throat, erysipelas
9.3 Peking Niu Huang Jie Du Pian	Acute toxic heat patterns of the upper body, mouth and throat, including superficial infections, sore throat, conjunctivitis, abscess and otitis
9.4 Huang Lien Shang Qing Pien	Toxic heat patterns of the upper body, mouth skin and throat, including superficial infections, sore throat, conjunctivitis, abscess and otitis
6.6 Long Dan Xie Gan Wan	Damp heat or fire in the Liver system
6.7 Da Chai Hu Wan	Damp heat in the Liver and Gallbladder systems; *shào yáng – yáng míng* syndrome
6.11 Lidan Tablets	Acute or chronic damp heat in the Liver and Gallbladder systems. Used for acute and chronic cholecystitis and hepatitis
1.36 Fu Yan Qing Tablets	Damp heat in the reproductive system and genitals
1.37 Bi Xie Sheng Shi Wan	Damp heat in the reproductive system, genitals and skin
1.38 Yu Dai Wan	Damp heat in the reproductive system with underlying blood deficiency

DAMP HEAT, PHLEGM HEAT, TOXIC HEAT, FIRE (cont.)	
1.39 Chien Chin Chih Tai Wan	Chronic damp heat in the reproductive system with Kidney deficiency
2.29 Mu Xiang Shun Qi Wan	Chronic damp heat dysenteric disorder
3.15 Qing Qi Hua Tan Wan	Acute and chronic phlegm heat in the Lungs
3.16 Ching Fei Yi Huo Pien	Acute Lung fire
3.19 Ding Chuan Wan	Phlegm heat in the Lungs causing wheezing
4.6 Ba Zheng San Wan	Acute damp heat in the Bladder causing dysuria and urinary tract infection
4.8 Tao Chih Pien	Heart fire invading the Small Intestine type dysuria
8.8 Wen Dan Wan	Phlegm heat affecting the Heart and *shén*, systemic phlegm heat, post febrile phlegm heat
8.9 Chai Hu Long Gu Mu Li Wan	Phlegm Heat and Liver fire type *shén* disturbances; withdrawal from drugs of addiction; mania; palpitations
9.8 Qing Wei San Wan	Heat in the Stomach causing oral and gingival inflammation
9.14 Bi Ye Ning Capsule	Phlegm heat in the sinuses
9.19 Cang Er Zi Wan	Wind heat and phlegm heat in the sinuses
9.21 Ming Mu Shang Ching Pien	Fire type eye disorders; also used for damp heat in the Bladder causing dysuria or hematuria
10.9 Xuan Bi Tang Wan 10.10 Guan Jie Yan Wan	Damp heat in the joints
11.1 Qian Lie Xian Capsule 11.2 Prostate Gland Pills	Damp heat and blood stasis in the prostate gland; chronic prostatitis
12.2 King Fung Powder	Phlegm heat infantile fever and convulsions
13.4 Ke Yin Wan	Stubborn damp heat in the skin
13.10 Zhen Zhu An Chuang Tablets	Toxic heat and damp heat type acne
13.12 Chuan Xin Lian Cream	Topical ointment for toxic heat and damp heat type skin lesions
15.1 Po Lung Yuen Medical Pills	Phlegm heat and wind type tics, tremors and seizures; febrile convulsions
15.2 Niu Huang Qing Xin Wan	Phlegm heat and wind type movement disorders and post stroke syndrome

DEFICIENCY - QI	
2.7 Si Jun Zi Wan	The base formula for Spleen and systemic qi deficiency, and the fundamental unit from which all other qi tonic formulas are built. Can be added to any other constitutional formula when a degree of qi tonification is desired
2.8 Liu Jun Zi Wan	Spleen qi deficiency with phlegm damp
2.9 Xiang Sha Liu Jun Wan	Spleen qi deficiency with phlegm damp and qi stagnation disrupting the qi dynamic
2.11 Bu Zhong Yi Qi Wan	Spleen qi deficiency with sinking qi. An important formula for prolapse, defensive qi deficiency, sweating disorders and immune weakness
2.12 Shen Ling Bai Zhu Wan	Spleen qi deficiency with damp pouring downwards as diarrhea
2.16 Zi Sheng Wan	Spleen qi deficiency with food stagnation, and chronic dysenteric disorder with diarrhea and food sensitivities
2.17 Jian Pi Wan	Spleen qi deficiency with food stagnation
3.38 Sheng Mai San Wan	Lung and Spleen qi and yin deficiency chronic respiratory problems and post febrile weakness
3.40 Bu Fei Wan	Lung qi and defensive qi deficiency chronic respiratory problems
3.41 Xu Han Ting	Defensive qi deficiency type spontaneous sweating
4.12 San Yuen Medical Pills	Kidney qi deficiency urinary dysfunction
7.22 Shen Qi Da Bu Wan	Spleen and defensive qi deficiency. Can be added to any other constitutional formula when a degree of qi tonification is desired
7.23 Yu Ping Feng Wan	Defensive qi deficiency type spontaneous sweating and weakness; immune weakness, frequent colds; allergies
7.24 Panax Ginseng Extractum	Lung and Spleen qi deficiency

DEFICIENCY - QI AND BLOOD	
1.1 Ba Zhen Wan	The fundamental qi and blood tonic formula; for all qi and blood deficiency patterns
1.3 Ba Zhen Yi Mu Wan	Similar to 1.1 Ba Zhen Wan with the addition of the mild blood regulating action of motherwort. Good for qi and blood deficiency with mild blood stasis
7.16.1 Shi Quan Da Bu Wan	Similar to 1.1 Ba Zhen Wan with the addition of the warming herbs. For qi and blood deficiency with cold, and chronic non healing ulcers and sores
1.31 Tangkwei Essence of Chicken	Powerful qi and blood tonic with black boned chicken for extra richness. Excellent for insufficient lactation, anemia, fatigue, convalescence and postpartum recovery
1.6 Bai Feng Wan	A general qi and blood tonic with black boned chicken for extra richness. Excellent for anemia and fatigue during pregnancy
1.7 Wu Ji Bai Feng Wan	Similar to 1.6 Bai Feng Wan with the addition of the yang and blood enriching deer horn for extra warmth and yang tonification
1.8 Tong Ren Wu Ji Bai Feng Wan	Similar to 1.6 Bai Feng Wan with the addition herbs to clear heat from deficiency. For heat symptoms such as flushing and sweats following childbirth
1.9 Gui Pi Wan	Spleen qi and Heart blood deficiency type bleeding, weakness and fatigue, *shén* disturbances and menstrual disorders
1.10 Dang Gui Jing	Similar to 1.1 Ba Zhen Wan in liquid extract
1.19 Yang Rong Wan	Qi and blood deficiency with Kidney yang deficiency type menstrual disorders and infertility
1.32 Shih San Tai Pao Wan	Qi and blood deficiency during pregnancy and for wind cold type common cold in patients with qi and blood deficiency
5.5 Zhi Gan Cao Wan	Heart qi and blood deficiency arrhythmias
7.6 Yang Xue Sheng Fa Capsule 7.7 Qi Bao Mei Ran Dan	Qi and blood deficiency and Liver and Kidney deficiency type alopecia and hair disorders
7.18 Yang Ying Wan	Similar to 7.16.1 Shi Quan Da Bu Wan with the addition of herbs to calm the Heart and *shén*
7.26 Reishi Mushroom	Immune enhancing and regulating herb for allergic, auto-immune and neoplastic disorders

8.3 An Shen Ding Zhi Wan	Qi and blood deficiency *shén* disturbances
8.6 Suan Zao Ren Tang Pian	Liver blood and yin deficiency *shén* disturbances. Also useful for night sweats from the same etiology
1.2 Si Wu Wan	The fundamental blood tonic formula, and the base unit from which all blood tonics are built. Good for combining with a constitutional formula when an enhanced degree of blood tonification is desired
13.3 Dang Gui Yin Zi Wan	Blood deficiency with wind in the skin
DEFICIENCY - YIN	
7.1.1 Liu Wei Di Huang Wan	Kidney yin deficiency. The base formula for all Kidney deficiency patterns. Wide application in general Kidney yin deficiency patterns and as a preventative for those at risk of yin depletion
1.23 Zhi Bai Di Huang Wan	Kidney yin deficiency with heat causing flushing, night sweats and low grade fever. Also for Kidney yin deficiency with chronic damp heat in the lower burner. A variation of 7.1.1 Liu Wei Di Huang Wan
7.2.2 Qi Ju Di Huang Wan	Kidney and Liver yin deficiency. A variation of 7.1.1 Liu Wei Di Huang Wan used for a wide variety of problems including dizziness, headaches and eye disorders
9.22 Ming Mu Di Huang Wan	Lung and Kidney yin deficiency chronic visual and eye disorders. A variation of 7.1.1 Liu Wei Di Huang Wan
3.35 Mai Wei Di Huang Wan	Lung and Kidney yin deficiency chronic respiratory disorders. A variation of 7.1.1 Liu Wei Di Huang Wan
9.1 Er Long Zuo Ci Wan	Liver and Kidney yin deficiency ear and hearing problems. A variation of 7.1.1 Liu Wei Di Huang Wan
7. 3 Zuo Gui Wan	Similar to 7.1.1 Liu Wei Di Huang Wan, without the draining components and with extra tonic herbs. More tonifying to yin generally
1.25 Er Xian Wan	Kidney yin and yang deficiency with heat, flushing and night sweats. An important formula for the symptoms of menopause
2.35 Yu Quan Wan	Spleen, Stomach and Kidney yin and qi deficiency. Used to assist in the treatment of type 2 diabetes
3.33 Yang Yin Qing Fei Wan	Lung and Kidney yin deficiency and dryness chronic throat and respiratory disorders

DEFICIENCY - YIN (cont.)	
3.34 Bai He Gu Jin Wan	Lung and Kidney yin deficiency chronic respiratory disorders; hemoptysis
3.38 Sheng Mai San Wan	Lung qi and yin deficiency chronic respiratory disorders; wheezing
5.5 Zhi Gan Cao Wan	Heart yin, qi and blood deficiency arrhythmias
6.8 Yin Guan Jian Wan	Liver yin deficiency with qi constraint. Good for chronic reflux and upper abdominal pain patterns
7.4 Da Bu Yin Wan	Kidney yin deficiency with bone steaming fever and chronic consumptive disorders
7.5 Gu Ben Wan	Lung, Stomach and Kidney yin deficiency with dryness and insufficient fluids
8.1 Tian Wang Bu Xin Dan	Heart and Kidney yin deficiency; also known as Heart and Kidney not communicating; chronic *shén* disturbances, insomnia, palpitations, anxiety
8.2 Bai Zi Yang Xin Wan	Yin and blood deficiency *shén* disturbances
8.4 An Shen Bu Xin Wan	Heart yin and blood deficiency with rising yang type *shén* and *hún* disturbances
8.6 Suan Zao Ren Tang Pian	Liver yin and blood deficiency *shén* disturbances. Also useful for night sweats from the same etiology
15.5 Tian Ma Wan	Liver yin deficiency with ascendant Liver yang type headaches, hypertension, dizziness and tinnitus
15.6 Zhen Gan Xi xsFeng Wan	Yin deficiency with ascendant yang type headaches, hypertension, transient ischaemic attacks, dizziness and tinnitus
DEFICIENCY - YANG	
7.9 Fu Gui Ba Wei Wan	The base formula for warming and tonifying Kidney yang. Widely applicable for all Kidney yang deficiency patterns
7.10 You Gui Wan	Tonifies and warms Kidney yang and essence
1.20 Cu Yun Yu Tai Wan 1.21 Tiao Jing Cu Yun Wan	Warms Kidney yang for infertility and menstrual disorders; weak progesterone phase and anovulation disorders
2.13 Li Zhong Wan	Spleen yang deficiency
2.14 Li Chung Yuen Medical Pills	Spleen yang deficiency. Very warming formula for relatively severe cold and very weak digestion
2.15 Xiao Jian Zhong Wan	Spleen yang deficiency with abdominal pain and yang deficiency type low grade fever

3.39 Yulin Bu Shen Wan	Lung and Kidney yang deficiency respiratory problems; Kidney not grasping Lung qi; chronic wheezing
4.1 Zhen Wu Tang Wan	Heart and Kidney yang deficiency fluid metabolism disorders, urinary dysfunction and edema
4.11 Ba Ji Yin Yang Wan 4.13 Zi Shen Da Bu Capsule	Kidney yang deficiency urinary dysfunction; nocturia, frequency, incontinence
7.11 Deer Velvet 7.12 Lu Rong Jiao	Kidney yang and essence deficiency. Usually combined with an appropriate constitutional formula for developmental problems or infertility
2.34 Cong Rong Bu Shen Wan	Yang deficiency chronic atonic constipation and impotence
7.13 Huan Shao Dan	Heart and Kidney qi and yang deficiency type memory disorders and disorders of aging
7.20 Cordyceps Essence of Chicken	Yang and yin tonic for Kidney and Lung deficiency patterns

Glossary

Abdominal masses (*jī jù* 积聚)

Abdominal masses are masses and lumps that can be palpated in the abdomen. They are classified into two types, *jī* and *jù* masses.

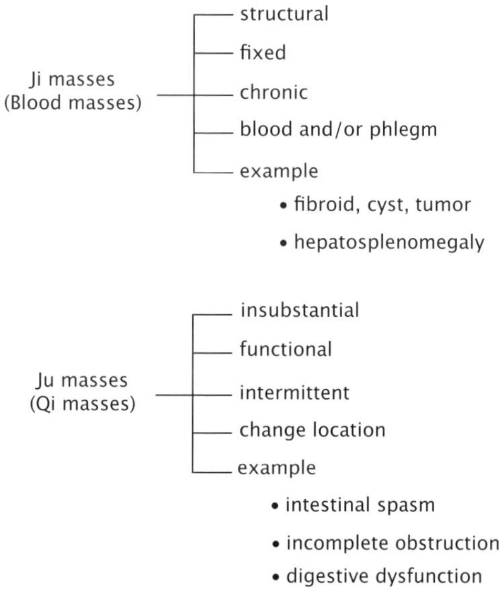

Jī masses are obvious and firm, clearly defined, fixed in location and often painful. *Jī* masses (commonly known as blood masses) are a deeper level of disharmony than *jù* masses, and are usually associated with chronic disease states involving the blood and elements of blood stasis. In general, they are associated with disorders of the yin organ systems organs. *Jī* masses are associated with structural change in tissues, for example, the proliferative growth of benign and malignant tumors, enlargement or swelling of organs, or inflammatory masses such as chronic appendicitis and diverticulitis.

Jù masses (commonly known as qi masses) are soft, ill defined on palpation, may or may not be painful, and tend to be intermittent. When present they move around, or come and go depending on the emotional state of the patient. They are associated with the qi and disorders associated with qi stagnation. *Jù* masses are generally functional disorders, that is, they are the result of functional changes in the tissues involved. They affect the yang organ systems organs, primarily the Stomach and Intestines.

Accumulation disorder (*gān jī* 疳积)

Accumulation disorder is a feeding disorder underling a large number of infant illnesses, and at its most basic is simply the inability of the delicate digestive system of the child to cope with the amount of food it is called on to process. When very small, infants are essentially feeding tubes dedicated to converting food into baby at an remarkable rate. Their digestive systems are working at capacity and are easily overtaxed. Feeding too much food too quickly, or giving hard to digest foods (as in weaning to solids too early) can cause a backlog of partially digested materials that accumulate and ferment in the gut. As a by-product of this accumulation, phlegm is produced. Once phlegm is present, a variety of other pathologies arise. Phlegm gums up the digestive process causing further gastrointestinal complaints. It causes obstruction, pressure build up and the generation of heat and fever. It can accumulate in the Lungs, ear or sinuses.

Many common, and some not so common, symptoms and disorders of infants such as fevers, convulsions, epilepsy, sleep and feeding problems, colic, reflux, vomiting, diarrhea and mucus congestion and its various complications (for example glue ear, asthma and allergies), have their beginnings in accumulation disorder.

Atrophy and muscular weakness syndrome (*wěi zhèng* 痿证)

Atrophy and muscular weakness characterized by wasting and weakness of the muscles of the extremities. There is usually no pain associated with the wasting. Disorders such as multiple sclerosis, muscular dystrophy and polio may be diagnosed as atrophy and muscular weakness syndrome.

Basal Body Temperature (BBT)

The basal body temperature is a method of graphically representing the hormonal changes of the menstrual cycle, and serves as a relatively accurate diagnostic tool for detecting problems in either the follicular (yin) or luteal (yang) phase. During the yin phase (day 4–14) the channels most closely associated with reproduction, the *chōng mài* and *rèn mài*, fill with blood (analogous to the thickening endometrium), and fertile mucus develops, a physical manifestation of the growing yin. The BBT remains steady around 36.1°C–36.6°C. At mid-cycle the resting body temperature of a normally ovulating woman rises by about 0.4°C, signaling the transformation of yin into yang, and the start of the yang phase. The elevation in temperature is maintained for 10–12 days, falling again with the onset of menstruation. Fertility relies upon sufficient yin and adequately maintained yang, and variations in the balance of these elements can contribute to infertility and other menstrual disorders. Charting variations from the normal pattern enables a very focused diagnosis and clear response, and is particularly useful when no clear pattern emerges from standard diagnostic methods.

Blood (*xuè* 血)

Blood in Chinese medicine is a technical term describing the function and structure of the fluid that circulates with qi through the channel and vessel network. While blood shares many features in common with the biomedical understanding of blood, it has unique characteristics. In addition to its general nutritive, lubricating and distributive function, blood has a special relationship with certain parts of the body, in particular the eyes, the sinews, skin and hair. A variety of visual, neurological and dermatological diseases are associated with blood problems. Blood anchors qi, preventing it from 'floating' away. This is particularly important in relationship to the *shén*, the most rarefied form of qi, which relies on blood for its foundation. Blood deficiency often causes *shén* disturbances such as insomnia, anxiety states and palpitations.

Blood stasis (*xuè yū* 血瘀)

Blood stasis refers to a continuum of states in which the movement of blood is in some way impeded or slowed. Blood stasis describes states ranging from poor or obstructed blood circulation in which drainage or supply of blood to a particular area is poor and the flow sluggish, to actual stasis, where blood circulation at some locus has ceased and a physical obstruction has formed, further impeding circulation.

Blood stasis can be localised or systemic, with a multitude of presentations depending on site and severity, and can be the result of a large variety of pathological processes. Trauma is a common cause of localised blood stasis, however constrained qi, obstruction to circulation by external pathogens (especially cold), insufficient motive force behind the circulation, emotional factors and surgery can all contribute.

Herbs for treating static blood are of varying strengths, designated by different terms in Chinese. The mildest are those that invigorate blood, suitable for mild blood stasis patterns characterized primarily by sluggish blood flow. Herbs that invigorate the blood are gentle in action, well tolerated, have a low incidence of side effects and are suitable for prolonged use. Invigorating implies not only restoring correct flow, but also promoting the normal physiological ability of the blood to nourish and moisten. Stronger are the herbs that disperse or dispel stagnant blood. These herbs are more dynamic in invigorating blood flow and clearing obstructions from stopped blood. Blood invigorating and stasis dispersing herbs have the potential for side effects. The strongest are herbs that break up blood stasis. These are powerful and dispersing to normal qi as well as pathological accumulation of blood, and are usually reserved for severe stasis patterns and masses. They have a high potential for side effects in inexperienced hands.

In biomedical terms, blood stasis is associated with a wide variety of disorders, in particular those associated with diseases of the hepatic and cardiovascular systems, connective tissue diseases, sclerotic disorders and tumors.

Burner (*jiāo* 焦)

The trunk of the body is divided into three functional units or burners, each with its own specific contents and physiological activity. The translation of the character is usually rendered as 'burning space' or 'heater'. This implies that dynamic physiological activity, including the generation and maintenance of body heat, occurs within these distinct units. The Heart and Lungs are located in the upper burner above the diaphragm, and as a unit are responsible for the motive force behind the circulation of qi and blood. The Spleen and Stomach are located in the middle burner, and the functional activity of digestion and acquisition of qi, and thus the Spleen and Stomach, is often referred to as middle burner qi. The Liver and Kidneys are situated, in a functional sense, in the lower burner and are the foundation of the constitutional strength of the individual.

Cold (*hán* 寒)

Cold in Chinese medicine is a technical term describing the physical response of the body to environmental cold or insufficient generation of body heat due to yang deficiency. Cold 'freezes and constricts', narrowing vessels and channel pathways, impeding the smooth circulation of qi and blood. The typical features of a cold pattern are cold intolerance, coldness in the body either perceived by the patient or felt by the examining hand, fairly severe localised pain that is significantly improved with heat and thin, clear, watery discharges.

Common cold (*gǎn mào* 感冒)

Gan mao is the Chinese expression for the common cold. In Chinese medical terms it can refer to any external invasion that causes acute symptoms consistent with colds or flu – fever and chills, sneezing, cough, sore throat and myalgia.

Cyclical treatment

Cyclical treatment is the technique aimed at restoring the menstrual cycle to normality, based on promoting the normal physiological event at the right time. For example, based on an average 28 day menstrual cycle, the main principle of treatment in the pre-ovulation phase (day 4-14) is to tonify qi and blood, as qi and blood are relatively deficient following menstruation and need to be replaced. At ovulation around day 14, the aim of treatment is to assist the transformation of yin into yang. The normal post ovulation phase (day

15-28) is characterized by an abundance of yang, qi and blood until menstruation begins around day 28, therefore the general principle of treatment is to support yang, regulate qi and facilitate blood flow.

Damp (*shī* 湿)

Damp in Chinese medicine is a technical term describing a pathological entity that results in a variety of gastrointestinal disorders, various swellings and discharges and a host of chronic and often difficult disease patterns. Damp has two origins; it can seep into the body from the environment or it can be manufactured internally by internal organ dysfunction. In either case, damp seeps into muscles and cavities obstructing the circulation of qi and blood and clogging the channels with its wet, heavy, cloying nature.

External damp is usually an acute disorder, similar to summerdamp and is associated with exposure to humid or wet environments, including damp housing. External damp can also seep into the joints causing pain and swelling. Internally generated damp is the product of poor digestive function, being the residue remaining from inefficient digestion and distribution of ingested material. Internal and external damp causes symptoms such as abdominal distension, indigestion, flatulence, loss of appetite, nausea, heaviness, lethargy, poor concentration, slippery pulses and a thick, greasy tongue coat. Damp is heavy and sinks downwards, preferentially affecting the gastrointestinal and reproductive systems, and lower body. Discharges such as heavy leukorrhea and diarrhea are physical manifestations of damp.

There are several methods of dealing with damp, depending on it's nature and location. Damp in the lower body can be eliminated through the urine. Damp affecting the Spleen and Stomach is dried with bitter parching herbs, or broken up and transformed. Damp is generally dried when it is introduced into the body by damp natured food or by invasion of a damp pathogen. Transformation of damp involves strengthening the function of the Spleen in processing food and fluids so damp is not created. Damp in the upper body can be dispelled. Dispelling damp involves the use of fragrant or acrid herbs that stimulate the diffusing function of the Lungs, and the Lungs regulatory control of the 'water passages'. By stimulating the Lungs, damp is sent down to the Kidneys for reprocessing and to the exterior to be eliminated with sweat.

Damp heat (*shī rè* 湿热)

Damp heat is a pathogenic entity with the cloying nature of damp intermingled with the inflammatory stimulus of heat. Damp heat patterns are characterized by having symptoms of both damp (discharge, swellings, thick tongue coat) and heat (redness, fever, inflammation). Damp heat disorders are often associated with problems that cause offensive, colored discharges.

Damp heat can invade from the environment, in which case the associated disorder is typically acute and seasonal, or it can be generated internally by internal organ dysfunction or by ingestion of an excess of damp heat generating substances, such as alcohol and rich fatty foods.

Biomedical conditions that are frequently diagnosed as damp heat include acute hepatitis and cholecystitis, pelvic inflammatory disease, acute inflammatory arthritis, dysentery, cystitis and suppurative skin diseases.

Dysenteric disorder (*lì jí* 痢疾)

Dysenteric disorder refers to a variety of patterns characterized by acute or chronic diarrhea with pus and/or blood in the stool. Dysenteric disorder overlaps with biomedical conditions such as amoebic and bacterial dysentery, as well as chronic disorders such as ulcerative colitis and Crohn's disease.

Deficient patterns (*xū zhèng* 虚证)

Deficient patterns in Chinese medicine are characterized by insufficiency of a normal physiological substrate (qi, blood, yin or yang, essence, body fluids), or hypofunction of an organ or metabolic system. Deficient patterns are usually chronic. In practice, deficient patterns are often complicated by excess patterns. For example, deficiency of Lung and defensive qi enables the penetration and lodgment of external pathogenic wind into the body; deficiency of Liver blood causes to a tendency to Liver qi constraint; Spleen qi deficiency often leads to the accumulation of damp.

Essence (*jīng* 精)

Essence is the fundamental substance inherited from parents that confers the ability to grow, develop and reproduce. The quality and quantity of essence inherited determines the constitutional strength, and to a certain extent, the duration of life of an individual. Essence also provides the ground substance from which the bones and 'marrow' (here the brain and spinal cord) are formed. Essence is stored in the Kidney system and is closely associated with Kidney function. Deficiency of essence leads to disorders characterized by bony deformity, learning difficulties, failure to thrive, growth problems, infertility and disorders of aging.

Excess patterns (*shí zhèng* 实证)

Excess patterns are characterized by the presence of a pathogen of some type in the body (wind, heat, cold, damp, phlegm or fire), or by a pathological accumulation of normal physiological substrates, i.e. qi and/or blood, either systemically or at some locus. Excess patterns are often acute but may be chronic. Excess patterns often have a degree of deficiency at their root, for example, Spleen qi deficiency easily gives rise to an accumulation of damp or phlegm.

Food stagnation (*shí jī* 食积)

Food stagnation is an important and often overlooked etiological component in a host of gastrointestinal and other disorders. Food stagnation patterns have traditionally been underrated in Chinese medical textbooks, disregarded as a mechanical event related to a single episode of overeating. In reality, food stagnation is usually more insidious and patients can become conditioned to ignoring, or may not even be conscious of, the traditional symptoms–abdominal and epigastric distension and discomfort, nausea and vomiting, belching, bad breath and flatulence. The eating patterns that give rise to food stagnation may be so ingrained that patients cease to be aware of the symptoms, or the symptoms experienced are considered to be normal.

By habitually overloading the Spleen and Stomach and exceeding their capacities to process the food ingested, a cycle is begun that can have profound ramifications. Firstly, instead of being sent through the intestine, the food lingers longer than it should, clogging the digestive system. The stagnant food may produce heat. The Spleen and Stomach are weakened, further inhibiting their abilities to perform their digestive tasks efficiently. The weakened Spleen produces damp which in turn may be congealed into phlegm by the heat. The phlegm or phlegm heat so produced can then affect other systems. For example, phlegm accumulation (with or without the frequently complicating blood stagnation) in the chest and cardiovascular system is a major cause of angina and heart disease; phlegm in the respiratory system can contribute to asthma, allergies and sinus problems. In addition, some neurological conditions such as tremors, anxiety states, insomnia, vertigo and paralysis, and dermatological disorders such as cysts, ulcerations, and chronic sores and swellings may be linked to phlegm, phlegm heat and other complicating pathogens produced by food stagnation.

Gu syndrome (*gŭ zhèng* 蛊症)

Gu syndrome is a complex type of systemic infection involving a host with a weakened constitution in a pathological equilibrium with a lingering pathogen, either viral, amoebic, vermiform, bacterial or fungal. *Gu* pathogens have been likened to 'oil seeping into flour–they are everywhere and cannot be separated out' (Fruehauf 1998). Treatment of *gu* syndrome is frequently lengthy, requiring months or even years. Clinically, patients with this type of problem often appear to be clearly qi deficient, or qi deficient with accumulated damp, but they typically get worse with standard qi tonic therapies. The symptoms are typical of Spleen disorder–chronic diarrhea or alternating bowel habits, abdominal distension and pain, nausea, loss of appetite or ravenous hunger or odd food cravings, muscle aches, weakness and physical and mental exhaustion.

Heart (*xīn* 心)

The organ system referred to as the Heart incorporates the cardiovascular system and certain aspects of the neurological system and higher consciousness. Functional weakness of the Heart (qi or yang deficiency) causes circulatory problems and various types of arrhythmia. In addition, the Heart is closely associated with maintenance of the *shén*, and disturbances of Heart function may give rise to various disturbances of consciousness, including manic behavior, anxiety, panic attacks, palpitations, depression and insomnia.

Hún 魂

The *hún* is the animus associated with the Liver. Anchored by Liver yin and blood, it is involved with creativity, artistic endeavor, intuition, the unconscious, the making of plans and the courage to follow them through. A balanced and grounded *hún* enables forward planning with creativity, vision and insight. It is active in dreams, and is the creative impulse drawn upon when a problem is solved by 'sleeping on it'. When the *hún* and *shén* are balanced, wisdom results; when unbalanced the person may have many dreams yet never accomplish anything.

A constrained *hún* leads to depression with a lack of inspiration and direction, diminished creativity and loss of insight. Patients feel themselves hemmed in by insurmountable barriers. A heated or overly stimulated *hún* results in manic or irrational behavior. A destabilized *hún*, cast adrift by deficiency of blood or yin, leads to aimlessness, lack of courage and resolve, indecisiveness and sleep walking.

Indefinable epigastric discomfort (*cáo zá* 嘈杂)

Indefinable epigastric discomfort is an uncomfortable sensation in the epigastric region that mimics hunger without the patient wanting to eat. Patients will often wake in the middle of the night with a nagging discomfort in the pit of the stomach, feeling the need to eat something but not knowing what. Often associated with peptic ulcer disease or chronic gastritis.

Kidneys (*shèn* 肾)

The organ system referred to as the Kidneys incorporates the genitourinary system, fluid metabolism, the ability to reproduce, and the development and maintenance of the bones, central nervous system and ears. The Kidneys are the foundation of constitutional health, the source of the body's yin and yang and the storehouse of inherited essence. The yang aspect of Kidney function underwrites all dynamic yang physiology, including fluid metabolism, digestion and circulation. The complement of yang, Kidney yin, maintains the integrity of the structural components upon which the yang acts and is the basis of the body's lubricating and moistening fluids, including fertile mucus, vaginal lubrication, prostatic and synovial fluids. Kidney deficiency problems include those associated with the aging process, disorders of fluid metabolism and reproduction, energy weakness, some skeletal, neurological and aural disorders, loss of structural integrity as occurs in some atrophic disorders, and congenital abnormalities.

Painful urination syndrome (*lín zhèng* 淋证)

Painful urination syndrome refers to a variety of disorders characterized by pain associated with urination. The key feature is pain, and it is the presence of pain that differentiates this group of disorders from other urinary disorders. Biomedically, painful urination syndrome includes such diseases as urinary tract infections, urinary calculi, pyelonephritis, tumors of the urogenital system, prostatic diseases, chyluria and albuminuria. There are six classifications of painful urination syndrome.

1. Heat or damp heat painful urination is clinically the most common variety, and is characterized by being acute and by rather intense burning pain upon urination.
2. Stone (or sand) painful urination is characterized by the presence of urinary calculi, and, depending on their location, intense radiating pain and/or obstructed urination.
3. *Qi* painful urination is traditionally divided into two types, deficiency (of qi) and excess (qi stagnation). The deficiency type is associated with Spleen qi deficiency and often follows recurrent heat types that have not been treated, or have been treated with antibiotics or excessively cold natured herbs. It is characterized by a dragging discomfort which is relieved by pressure, or a feeling of burning that improves with warmth and pressure. The excess type is characterized by discomfort during or following urination aggravated or initiated by stress and emotional upset.
4. Blood painful urination is painful urination with bleeding.
5. Cloudy or turbid painful urination is painful urination with cloudy or milky urine.
6. Exhaustion painful urination is chronic and recurrent, initiated or aggravated by sex, overexertion and fatigue. It is characterized by incomplete or dribbling urination, lumbar pain and weakness and mild dysuria that is often worse following urination.

Liver (*gān* 肝)

The organ system referred to as the Liver incorporates the functional activity of the Liver, as well as the tissues and structures traversed by the channel pathways of the Liver and it's partner, the Gallbladder. These structures include the reproductive system, external genitals, flanks, breasts, throat and eyes. Functionally, the Liver is responsible for the regular and uninterrupted distribution of qi and blood. It is the coordinator of the other organ systems, ensuring a steady supply of qi where and when it is needed. Failure of qi distribution leads to localised accumulations and obstructions. In pathological terms this results in hypertonicity of the affected tissues with consequent decrease in perfusion and nutrition. The Liver is very susceptible to emotional turmoil and stress, and conversely, malfunction of the Liver can give rise to various emotional or psychological problems, most notably depression and mood swings.

Lungs (*fèi* 肺)

The organ system referred to as the Lungs incorporates the respiratory system, the skin and large intestine. The Lungs perform the function of respiration and as such are part of the energy generating system of the body, in concert with the Spleen. The Lungs are a fundamental component of the immune system via the media of defensive qi. Healthy Lung function facilitates elimination of waste products. Weakness of the Lungs leads to various respiratory and energy problems, immune weakness, poor elimination, sweating disorders, some skin disorders and problems of the large intestine.

Malarial Disorder (*nüè ji* 疟疾)

Malarial disorders are a collection of conditions characterized by alternating fever and chills or a cyclical fever pattern. The diseases that fall into this category include true *Plasmodium* malaria, but also Dengue fever, Ross River fever and other fevers of the subtropic and tropical regions.

Masses and nodules

There are three main types of mass defined by Chinese medicine, qi, phlegm and blood stasis. They may occur anywhere in the body.

Qi masses are intermittent, can vary in location, are quite soft upon palpation and will generally dissipate with prolonged pressure. They are usually associated with a functional disorder of an organ or tissue.

Phlegm masses do not move location, feel smooth, rubbery and round on palpation, and are usually not painful. Phlegm masses often occur in the neck, extremities and gynecological system.

Blood masses are hard, fixed in location and feel very firm or irregular on palpation. They are often painful, especially when palpated. Blood masses can be associated with relatively benign lesions such as benign gynecological tumors, chronic inflammatory masses like diverticulosis, chronic salpingitis, ulcerative colitis, chronic appendicitis and more sinister problems including malignant tumors.

Painful obstruction syndrome (*bì zhèng* 痹证)

Painful obstruction syndrome is a class of disorders characterized by pain, stiffness, numbness and paresthesia of muscles and joints, usually due to an invasion of the channel system by pathogenic wind, cold, damp and/or heat. Usually a chronic disorder, but may be acute or have occasional acute flare-ups. *Bi* literally means to obstruct or block, and the term refers to the statement 'where there is obstruction there is pain'. It corresponds to biomedical conditions characterized primarily by pain, such as osteoarthritis and rheumatoid arthritis, sciatica, infectious arthritis, lumbago, cervical and lumbar spondylosis, ankylosing spondylitis, rheumatic fever, systemic lupus erythematosus and polymyositis.

Paradoxical pulse

The paradoxical pulse is so called because it is the opposite of the pulse expected for the pattern it reflects. The paradoxical pulse is a very clear indicator of Liver invading Spleen and Stomach patterns, where the expected pulse is an excess pulse–wiry, strong etc., at the left middle position (Liver) and a deficient pulse–weak, fine etc., at the right middle position (Spleen/Stomach). The paradoxical pulse presents as a large bulge at the right middle position and a clear dip at the left middle position.

Primary Pathological Triad (PPT)

The Primary Pathological Triad represents three patterns of pathology which are frequently found to occur simultaneously, are tightly interlinked and mutually engendering. The triad comprises Spleen deficiency and Liver qi constraint with heat or damp heat. In addition to the basic triad of pathology, there may be further complication by blood and/or yin deficiency, blood stasis, disruption to communication between the Heart and Kidney, and phlegm.

The three main patterns of the PPT reinforce each other in the following way. Liver qi constraint impacts on the Spleen, weakening it and encouraging the generation of damp. Damp is heavy and tends to sink downwards to the lower body and depths of the gastrointestinal system. Constrained qi, with the increase in qi pressure behind an obstruction, generate heat. Heat, once present and applied to preexisting damp, creates damp heat. Damp on its own, as a sticky obstructing pathogen, can also generate heat and become damp heat.

The Western lifestyle is adept at producing and maintaining the PPT. A combination of stress, inappropriate diet and eating habits, alcohol, sedentary occupations, and overuse of pharmaceuticals can all contribute.

The frequency of this combination of pathologies and the complex interactions between them is the reason the 'harmonizing' category of prescriptions is the most widely used group of formulations worldwide. Harmonizing prescriptions combine herbs with several different, often opposing, actions. They are typically complex, utilizing acrid hot, bitter cold and sweet warm substances to relieve constraint, clear heat and tonify qi. As a group, the harmonizing formulas work on various aspects of the PPT, with varying degrees of emphasis.

Successful treatment of the triad of pathological patterns requires that each pattern be addressed at the same time, otherwise the condition will either not improve or will quickly relapse. For example, if only the Spleen is treated, repeated insult by invasive Liver qi will continue to weaken it and the Spleen will be damaged again. If only damp heat is treated, the weakened Spleen will continue to produce damp and will likely be damaged by the bitter cold herbs or substances used to clear the damp heat.

The major prescriptions for treating the various elements of the PPT can be mapped according to the hierarchy of therapeutic features they display. Figure 1 charts a selection of prescriptions commonly used for this purpose. Their position inside the triangle indicates the relative balance of the formula's activity on Spleen qi deficiency, Liver qi constraint and the heat component. For example, **6.1 Xiao Chai Hu Wan** can be mapped in the center of the triangle, as it is equally balanced between the three major principles of treatment. It strengthens the Spleen and tonifies qi, regulates Liver qi and clears damp heat, in about equal proportions.

Figure 1. Map of selected formulae according to their relative action on the PPT

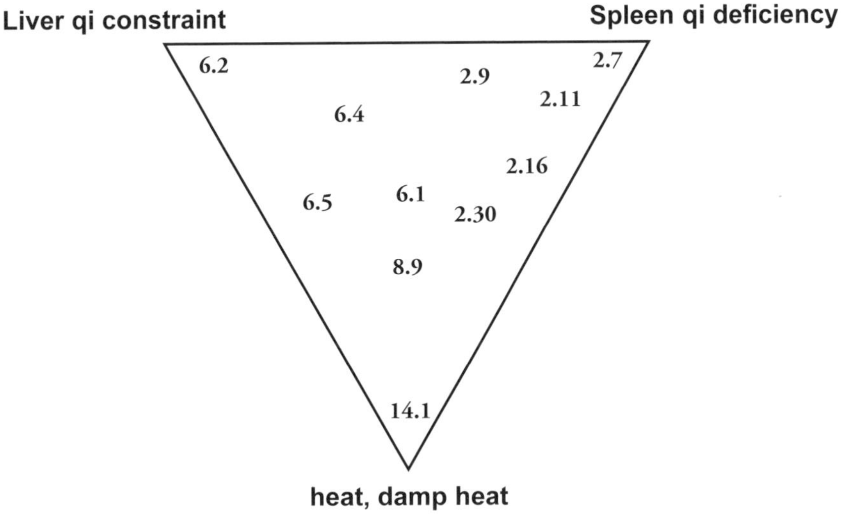

6.1 Xiao Chai Hu Wan
8.9 Chai Hu Long Gu Mu Li Wan
6.4 Xiao Yao Wan
6.5 Jia Wei Xiao Yao Wan
2.11 Bu Zhong Yi Qi Wan
2.9 Xiang Sha Liu Jun Wan
14.1 Huang Lian Jie Du Wan
6.2 Si Ni Wan
2.7 Si Jun Zi Wan
2.16 Zi Sheng Wan
2.30 Chen Xiang Hua Qi Wan

Phlegm (*tán* 痰)

Phlegm in Chinese medicine is a technical term describing a pathological product resulting from the stagnation and congealing of body fluids or damp. There are two broad types of phlegm, material (or substantial) and latent (or insubstantial). Material phlegm has physical form and can be observed in the thin or thick sputum of acute and chronic respiratory problems, the congesting mucus of sinus disease, and the rounded rubbery masses of various benign nodules, such as lipomas and thyroid nodules. Latent phlegm has no physical form, instead it is detected through the symptoms and constitutional patterns it produces. The symptoms of latent phlegm are mostly associated with its inhibiting effect on the clear expression of the *shén*–disturbances of consciousness, anxiety states, insomnia, foggy head and palpitations–and its cloying effects on the circulation and distribution of yang, qi and blood.

Several methods are employed for dealing with phlegm, depending on its nature and location. Phlegm in the Lungs is expelled by promoting expectoration. Phlegm can be transformed by strengthening fluid metabolism and the organ systems responsible for production of the phlegm in the first place. Phlegm that accumulates in masses and lumps can be dispersed with acrid herbs, or, if particularly hard, softened first with salty substances.

Qì 气

Qi is the functional component of Chinese physiology. Qi is required and necessary to enable people to perform the various tasks associated with life; gathering and harvesting food, transforming the qi of the raw materials into a form the human body can use, performing the daily maintenance tasks of respiration, protection from pathogens and generation of body heat. All the organ systems rely on a steady supply of qi in order to be able to perform their various functions. An inadequate supply of qi usually means that one or more systems is in a state of hypofunction.

Qi can be tonified by strengthening the source of qi, the Spleen and Lungs. The distribution of qi can be facilitated by using acrid herbs to regulate qi, spread Liver qi, invigorate qi or break up stagnant qi. Regulating qi is the mildest method and generally applies to stagnant qi in the Spleen, Stomach and Intestines. Spreading Liver qi and invigorating qi are stronger, and utilized when Liver dysfunction leads to uneven distribution of qi in the structures of the Liver and Gallbladder organ systems. Breaking up stagnant qi is the strongest, utilizing intensely acrid herbs to powerfully disperse pathological accumulation of qi, often in the form of knots or clumps.

Qì dynamic (*qì jī* 气机)

The qi dynamic is one of the fundamental axes of normal physiological function in the body. Essentially, it is the dynamic created by the natural tendency of Spleen qi to rise ('the raising of the pure'), and Stomach qi to descend ('descent of the turbid'). Spleen and Stomach qi acts as the dynamo, or pivot, of ascent and descent throughout the body, thus the qi dynamic facilitates the general movement and distribution of qi throughout the body. Disruption to the qi dynamic features prominently in many gastrointestinal problems. Nausea and vomiting are associated with blockage to, and consequent rising of, Stomach qi; abdominal distension occurs when qi fails to descend and accumulates in the middle burner. Constipation often reflects a failure of the descent of Stomach qi.

There are two main types of disruption to the qi dynamic, excess and deficient. The excess type of qi blockage is usually related to Liver qi constraint and its obstructing action on the movement of Spleen and Stomach qi. Pathogenic accumulations, such as damp, phlegm or stagnant food can obstruct qi movement and disrupt the qi dynamic. Less commonly, excess qi blockage can be associated with obstruction of Lung qi. Lung qi diffuses to the surface and descends. When this process is blocked by a pathogen, the subsequent accumulation of qi in the Lungs has a disruptive effect on the ascent of Spleen qi. The result is disruption of the qi dynamic, the natural movement of qi, and consequent accumulation of qi in the middle burner.

The deficient type of qi dynamic dysfunction is due to a weakness of middle burner qi. Put simply, there is insufficient motive force behind the rising of Spleen qi, or the descent of Stomach qi. Deficient type qi blockage will often be further complicated by excess accumulation. The obstruction in this case occurs because the qi is too feeble to move adequately, or the weakened Spleen/Stomach invite the attention and over-control of Liver qi, or because they are too weak to process food adequately so that food or dampness and phlegm accumulate.

Restless organ disorder (*zàng zào* 脏躁)

An emotional condition, neurosis or hysteria, predominantly seen in women but occasionally also in men, characterized by emotional instability, sadness and crying for no apparent reason, frequent yawning or sighing, melancholy, nervous excitability, hypersensitivity, confusion and absent mindedness. In some cases, sudden loss of speech, hearing or vision may occur. In between episodes patients may appear normal. This is a form of Heart and Spleen deficiency brought about by obsessive worry or prolonged anxiety, or as result of damage from a prior illness or chronic blood loss. It is considered a relatively rarefied species of deficiency, affecting the *shén* rather than the physical body, so a gentle touch, rather than powerful and potentially cloying tonic herbs, is the aim of treatment. The classical indications in the source text (Discussion of Cold Induced Disorders, Han dynasty, circa 200AD) note a red tongue and rapid pulse (suggesting yin deficiency) are part of the picture, but in practice the tongue and pulse findings are more variable. A pale tongue is a common observation.

Shào yáng syndrome (*shào yáng bìng* 少阳病)

Shào yáng syndrome is a pattern of disharmony characterized by the residence of a pathogen in the second of the six levels (*see* below), the *shào yáng* level. The *shào yáng* is considered to be neither external, that is, on the surface of the body, the *tài yáng* level, nor internal, affecting the internal organs, *yáng míng* and the three yin levels. It represents a transitional zone where pathogens can hide and get locked away, sometimes for prolonged periods. From a clinical perspective, numerous common post acute and chronic infections, as well as a host of hepatic and gastrointestinal disorders may manifest as variations of *shào yáng* syndrome.

Shén 神

The *shén* is the animus associated with the Heart. Usually translated as 'spirit' or 'mind', the *shén* is at the most rarefied end of the spectrum of qi. The most condensed is essence; in between are the various functional types of qi (gathering qi, defensive qi, organ system qi etc.). These three aspects of qi (essence, qi, *shén*, the 'three treasures' [*sān bǎo* 三宝]) are the foundation of Chinese physiology and at the root of Taoist meditation techniques. Indeed, it is the transformation of essence into *shén* that preoccupies some of the Taoist and other esoteric schools of Chinese philosophical thought and practice. The *shén* plays a key role in higher mental functions, including many of the intellectual and spiritual aspects of consciousness. In practical terms, the *shén* is most closely associated with our conscious awareness, and is essentially our ability to perceive, interact and communicate with our world clearly. In addition, the *shén* and the Heart share an intimate and interdependent relationship. Chinese medicine describes the Heart as the residence of the *shén*. *Shén* pathology is associated with disturbances of consciousness and perception, sleep, higher mental function and some aspects of Heart function.

Six level disease differentiation (*liù jīng biàn zhèng* 六经辨证)

Six level theory, elucidated in the *Shāng Hán Lùn* (Discussion of Cold Induced Disorders, Han dynasty, circa 200AD) by Zhang Zhong-Jing, describes the events that occur as a pathogen, usually wind cold, drives into the body, interacting with the body's normal qi. The *Shang Han Lun* systematized the prevailing concepts of feverish diseases, the most significant cause of mortality of the time, into a series of levels through which a pathogen can penetrate, each successive level deeper in the body than the one preceding it. In the three yang levels, the body's qi is generally intact and able to put up a defense against the pathogen, hence the key manifestation of this stage of the conflict, the fever. By the time a pathogen reaches the internal organs, the normal qi has been significantly weakened, and the remaining levels represent various aspects of internal organ deficiency. The symptoms characteristic of each level are due to the interaction and relative strengths of the pathogen and the body's normal qi. Zhang clearly laid out the clinical features of the interaction between the pathogen and the body at each level, with common variations, and designed diagnostic strategies and treatments which are still in use today.

The six levels are the *tài yáng*, *shào yáng*, *yáng míng*, *tài yīn*, *shào yīn* and *jué yīn*. The *tài yáng* level is the most superficial, generally the first point of contact between a pathogen and the body, and corresponds anatomically to the channel system, skin and muscles. The *shào yáng* level represents a transitional zone between the interior of the body and the exterior (*see* above). The *yáng míng* is the most superficial part of the interior, corresponding to the yang organ systems of the Stomach and Large Intestine. The *tài yīn* level is the first internal level as it represents the yin organ systems of the Spleen and Lungs. Although yin organs, they are still relatively shallow compared to those that follow, and retain some connection with the exterior. The *shào yīn* is fully internal, representing the vulnerable and critical Heart and Kidneys. A pathogen gaining access to the *shào yīn* level can wreak havoc. The final level, the *jué yīn* involves the Liver and Pericardium. If a pathogen manages to reach the *jué yīn*, the situation is dangerous, potentially giving rise to wind, convulsions, coma and death.

Zhang's achievement was far reaching – of the 100 or so formulas he describes, a significant number are still being used today, including many in this book, and are among the most popular and effective.

Spleen (*pí* 脾)

In Chinese medicine the organ system referred to as the Spleen incorporates the functions attributed to the Spleen organ, as well as the tissues and structures along the pathway of the Spleen channel, smooth and skeletal muscle and the oral cavity. The Spleen performs several fundamental processes that are critical to daily functional maintenance and metabolism. The Spleen is the basis of digestion, the harvesting of nutrients and the transformation of the raw materials of food into usable physiological qi. The Spleen plays a crucial role in maintaining vascular integrity and preventing leakage of blood from the circulatory system. Healthy Spleen function maintains muscular tone and bulk and provides the complimentary force to counter the relentless pull of gravity. Spleen weakness can lead to a variety of digestive, metabolic and energy problems, bleeding disorders, muscular weakness and wasting and prolapse of various structures.

Sudden Turmoil (*huò luàn* 霍乱)

Characterized by acute, violent vomiting and diarrhea. There may or may not be abdominal pain. The most common cause is invasion of a strong, epidemic or pestilential pathogen that disrupts the qi dynamic. As the pressure builds up due to the obstruction in the middle burner, the conglomerate of turbid untransformed materials and pathogen is forcefully ejected upwards and downwards.

Even though the pathogenic influence is usually quite strong, patients with sudden turmoil disorder can present with varying degrees of disharmony, from mild to severe. The common types in the Western clinic are generally relatively mild and self limiting, but should always be treated to fully clear the offending pathogen, and thereby preventing recurrence. Patients with sudden turmoil disorder may be diagnosed with biomedical conditions such as acute gastroenteritis associated with infection by numerous bacterial, viral or parasitic agents, including *Campylobacter*, *Salmonella*, *Shigella*, *Giardia* and *Cryptosporidium*, gastric 'flu', food poisoning or cholera.

Summerdamp (*shǔ bìng* 暑病)

Summerdamp is an acute disorder primarily affecting the gastrointestinal system. It tends to be seasonal, most frequently occurring during the humid months of late summer or during periods of hot humid weather. Summerdamp is always an external environmental pathogen and is often epidemic, sweeping through offices and schools. It has a tendency to linger or recur if not promptly or correctly resolved. The typical features are nausea and vomiting, urgent diarrhea, muscle aches, foggy head and malaise.

Surgery, using prepared medicines in association with

Certain prepared medicines can be used to enhance recovery from, and decrease the risk of complications of, surgical procedures. Surgery of any type disrupts the circulation of qi and blood and leaves a residue of stagnant blood. Certain surgical procedures appear to damage yang qi. There are two main groups of prepared medicines that are frequently used, depending on the constitution and medical condition of the patient, and the nature of the surgery. These are the tonic and the blood invigorating medicines. For patients who are weakened from illness or in some way deficient in the lead up to a surgical procedure, building qi, blood or yang can be useful to help them to better weather the trauma of the procedure and to hasten recovery during convalescence. This is especially the case in the elderly and debilitated, and those who tend to heal slowly. A gentle yang qi tonifying approach, used both before and after a procedure is also useful for those undergoing abdominal surgery, which can in some cases damage Spleen yang qi. Common preparatory formulas include **1.1 Ba Zhen Wan**, **1.6 Bai Feng Wan**, **2.11 Bu Zhong Yi Qi Wan**, **2.12 Shen Ling Bai Zhu Wan** and **2.13 Li Zhong Wan**.

For robust patients, those having surgery following a traumatic injury or broken bones, and for those prone to keloid scarring, regulating and invigorating the blood accelerates healing, promotes osteogenesis and decreases the likelihood of excessive fibrosis. The famous hemostatic medicine **10.1 Yunnan Paiyao** has been used and studied extensively in China in this regard, and has been found to significantly decrease post-surgical blood loss, while improving circulation to encourage and accelerating healing. Other suitable medicines, drawn mostly from the Cardiovascular and Pain and Trauma sections of the text, can be found under the relevant headings in the index.

Tonic and blood invigorating formulas are the most commonly used medicines to enhance healing and recovery around surgery, however, practitioners are not restricted to these groups. Other medicines can be utilized as appropriate. For example, prepared medicines that clear damp heat from the Gallbladder are often useful in the run up to a cholecystectomy or keyhole gallstone removal.

In all cases however, prepared medicines should be discontinued at least one week prior to the surgical procedure. This is especially important for medicines which influence blood viscosity and clotting time. This includes not only blood regulating medicines, but also those with high doses of ginseng. The appropriate medicine can be resumed once the patient is able to ingest the medicine in the convalescent stage.

Toxic heat (*rè dú* 热毒)

Toxic heat refers to two types of disorder. The first is a severe localised accumulation of heat or damp heat that reaches a level of intensity sufficient to destroy tissue and create pus. Abscesses and carbuncles, acute appendicitis or diverticulitis and suppurative tonsillitis are all examples of localised Toxic heat disorders. Toxic heat patterns may also be systemic, in which case they are observed in generalized malaise, sickness, nausea and vomiting that accompanies serious infections like lymphangitis, lymphadenitis, bacteremia and septicemia.

Warm disease (*wēn bìng* 温病)

Warm diseases are acute disorders caused by invasion of powerful external pathogens, usually occurring in epidemics and affecting the weak and strong alike. They superficially resemble simple wind heat patterns in the early stages. Unlike simple wind heat disorders however, quick intervention does not always bring a quick cure, and the pathogen often swiftly penetrates deep into the body through the theoretical four levels into the deepest reaches of the body. The four levels are the defensive level, corresponding to the surface, an external disorder, the qi level involving the Lungs, chest, Stomach and Intestines, the nutritive level, and the blood level. By the time a pathogen has entered the nutritive and blood levels, the disorder is serious, and is characterized by febrile rashes, disordered consciousness and convulsions. Warm diseases include biomedical conditions such as meningitis and encephalitis, febrile rashes, scarlet fever, measles, chicken pox and numerous tropical fevers.

Wasting and thirsting disorder (*xiāo kě* 消渴)

Wasting and thirsting disorder describes conditions characterized by intense thirst, copious urination, frequent hunger and weight loss. In biomedical terms wasting and thirsting disorder is broadly analogous to diabetes mellitus and diabetes insipidus.

Wind (*fēng* 风)

Wind in Chinese medicine is a pathological entity that gives rise to disorders characterized by sudden onset, rapid development, mobile symptoms and involuntary movements and spasms. There are two types of wind defined by Chinese medicine, external and internal. External wind invades the body from the environment, usually in combination with cold, heat or dampness, and is implicated in acute colds, influenza, gastric flu and some skin disorders. External wind is usually dispelled from the body with diaphoretic herbs. Internal wind is a more complex phenomena, being generated by pathological processes within the body. There are three common mechanisms that can create internal wind, yin deficiency, blood deficiency and extreme heat. Internal wind is extinguished.

- **Yin deficiency**: The body's yin is the anchor that secures yang and provides a counterweight to the active and rising nature of yang. At a critical point of deficiency, yin is unable to restrain yang which ascends, and at a certain point of chaotic volatility and movement, becomes wind. This type of wind can be sudden and catastrophic–it is the type of wind that can cause severe dizziness to the point of wind stroke, potentially leading to hemiplegia or death. It typically follows years of yin depletion.
- **Blood deficiency**: This type of wind is similar in etiology to the yin deficiency in that the wind is generated by failure of the blood to anchor qi–when qi moves without the grounding control of blood, a mild form of wind is generated. Blood deficient wind is more likely to cause mild rhythmic tics, tremors, fasciculations and spasms.
- **Extreme heat**: Because heat and movement are closely related physiologically, at a certain

level of intensity, internal heat can generate sufficient movement to become wind. This most frequently manifests as the convulsions of a high fever.

Wind edema (*fēng shuǐ* 风水)

Wind edema is due to wind disrupting the normal fluid descending and dispersing function of the Lungs. The fluids that should be directed to the skin and the Kidneys though the 'water passages', back up and accumulate, primarily in the face and upper burner. The main feature is sudden onset of orbital and facial edema. In the early stages the eyes, then the face, become swollen and puffy. Swelling of the limbs and rest of the body may follow. The edema generally develops quickly. This is a yang type of edema. The wind can combine with either cold, heat or dampness producing a variable secondary symptom picture. With cold, there are generalized muscle and joint aches, cold and wind intolerance, no sweating, chills, mild fever, scanty urination, dyspnea or wheezing, cough, a thin, white tongue coat and a floating, tight pulse. With heat, there is fever, aversion to wind, sore throat, cough, scanty concentrated urine, a red tipped tongue with a thin, yellow coat and a floating, rapid pulse. With damp, there is heaviness and lethargy, swelling in the lower body and a floating, soggy pulse.

Edema of this type may follow an acute upper respiratory tract infection, or disorders such as acute boils and sores, acute (post streptococcal) glomerulonephritis, or tooth extraction. It tends predominantly to affect young people, although older people may also be affected.

Wind stroke (*zhōng fēng* 中风)

The Chinese medical classification of wind stroke is closely analogous to the biomedically defined cerebrovascular accident (CVA), although it also incorporates some non central nervous system conditions such as Bell's Palsy. There are two main classifications of wind Stroke:

- **Channel stroke** is a mild type of wind stroke that only affects the channels and does not cause loss of consciousness. The main manifestations are facial paralysis, dysphasia and hemiplegia. The general prognosis for recovery is good, or at least better than when consciousness is lost.
- **Organ stroke** is a serious disorder thought to involve severe damage to the internal organs. This type causes loss of consciousness as well as hemiplegia, facial paralysis and dysphasia. This type frequently leads to permanent disability or death.

Yang 阳

Yang is a technical term describing all the functional activity of body's tissues and organ systems, and the energetic principle responsible for generation of body heat. Insufficient yang leads to problems associated with severe hypofunction of tissues and organ systems and insufficient thermogenesis. Patients tend to be weak, sluggish and cold. Many disorders may be associated with insufficient yang, in particular reproductive problems, fluid and urinary disorders, circulatory and some endocrine disorders.

Yáng míng syndrome (*yáng míng bìng* 阳明病)

Yáng míng syndrome refers to a variety of disorders characterized by an accumulation of excess heat in the Stomach and Intestines. The main symptoms are fever, thirst, sweating and a large rapid pulse. If the *yáng míng* organ is involved there will be constipation. *Yáng míng* syndrome may begin as an acute invasion of wind cold or heat that penetrates through the surface into the interior (*see* Six level disease differentiation, p.639), or may occur due to heat generated by some pathological process internally. In biomedical terms, *yáng míng* syndrome may correspond to disorders as diverse as meningitis, pneumonia, acute appendicitis, heat stroke and dysentery.

Yin 阴

Yin is a technical term describing the structural components of the body upon which the functional yang acts, and the cool moistening fluid components that contain, balance and cool the heat and activity of the yang elements. Many problems associated with weakness of yin involve a loss of structural integrity, actual atrophy or deterioration of tissues (such as chronic atrophic gastritis and glossitis), decrease in fluids or an increase in fluid viscosity. Yin deficiency also leads to overheating in much the same way as a car engine with insufficient water in the radiator tends to overheat. Yin deficient patients tend to be hot, dry and agitated. Disorders that may have a component of yin deficiency include menopausal syndrome, sleep disturbances, chronic inflammatory states such as interstitial cystitis, pelvic inflammatory disease and prostatitis, hearing or visual weakness, some endocrine problems such as diabetes and hyperthyroidism, and chronic respiratory disorders.

Symptom index

A

B

E

F

G

H

Heat pathology

Heart pathology

Large Intestine pathology

M

N

O

P

Phlegm pathology

S

T

U

V

W

Wind pathology

Prepared medicine Index

T

U

Bibliography and references

Bensky D and Gamble A (2004) Chinese Herbal Medicine: Materia Medica, 3rd ed., Eastland Press, Seattle, WA

Bensky D and Barolet R (2015) Chinese Herbal Medicine: Formulas and Strategies, Portable 2nd ed., Eastland Press, Seattle, WA

Beers M and Berkow R, et al. (1999) The Merck Manual, 17th ed., Merck Research Laboratories, Whitehouse Station, New Jersey

Chen J (1999) Recognition and Prevention of Herb-Drug Interaction. Medical Acupuncture Journal 10(2)

Chu Han Zhu (1989) Clinical Handbook of Chinese Prepared Medicines, Paradigm Publications, Brookline, Mass.

Clavey S (1995) Fluid Physiology and Pathology in Traditional Chinese Medicine, Churchill Livingstone, Melbourne

Walker BR et al. (2014) Davidson's Principles and Practice of Medicine, 22nd ed., Churchill Livingstone, Edinburgh

Fratkin J (2001) Chinese Herbal Patent Formulas, The Clinical Desk Reference, Shya Publications, Boulder, CO

Fruehauf H (1998) Gu Syndrome. The Journal of Chinese Medicine, 57:10-17

Fugh-Bergman A (2000) Herb-Drug Interactions. Lancet 355:134-138

Ko RJ (1998) Adulterants in Asian Patent Medicines. N Engl J Med 339:847

Maclean W, Lyttleton J, Bayley M, Taylor K (2018) Clinical Handbook of Internal Medicine, The Treatment of Disease with Traditional Chinese Medicine. Eastland Press, Seattle

Miller LG (1998) Herbal Medicinals: Selected Clinical Considerations Focusing on Known or Potential Drug-Herb Interactions. Arch Intern Med 158(20):2200-2211

Naeser M (1992) Outline to Chinese Herbal Patent Medicines in Pill Form (2nd ed.), Boston Chinese Medicine

Shi Yong Fang Ji Xue 实用方剂学 (1989) Practical Chinese Herbal Formulas, Zhou Feng-Wu (ed.), Shandong Science and Technology Press, Shandong

Townsend P (1997) Chinese Herb and Modern Drug Interactions. (Unpublished)

Zhong Yi Nei Ke Xue 中医内科学 (1999) Traditional Chinese Internal Medicine, Wang Yong–Yan, Lu Zhao–Lin (eds.), Peoples Medical Publishing House, Beijing

Zui Xin Fang Ji Shou Ce 最新方剂手册 (1998) Handbook of the Latest Prescriptions, Fan Wei-Hong (ed.), Central Plains Publishing Company, Henan

About the Authors

William Maclean is a graduate of the New South Wales College of Natural Therapies (Diploma of Traditional Chinese Medicine, 1987) and the University of Technology Sydney (M.Sc Traditional Chinese Medicine, 2004). Will interned at the Red Cross Hospital in Hangzhou, China, and apprenticed for several years under the renowned Chris Madden. Will is the author of the Clinical Handbook of Chinese Herbs. He is also the co-author of Clinical Handbook of Internal Medicine: The Treatment of Disease with Traditional Chinese Medicine (2nd Ed). Will has taught widely in Australia, Europe and the U.S., and while recently retired from nearly thirty years of clinical practice, maintains an ongoing interest in the development of strategies for the understanding and treatment of chronic infection (lingering pathogens) and chronic inflammatory disorders.

Kathryn Taylor is a graduate of the University of Technology Sydney (Bachelor of Health Science in Acupuncture, 1997), Sydney College of Chinese Medicine (Diploma of Traditional Chinese Medicine, 1999), University of Western Sydney (Masters of Traditional Chinese Medicine, 2004; Bachelor of Nursing, 2015) and Charles Sturt University (Graduate Diploma of Midwifery, 2017). She is the co-author of Clinical Handbook of Internal Medicine: The Treatment of Disease with Traditional Chinese Medicine (2nd Ed). She practiced as a women's and children's health care clinician for over 20 years. Kathryn currently works as a midwife in a Sydney tertiary public hospital integrating evidence-based acupuncture and complementary medicine into maternity care, and maintains a private Chinese medical practice in the beautiful Blue Mountains to the west of Sydney.